Thieme

Clinical Laryngology

Marvin P. Fried, MD, FACS
Professor and University Chairman
Department of Otorhinolaryngology–Head and Neck Surgery
Montefiore Medical Center
The University Hospital for Albert Einstein College of Medicine
Bronx, New York

Melin Tan, MD
Assistant Professor
Department of Otorhinolaryngology–Head and Neck Surgery
Montefiore Medical Center
The University Hospital for Albert Einstein College of Medicine
Bronx, New York

Thieme
New York • Stuttgart • Delhi • Rio de Janeiro

Thieme Medical Publishers, Inc.
333 Seventh Ave.
New York, NY 10001

Executive Editor: Timothy Y. Hiscock
Managing Editors: Owen J. Zurhellen and Kenny Chumbley
Editorial Assistant: Heather Allen
Senior Vice President, Editorial and Electronic Product Development: Cornelia Schulze
Production Editor: Sean Woznicki
International Production Director: Andreas Schabert
International Marketing Director: Fiona Henderson
Director of Sales, North America: Mike Roseman
International Sales Director: Louisa Turrell
Vice President, Finance and Accounts: Sarah Vanderbilt
President: Brian D. Scanlan
Printer: Replika Press Pvt. Ltd.

Library of Congress Cataloging-in-Publication Data

Clinical laryngology : the essentials / [edited by] Marvin P. Fried, Melin Tan.
p. ; cm.
Includes bibliographical references.
ISBN 978-1-60406-749-1 (hardback : alk. paper) – ISBN 978-1-60406-750-7 (eISBN)
I. Fried, Marvin P., editor. II. Tan, Melin, editor.
[DNLM: 1. Laryngeal Diseases. 2. Larynx–pathology. WV 500]
RF510
616.2'2–dc23 2014007023

Thieme Publishers New York
333 Seventh Avenue, New York, NY 10001 USA
+1 800 782 3488, customerservice@thieme.com

Thieme Publishers Stuttgart
Rüdigerstrasse 14, 70469 Stuttgart, Germany
+49 [0]711 8931 421, customerservice@thieme.de

Thieme Publishers Delhi
A-12, Second Floor, Sector-2, Noida-201301
Uttar Pradesh, India
+91 120 45 566 00, customerservice@thieme.in

Thieme Publishers Rio, Thieme Publicações Ltda.
Argentina Building 16th floor, Ala A, 228 Praia do Botafogo
Rio de Janeiro 22250-040 Brazil
+55 21 3736-3631

Printed in India
5 4 3 2 1

ISBN 978-1-60406-749-1

Also available as an ebook:
eISBN 978-1-60406-704-0

Important note: Medicine is an ever-changing science undergoing continual development. Research and clinical experience are continually expanding our knowledge, in particular our knowledge of proper treatment and drug therapy. Insofar as this book mentions any dosage or application, readers may rest assured that the authors, editors, and publishers have made every effort to ensure that such references are in accordance with **the state of knowledge at the time of production of the book.**

Nevertheless, this does not involve, imply, or express any guarantee or responsibility on the part of the publishers in respect to any dosage instructions and forms of applications stated in the book. **Every user is requested to examine carefully** the manufacturers' leaflets accompanying each drug and to check, if necessary in consultation with a physician or specialist, whether the dosage schedules mentioned therein or the contraindications stated by the manufacturers differ from the statements made in the present book. Such examination is particularly important with drugs that are either rarely used or have been newly released on the market. Every dosage schedule or every form of application used is entirely at the user's own risk and responsibility. The authors and publishers request every user to report to the publishers any discrepancies or inaccuracies noticed. If errors in this work are found after publication, errata will be posted at www.thieme.com on the product description page.

Some of the product names, patents, and registered designs referred to in this book are in fact registered trademarks or proprietary names even though specific reference to this fact is not always made in the text. Therefore, the appearance of a name without designation as proprietary is not to be construed as a representation by the publisher that it is in the public domain.

FSC www.fsc.org
MIX
Paper from responsible sources
FSC® C021256

We wish to dedicate this book to our respective spouses, Rita and David, and to our children and grandchildren.

Contents

Preface

Laryngology has evolved over more than a century. Indeed, in the United States it is one of the earliest recognized medical specialties as reflected in the scientific organizations that have been created focused on this unique structure. The New York Laryngological Society was formed in 1873, subsequently giving rise to the American Laryngological Association in 1878. Although the early activities in the field now appear rudimentary, they developed an understanding of the structure and function of the larynx. Further work by notable physicians and scientists worldwide helped define the myriad of disease processes that affect the larynx and methods for treatment. The interest in laryngology has burgeoned over recent decades. Young otolaryngologists have become fascinated by the larynx. It is this fascination, shared with a well-established foundation, that propels ongoing diligent investigation. Expansion of our knowledge through basic research and advanced diagnostic techniques has led to improved and more sophisticated treatments.

Our purpose in this text is to have a resource for the practitioner and resident in this exciting specialty. As editors, we have engaged some of the most respected laryngologists and speech pathologists to share their knowledge and insights into a rapidly expanding field. Not only are the basic tenets covered, but also the newest treatments and interventions.

Acknowledgments

We are grateful to all the contributors to this effort who were so willing to share their expertise with their colleagues. We also have had outstanding assistance from the Thieme Publishers editorial staff, including Timothy Hiscock, J. Owen Zurhellen, and Heather Allen. But most of all, we wish to thank our families for their encouragement and support with this effort and in our professional lives.

Contributors

Ahmad I. Al Omari, MD
Laryngology Clinical Instructor
Department of Otolaryngology–Head and Neck Surgery, Laryngoglogy
Stanford University
Palo Alto, California

Kenneth W. Altman, MD, PhD, FACS
Professor of Otolaryngology
Director
Eugen Grabscheid MD Voice Center
Director, Laryngology Fellowship
The Icahn School of Medicine at Mount Sinai
New York, New York

Gerald S. Berke, MD
Professor and Chair
Department of Head and Neck Surgery
Medical Director
UCLA Voice Center for Medicine and the Arts
Department of Head and Neck Surgery
David Geffen School of Medicine at UCLA
Los Angeles, California

Craig Berzofsky, MD, MHS
Laryngology Fellow
Department of Surgery
Southern Illinois University
Springfield, Illinois

Andrew Blitzer, MD, DDS
Emeritus Professor of Clinical Otolaryngology
Columbia University College of Physicians and Surgeons
Adjunct Professor of Neurology
Mt. Sinai School of Medicine
Director
New York Center for Voice and Swallowing Disorders
New York, New York

Linda M. Carroll, PhD, CCC-SLP
Speech-Language Pathologist, Private Practice
New York, New York
Senior Voice Scientist
The Children's Hospital of Philadelphia
Philadelphia, Pennsylvania
Research Scientist
Department of Otorhinolaryngology
Montefiore Medical Center
Bronx, New York

Roger L. Crumley, MD, MBA
Interim President
University Physicians and Surgeons
Interim Senior Associate
Dean for Clinical Affairs
University of California–Irvine School of Medicine
Irvine, California

Seth H. Dailey, MD
Associate Professor, Chief of Laryngology
Department of Surgery
Division of Otolaryngology–Head and Neck Surgery
University of Wisconsin School of Medicine and Public Health
Madison, Wisconsin

Edward J. Damrose, MD, FACS
Associate Professor, Chief of Laryngology
Department of Otolaryngology/Head and Neck Surgery
Stanford University School of Medicine
Stanford, California

Marvin P. Fried, MD, FACS
Professor and University Chairman
Department of Otorhinolaryngology–Head and Neck Surgery
Montefiore Medical Center
The University Hospital of Albert Einstein College of Medicine
Bronx, New York

Lowell E. Gurey, MD
Director of Voice and Swallowing
Department of Otorhinolaryngology–Head and Neck Surgery
Summit Medical Group
Berkeley Heights, New Jersey

Christopher Hartnick, MD
Professor
Department of Otology and Laryngology
Harvard Medical School
Division Director, Pediatric Otolaryngology
Director, Pediatric Airway, Voice and Swallowing Center
Chief Quality Officer for Otolaryngology
Massachusetts Eye and Ear Infirmary
Boston, Massachusetts

Mary J. Hawkshaw, RN, BSN, CORLN
Research Associate Professor
Department of Otolaryngology–Head and Neck Surgery
Drexel University College of Medicine
Philadelphia, Pennsylvania

Chandra M. Ivey, MD
Director, Division of Laryngology
Department of Otolaryngology–Head and Neck Surgery
Columbia University Medical Center
New York, New York

Nausheen Jamal, MD
Assistant Professor
Department of Otolaryngology–Head and Neck Surgery
Temple University School of Medicine
Philadelphia, Pennsylvania

William E. Karle, MD
Department of Otolaryngology–Head and Neck Surgery
The New York Eye and Ear Infirmary
New York, New York

Cathy L. Lazarus, PhD, FASHA
Associate Professor
Icahn School of Medicine at Mount Sinai
Research Director
Thyroid Head and Neck Functional Outcomes Center Foundation
Department of Otolaryngology Head and Neck Surgery
Mount Sinai Beth Israel
New York, New York

Pavan S. Mallur, MD
Instructor
Department of Otology and Laryngology
Harvard Medical School
Beth Israel Deaconess Medical Center
Boston, Massachusetts

Hiroumi Matsuzaki, MD, PhD
Assistant Professor
Department of Otorhinolaryngology–Head and Neck Surgery
Nihon University School of Medicine
Tokyo, Japan

Albert L. Merati, MD, FACS
Professor and Chief, Laryngology
Department of Otolaryngology–Head and Neck Surgery
School of Medicine
Adjunct Associate Professor
Department of Speech and Hearing Services
College of Arts and Sciences
University of Washington
Seattle, Washington

Ashli O'Rourke, MD
Assistant Professor
Evelyn Trammell Institute for Voice and Swallowing
Department of Otolaryngology–Head and Neck Surgery
Medical University of South Carolina
Charleston, South Carolina

Sapna A. Patel, MD
Department of Otolaryngology
University of Washington
Seattle, Washington

Michael Jay Pitman, MD
Associate Professor of Otolaryngology
Department of Otolaryngology
New York Eye and Ear of Mount Sinai
New York, New York

Gregory N. Postma, MD
Professor
Department of Otolaryngology
Director
Center for Voice, Airway and Swallowing Disorders
Georgia Regents University
Augusta, Georgia

Clarence T. Sasaki, MD
The Charles W. Ohse Professor
Department of Surgery
Yale School of Medicine
New Haven, Connecticutt

Johnathan B. Sataloff
Amherst College
Amherst, Massachusetts
Research Associate
American Institute for Voice and Ear Research
Department of Otolaryngology–Head and Neck Surgery
Drexel University College of Medicine
Philadelphia, Pennsylvania

Robert T. Sataloff, MD, DMA, FACS
Professor and Chairman
Department of Otolaryngology–Head and Neck Surgery
Senior Associate Dean for Clinical Academic Specialties
Drexel University College of Medicine
Philadelphia, Pennsylvania

Bradley A. Schiff, MD
Associate Professor
Department of Otorhinolaryngology–Head and Neck Surgery
Albert Einstein College of Medicine
Montefiore Medical Center
The University Hospital of Albert Einstein College of Medicine
Bronx, New York

Jennifer Setlur, MD
Connecticut Pediatric Otolaryngology
Madison, Connecticutt

Jo Shapiro, MD
Chief
Division of Otolaryngology
Director
Center for Professionalism and Peer Support
Brigham and Women's Hospital
Boston, Massachusetts

Catherine F. Sinclair, BSc, BMBS, FRACS
Director, Division of Head and Neck Surgery,
St. Luke's and Roosevelt Hospitals
Assistant Clinical Professor
Albert Einstein College of Medicine
New York, New York

Richard V. Smith, MD, FACS
Professor and Vice-Chair
Department of Otorhinolaryngology–Head and Neck Surgery
Professor of Surgery and Pathology
Albert Einstein College of Medicine
Montefiore Medical Center
Bronx, New York

Manikandan Sugumaran, MD
Laryngology, Voice, and Swallowing Disorders
Department of Otolaryngology
Arizona Otolaryngology Consultants
Phoenix, Arizona

C. Kwang Sung, MD, MS
Assistant Professor
Department of Otolaryngology–Head and Neck Surgery
Stanford University School of Medicine
Stanford, California

Melin Tan, MD
Assistant Professor
Department of Otorhinolaryngology–Head and Neck Surgery
Montefiore Medical Center
The University Hospital for Albert Einstein College of Medicine
Bronx, New York

Andrew B. Tassler, MD
Assistant Professor
Department of Otorhinolaryngology–Head and Neck Surgery
Albert Einstein College of Medicine
Montefiore Medical Center
The University Hospital of Albert Einstein College of Medicine
Bronx, New York

Mai Thy Truong, MD
Clinical Instructor
Department of Otolaryngology–Head and Neck Surgery
Stanford School of Medicine
Stanford, California

Sunil P. Verma, MD
Director
Univerisity Voice and Swallowing Center
Medical Director
Department of Otolaryngology–Head and Neck Surgery
University of California–Irvine School of Medicine
Irvine, California

Philip A. Weissbrod, MD
Assistant Professor of Otolaryngology
Director, Center for Voice and Swallowing
Division of Otolaryngology
University of California—San Diego Health System
La Jolla, California

Peak Woo, MD
Clinical Professor
Department of Otolaryngology
Icahn School of Medicine at Mount Sinai
New York, New York

Nwanmegha Young, MD
Assistant Professor
Surgery Section of Otolaryngology
Yale School of Medicine
New Haven, Connecticutt

Steven M. Zeitels, MD, FACS
Eugene B. Casey Professor of Laryngeal Surgery
Harvard Medical School
Chief
Division of Laryngeal Surgery
Massachusetts General Hospital
Boston, Massachusetts

1 Anatomy of the Larynx

Nwanmegha Young, Hiroumi Matsuzaki, and Clarence T. Sasaki

In the midline of the neck lies the larynx, a multitask organ that functions as the gateway between the respiratory and the upper digestive systems. Acting as a complex biological sphincter, the larynx serves the important role of balancing the often conflicting functions of respiration, deglutition, and phonation. Specific anatomical and complex neural adaptations have transpired that are critical for this ability. In this chapter, the authors discuss laryngeal anatomy related to these functions.

1.1 Basic Anatomy of the Larynx

The laryngeal exoskeleton is comprised of a series of cartilages connected by ligaments, membranes, and muscles. Superiorly, the larynx communicates with the oropharynx; inferiorly, it connects with the trachea and the remainder of the lower respiratory tract. Directly posterior to the larynx lies the beginning of the upper esophageal sphincter, the entrance to the lower digestive system (▶ Fig. 1.1).

1.1.1 Cartilages of the Larynx

The larynx has nine cartilages (▶ Fig. 1.2). Three of the nine cartilages are individual cartilages; the remainder are paired.

1.1.2 Thyroid Cartilage

The thyroid cartilage is the largest of the laryngeal cartilages and forms the anterior wall of the larynx. It is a single wedge-shaped structure composed of two lateral wings that fuse anteriorly to form the laryngeal prominence ("Adam's apple"). In males, the wings meet at an acute angle of approximately 90 degrees. In females, the angle is more obtuse, approximately 120 degrees. Superiorly, the juncture point forms the thyroid notch. Laterally, the wings fan out from above and below to form the superior greater and inferior lesser horns, respectively. The superior horn of the thyroid attaches to the greater horn of the hyoid bone. The inferior thyroid horn cornu articulates with a facet on the cricoid cartilage to form the cricothyroid joint. The thyroid cartilage is attached to the hyoid bone superiorly via the thyrohyoid membrane.

An understanding of the laryngeal surface anatomy and its relationships to its internal structures is vital for the otolaryngologist. The midline vertical distance from the thyroid notch to its inferior border ranges from 20 to 47 mm in men and 15 to 38 mm in women.[1] The midpoint between these two landmarks houses the anterior commissure.

1.1.3 Cricoid Cartilage

The cricoid cartilage forms the foundation of the larynx. It is the only complete ring in the airway. It has the shape of an asymmetric signet ring, with a narrow anterior arch 0.5 to 1 cm in height and a broader posterior portion 2 to 3 cm in height. On the superior surface of the posterior lamina are articulations for the arytenoid cartilages. On the posterolateral aspect are articulations for the cricothyroid joint. The horizontal inferior border is attached to the first tracheal cartilage by the cricotracheal ligament.[2] Anteriorly, along the superior surface of the arch, the cricothyroid ligament is attached.

1.1.4 Arytenoid Cartilages

Arytenoid cartilages are paired cartilages shaped like three-sided pyramids. Each cartilage has a base with a muscular process laterally, a vocal process anteriorly, and inferiorly an articular facet. The vestibular ligament as well as the thyroarytenoid muscles attach to the anterolateral surface. The posterior surface contains muscular attachments and the posterior cricoarytenoid ligament is attached to the medial surface. The corniculate cartilage sits at the apex of the arytenoid.[3]

1.1.5 Corniculate and Cuneiform Cartilages

The corniculate and cuneiform cartilages are small fibroelastic cartilages that are thought to be rudimentary and vestigial. The corniculate (Santorini) cartilages are in the posterior aspect of

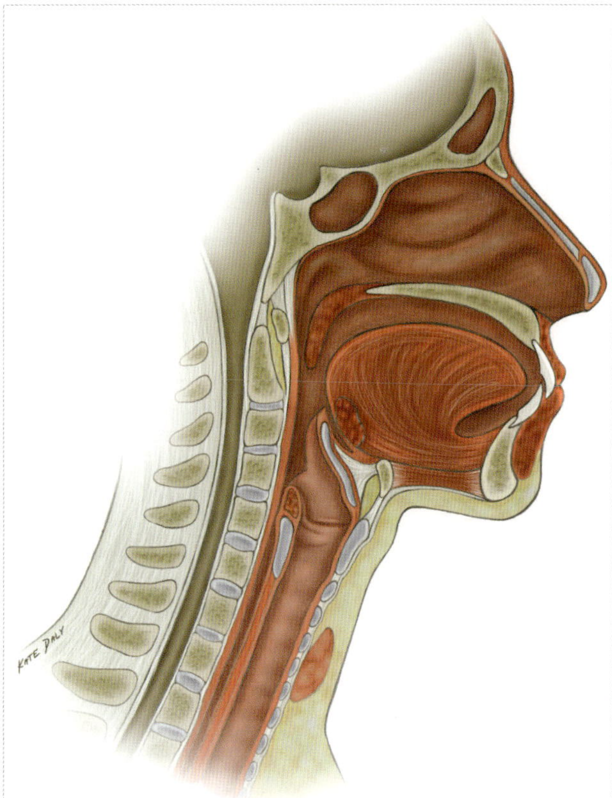

Fig. 1.1 The upper aerodigestive tract.

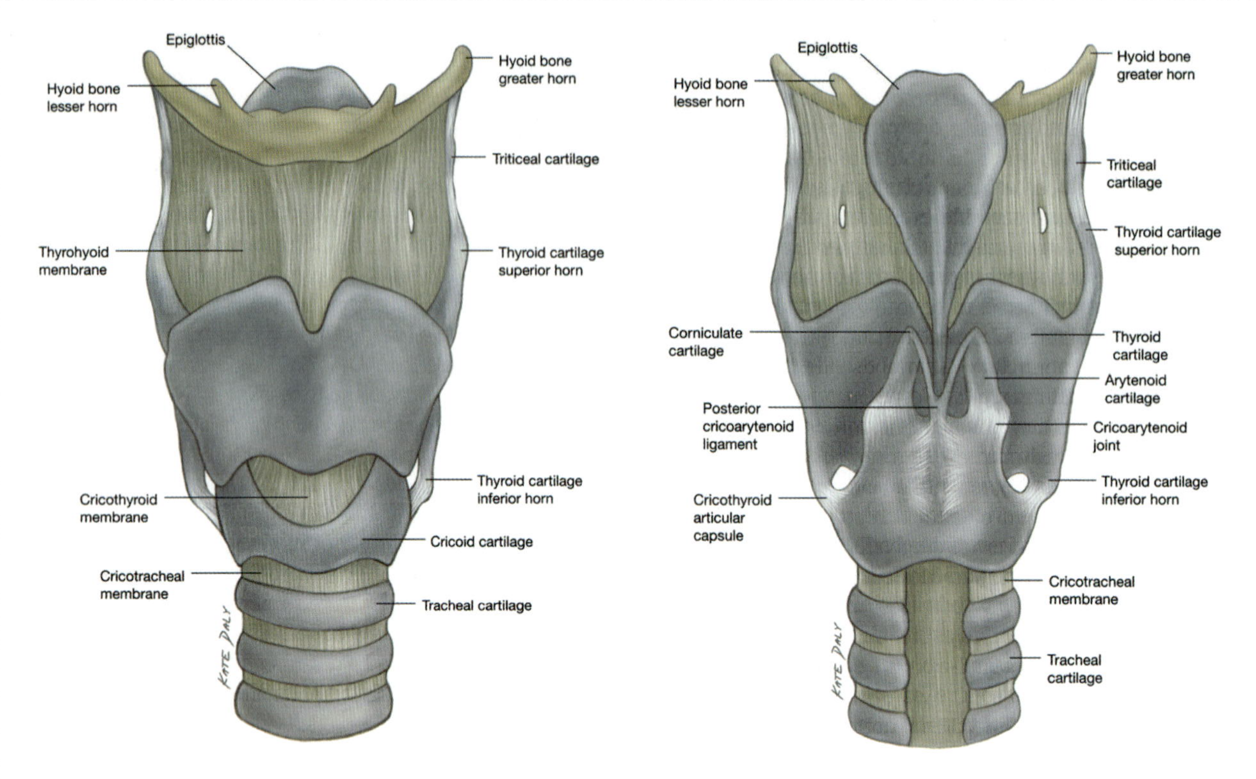

Fig. 1.2 The laryngeal exoskeleton. (a) Anterior view. (b) Posterior view.

the aryepiglottic folds and articulate with the apices of the arytenoid cartilages. The cuneiform (Wrisberg) cartilages lie within the aryepiglottic folds and are approximated to the tubercle of the epiglottis when the inlet of the larynx is closed during swallowing. They are thought to add rigidity to the aryepiglottic folds during swallowing.[4]

1.1.6 The Epiglottic Cartilage

The epiglottis is a thin piece of cartilage that is shaped like a leaf. It is situated posterior to the root of the tongue and hyoid bone and anterior to the inlet of the larynx. It forms the superior part of the anterior wall of the larynx as well as the superior margin of the inlet of the larynx. It can be divided into a suprahyoid and an infrahyoid portion. The laryngeal and lingual surfaces of the broad suprahyoid portion are free and unattached. Only the laryngeal surface of the tapered infrahyoid epiglottis is free and unattached. The lingual surface of the infrahyoid portion is attached to the thyroepiglottic ligament, located in the angle formed by the thyroid laminae. The laryngeal mucosa is more adherent to its surface than the lingual side.

The anterior surface of the epiglottic cartilage is attached to the hyoid bone by the hyoepiglottic ligament. The inferior part of the posterior surface of the epiglottic cartilage that projects posteriorly is called the epiglottic tubercle. It is unique among the laryngeal cartilages as it is comprised of elastic rather than hyaline cartilage, which enables its flexibility throughout life without the ossification seen in the other laryngeal cartilages.

1.2 Extrinsic Muscles

The extrinsic muscles of the larynx, also referred to as the strap muscles, function to raise, lower, or stabilize the larynx. The infrahyoid group includes the omohyoid, sternothyroid, thyrohyoid, and sternohyoid muscles, which are innervated by the ansa cervicalis. These muscles depress the larynx, displacing it downward during inspiration. The suprahyoid group of muscles includes the digastrics, stylohyoid, geniohyoid, mylohyoid, and stylopharyngeus. These muscles elevate and anteriorly displace the larynx during swallowing and suspend the larynx from the skull base and mandible via the hyoid bone. The middle and inferior constrictors, as well as the cricopharyngeus muscles, are also extrinsic muscles that play an imperative role in the precisely timed act of deglutition.[5]

1.3 Intrinsic Muscles

The intrinsic laryngeal muscles act in synchrony to modify the size of the glottic opening, as well as both the length and tension of the vocal folds (▸ Fig. 1.3). These muscles are restricted to the internal larynx; they consist of numerous adductors and a single abductor. The intrinsic muscles are paired, with the exception of the interarytenoid (▸ Fig. 1.4).

1.3.1 Posterior Cricoarytenoid Muscle

The posterior cricoarytenoid muscle (PCA) is a broad muscle that originates from the shallow depression on the posterior

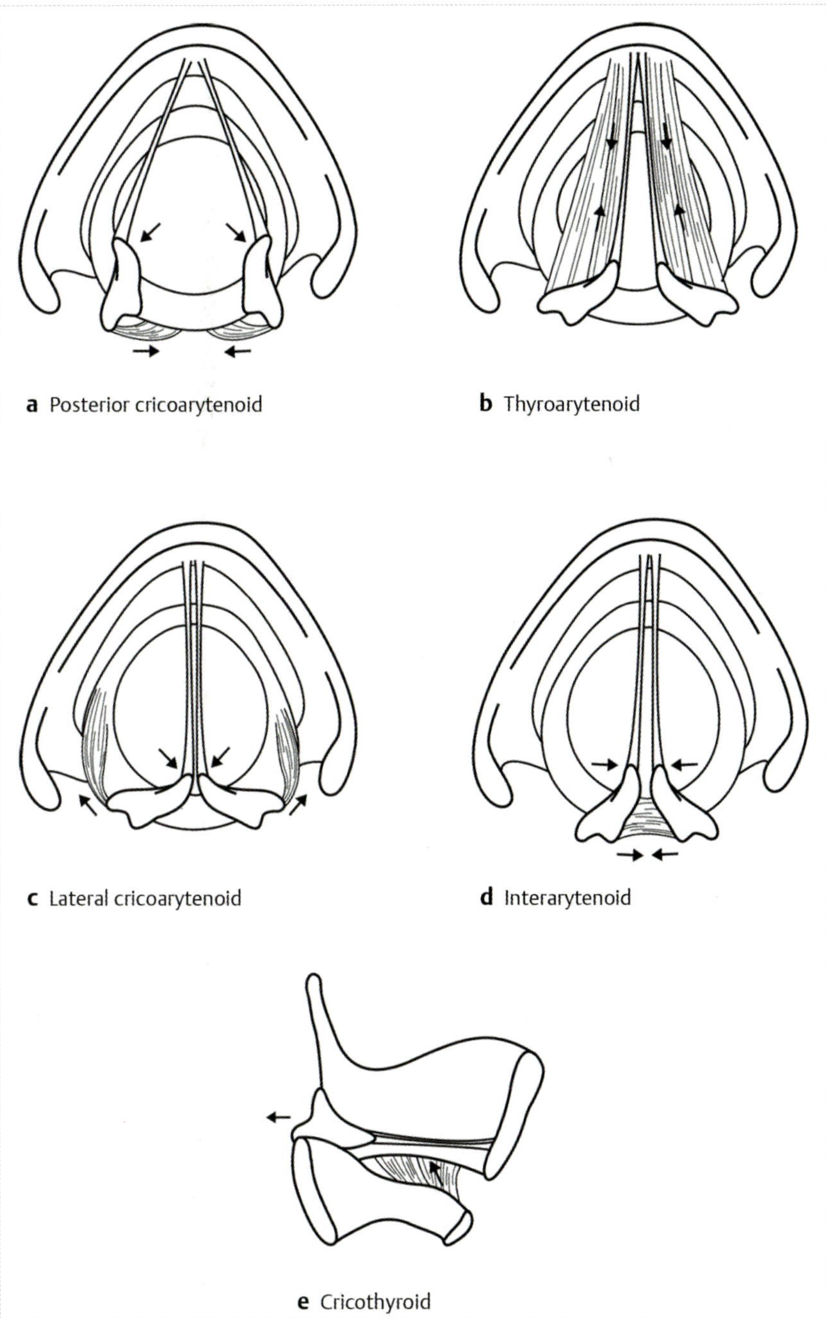

Fig. 1.3 Basic modifications of the glottis. **(a)** Posterior cricoarytenoid. **(b)** Thyroidarytenoid. **(c)** Lateral cricoarytenoid. **(d)** Interarytenoid. **(e)** Cricothyroid.

surface of the quadrate lamina. It inserts into the muscular process of the arytenoid cartilage on the same side. It is described as having a fan-shaped medial part and a vertical lateral part. This muscle is the only abductor of the vocal cords.

Contraction slides the arytenoid cartilage inferiorly and laterally on the cricoid cartilage in a posteromedial direction. Therefore, it abducts and elevates the tip of the vocal process, elongating and thinning the vocal fold, causing its edge to be rounded.

1.3.2 Lateral Cricoarytenoid Muscle

The lateral cricoarytenoid muscle is a slightly fan-shaped muscle, which originates along the upper border of the arch of the cricoid cartilage. Its fibers course upwards and backwards to insert on the muscular process and anterior border of the arytenoid cartilage. During contraction it slides the arytenoid cartilage superiorly and medially on the cricoid with an anterolateral pull. It acts as the antagonist to the PCA.

1.3.3 Interarytenoid/Aryepiglottic Muscle

The unpaired interarytenoid muscle is a complex of muscle fibers located on the posterior surfaces of the arytenoid cartilages. Its transverse fibers attach to the lateral margins and posterior surfaces of the arytenoid cartilages. Its oblique fibers originate from the posterior surface of the muscular process of one arytenoid cartilage and insert near the apex of

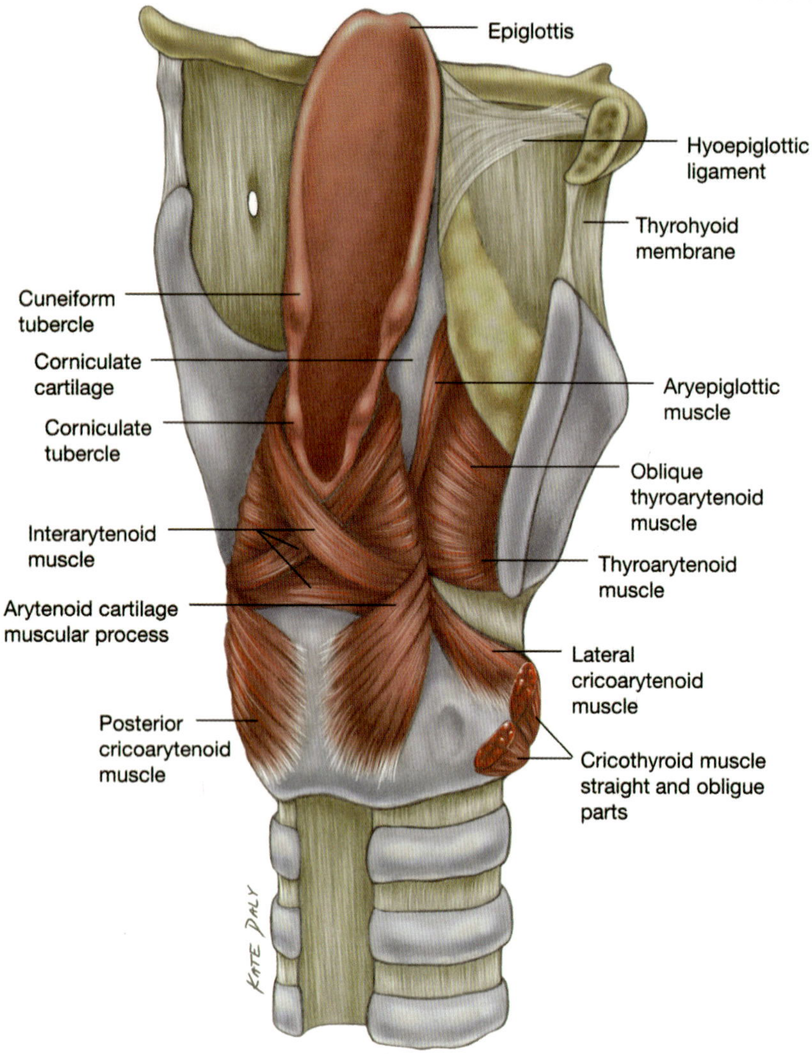

Fig. 1.4 Intrinsic laryngeal muscles.

the other arytenoid cartilage. Together, the oblique fibers form an "X" on the posterior surface of the transverse fibers. Contraction of the arytenoids draws the two arytenoid cartilages toward each other, i.e., it adducts the vocal cords during phonation.

Some of the oblique fibers do not insert on the apex of the contralateral arytenoid; instead they fan out in the quadrangular membrane, forming the aryepiglottic muscle.

1.3.4 The Cricothyroid Muscle

The cricothyroid muscle originates on the arch of the cricoid cartilage and inserts on the inferior border of the thyroid lamina. It is described as having two parts: a pars recta, whose fibers course vertically, and a pars oblique, whose fibers course upward and backward. Contraction of its fibers rotates the anterior part of the thyroid cartilage downward, causing rotation at the cricothyroid joint. The net result is that the anterior attachment of the vocal cords is pulled away from the arytenoid cartilages, thereby stretching (tensing) the vocal cords. The cricothyroid muscle is innervated by the external laryngeal nerve.

1.3.5 The Thyroarytenoid Muscle

The thyroarytenoid muscle arises from a narrow, vertically oriented region of the inner surface of the angle of the thyroid cartilage. It then courses posteriorly, to insert into the lateral and inferior aspect of the vocal process of the arytenoid cartilage. The medial fibers form the vocalis muscle. The lateral fibers form the thyromuscularis. Contraction adducts, shortens, and thickens the vocal fold by rotating the arytenoid cartilages anteromedially.

1.4 Joints of the Larynx

1.4.1 Cricothyroid Joints

The cricothyroid joint is formed between the inferior horns of the thyroid cartilage and the posterior cricoid arch. It is a synovial joint with a fibrous capsule. Thickenings in the capsule are named the anterior, lateral, and posterior ceratocricoid ligaments. The joint plays an important role in adjusting pitch by changing/altering the tension of the vocal cords. The joint movement is controlled by the cricothyroid muscle, as well as

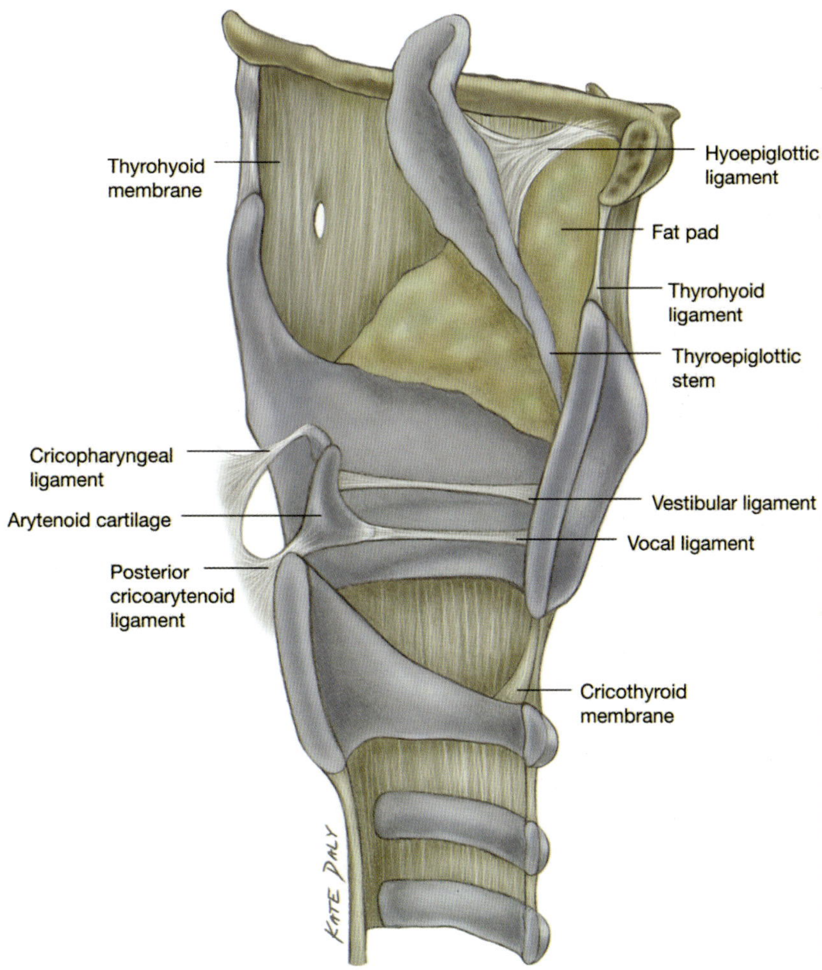

Fig. 1.5 Membranes of the larynx.

the vocalis/thyroarytenoid muscle. The main movements at these joints are rotation and gliding of the thyroid cartilage in both horizontal and vertical directions. This results in narrowing of the cricothyroid space, with a resultant increase in the length of the vocal fold between the anterior commissure and the vocal process, effectively tensing the fold.

1.4.2 Cricoarytenoid Joints

The cricoarytenoid joints are formed between the cricoid cartilage and the arytenoid cartilages. They are synovial joints. On the dorsal medial aspect of the joint capsule, there is a thickening that is the cricoarytenoid ligament. The movement at the joint is described as a rocking–gliding motion. The net result of the complex movement is that the vocal processes of the arytenoid cartilages swing downward and inward, or upward and outward. The cricoarytenoid ligament limits the anterior movement of the arytenoid cartilages. These movements are important in approximating, tensing, and relaxing the vocal folds.

1.4.3 Membranes of the Larynx

The components of the laryngeal apparatus are connected to each other and the external environment by extrinsic (connecting the larynx to the hyoid bone and/or trachea) and intrinsic (connecting the laryngeal cartilages with each other) membranes. The extrinsic membranes include the thyrohyoid membrane, the hyoepiglottic membrane, and the cricotracheal membrane (▶ Fig. 1.5). The thyrohyoid membrane attaches the thyroid cartilage to the hyoid bone. It is made up of a thickened middle portion and a thinner lateral portion named the median and lateral thyrohyoid membrane, respectively. In the lateral portion there are often small triticeal cartilages where the superior cornu attaches to the greater cornu of the hyoid bone. The thyrohyoid membrane has an opening in its lateral aspect to admit the internal laryngeal nerve and artery. The hyoepiglottic membrane extends from the anterior surface of the epiglottis to the upper border of the body of the hyoid bone. It forms the roof of the pre-epiglottic and paraglottic spaces. The cricotracheal ligament is a fibrous membrane that connects the first ring of tracheal cartilage with the inferior border of the cricoid cartilage.

The intrinsic membranes of the larynx connect the laryngeal cartilages with each other and are critical in allowing the larynx to function as a complex biological sphincter. There are two parts that comprise this intrinsic system: the conus elasticus and the quadrangular membranes (▶ Fig. 1.6). The quadrangular membranes are paired membranes extending from the lateral margins of the epiglottic cartilage. They course posteriorly to attach to the corniculate and lateral aspect of the arytenoid

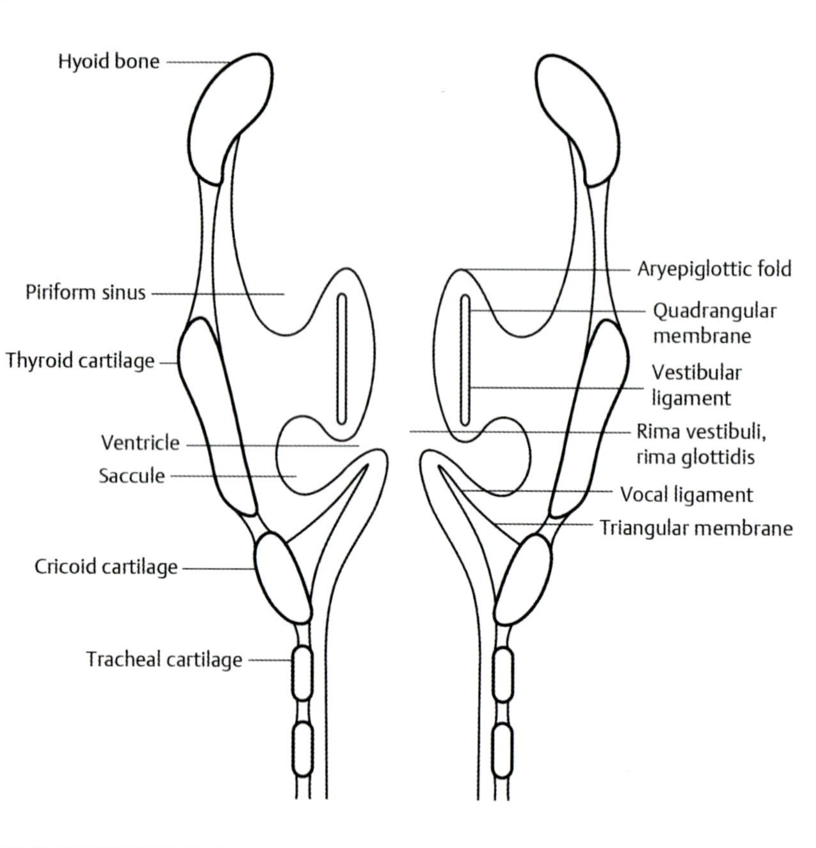

Fig. 1.6 Coronal view of the intrinsic membrane.

cartilages. Superiorly, the free margin forms the aryepiglottic fold with the mucous membrane overlying it. Inferiorly, the quadrangular membrane forms the vestibular ligament that helps produce the false vocal folds.

The conus elasticus connects the cricoid cartilage with the thyroid and arytenoid cartilages. It is composed of dense fibroconnective tissue with abundant elastic fibers. The conus elasticus has a more strongly developed layer of elastic tissue than the quadrangular membrane. Its inferior attachment is at the superior border of the cricoid cartilage. It has both superior and medial projections attaching superiorly to the anterior commissure of the thyroid cartilage and the vocal processes of the arytenoid. It thickens between these attachments to form a vocal ligament. The cricothyroid membrane, with its midline thickening into the cricothyroid ligament, is formed by the conus anteriorly. The thyroglottic membrane, which parallels the superior surface of the true vocal fold, is the superior extension of the conus. The thyroglottic membrane forms an incomplete barrier to the extension of transglottic cancer due to normal dehiscence in the membrane.[3,6]

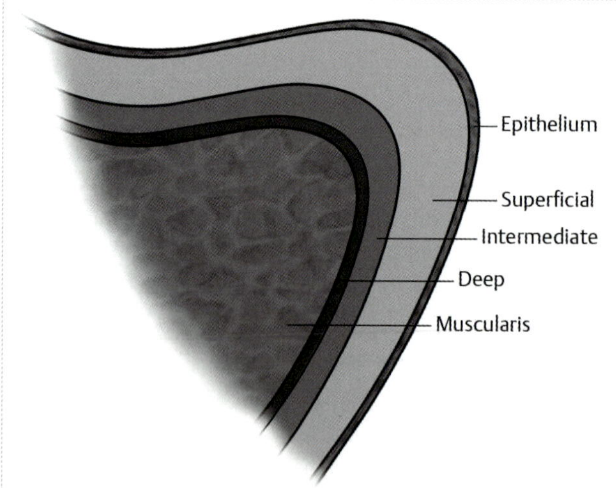

Fig. 1.7 The layers of the vocal fold.

1.5 Vocal Ligaments

The free edge of the conus elasticus forms the true vocal cords (▶ Fig. 1.7). The vocal folds form the glottis, the narrowest portion of the larynx. The anterior membranous three-fifths of the true vocal fold (rima glottis vocalis) is formed by the vocal folds, comprised of a ligament and covering epithelium. The posterior cartilaginous two-fifths (respiratory portion) is formed by the vocal process of the arytenoid cartilages. The membranous (vibratory) portion can be divided structurally into three layers.[7,8] The most superficial layer is made up of stratified squamous epithelium. This layer maintains the shape of the vocal folds and protects the underlying tissue from trauma. Immediately deep is the second layer, the lamina propria. The lamina propria has three components: (1) the superficial lamina propria (SLP), also known as the Reinke space, composed mostly of loose fibrous and elastic components in a matrix similar in texture to soft gelatin; (2) the intermediate lamina propria (ILP), composed of mostly elastic fibers; and (3) the deep lamina propria (DLP), composed of mostly collagenous fibers. The third structural layer is the vocalis muscle. In relation to phonation, the vocal cord functions as two layers, a "cover" made up of squamous epithelium and the SLP. This structure overlies the "body" made up of the vocalis. The deep lamina propria (intermediate and deep layers) functions as a transition zone. The body provides the rigid base on which the cover vibrates. The anterior and posterior macula flava at the anterior and posterior ends of the vocal folds are a thickening of the intermediate elastic layer. They are thought to protect the ends of the vocal folds from vibratory damage. The pediatric larynx lacks this protective cushion, as well as the cover-body microanatomy, due to a single-layered lamina propria. The geriatric larynx develops a thickened and edematous cover with age-related changes in the superficial lamina propria, while the vocalis muscle atrophies.[8,9]

1.6 Compartments of the Larynx

1.6.1 Pre-epiglottic Space

The epiglottis is the posterior boundary of the pre-epiglottic space, which lies anterior to it (▶ Fig. 1.8). The thyrohyoid membrane and inner surface of the thyroid lamina are the anterior borders. The hyoepiglottic ligament and mucosa of the vallecula and thyroepiglottic ligament are the superior and inferior borders, respectively. The pre-epiglottic space opens into the paraglottic space laterally.

1.6.2 Paraglottic Space

This space is superior and inferior to the true and false vocal folds on both sides of the glottis (▶ Fig. 1.8). The cricothyroid membrane and perichondrium of the thyroid lamina define the space laterally, while the quadrangular membrane, ventricle, and conus elasticus serve as medial borders. The space opens into the posterior pre-epiglottic space anterosuperiorly. Pyriform sinus mucosa forms the posterior boundary.

1.7 Vessels

1.7.1 Arteries and Veins

The paired superior and inferior laryngeal arteries are the main arterial supply to the larynx. The superior thyroid artery is the first branch off the external carotid artery, and after coursing lateral to the laryngohyoid complex, the superior laryngeal artery branches off at about the hyoid level. The superior laryngeal artery runs horizontally across the posterior portion of the thyroid membrane, along with the internal branch of the superior laryngeal nerve. The artery penetrates the thyrohyoid membrane inferior to the nerve, entering the submucosa of the pyriform sinus, where it supplies the mucosa and musculature

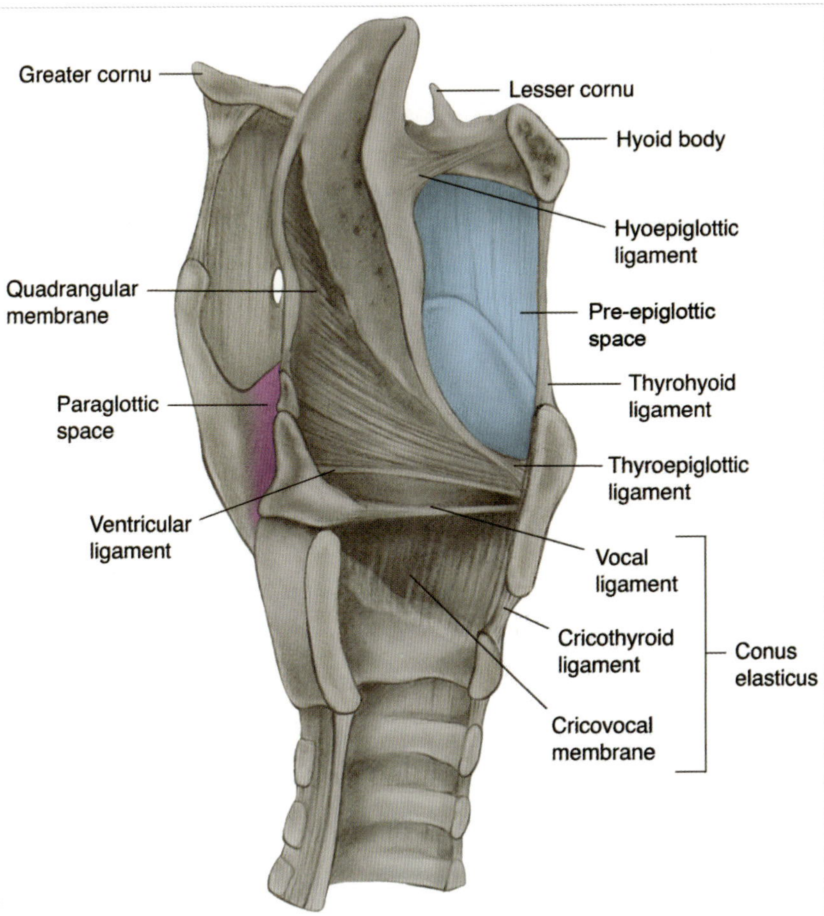

Fig. 1.8 The pre-epiglottic and paraglottic spaces.

of the larynx. At the level of the cricothyroid membrane, the superior thyroid artery gives off a small cricothyroid artery, which passes horizontally below the cricoid cartilage. The inferior laryngeal artery, a branch of the inferior thyroid artery that emanates from the subclavian artery via the thyrocervical trunk, takes a course posterior to the cricothyroid joint with the recurrent laryngeal nerve. The inferior thyroid artery accesses the larynx through a gap in the inferior constrictor muscle known as the Killian-Jamieson area. Within the larynx, the artery branches and supplies mucosa and musculature, anastomosing with the superior laryngeal artery.

Superior and inferior laryngeal veins parallel the arteries, joining the superior and inferior veins, respectively.

1.8 Lymphatics

The lymphatics of the larynx have numerous divisions, an understanding of which is essential in contemplating the spread of laryngeal cancer and its treatment modalities. The divisions start with superficial (intramucosal) and deep (submucosal) groups, which are further divided into right and left halves, broken down into supraglottic, glottic, and subglottic. The deep portion is more important in the spread of cancer. The supraglottic region (false cords and aryepiglottic folds) flows to the deep jugular chain near the carotid bifurcation, as the lymphatic channels follow the superior laryngeal and superior thyroid vessels from the pyriform sinus through the thyrohyoid membrane. The epiglottis, as a midline structure, has bilateral drainage. The ventricle is drained through the cricothyroid membrane and ipsilateral thyroid lobe. There are two systems in the lymphatic drainage of the subglottic larynx. The first system ends in the subclavian, paratracheal, and tracheoesophageal chains, as well as the lower portion of the deep jugular chain by following the inferior thyroid vessels. The other system drains bilaterally to the middle deep cervical nodes and prelaryngeal (Delphian) nodes by piercing the cricothyroid membrane. Cancer localized to the true vocal folds has a high curability rate because there is no lymphatic drainage of this structure.[10,11]

1.9 Conclusion

The larynx sits at the crossroads of the upper respiratory and digestive systems. It is made up of a series of cartilages, ligaments, muscles, and membranes. These structures divide the larynx into compartments, which have important implications surgically as well as pathologically.

References

[1] Sasaki CT, Young-Ho K, LeVay AJ. Development, anatomy, physiology of the larynx. In: Snow JB, Wackym PA, eds. Ballenger's Otorhinolaryngology Head and Neck Surgery. 17th ed.Shelton, CT: BC Decker; 2009:73–98

[2] Maue WM, Dickson DR. Cartilages and ligaments of the adult human larynx. Arch Otolaryngol 1971; 94: 432–439

[3] Tucker HM. Anatomy of the larynx. In: Tucker HM, ed. The Larynx. 2nd ed. New York, NY: Thieme Medical Publishers; 1993

[4] Negus VE. The Comparative Anatomy and Physiology of the Larynx. London: Heinemann; 1949

[5] Hollinshead WH. The pharynx and larynx. In: Hollinshead WH, ed. Anatomy for Surgeons. Volume 1: The Head and Neck. 3rd ed. Philadelphia, PA: JB Lippincott; 1982:389–441

[6] Spector GJ. Anatomy of the larynx. In: Ballenger JJ, ed. Diseases of the Nose, Throat, Ear, Head and Neck. 13th ed. Philadelphia, PA: Lea & Febiger; 1985:376–385

[7] Hirano M. Outline of voice production and its examination. In: Hirano M, ed. Clinical Examination of Voice. New York, NY: Springer-Verlag; 1981:1–100

[8] Boseley ME, Hartnick CJ. Development of the human true vocal fold: depth of cell layers and quantifying cell types within the lamina propria. Ann Otol Rhinol Laryngol 2006; 115: 784–788

[9] Sanders I. The microanatomy of the vocal fold musculature. In: Rubin JS, Sataloff RT, & Korovin GS, eds. Diagnosis and Treatment of Voice Disorders. Clifton Park, NY: Delmar Learning; 2003: 49–68

[10] Johner CH. The lymphatics of the larynx. Otolaryngol Clin North Am 1970; 3: 439–450

[11] Hanafee WN, Ward PH. Anatomy and physiology. In: Hanafee WN, Ward PH, eds. Clinical Correlations in the Head and Neck. Volume 1: The Larynx. New York, NY: Thieme Medical Publishers; 1990:1–7

2 Physiology of the Larynx

Nwanmegha Young, Hiroumi Matsuzaki, and Clarence T. Sasaki

2.1 Functional Anatomy

The larynx has three basic functions that are inherently in conflict with one another. Understanding the structural as well complex neuromuscular adaptations that have occurred to resolve these conflicts is essential to the management of the myriad of diseases besetting this complex organ.

2.2 Phylogeny

Comparative analysis of larynges from several species gives unique insight into the laryngeal adaptations. Negus carried out a comprehensive study. He postulated that as animals migrated from an aquatic to a terrestrial existence, their respiratory requirements changed. These were reflected in certain contemporary species of fish that developed unique respiratory modifications to allow intermittent sojourns on dry land. Notably, the climbing perch (*Anabas scandens*) possessed a respiratory diverticulum located above its gills. The most primitive larynx may be found in the bichir lungfish (*Polypterus*), which inhabits the Nile River. The larynx of this fish consists simply of a muscular sphincter to guard against the entrance of water. However, the African lungfish (*Protopterus*) and Australian lungfish (*Neoceratodus*) both possess, in addition to sphincteric musculature, discrete muscle fibers that effectively draw the margins apart to produce active dilatation. The muscular sphincter therefore remains contracted when the fish is in the water, but, during a drought, the sphincter is actively opened to allow air to be gulped into the lungs by a swallowing maneuver. This capacity provides obvious advantages for survival when the supply of water is limited or undependable.

2.3 Nasolaryngeal Relations

Many mammalian species are provided with a relatively high-riding larynx, affording its close approximation with structures of the posterior nasal cavities. The intracranial position of the larynx, which secures a continuous airway from the nose to the bronchi, decreases the risk of pulmonary contamination by swallowed matter. Secondarily, the epiglottis serves in an olfactory capacity, ensuring that inspired air enters exclusively through the nose. Negus' work supported this contention by a series of anatomic demonstrations in macrosomatic animals. Histological evidence also demonstrates epiglottic chemoreceptors similar in structure to taste buds of the oral cavity, implying epiglottic participation in chemosensory perception as well.[1] The human newborn exhibits a similar nasolaryngeal connection by the approximation of the epiglottis with the posterior surface of the palate, thus ensuring against aspiration. The observation of obligate nasal breathing in the newborn period may be related to this anatomic configuration, which is lost between 4 and 6 months postnatally.[1] In the adult, the larynx rides low in the neck, and the characteristic flat, shield-like configuration of the epiglottis serves to direct swallowed food laterally into the piriform sinuses, away from the midline laryngeal aperture. Furthermore, in adults, elevation of the larynx toward the nasal cavity during the height of deglutition exaggerates this protective function. The aryepiglottic folds act as ramparts to the larynx, allowing food to pass on either side of the epiglottis along the gutter produced between each fold and the lateral pharyngeal wall. It appears that the primary function of the supraglottic larynx is its protection of the lower airway.

2.4 Valve Actions

Due to their unique configuration, the false and true cords have the ability to function as valves. The ventricular folds, which are located superiorly, act as an exit valve, preventing the escape of air from the lower respiratory tract. When medialized by muscular contraction, these false cords seal even more tightly as tracheal pressure is increased below. This feature of adducted false cords is attributable to their unique shape, characterized by the down-turned direction of their free margins.

Conversely, the true cords behave as a one-way valve in the opposite direction, obstructing the ingress of air or fluid. The false cords prevent the egress of air from the lungs, and the true cords, with their upturned margins, are capable of arresting its ingress. These features of the larynx are exploited in several essential bodily functions, such as coughing and elimination.[2]

2.5 Neuromuscular Physiology

The larynx has developed complex polysynaptic reflex arcs to adjust to its need to be dynamic in fulfilling its three basic functions. We briefly discuss the afferent and efferent components of the arcs and then the reflexes themselves.

2.5.1 Afferent System

Sensory nerve fibers to the larynx are derived from the internal branches of the superior laryngeal nerve (SLN). Each nerve innervates the ipsilateral upper half of the larynx to the level of the true vocal cord. Likewise, below the level of the true cords, ipsilateral sensation is mediated by each recurrent laryngeal nerve (RLN). However, Suzuki and Kirchner[3] demonstrated that a diamond-shaped area in the anterior midline of the subglottic space in the cat is innervated by both external branches of the SLN. Afferent impulses from deep muscle receptors and cricothyroid joints also travel cephalad in this nerve branch (▶ Table 2.1). The density of sensory innervation is greatest in the laryngeal inlet. When nerve-staining techniques are used, the laryngeal surface of the epiglottis appears to contain the most compact innervation, whereas the true cords exhibit lesser degrees of sensory density.[3] Specifically, the posterior half of the true cord is more heavily furnished with touch receptors than its anterior portion. The distributions of chemical and thermal sensors differ as well. These sensors appear to be limited to the supraglottic larynx and are sensitive to a variety of noxious substances. This is logical because the entrance to the larynx is thought to serve as a protective zone for more distal parts of

Table 2.1 Sensory innervation of the larynx

Nerve	Distribution
Superior laryngeal nerve (external branch)	Supraglottic mucosa, thyroepiglottic and cricocothyroid joints
Superior laryngeal nerve (internal branch)	Anterior subglottic mucosa
Recurrent laryngeal nerve	Subglottic mucosa, muscle spindles
Nerve of Galen	Aortic arch

Table 2.2 Motor innervation of the larynx

Nerve	Distribution	Action
Superior laryngeal nerve (external)	Cricothyroid muscle	Isotonic tensor adduction
Recurrent laryngeal nerve	Intrinsic muscles of the larynx	Adduction, abduction, and isotonic tension
Nerve of Galen (communicating)	Tracheal smooth muscle and mucosa	Autonomic

the respiratory system. Some of these afferent signals are part of a reflex arc that can affect important physiological functions. Water chemoreceptors on the epiglottis have been implicated experimentally in the production of prolonged apnea.[4] Furthermore, it has been demonstrated that the respiratory response to water–aerosol inhalation for treatment of croup and other upper-airway obstruction may be related to the exquisite water sensitivity of these epiglottic receptors. The respiratory effect produced consists of slowing of breathing and a concomitant increase in tidal volume. This effect is beneficial in the setting of partial airway obstruction. In addition, this centrally mediated respiratory response appears to be greater in early life than in adulthood.[5]

It is generally agreed that sensory components of the SLN include representation from mucosal touch receptors, epiglottic chemoreceptors, joint receptors, aortic baroreceptors, and stretch receptors from the intrinsic laryngeal muscles.[6] Afferent impulses are delivered through the ganglion nodosum to the brainstem tractus solitarius. In sum, laryngeal sensation is extremely complex.

2.5.2 Efferent System

Motor innervation of the larynx is no less complex (▶ Table 2.2). It is generally agreed that the motor distribution of the intrinsic laryngeal musculature originates in the nucleus ambiguus. This motor nucleus is topographically divided into abductor and adductor zones. Each RLN innervates all muscles ipsilaterally except the cricothyroid muscle, which receives its motor impulses from the external division of its ipsilateral SLN. The interarytenoid muscle, however, receives bilateral innervation from both RLNs.

2.6 Laryngeal Reflexes

Basic functions of the larynx (protective, respiratory, and phonatory) are derived from a complex interrelationship of diverse polysynaptic brainstem reflexes. The protective function is entirely reflexive and involuntary, whereas the other two can be modulated with voluntary input.

2.6.1 Protective Reflex

Stimulation of the upper respiratory tract, especially the larynx, evokes a strong glottic closure reflex (GCR). The afferent sensory impulses via the internal branch of SLN project to the ipsilateral nucleus ambiguus after synapsing in the nucleus tractus solitarius. The motor neurons within the nucleus ambiguus then project through the RLN, completing the efferent limb of the ipsilateral GCR (▶ Fig. 2.1). The functional analog of this reflex is reproduced as protective glottic closure during deglutition. Touch and chemical and thermal stimulation of the laryngeal aditus produce the same response as seen experimentally with electrostimulation of the SLN. In an experimental setup, it has been observed that stimulation of ipsilateral internal SLN elicits three categories of protective laryngeal responses. First, an early response involves adduction of the ipsilateral vocal cord with a latency of approximately 10 to 18 ms in an anesthetized cat, dog, and pig.[7,8] This short-latency, R1 evoked response, has been consistently noted in anesthetized humans. A second category of short-latency R1 response involves simultaneous contralateral adduction also known as the crossed adductor reflex (▶ Fig. 2.2). In anesthetized human subjects, this reflex is suppressed (▶ Fig. 2.3).[9] Clinically, this may manifest as increased incidence of life-threatening aspiration in sedated patients. Still, a third category of adductor response involving a longer-latency reflex, termed R2, has been observed to produce bilateral vocal fold responses, but its presence appears to be most readily noted in awake human subjects; it has a latency of 50 to 80 ms.[10]

Bilateral SLN stimulation results in sphincteric closure of the upper airway of its three muscular tiers within the laryngeal framework. The highest occurs at the level of the aryepiglottic folds, which contain the superiormost divisions of the thyroarytenoid muscle. The contraction of these fibers approximates the aryepiglottic folds to cover the superior inlet of the larynx, and with the arytenoid cartilages in the posterior gap, completes the first of the three sphincteric tiers of protection. The second tier of protection occurs at the level of the false cords, consisting of bilateral folds forming the roof of each laryngeal ventricle. The third tier of protection occurs at the level of the true vocal cords, which are shelf-like with a slightly upturned free border.

The inferior division of the thyroarytenoid muscle forms the bulk of this shelf, and with the passive valvular effect of the upturned border or the true cord margin, the true vocal cord folds are perhaps the most significant of the three barriers to aspiration.

Mechanical stimulation applied to the upper respiratory tract, which is innervated by the trigeminal and glossopharyngeal nerves, or the electrical stimulation of all major cranial afferent nerves produces strong laryngeal adductor responses. In the cat, reflex action potentials in the adductor branch of the RLN can be elicited by electrostimulation of the optic, acoustic, chorda tympani, trigeminal, splanchnic, vagus, radial, and intercostal nerves.[11] The susceptibility of this reflex response to such diverse sensory stimulation is unique and emphasizes its primitive role in respiratory protection of the organism from a wide variety of potentially noxious influences.

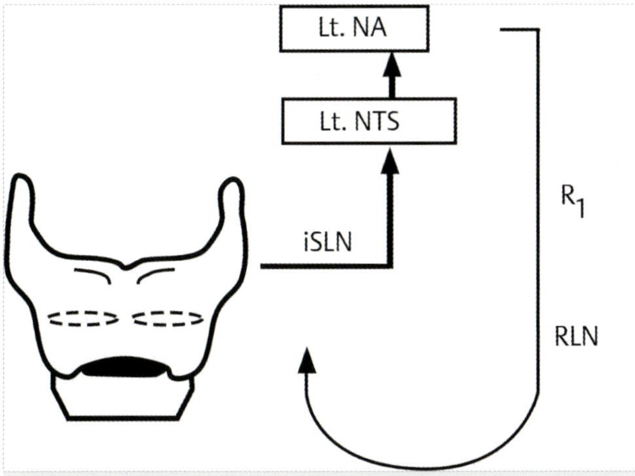

Fig. 2.1 Organizational model of the ipsilateral glottic closure reflex. Lt. NA, left nucleus ambiguus; Lt. NTS, left nucleus tractus solitarius; iSLN, ipsilateral superior laryngeal nerve; RLN, recurrent laryngeal nerve.

Physiologic exaggeration of the GCR is called laryngospasm, which is clinically observed as a strong prolonged closure of the glottis when the adductor muscle is tonically contracted and maintained well beyond the cessation of mucosal irritation. From neurophysiologic analysis, laryngeal spasm consists of prolonged tonic adductor spike activity in the RLN that bears no precisely reproducible temporal relationship or latency to its initiating stimulus. This observation is based on the fact that laryngeal spasm is solely mediated by stimulation of the SLN. In fact, high-frequency stimulation of other afferent nerves, capable of eliciting simple glottic closure, produces little adductor after-discharge activity that is characteristic of laryngospasm.

Adductor motor depression caused by hypoventilation is supported by other experimental data indicating preferential abolition of postsynaptic potentials by hypoxia.[12] This experimental evidence further indicates that, in hypoxic states, postsynaptic recovery lags behind the presynaptic recovery, producing a net depressive effect on all reflex neural activity. Therefore, hypoventilation understandably impairs the output capability of the brainstem adductor motor aggregate to repetitive SLN stimulation. Such experimental data seem to support the clinical observation that laryngeal spasm occurs more often in well-ventilated rather than cyanotic patients. Aside from the variety of excitatory adductor responses it produces, SLN stimulation also exerts an inhibitory effect on the medullary inspiratory motor neurons. Not only does laryngeal abductor activity cease, but phrenic activity is also inhibited, resulting in various degrees of reflex apnea.

2.6.2 Respiratory Reflex

The respiratory contribution of the larynx, however, was not appreciated until 1949, when Negus noted that the glottis opened a fraction of a second before air was drawn in by the

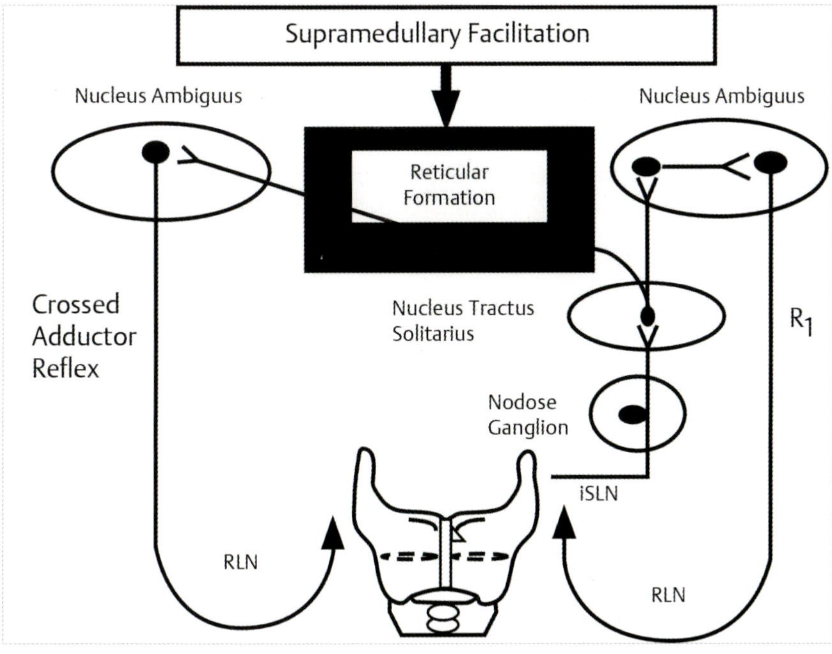

Fig. 2.2 Organizational model of the ipsilateral and crossed adductor reflex pathway in humans.

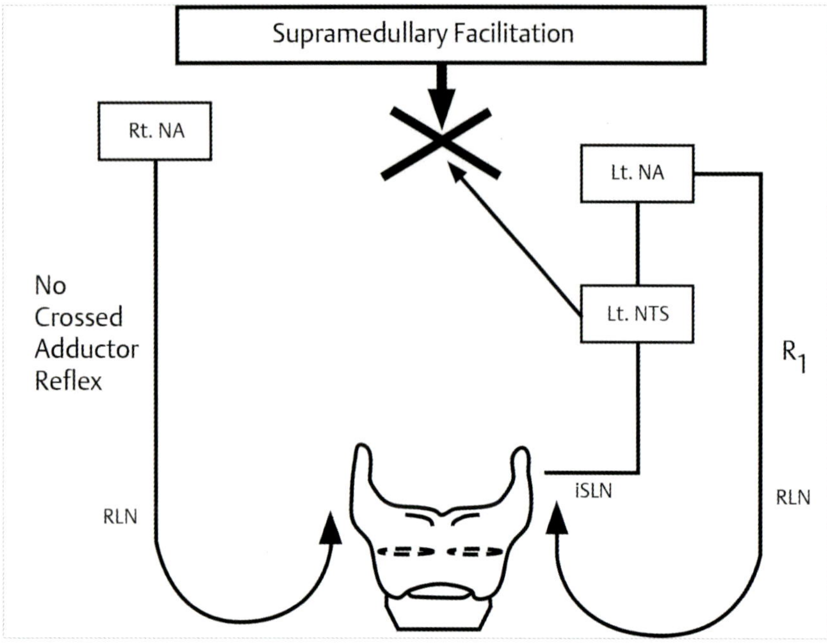

Fig. 2.3 Organizational model demonstrating the loss of contralateral R1 under deep anesthesia. Rt. NA, right nucleus ambiguus; Lt. NA, left nucleus ambiguus; Lt. NTS, left nucleus tractus solitarius; iSLN, ipsilateral superior laryngeal nerve; RLN, recurrent laryngeal nerve.

descent of the diaphragm. The neurophysiology behind this observation was clarified by Suzuki and Kirchner, who established this activity as a direct effect of the medullary respiratory center. Having shown that widening of the glottis occurred with rhythmic bursts of activity in the RLN, Suzuki and Kirchner then demonstrated that, like phrenic activity, this rhythmicity was accentuated by hypercapnia and ventilatory obstruction and depressed by hyperventilation and resultant hypocapnia.[14]

Likewise, as phrenic activity is modified by ventilatory resistance, it would seem reasonable that glottic widening, influenced by the respiratory center, would be similarly modified. From a structural perspective, the true vocal folds passively act to obstruct the ingress of air to the lungs. Therefore, to relieve obstruction of active inspiratory abduction, the posterior cricoarytenoid muscle must contract. Further, this activity has been demonstrated to be synchronous with inspiration. Electromyography (EMG) of the posterior cricoarytenoid muscle has shown that phasic inspiratory abduction is synchronous with inspiration (▶ Fig. 2.4).[14] The degree of abductor activity appears to vary directly with ventilatory resistance, disappearing entirely when inspiratory resistance is removed and returning when resistance to ventilation is re-established. Because vagotomy abolishes this response, it is thought that the afferent limb for the reflex regulation of phasic inspiratory abduction lies within the ascending vagus nerve.[15] End-organ receptors contributing to this reflex presumably lie within the thorax, although their exact nature and location remain unknown.

The cricothyroid muscle behaves in an unusual way as a respiratory muscle. It is known to be a vocal cord adductor and isotonic tensor. It is odd, then, that it is seen to contract during inspiration, when adduction would seem counterproductive.[16] In fact, its role in cord lengthening actually enhances the cross-sectional diameter of the glottis by increasing its anteroposterior dimension. Thus, the posterior cricoarytenoid and cricothyroid muscles act together to widen and lengthen the glottic chink.[17]

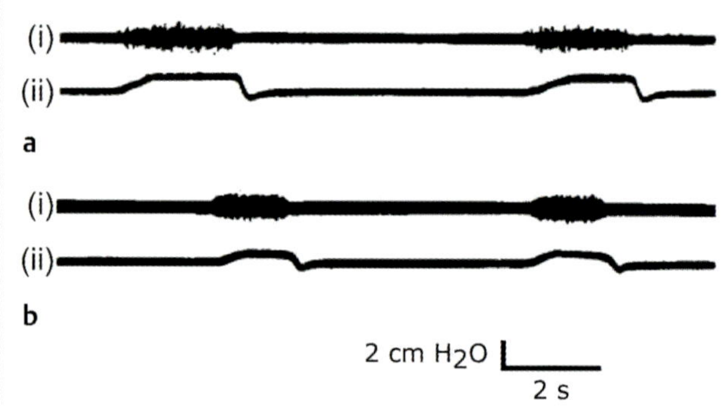

Fig. 2.4 (a) Nose breathing. (b) Mouth breathing. i, Posterior cricoarytenoid electromyography; ii, intratracheal pressure. (Upward deflection represents negative pressure change.)

2.6.3 Phonatory Reflex System

The phonatory function of the larynx is probably the least well understood of its three basic functions. With advances in investigative technique, many established hypotheses based on animal models have been challenged, a result in large measure to the advent of more specialized technology based on human study. High-speed cinematography, electro- and photoglottography, improved endoscopic techniques using the video stroboscope, and direct human EMG measurements made possible by hooked-wire electrodes, combined with advanced aerodynamic measurements, are largely responsible for these newer additions.

It is generally agreed that speech results from the production of a fundamental tone at the larynx and is modified by resonating chambers of the upper aerodigestive tract. Therefore, intelligible speech represents the combined effect of the larynx, tongue, palate, and related structures of the oral vestibule. The

Table 2.3 The influence of each of the intrinsic muscles on the shape and tension of the glottis during phonation

	Cricothyroid	Vocalis	Lateral cricoarytenoid	Interarytenoid	Posterior cricoarytenoid
Position	Paramedian	Adduct	Adduct	Adduct	Abduct
Level	Lower	Lower	Lower	X	Elevate
Length	Elongate	Shorten	Elongate	(Shorten)	Elongate
Thickness	Thin	Thicken	Thin	(Thicken)	Thin
Edge	Sharpen	Round	Sharpen	X	Round
Muscle (body)	Stiffen	Stiffen	Stiffen	(Slacken)	Stiffen
Mucosa (cover and transition	Stiffen	Slacken	Stiffen	(Slacken)	Stiffen

Table 2.4 Factors that regulate vibratory pattern of the vocal fold

			Factors that specify vibratory pattern	Factors that specify sound generated	
Level	Physiologic	Physical	Physical	Acoustic	Psycho-acoustic
Parameters	Neuromuscular control Respiratory muscles Laryngeal muscles Articulatory muscles	(Primary) Expiratory force Vocal position, shape, and size Elasticity Viscosity State of vocal tract (Secondary) Pressure drop across glottis Volume velocity Glottal impedance	Fundamental period Symmetry Periodicity Uniformity Glottal closure Amplitude Mucosal wave Speed of excursion Glottal area waveform	Fundamental frequency Amplitude (intensity) Waveform Acoustic spectrum fluctuations	Pitch loudness Quality fluctuations

fundamental tone is produced by vibration of the vocal folds against each other, powered by the passage of air between them. The passive nature of vocal cord vibration forms the basis of the aerodynamic theory of sound generation. Such a theory is supported by the observation that a completely paralyzed larynx is capable of producing sound, as is the cadaver larynx when air is blown through it. Furthermore, vocal cord vibration ceases when a tracheostomy is performed for diversionary purposes. The aerodynamic theory of sound production replaces the neurochronaxic theory proposed by Husson, who postulated that the central generation of RLN impulses produces cord vibrations by active contraction of the thyroarytenoid muscles.[18] According to this theory, each vibration represented the result of beat-by-beat impulses through the RLN. This concept is no longer accepted as tenable on acoustic or neurophysiological grounds.

Although sound production may be considered a passive function, the regulation of its acoustic quality is not. Rather, vocal cord shaping and positioning are under active neurophysiological regulation. During phonation, the vocal folds are positioned near the midline by isotonic tensing provided by the cricothyroid muscles. Additionally, the thyroarytenoid muscles provide finer shaping of the vocal folds. The effect of shaping may be appreciated when the vocal folds are viewed in the frontal plane during phonation. During the production of high-pitched notes, the folds seen on cross section appear thin, but during low pitches the folds appear thickened considerably. Thus, the frequency of vibration depends on the vibratory mass of both cords, their anteroposterior tension, functional damping at high pitches, and subglottic pressure. As pitch increases, the true cords lengthen and tense isotonically through the action of the cricothyroid muscles. Although cord lengthening alone might serve to lower pitch, cord thinning produced by thyroarytenoid action, which also increases the internal tension of the true cord, offsets this effect. It must also be recognized that the activity of the extrinsic laryngeal muscles affects pitch by altering the spatial relationship between the cricoid and the thyroid cartilages. The sternothyroid muscle is felt to influence pitch in this way.[18] ▸ Table 2.3 summarizes the influence of each of the intrinsic muscles on the shape and tension of the glottis during phonation. In considering the phonatory process, a variety of factors necessarily contribute to the acoustic product; they are defined in ▸ Table 2.4.

A variety of feedback mechanisms aid in the fine tuning of the voice. The contribution of auditory input is demonstrated by observing a nonprofessional singer's ability to hit a desired note when hearing is masked by white noise. Mucosal receptors in the pharynx and larynx also supply important information, the transmission of which can be blocked by topical anesthetics. Finally, stretch receptors in the laryngeal joint capsules give critical proprioceptive information.[19,20]

2.7 Conclusion

The larynx is a complex organ that serves to protect the lower airways and to facilitate respiration, and deglutition; it also plays a key role in phonation.

References

[1] Shin T, Watanabe S, Wada S, Maeyama T. Sensory nerve endings in the mucosa of the epiglottis—morphologic investigations with silver impregnation, immunohistochemistry, and electron microscopy. Otolaryngol Head Neck Surg 1987; 96: 55–62

[2] Pressman JJ. Sphincters of the larynx AMA. Arch Otolaryngol 1954; 59: 221–236

[3] Suzuki M, Kirchner JA. Afferent nerve fibers in the external branch of the superior larygneal nerve in the cat. Ann Otol Rhinol Laryngol 1968; 77: 1059–1070

[4] Koizumi H. On sensory innervation of larynx in dog. Tohoku J Exp Med 1953; 58: 199–210

[5] Downing SE, Lee JC. Laryngeal chemosensitivity: a possible mechanism for sudden infant death. Pediatrics 1975; 55: 640–649

[6] Sasaki CT, Suzuki M. The respiratory mechanism of aerosol inhalation in the treatment of partial airway obstruction. Pediatrics 1977; 59: 689–694

[7] Bowden REM. Innervation of intrinsic laryngeal muscles. In: Wyke B, ed. Ear Drainage: Ventilatory and Phonatory Control Systems. London: Oxford University Press, 1974; 370-382

[8] Sasaki CT, Suzuki M. Laryngeal reflexes in cat, dog, and man. Arch Otolaryngol 1976; 102: 400–402

[9] Goding GS, Richardson MA, Trachy RE. Laryngeal chemoreflex: anatomic and physiologic study by use of the superior laryngeal nerve in the piglet. Otolaryngol Head Neck Surg 1987; 97: 28–38

[10] Ludlow CL, Van Pelt F, Koda J. Characteristics of late responses to superior laryngeal nerve stimulation in humans. Ann Otol Rhinol Laryngol 1992; 101: 127–134

[11] Chang HT. Activation of internuncial neurons through collaterals of pyramidal fibers at cortical level. J Neurophysiol 1955; 18: 452–471

[12] Suzuki M, Sasaki CT. Effect of various sensory stimuli on reflex laryngeal adduction. Ann Otol Rhinol Laryngol 1977; 86: 30–36

[13] Chang HT. Activation of internuncial neurons through collaterals of pyramidal fibers at cortical level. J Neurophysiol 1955; 18: 452–471

[14] Suzuki M, Kirchner JA. The posterior cricoarytenoid as an inspiratory muscle. Ann Otol Rhinol Laryngol 1969; 78: 849

[15] Sasaki CT, Fukuda H, Kirchner JA. Laryngeal abductor activity in response to varying ventilatory resistance. Trans Am Acad Ophthalmol Otolaryngol 1973; 77: ORL403–ORL410

[16] Fukuda H, Sasaki CT, Kirchner JA. Vagal afferent influences on the phasic activity of the posterior cricoarytenoid muscle. Acta Otolaryngol 1973; 75: 112–118

[17] Suzuki M, Kirchner JA, Murakami Y. The cricothyroid as a respiratory muscle. Its characteristics in bilateral recurrent laryngeal nerve paralysis. Ann Otol Rhinol Laryngol 1970; 79: 976–983

[18] Husson R. Etude des Phénomènes Physiologiques et Acoustiques Fondamentaux de la Voix Chantée. Paris, France: These Fac Sc; 1950

[19] Gracheva MS. [On sensory innervation of the framework of the motor apparatus of the larynx][in Russian] Arkh Anat Gistol Embriol 1963; 44: 77–83

[20] Sanders I, Aviv J, Biller HF. Transcutaneous electrical stimulation of the recurrent laryngeal nerve: a method of controlling vocal cord position. Otolaryngol Head Neck Surg 1986; 95: 152–157

3 Evaluation and Management of the Dysphonic Patient

Peak Woo

Evaluation and management of the patient with dysphonia can be easy or hard. It is easy if a lesion, motion impairment, or inflammation is found and is the presumed cause of the patient's symptom. It is hard if a voice complaint is present but there is no obvious cause. Unfortunately, for the general otolaryngologist, more often than not, it is the latter. This chapter will serve to guide the general otolaryngologist in a systematic approach to the evaluation and management of the patient with dysphonia. From the simple to the complex, there are now many new tools in the physician's tool chest for the evaluation and management of these patients. With a minimum of training, the diagnosis in almost all patients with complaints of dysphonia can be shifted from "I see nothing wrong" to "I believe this is the cause or causes of your difficulty."

Patients presenting with a voice disorder come from a variety of backgrounds with varying needs. Some patients are voice professionals for whom simple dysphonia represents significant functional and job-related quality of life (QOL) disturbance. Others have concerns regarding the possibility of neoplasm. The otolaryngologist may need to tailor the diagnostic and treatment effort to the patients' needs when there is no obvious mass lesion or medical illness.

The causes of voice disorder are quite variable. They include inflammation, benign mucosal conditions, malignancies, and functional disorders. Sometimes, multiple factors contribute to the patient's dysphonia. Obvious lesions and vocal fold motion impairment are often not present on initial examination. In the absence of an obvious lesion, the otolaryngologist must consider other potential etiologies, such as low-grade laryngitis (possibly due to environmental irritants), reflux laryngitis, allergies, and functional problems, such as muscle tension dysphonia. Initial treatment in a patient without obvious lesions may include empirical treatment for reflux or inflammation using a proton pump inhibitor (PPI), or steroid or antiallergy medications. In the approach to the adult patient with normal vocal fold movement and no obvious vocal lesion, additional management steps may include referral for a speech-language pathology consultation, an empiric trial of PPI, a stroboscopy, referral to a laryngologist, an oral-steroid trial, and other testing, such as pH probe testing and a computed tomography (CT) scan.[1,2]

3.1 History

A history template and review of systems are useful for dysphonia complaints. With today's computer records, the key word in the chief complaint can prompt the generation of questions to be answered by the patient before the physician encounter. This can save time. These questions are specific for the dysphonic patient and are done in addition to the general review of systems. Some sample symptoms that deserve inquiry are given in ▶ Table 3.1.

There are three special areas of inquiry in the assessment of dysphonia: assessment of risk factors, significance of the voice disturbance to the patient, and associated throat symptoms.

3.2 Risk-Factor Assessment

A good place to start in the assessment of risk factors is to inquire about the voice use history. Much of voice use is taken for granted and subtle environmental and voice-over use patterns are not recognized by the patient unless specific inquiry is performed. Risk factors for voice disturbance include recent heavy voice use history. Pediatric dysphonia occurs more in large families with younger siblings. For the professional speaker or singer, the history should focus on recent change in the voice exposure. Has there been a change in the environment where speaking or singing has occurred? Has there been recent travel and environmental change? For the speaker or teacher, is there a history of performance or speaking in loud background or public speaking?

Chronic allergic rhinitis and upper airway reactive airway disease, such as asthma and chronic adenoiditis, may contribute to chronic hoarseness by activating inflammatory cascade that results in a chronic hoarse voice. A careful inquiry into the patient's allergic history, postnasal discharge history, and asthma history should be done as part of the review of systems.

Reflux laryngitis has received much attention as a cause of throat clearing, voice disturbance, and increased mucus. This often occurs without the classic signs and symptoms of heartburn. Morning voice, fluctuating voice disturbance, and dysphonia associated with increased phlegm and throat clearing are the usual complaints of patients with suspected reflux laryngitis.

3.2.1 Severity of Voice Handicap for the Patient and the VHI QOL Score

The implication of the voice loss to the patient should be assessed early in the patient visit. The psychological effects and the significance of the presenting problem must be factored into the equation before the examination and may impact how much effort and resources are to be devoted to the patient. For example, the patient with concern about cancer of the larynx and mild laryngitis may need nothing more than a simple laryngoscopy. The singer with singing voice fluctuation who is no longer able to sing may need laryngeal electromyography and neurologic, endocrine, and singing-voice therapy evaluation.

At the beginning of any medical or voice therapy evaluation, it is helpful to assess the impact of the voice disturbance on the

Table 3.1 Symptoms commonly experienced by the dysphonic patient

Voice symptoms	Associated symptoms
Runs out of air with speaking	Throat pain with speaking
Cannot be heard over others	Chronic throat clearing with speaking
Loss in voice range and volume	Excessive phlegm
Has to strain to talk	Short of breath with voice use
Voice fluctuates all the time	Swallow is effortful

patient using validated instruments for voice function assessment.[3] Common evaluation instruments include the Voice Handicap Index (VHI), Voice-Related Quality of Life (V-RQOL),[4] the short form VHI-10, the pediatric VHI, the singer VHI, and others. These are now available in short-form versions and in many languages. They have also been validated for singers and for the pediatric population.[5,6,7,8] Changes in VHI with treatment have also been well documented.[9] A review of the QOL-content development was recently published.[10] These validated QOL instruments serve two major functions. The first is an estimate of the meaning of voice disturbance for the patient. The subscales in the standard VHI divide the questions into psychological, functional, and physiological domains. It is useful for the examiner to understand the impact of the patient's voice disorder on the patient. In general, severity should be equal in distribution of scores among the subscales. Severity should correlate with the examiner's perception of the voice based on mild–moderate–severe ratings. If there is a large discrepancy in the rating scales based on the patient's and the examiner's perceptions, further investigation into the functional, psychological, and social impact of the patient's voice disorder should be pursued. In a study using meta-analysis of VHI and impact on QOL in patients with nonneoplastic voice disorders, voice disturbance was found to adversely impact patients' voice-related and general QOL. Its impact was equivalent to having a chronic, debilitating illness. Patients with neurologic voice disorders experience the greatest impact.[11]

3.2.2 Assessment of the Associated Symptoms

Associated signs and symptoms, such as pain with speaking (odynophonia), dysphagia, throat clearing, dyspnea, and associated throat symptoms, should be elicited in the history (▶ Table 3.1). In patients with associated symptoms, it may be appropriate to administer the Reflux Symptom Index questionnaire.[12] Vocal fatigue with throat pain may be an early indication of contact ulcer or vocal fold paresis. Chronic thick phlegm and coughing with speaking may reveal associated laryngitis on examination. If there is unilateral throat pain or pain on swallowing, a careful search for ulceration and neoplasm should be done with reference to the side of the experienced pain.

3.2.3 Review of Systems

General health should be reviewed. A patient who has been recently hospitalized and has lost weight may present with an asthenic voice that is unrelated to the vocal apparatus. The aging population is a rich source of voice complaints.[13,14] Many of the causes of voice disturbance in the aging population are multifactorial. In this group of patients, medication history and their side effects, physiological aspects of breath support and physical fitness for sustained flow during phonation should be assessed. A neurologic history including memory, gait, and swallowing history should be obtained. The history should especially inquire as to the changes of voice with menses in the adult female singer.[15] If the voice range is changing, endocrine etiology should be considered in the female undergoing menopause, in the pediatric patient, and in patients with history of thyroid or adrenal endocrinopathy.[16]

3.3 Office Examination

Evaluation of the patient starts with a general ear, nose, and throat examination. Screening of hearing, nasal pathology, tonsil size, and neck masses should be performed prior to a detailed examination of the phonatory apparatus. Examination of the dysphonic patient goes beyond laryngoscopy. If otolaryngologists are to be the entry point for the evaluation of the patient with dysphonia, they must have the skills to do rudimentary evaluation of the phonation process. Laryngoscopy and evaluation of phonation by examination of the voice production process should be incorporated into the examination.

3.3.1 Listening to the Voice and Rating the Voice

Rating the voice before an examination is helpful to guide the type of instrumentation to be considered. For example, a rough voice quality suggests lesions on the vocal fold edge, whereas a breathy voice quality suggests glottal incompetence. Rigid endoscopy is usually preferred for patients presenting with rough voice quality; fiberoptic examination of the vocal function is preferred in patients with dysphonia and dysarthria.

Prior to examination of the patient by instrumentation, it is important to note the quality of the voice. The GRBAS Scale is useful for determining what instrument and what visualization tests to perform. The GRBAS Scale rates the voice based on perceptual qualities of grade, roughness, breathiness, asthenia, and strain.[17] As part of the general examination of the singer's speaking and singing voice, perceptual evaluation of the voice quality should be done beyond the GRBAS quality. The overall grade of the voice is rated as normal (0), mild (1), moderate (2), severe (3), or aphonia (4). The voice is then rated as to the presence or absence of roughness, asthenia, breathiness, and strain as normal (0), mild (1), moderate (2), or severe (3). While listening to the voice, the examiner should have some judgment as to the speaker's breath support and the resonance of voice. An excessively high tonal placement will give the voice a twangy and bright sound. A low tonal focus will give the voice a covered, often muffled quality.[18] These tonal qualities may be faulty due to laryngeal placement, large tonsils, and incorrect palatal position or tongue position.

As part of the initial examination, the speaking fundamental frequency should be noted as to whether it is appropriate. If there is excessive hard glottal attack or if there is prephonatory spasm with strain, the examiner should investigate functional or neurogenic causes, such as muscle tension dysphonia (MTD) or spasmodic dysphonia. If the voice quality is breathy or asthenic, investigation into vocal fold paresis or neurogenic causes of dysphonia may be considered.

3.3.2 Palpation

In the examination of the neck and larynx, palpation should be done before visual inspection. Palpation of the larynx allows for evaluation of appropriate laryngeal position and movement, softness of the larynx during phonation and confirmation of the presence of an easy posture without excessive tension. If there is pain or tenderness, the site and side are noted. The common causes of excessive tension that may be elicited by palpation are:

1. Base of tongue and suprahyoid muscle tension.
2. Short thyrohyoid distance with contracted, tight thyrohyoid distance. The thyroid to hyoid distance is shortened with a barely palpable thyrohyoid membrane. This corresponds to a tight, squeezed voice with a high larynx position.
3. Cricothyroid lock. Pitch glides in the patient with fixed cricothyroid distance are associated with a higher pitch, but with a strained quality. There is no closure of the cricothyroid membrane with pitch elevation and there is a lack of opening of the cricothyroid membrane with low phonation.
4. Lack of freedom of movement of the larynx with phonation.
5. Palpation of the base of the lesser horn of the hyoid bone and the superior cornu of the thyroid cartilage are used to elicit extrinsic laryngeal muscle tension. The cricothyroid membrane is palpated with pitch glides to feel for adequacy of laryngeal movement.

On palpation, the larynx should be supple. With manual rocking side to side, the larynx should give easily and show the normal laryngeal crepitance. Consistent findings of isolated muscle tenderness after voice usage are not normal. The most common findings are tenderness of the suprahyoid muscles.[19] Overactivation of the stylohyoid muscles, the sternohyoid muscles, and the laryngeal elevators will result in tenderness of the greater hyoid cornu and the superior horn of the thyroid cartilage. Laryngeal isometric tension may involve either the extrinsic laryngeal muscles or the intrinsic laryngeal muscles or both. This muscle tension results in protracted tenderness to palpation. It is usually associated with a throaty voice with other vocal faults, such as low-tone focus and lack of appropriate resonance.[20] In a systematic examination of extralaryngeal muscles by palpation, a strong relationship was found between thyrohyoid muscle tension and MTD.[21] ▶ Fig. 3.1 illustrates the site of maximal tenderness in patients with MTD.

In patients with vocal fold immobility, palpation of the cricoarytenoid joint may be carried out by slipping the finger behind the thyroid ala for direct palpation of the joint. The patient is asked to perform an "eee-sniff" gesture with the examiner's finger on the affected arytenoid. The paralyzed vocal fold will show no movement, while the innervated vocal fold will result in a gentle tap on the examiner's finger.[22] Circumferential palpation and the effect on MTD can also be performed as part of the diagnostic, therapeutic exploration. Popularized by Roy[23] and Aronson,[24] this technique is not often used by otolaryngologists in their diagnostic regimen, but it has distinct advantages in the evaluation and management of MTD. The manual technique consists of focal palpation to determine laryngeal elevation, tenderness, and voice effect of pressure over the superior border of the thyroid lamina. Voice improvement following circumlaryngeal massage is noted. In patients with history of laryngeal trauma, palpation may show marked asymmetry of the laryngeal skeleton.[25] These findings may then be further investigated by CT scanning. Similarly, palpation of the cricoarytenoid joint may induce pain in a patient with suspected cricoarytenoid joint dislocation, which may also be further investigated by CT scanning.

As part of the assessment, medial compression testing and anterior to posterior displacement for testing stiffness has been advocated by Isshiki.[26] Manual pressure on the thyroid cartilage during phonation can provide the examiner with useful information about the stiffness and competence of the vocal fold. A positive response to manual compression may be predictive of response to phonosurgery.

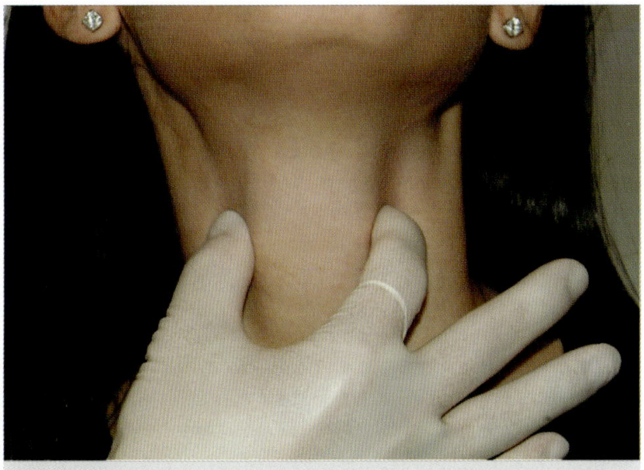

Fig. 3.1 Areas of palpation to elicit pain and tenderness in patients with muscle tension dysphonia. The maximum tenderness is at the superior thyroid horn and the oblique line.

3.3.3 Visual Examination of the Phonatory Apparatus and the Vocal Folds

Visual examination of phonation is divided into the examination of the larynx and laryngeal function without investigation into the vibratory function or examination of vocal fold vibratory behavior. Rigid endoscopy with a 70- or 90-degree endoscope, flexible fiberoptic laryngoscope, or the high-definition chip-tip scopes is used for laryngeal visualization.[27,28] With improved resolution, the chip charge-coupled device (CCD) scopes are now approaching the resolution of the rigid scopes.[29] For investigation of vocal fold vibratory behavior, the standard method has been by stroboscopy.[29,30,31,32] Recent commercial availability of high-speed color systems allows an alternative method for looking at vocal fold vibration without the need for the stroboscopy effect. Whether such tools will become commonly used in the clinic is still in question.[33,34]

3.4 Laryngeal Visualization: Instrument Differences

There are many instruments available for imaging of the vocal apparatus. There are cost and time considerations for each. The mirror examination is still preferred as a screening tool, but it has largely been replaced by endoscopes and cameras. The rigid endoscope is unfortunately not often used by most general otolaryngologists. Routine rigid endoscopy with visual recording is excellent for estimation of mucosal health, for detection of lesions on the vibratory margins, and for detection of gross

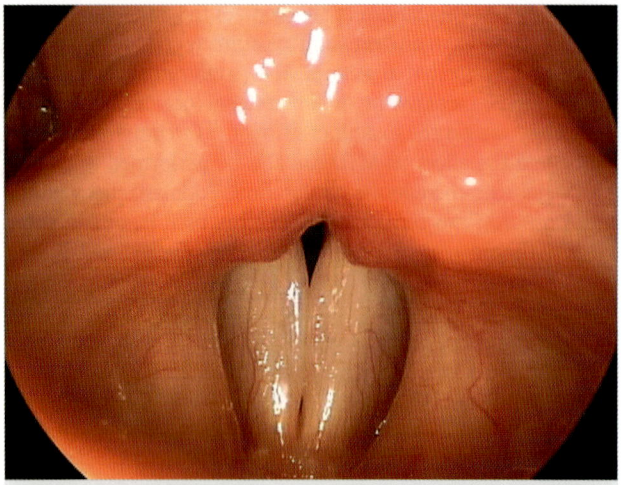

Fig. 3.2 Rigid endoscope examination can show excellent detail of the mucosa without the need for stroboscopy.

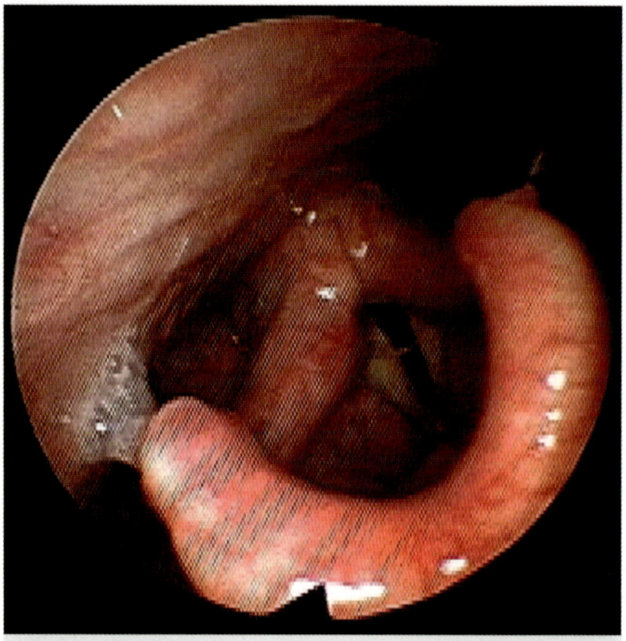

Fig. 3.3 The fiberoptic scope is small and convenient for visualization of vocal fold movement, but it shows less mucosal detail than the rigid scope due to the lower number of pixels that the fiberscope displays.

movement abnormalities of the vocal folds. ▸ Fig. 3.2 is a rigid endoscopy photograph. This is compared with a similar picture acquired with the fiberoptic laryngoscope in ▸ Fig. 3.3. The contrast between the details in each photo is clear. Yet most otolaryngologists use the fiberscope to make the majority of their diagnoses. The rigid endoscope examination reveals the anatomical details better, but it is not dynamic and requires the tongue to be held forward. In some patients, both a fiberscope and a rigid examination should be considered. A flexible examination of vocal fold function allows the examiner to view laryngeal dynamics without holding onto the tongue. Dynamic exploration of voice gestures and function is made easier by pernasal endoscopy. Flexible laryngoscopy is the preferred imaging modality in patients with asthenic voice, vocal tremor, and vocal strain. Patients suspected of functional voice disorders and neurogenic disorders, such as dystonia, Parkinson disease, and dysarthria, should also have a flexible laryngoscopy as the primary examination. The patient's perceptual qualities determined using the GRBAS Scale are helpful to decide how best to initially examine the patient. In general, patients presenting with a rough or breathy voice quality will benefit from rigid endoscopy first; patients with asthenia and strain will benefit from initial fiberoptic laryngoscopy.

3.5 Fiberscope Examination

Some voicing problems cannot be readily diagnosed by rigid stroboscopy alone; therefore, flexible endoscopy with or without stroboscopic light should always be entertained in an initial examination. Examination of the biomechanics of the speaking voice is best done by fiberoptic examination.[35] Fiberoptic examination should always be considered in the patient with suspected MTD. Once the diagnosis is clearly related to a vocal fold edge abnormality, follow-up examinations may be shortened to include only the rigid or the flexible endoscope alone.

Fiberoptic laryngoscopy should be routinely used in singers presenting with specific problems in areas of their singing. Pitch elevation is associated with specific changes in the pharynx, base of tongue, and laryngeal position.[36] Whether these are adaptive, maladaptive, or normal depends on the clinical scenario.

In patients with suspected spasmodic dysphonia or MTD, the difficulties may not occur during sustained vowels, but may occur only with rapid onset and offset of the voice. Thus, the examiner must ask for speech and singing tokens laden with voice gestures most likely to reveal the abnormality. For spasmodic dysphonia, voiced and voiceless consonant to vowel transitions are more likely to reveal adductor and abductor spasms than other words or sustained vowels. Words like "queen," "cake," "chew," "birthday," "rainbow," and "shoebench" are good at eliciting adductor or abductor spasms. These words can be strung into nonsense sentences by the patient while the video camera coupled to the laryngoscope records the speaking session. The postrecording review allows the examiner a separate time to review the laryngeal findings with the acoustic output. This type of repeated review can often confirm or make the diagnosis that cannot be made easily with a single viewing.

The fiberoptic testing protocol is divided into three key areas. These three key areas are divided into (1) anatomy and mucosal health, (2) laryngeal movement evaluation with vegetative gestures, and (3) voicing gestures. The fiberoptic testing protocol is outlined in the box "Tests for dynamic motion of laryngeal function (p. 19)."

Tests for dynamic motion of laryngeal function

Testing protocol with fiberoptic laryngoscopy

- Laryngeal anatomy and mucosal health
- Laryngeal movement with vegetative and nonvoicing gestures
  - Cough
  - "eee-sniff"
  - Whistle
  - Laugh
  - Deep inspiration
  - Rapid diadochokinesis evaluation with throat clearing
- Voice testing
  - Sustained phonation and speaking
    - Pitch and loudness range testing
    - Task-specific voicing
    - Speaking sentences

The fiberscope should be placed into the nostril on the side opposite the vocal side suspected of the lesion. Thus a patient with left side vocal fold lesions or paralysis should be examined through the right nostril. This takes the advantage of the fiberscope's ability to be turned to slightly look to the side, revealing more information than from the top-down view. A panoramic view of the larynx and pharynx is used to evaluate the anatomy and the function. The anatomy of the larynx and pharynx is evaluated as to symmetry and motion. Some simple questions remind the examiner to systematically inspect the structures beside the vocal folds during flexible laryngoscopy: Is the base of tongue forward enough to see the larynx? Are there lingual tonsils and pharyngeal tonsil tissue? Are the pharynx and larynx hydrated and without excessive mucus? Is there pharyngeal pooling?

After the anatomy and mucosal hygiene are evaluated, laryngeal movement is checked. The "eee-sniff" gesture is used to check for adduction and abduction. The symmetry of arytenoid cartilage motion and the symmetry of pharyngeal constriction are important to evaluate for pharyngeal or laryngeal paresis. Patients with vocal fold paresis may show excellent adduction and abduction, but subtle abnormalities may be revealed with gestures that require rapid diadochokinesis of the vocal folds. Thus whistle, laughter, and cough are used to evaluate the symmetry of motion of the vocal folds. Asymmetric vocal fold motion should raise the suspicion of vocal fold motion abnormality, such as paresis or ankylosis.

Muscle tension dysphonia may be categorized as primary or secondary. Primary muscle tension dysphonia presents with neck pain, voice disturbance, and vocal fatigue. Secondary muscle tension dysphonia presents as a compensatory mechanism of vocal hyperfunction to compensate for vocal fold lesions like scar, reflux laryngitis, or vocal fold paralysis.[37] The evaluation of muscle tension dysphonia is best done with a fiberoptic scope in place, with analysis of running speech. Fiberoptic laryngoscopy findings include medial compression of the false vocal fold, sphincteric closure of the supraglottic larynx, and base of tongue tension with anterior to posterior supraglottic compression. At the glottis level, there may be a wide open posterior glottic aperture signifying isometric glottic tension or excessive anterior to posterior shortening with associated vocal fry. Physical examination by palpation also reveals excessive submental tongue tension as well as excessive laryngeal elevation with speech. There may be tenderness over the strap muscle insertion on the hyoid horn, the oblique line of the thyroid cartilage, and at the base of the tongue. In patients with a habitual chest voice dominant pattern of speech, palpation of the cricothyroid membrane may demonstrate a cricothyroid lock with failure of closure of the cricothyroid visor with pitch glide, as the patient is asked to phonate with increasing pitch followed by decreasing pitch. This is often associated with laryngeal elevation and a squeezed strained quality.

Muscle tension dysphonia comes in many forms.[37] Observation of the patient and laryngoscopy examination may show evidence of MTD.[38] Extrinsic laryngeal muscles, such as the suprahyoid muscles and strap muscles, will tend to elevate the larynx and squeeze the pharynx. Base of tongue tension will push the epiglottis posteriorly and retroflex the epiglottis, obstructing the view of the vocal folds due to epiglottic hooding. Therefore, the finding of an elevated larynx during pitch glides, with retroflexion of the epiglottis would suggest the presence of excessive extralaryngeal neck muscle tension. Intrinsic muscles of the larynx may also be postured in a maladaptive way. There are typical laryngeal configurations due to intrinsic MTD. Some of these are (1) prephonatory ventricular adduction and constriction with release on phonation, (2) short thick vocal folds that fail to lengthen on pitch glide, (3) isometric tension with fixed vocal folds and a large posterior chink, and (4) false vocal fold phonation. Muscle tension dysphonia patterns have not been well studied by laryngeal electromyography (EMG) or laryngeal kinesthetic studies but are believed to exist on the basis of muscle imbalance during phonation. Some postulated abnormal patterns are (1) thyroarytenoid muscle hyperfunction (thyroarytenoid predominance pattern), (2) lack of engagement of the cricothyroid muscle (cricothyroid lock), or (3) isometric muscle tension pattern (posterior chink). Additional laryngeal research is needed to separate the different patterns.

The presence of MTD is indicative of adaptive or maladaptive functional compensation for the production of voice. The presence of MTD does not differentiate a primary MTD pattern from that of a compensatory MTD pattern. An example of secondary MTD is a pattern of muscle hyperfunction due to reflux laryngitis.[39] Primary MTD is the presence of MTD without organic disease or injury. Thus, a singer who has spent too long during a practice or lessons may show evidence of MTD after a long session. Compensation by MTD may be a consequence of adaptation after injury to the vocal folds by scar, hemorrhage, inflammation, or trauma. Therefore, a patient with an intubation injury to the larynx resulting in glottal incompetence may phonate with a MTD pattern that is an adaptive response to a need for greater generation of subglottic pressure to drive the vocal folds in vibration. A singer with chronic reflux laryngitis may sing in a maladaptive way with MTD in response to edematous inflamed vocal folds and not as a consequence of poor singing technique. After the examiner has identified the presence of MTD, the determination of the primary cause of the MTD—primary or compensatory MTD—is a challenge to the diagnostician.

Another application of fiberoptic laryngoscopy is in the identification of subtle vocal fold paresis. The degree of paresis may be variable and office fiberoptic laryngoscopy testing is the best way to elicit more subtle cases. The criterion for the clinical diagnosis of paresis is asymmetry of vocal fold movement compared to the contralateral vocal fold. The asymmetry may be obvious in differences in degree of abduction and adduction during phonation or respiration or it may only be[40]elicited by systematic testing.[41] Patients with vocal paresis may show asymmetry in pharyngeal squeezing during phonation, a lag of the affected vocal fold during laryngeal movements that require rapid movement, such as in a whistle or laughter. Superior laryngeal nerve paresis may be elicited as an axis shift of the larynx during a pitch glide and/or the presence of vocal fold bowing of the affected vocal fold.

3.5.1 Stroboscopy

Stroboscopy has been used by laryngologists for over 100 years. Yet only within the last 20 years has it become popular in the investigation of dysphonia.[42,43,44,45] Despite its clinical availability, not all otolaryngologists will have access to stroboscopy. Some prefer referral of voice patients to laryngologists; others will refer the patient to speech and language pathologists working in collaboration with a laryngologist.

Not all patients with voice disorders should have a video stroboscopic laryngoscopy (VSL) examination. Some pediatric patients cannot tolerate examination with this technique.[46] Candidacy for examination by VSL is based on the fact that the principle of stroboscopy is based on Talbot's law. Talbot's law states that there is retention of an image on the retina of 200 milliseconds after exposure. This optical illusion of apparent motion from a series of images presented with rapid succession is the basis for motion films. Thus, by exposing rapid microsecond flashes of light on a quasiperiodic vibratory source such as oscillating vocal folds, the image may be frozen. When the flashes of light are synchronized just off the fundamental frequency of vibration, the vocal folds may be seen to oscillate at 1.5 to 3 times per second. The multiple images from VSL recordings of vocal folds oscillating in slow motion are made up of hundreds of glottal cycles and are a montage of glottal vibration. Thus, based on the principle of stroboscopy, the best patients chosen for VSL examination should be those with a vibratory source that is quasiperiodic. The professional voice user, the singer with subtle dysphonia noticeable as a qualitative abnormality in the voice, the patient with a veiled husky voice, and the patient with intermittent voice abnormalities are considered ideal candidates for VSL. Low gag reflex and phonation time of greater than 5 seconds are desirable, but not mandatory. Ideally, the VSL patient should have enough insight and cooperation to produce phonation tasks directed by the examiner at sustained pitch and loudness.

For practical VSL recording in the office, four parameters are typically recorded. These are modal phonation at habitual pitch and loudness, high-pitched phonation at habitual loudness, low-pitched phonation at habitual loudness, and loud phonation at modal pitch frequency. On the VSL machines, this translates into: modal phonation—males (M): 125 Hertz (Hz), females (F): 225 Hz, 70 to 75 decibels (db); high phonation—M: 200 Hz, F: 300 Hz, 70 to 75 db; low phonation—M: 100 Hz, F: 190 Hz, 70 to 75 db; and loud phonation—M: 140 Hz, F: 250 Hz, 80 to 85 db. These are guidelines that are easily achievable by most patients. Although it does not evaluate the true vocal range in frequency and amplitude of vocal phonatory function, it does test the larynx and its function by using different subglottic pressures and laryngeal muscles. By adding specific tasks, such as pitch glides and loudness variation, different modes of phonation such as chest, falsetto, and flute register can be evaluated during the examination.

A co-operative patient can have the simple protocol examination done in 1 to 2 minutes. By recording the examination by VSL, the playback can be reviewed with the patient and interpretation and report generation based on oscillatory patterns of the vocal folds. A visual montage of the glottal cycle can be saved in hard copy in the patient's chart as a visual reference to the vibratory characteristic (▶ Fig. 3.4).

Interpretation of the VSL examination is done after the recording. It is used as part of the information for synthesis of the cause of the voice disorder by incorporation of all the data from the history through the video examination. As the VSL is viewed at regular speed and in slow motion, several features of vocal fold anatomy will be rated relative to normal vocal fold anatomy and physiology. The key features of VSL interpretation are listed in ▶ Table 3.2. After the VSL is reviewed with those features in mind, the clinician should be able to decide on the primary diagnosis of the phonatory disorder, make a functional assessment of vocal fold vibratory function, and, based on these, make decisions as to treatment. Great variations can occur in the normal larynx. This is true in normal voices without perceived dysphonia as well as in singers. For example, the presence of a small posterior chink that permits air leakage in females is normal. Elias and Sataloff investigated strobovideolaryngoscopy findings in normal professional singers without voice complaints. "Abnormal" strobovideolaryngoscopy findings occur in this asymptomatic population of "volunteers" with great frequency. These abnormalities might have been misinterpreted as causing dysphonia.[47] Therefore, it is a good rule to review any prior videos or prints of the larynx before a new diagnosis of nodule, edema, or scar is made. A great deal of latitude must be applied in determining the clinical interpretation of a specific laryngeal gesture as abnormal.

The interpretation of stroboscopy is subjective and has been well documented.[48,49,50] The features that should be rated are found in textbooks; they are even included in the software of stroboscopy systems. The key features include glottal configuration, closure, symmetry, edge, phase, phase shift, vibratory amplitude, and mucosal wave. Some ratings are for the glottis; others are performed for each vocal fold. From these ratings, one can make observations as to mass, stiffness, or tension effects on the vocal fold. Asymmetric change in the vibratory behavior may be the most obvious visual abnormality to indicate pathological change in tissue rheology of the vocal fold cover. Careful analysis of the stroboscopy video gives the clinician a power tool for understanding the effects of treatment on the vocal vibratory characteristic.

The clearest indication for stroboscopy is the examination of the vocal folds for vocal fold pathology, such as cysts, polyps, nodules, and inflammation. ▶ Fig. 3.5 is an example of scar on the left vocal fold with stiffness. The loss in amplitude and mucosal wave associated with loss in the translucent lamina

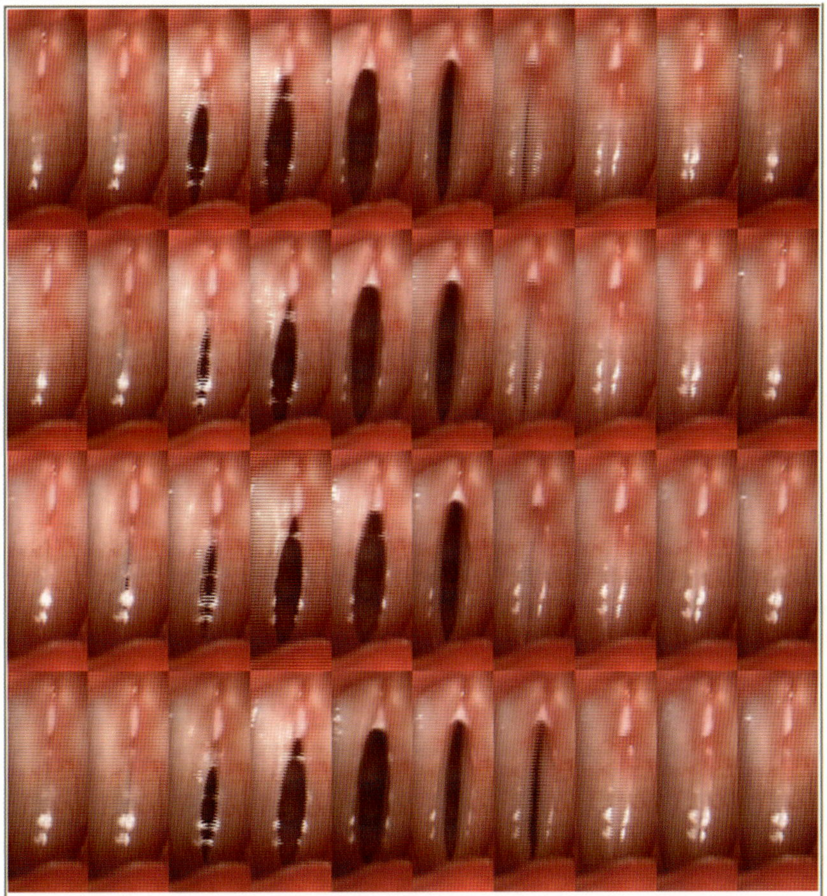

Fig. 3.4 A montage of three glottal cycles can be assembled from the stroboscopy for a visual record in the patient's chart.

Table 3.2 Stroboscopy features

Rating for the larynx	Rating for each vocal fold (right and left)
Configuration	Edge irregularity
Fundamental frequency	Amplitude
Out-of-phase vibration	Mucosal wave
Asymmetric vibration	Stiffness
Level difference	Nonvibrating segment
Phase closure	Mass

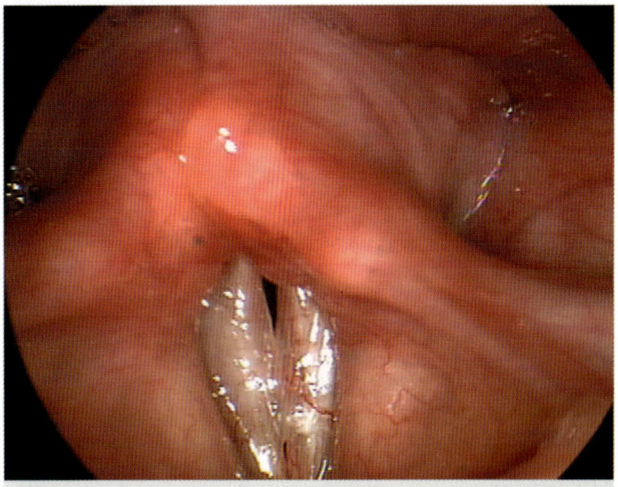

Fig. 3.5 Stroboscopy showing stiffness of left vocal fold due to scar.

propria is clearly seen. The second and sometimes as important indication is the evaluation of laryngeal phonatory gestures that accompany sound production.[38] VSL examination will open a new world for the understanding of dysphonia. From a paucity of findings in many patients with dysphonia, stroboscopy examination will show a plethora of new visual data, which can be confusing. Despite this confusing new abundance of information, proper understanding and interpretation of the stroboscopic examination will expand the understanding of phonation by the voice health professional. Much as a microscope will expand the understanding of vocal anatomy, stroboscopy allows the clinician a practical way to look at vocal fold vibration that was previously not visible. Errors and pitfalls that can be avoided by such evaluation include (1) organic lesions previously attributed to functional etiology, (2) scarring and vocal fold injury that was not recognized, and (3) unilateral polyp previously mistaken as nodules and vice versa. Clinical errors, such as failure to consider multiple sources for inflammation, failure to try conservative medical or voice therapy, and the

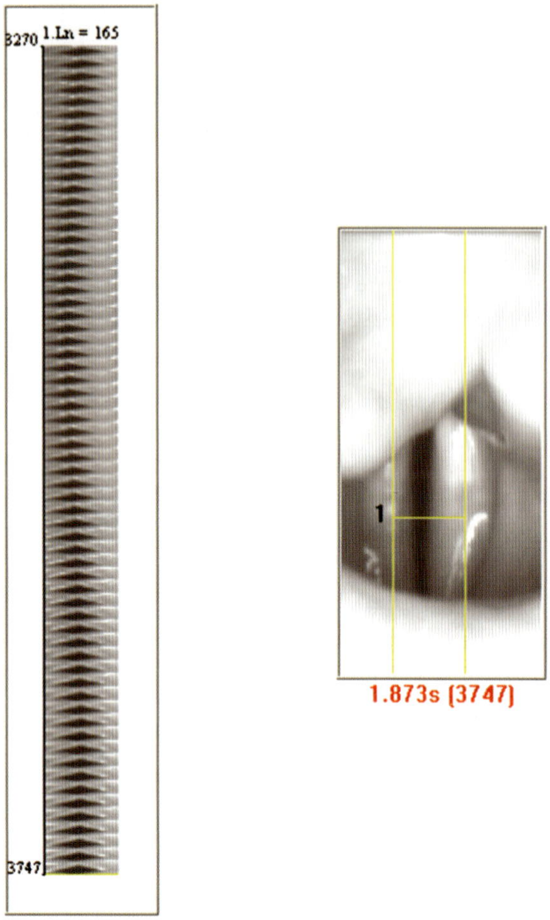

Fig. 3.6 Digital kymography plot of a high-speed video showing each glottal cycle at the line of interest.

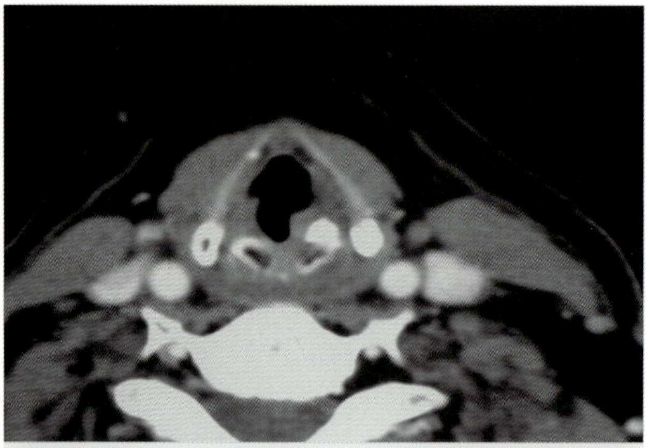

Fig. 3.7 Computed tomography scan of a small chondrosarcoma of the cricoid cartilage detected after observation of level difference between the vocal folds.

recommendation for speech therapy for voice disorders when there is no evidence it will be helpful, are far too common. Accurate stroboscopy evaluation can help to avoid such errors.

One of the best applications of VSL is identification of glottic insufficiency and vocal fold paresis. The paretic vocal fold will be difficult to identify as there will still be good movement. However, glottic insufficiency will be accompanied by stroboscopy signs, such as open-phase dominant pattern and lateral-to medial-phase shift with a glottal gap.

Clinical diagnosis of vocal fold motion impairment suggestive of paresis may be made by flexible laryngoscopy.[51] However, stroboscopy examination will often document the functional deficit that accompanies the complaint of vocal fatigue, loss of projection, and breathy phonation. Vocal fold paresis may be due to superior laryngeal nerve injury,[40] recurrent laryngeal nerve injury, or combined nerve injury. Paresis differs from paralysis in that there is preserved adduction and abduction in paresis, but not in paralysis.

Some features of the vocal fold vibratory behavior are not able to be tracked by stroboscopy. This is because a stroboscopy image is made up of a montage of many glottal cycles. The principle of stroboscopy presumes the presence of a quasiperiodic oscillation source that is present in normal vocal folds, but may not be present in patients with dysphonia. Some features of vocal fold behavior that cannot be imaged by stroboscopy are listed in the box, "Features of vocal fold behavior not able to be imaged with stroboscopy (p.22)." For this group of patients, high-speed video and digital kymography investigation may define the cause of the vibratory abnormality.[33,34,52,53] ▶ Fig. 3.6 demonstrates the digital kymography plot of the vocal fold vibration from the high-speed video shown on the right. Each vocal fold vibration is shown at the line of interest at the mid-membranous vocal fold of interest. This approach is useful for investigation of voice breaks, diplophonia, and voice strain.

Features of vocal fold behavior not able to be imaged with stroboscopy

(a) Voice breaks
(b) Diplophonia
(c) Vocal function during voice onset and voice offset
(d) Vocal tremor and spasms
(e) Extremely rough voice quality
(f) Alternate laryngeal and pharyngeal sources of oscillation

3.5.2 Computed Tomography Scan

Fine-cut CT of the larynx is an underutilized technology in the evaluation of the patient with dysphonia. Besides the obvious use of the CT scan to assess tumor or masses of the larynx, today's CT scan can be used to assess the fine details of laryngeal anatomy that can often be helpful. The CT scan can be done in 1-mm cuts with rapid sequence acquisition. These can be done in sufficiently fast scanners such that a specific phonation gesture can be imaged. The images can also be reformatted using software for three-dimensional reconstruction for direct comparison of the size of the arytenoid cartilage, the cricothyroid and thyroarytenoid joints, and compare level differences between the vocal folds. ▶ Fig. 3.7 is a CT scan of a patient with a small chondrosarcoma who presented with voice fatigue secondary to upward displacement of the cricoarytenoid joint by the cricoid tumor. CT scan of the larynx should be considered in the workup of patients with iatrogenic laryngeal trauma and laryngeal fracture, residual dysphonia after phonosurgery, level differences between the vocal folds, and in cases in which the vocal folds are obscured during laryngoscopy by the supraglottic structures.[54,55,56,57,58,59] The major indications for CT imaging in patients presenting with voice disturbance based on their laryngoscopy findings are

- Suspected laryngeal fracture or trauma
- Level difference between the vocal folds
- Contact ulcer or granuloma-recurrent
- False cord fullness not explained by MTD
- Vocal fold immobility or laryngeal stenosis

3.5.3 Laryngeal Electromyography

In patients with suspected paresis or paralysis, laryngeal EMG (LEMG) should be considered. LEMG is useful in differentiating between mechanical fixation and ankylosis, and between dislocation and denervation in unilateral or bilateral vocal fold motion impairment. In patients with vocal fold paralysis, testing at a predetermined period after the onset of the paralyzed vocal fold can guide the clinician to the site of the lesion and can provide valuable information regarding prognosis.[60] Some of the indications for LEMG are listed in the box, "Clinical applications of laryngeal electromyography (p.23)." The standard EMG of the laryngeal muscles tests four different muscles that are innervated by the four nerves of interest. The four muscles are the right and left cricothyroid muscle and the right and left thyroarytenoid muscles. These correspond to the right and left superior laryngeal nerve and the right and left recurrent laryngeal nerve.

Clinical applications of laryngeal electromyography

- Immobile vocal fold
  - Traumatic ankylosis versus paralysis
  - Prognosis for return of function
  - Site of lesion testing
- Laryngeal dystonia
- Myopathy versus neuropathy
- Motor neuron disease—Upper motor neuron versus lower motor neuron
- Amyotrophic lateral sclerosis, Parkinson disease, pseudobulbar palsy, and bulbar palsy
- Stroke, functional voice disorders
- Investigation of laryngeal spasm and vocal fold dysfunction
- Investigation of aberrant innervations
- Kinesiology of function in voice and swallow

The normal EMG signal is inherently a composite of many motor units; combined, they make up the interference pattern. The technical aspect of validating the needle insertion is sometimes complicated by a patient's movement and swallow. The motor unit territory is small, as is the size of the muscle to be sampled. The LEMG, like all laryngeal examinations, is open to subjective interpretation. Although subjective, interpretation has strict guidelines as to what is considered hard versus soft evidence of neural dysfunction. The interpretation of LEMG is divided into evidence of denervation potentials (fibrillation potentials, complex repetitive discharges, and spontaneous irritability), reinnervation potentials (polyphasic potentials, giant potentials, and nascent units) and insertional irritability. Voluntary motor unit firing and recruitment pattern are also analyzed for recruitment of larger motor units and unit-firing rate according to the size principle. Although identification of the denervation potentials and units associated with reinnervation is not difficult, interpretation of loss of recruitment and motor unit firing rate may be subjective. This is further complicated by the fact that the laryngeal muscle is neither a sphincter muscle nor a single pulley muscle with well-defined motor-unit endplate territory. Combine this with the fact that patients with the needle in their intrinsic laryngeal muscle often exhibit guarding and do not give supramaximal effort on the requested token. All of these factors often create a situation where the motor-unit-recruitment pattern is highly variable. An approach to overcome the subjective bias and reduce variability is quantitative laryngeal electromyography. Quantitative laryngeal electromyography has been used in other areas of electrophysiology for analysis of nerve disorders but is relatively uncommon in the larynx.

3.6 Phonatory Airflow and Phonatory Function Analysis

The modern voice laboratory has evolved such that physiological data is easily recorded and preserved for comparison and analysis. From the days when there were many physiological tools for assessment of voice, several clinical tools have become standard. The two major tools that are used today are based on the acoustic voice recording and analysis and those that are based on aerodynamics. The recording and analysis of the voice is not routinely done by the otolaryngologist–head and neck surgeon, but nevertheless should be considered in medical legal cases, in cases of high-profile patients, and in patients being studied as part of a research study protocol. Although some authors believe there is clinical data that can be derived from acoustic screening, the sensitivity of acoustic screening for pathology is poor. The main role of acoustic recording today is its value as an objective record of the voice outcome. ► Fig. 3.8 is a printout of a software graphic display of an acoustic analysis of common parameters from a popular commercially available acoustic analysis program (MVDP; Kay Pentax Corp., Montvale, NJ). Green represents the normative values; red indicates values beyond the norm. Acoustic recording and analysis allow the clinician to compare results based not on patient or examiner perception, but on computer-based analysis of the acoustic signal. There are many parameters that are used. The most common are the commercially available software for sustained vowel analysis based on jitter, shimmer, signal-to-noise ratio, and others. Unfortunately, routine recording and analysis of acoustic parameters based on sustained phonation have little validity in tracking dysphonic voices.[61] Running speech analysis and a score for dysphonia has also gained interest by using a cepstral analysis program. The consensus auditory-perceptual evaluation (CAPE V) is a clinical voice assessment tool developed by a consensus group sponsored by the American Speech-Language

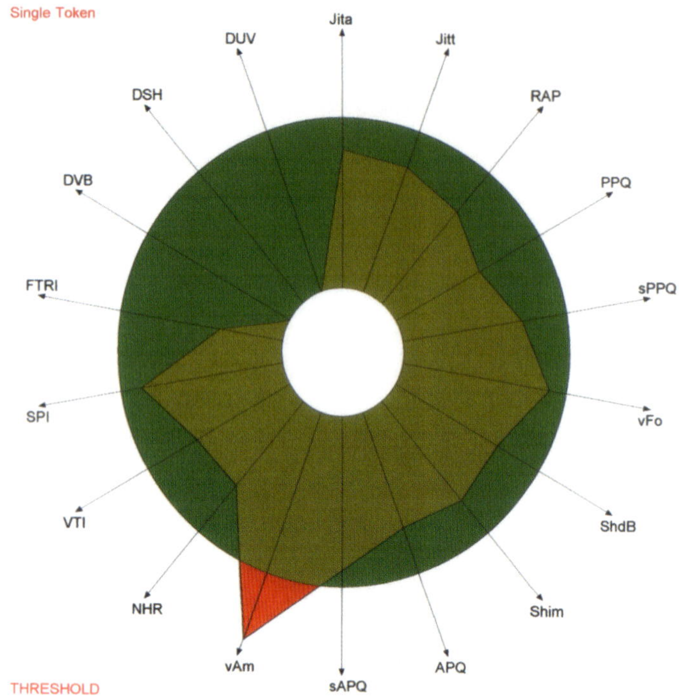

MDVPreport: Voice Report

Parameter	Name	Value	Unit
Average Fundamental Frequency	Fo	119.712	Hz
Mean Fundamental Frequency	MFo	119.700	Hz
Average Pitch Period	To	8.354	ms
Highest Fundamental Frequency	Fhi	122.761	Hz
Lowest Fundamental Frequency	Flo	116.191	Hz
Standard Deviation of Fo	STD	1.174	Hz
Phonatory Fo-Range in semi-tones	PFR	2	
Fo-Tremor Frequency	Fftr	2.222	Hz
Length of Analyzed Sample	Tsam	3.750	s
Absolute Jitter	Jita	67.588	µs
Jitter Percent	Jitt	0.809	%
Relative Average Perturbation	RAP	0.477	%
Pitch Perturbation Quotient	PPQ	0.487	%
Smoothed Pitch Perturbation Quotient	sPPQ	0.742	%
Fundamental Frequency Variation	vFo	0.981	%
Shimmer in dB	ShdB	0.246	dB
Shimmer Percent	Shim	2.850	%
Amplitude Perturbation Quotient	APQ	2.192	%
Smoothed Ampl. Perturbation Quotient	sAPQ	3.808	%
Peak-to-Peak Amplitude Variation	vAm	11.602	%
Noise to Harmonic Ratio	NHR	0.122	
Voice Turbulence Index	VTI	0.040	
Soft Phonation Index	SPI	12.362	
Fo-Tremor Intensity Index	FTRI	0.372	%
Degree of Voice Breaks	DVB	0.000	%
Degree of Sub-harmonics	DSH	0.000	%
Degree of Voiceless	DUV	0.000	%
Number of Voice Breaks	NVB	0	
Number of Sub-harmonic Segments	NSH	0	
Number of Unvoiced Segments	NUV	0	
Number of Segments Computed	SEG	124	
Total Number Detected Pitch Periods	PER	448	

Fig. 3.8 Multidimensional voice program plot of a mildly dysphonic patient with the normative values in green and the patient value in red.

Hearing Association, designed to score dysphonia based on tasks including sustained vowels, a series of six sentences to elicit various laryngeal behaviors, and running speech. The clinician rates the voice based on these tasks, creating a score that seems to correlate well with the degree of dysphonia. Routine use of this measure can give the clinician an objective score to follow in his or her patient, with rough voice quality. Other software that has been used to map out the functional phonatory envelope is the phonetogram. More popular in Europe than in the United States, the phonetogram requires some experience on the part of the clinician as an automated phonetogram has not proven to be clinically possible.

The need for objective recording and analysis in addition to QOL score alone needs to be highlighted. The objective recording and analysis of the voice do not correlate well with the VHI. In a study of mildly disordered voices analyzed by objective testing and VHI, there was poor correlation between fundamental frequency, jitter percentage, shimmer percentage, signal-to-noise ratio, mean root-mean-square intensity, fundamental frequency standard deviation, and aphonic periods; breath groups were predictive of overall VHI score. No cohesive or predictable pattern was identified when comparing individual measures with overall VHI or with each subscale item.[62] In the review of measuring voice outcomes, Carding[61] concluded that an expert rating of voice quality using the GRBAS rating scale and rating with a self-reporting tool have high validity and reliability with good sensitivity to change.

Physiological data on voice function are available and may be simple or complex. Simple phonation time and phonatory vital capacity can be obtained by a simple spirometer and a

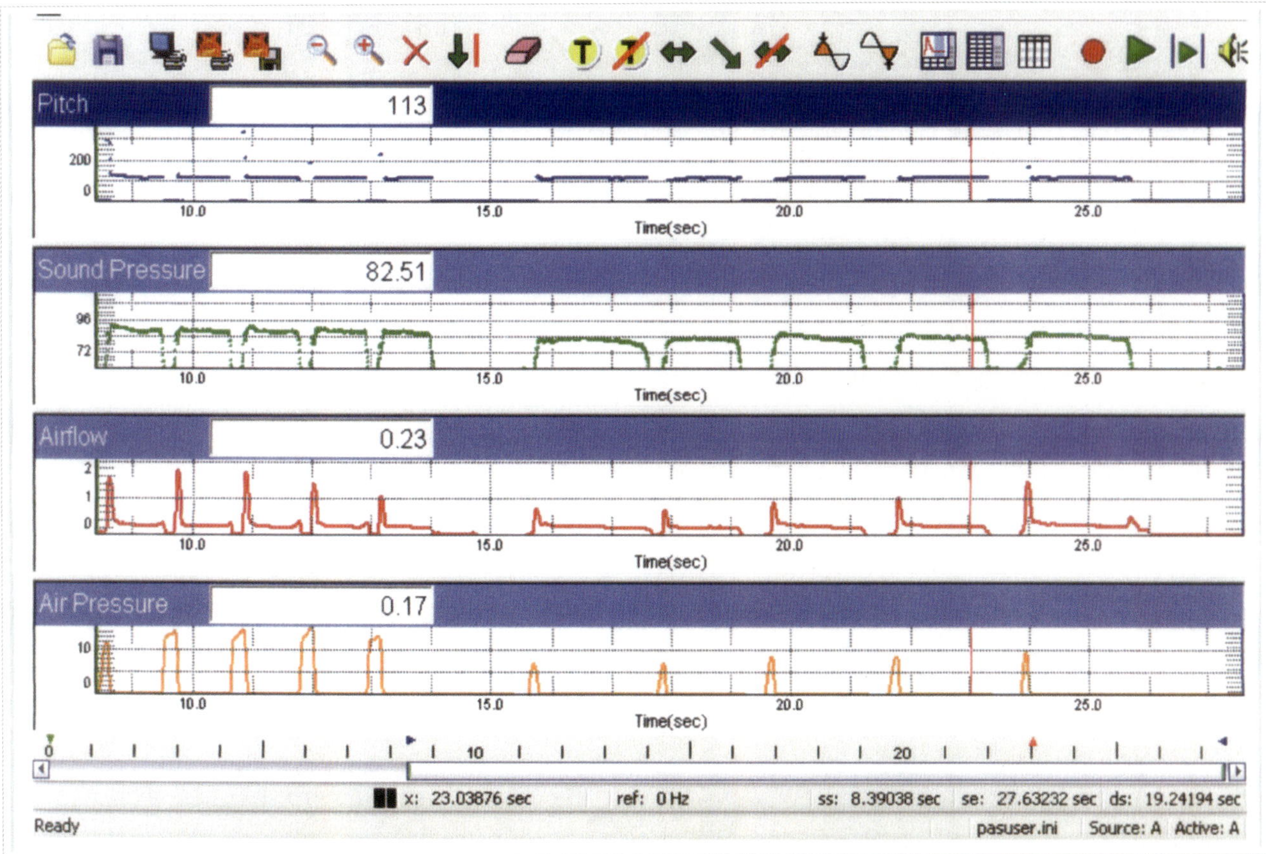

Fig. 3.9 Fundamental frequency, decibel output, subglottic pressure, and phonatory airflow are plotted over time in this phonatory function analysis.

stopwatch. This is an investment of less than $1,000 in the clinic setting. From the phonation time and the phonatory vital capacity, the mean phonatory airflow rate can be derived by dividing the phonatory vital capacity by the phonation time. Mean phonatory airflow is a good indicator to see if injection laryngoplasty or voice therapy alone can be adequate or whether more aggressive surgery, such as thyroplasty and arytenoid adductions, should be considered in the correction of glottic insufficiency.

Commercially available phonatory function analyzers are available and cost effective and utilize the personal computer, allowing relatively easy integration into the clinical setting. From the recordings, one can obtain the phonatory subglottic pressure, the acoustic output, and the phonatory airflow rates. The aerodynamic data, the subglottic pressure plot, the sound pressure, and the fundamental frequency plots are shown in ▶ Fig. 3.9. The software can automatically derive measures like glottal efficiency, glottal resistance, and other measures relevant to the physiology of the phonation production. Its use is becoming popular in the voice laboratory, but it is not commonly applied by the clinical otolaryngologist.

3.7 Empirical Treatment and Allergy Consultation

A medication trial is a common approach to use for patients without obvious laryngeal abnormality. Proton pump inhibitor trials for presumed laryngeal reflux have been used with variable duration. In one study, five times as many respondents prescribed PPIs as opposed to other medications.[1] Although some favor high-dose PPI treatment followed by tapering of medications, others use an escalating regimen to control symptoms and signs. Many otolaryngologists rely on the severity of the signs and symptoms as well as their patients' clinical response to empiric PPI trials without any objective evidence of acid reflux on testing.

Dysphonic patients may also present with throat symptoms, such as throat clearing, postnasal drip, and throat pain. There is also an overlap of throat symptoms and findings with allergic and nonallergic rhinitis, allergic laryngitis, and laryngeal pharyngeal reflux. A patient who has failed treatment with PPI should be considered for allergy evaluation and testing.

3.8 Speech Pathology Consultation

Probably one of the most underappreciated factors in the evaluation and management of the patient with dysphonia is the impact of form on function and function on form in the production of normal and abnormal voice. The dynamic interplay between form and function is often clearly displayed in the patient with laryngitis who recovers but cannot gain the voice back. The opposite is true in the patient who habitually overuses the voice and forms recurrent nodules and polyps that fail

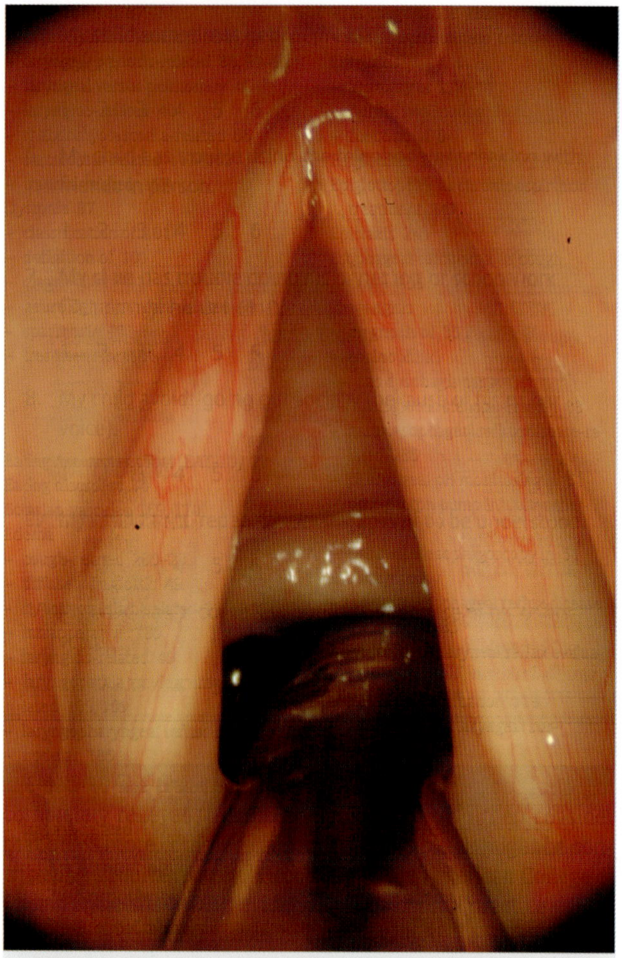

Fig. 3.10 Intraoperative photo of a small cyst on the left and scar on the right that could not be appreciated well except upon surgical exploration.

to be treated by surgery alone. This is because an otolaryngologist's training is generally focused on the form, whereas a speech-language pathologist is generally focused on restoring function. Communication and understanding of each other's role in diagnosis and treatment of the dysphonic patient are mandatory. Unfortunately, the concept of form and function is both underutilized and overutilized. The general otolaryngologist is primarily interested in the medical aspect of laryngeal disease as it relates to form. Is there a mass present? Is there inflammation? Is there paralysis? In patients with dysphonia, early evaluation and management by members of the voice team, such as a speech-language pathologist and a singing specialist, can identify maladaptive voice use patterns that can be instituted as a diagnostic paradigm. Reduction of muscle tension, improved mucosal hygiene, and improved breath support with better resonance can often reverse mucosal-based lesions like polyps, nodules, and granuloma so as to avoid surgery. In the postoperative period, close monitoring and rehabilitation can mean the difference between surgical success and failure. In the patient with compensated muscle tension, exploratory voice therapy consultation can yield positive results by unloading the patient and allow a truer picture of the organic disorder.[35,63]

3.9 Surgical Exploration

Most otolaryngologists do not consider examination under anesthesia in the management of adult dysphonic patients who present with no obvious mass lesions. The barrier to this may be due to the assumption that office endoscopy and radiographic examination are sufficient to rule out pathological entities that would justify general anesthesia. Exploratory surgical examination should be considered in the patient with suspected vocal fold lesions.[64,65,66] This is not usually necessary with the patient with exophytic lesions, such as polyps and papilloma, but should be considered in the patient with infiltrative lesions of the vocal folds, scarring, or suspected sulcus vocalis. Sulcus vocalis, fibrovascular deposit lesions, and mucosal bridges are common causes of dysphonia, but may not present with an obvious mass lesion. The clinical indicators for surgical exploration depend on the finding of glottic insufficiency and stiffness. This is most often seen as a vibratory abnormality and asymmetry between the vocal folds. In patients with infiltrative lesions like granuloma and systemic diseases of the larynx (tuberculosis, fungal laryngitis, sarcoidosis, myeloma, amyloid, and lymphoma), exploration, biopsy, and culture should be considered even in the absence of an obvious mass lesion of the larynx. Under high-power microscopy, the examination is systematically carried out by microscopy and by using 30-degree and 70-degree angled telescopes. This allows examination of the undersurface of the vocal fold as well as areas of the subglottis, ventricles, and the posterior and anterior commissures. These areas are difficult to examine in the office and may harbor a small tumor or mass lesion. Under anesthesia, palpation of the vocal fold can be done using a fine blunt probe. This will give the examiner appreciation for scar, fibrovascular deposits, sulcus, or a mucosal bridge that may be the cause of dysphonia. Subtle rheological differences between the vocal fold can be appreciated only with routine palpation of the vocal fold under anesthesia. ▶ Fig. 3.10 is a photograph of a small vocal fold cyst that could not be identified by stroboscopy except as an area of stiffness. Using modern phonosurgery techniques, these lesions can be addressed.

References

[1] Cohen SM, Pitman MJ, Noordzij JP, Courey M. Evaluation of dysphonic patients by general otolaryngologists. J Voice 2012; 26: 772–778

[2] Cohen SM, Pitman MJ, Noordzij JP, Courey M. Management of dysphonic patients by otolaryngologists. Otolaryngol Head Neck Surg 2012; 147: 289–294

[3] Benninger MS, Ahuja AS, Gardner G, Grywalski C. Assessing outcomes for dysphonic patients. J Voice 1998; 12: 540–550

[4] Morzaria S, Damrose EJ. A comparison of the VHI, VHI-10, and V-RQOL for measuring the effect of botox therapy in adductor spasmodic dysphonia. J Voice 2012; 26: 378–380

[5] Zur KB, Cotton S, Kelchner L, Baker S, Weinrich B, Lee L. Pediatric Voice Handicap Index (pVHI): a new tool for evaluating pediatric dysphonia. Int J Pediatr Otorhinolaryngol 2007; 71: 77–82

[6] Degroote G, Simon J, Borel S, Crevier-Buchman L. The French version of Speech Handicap Index: validation and comparison with the Voice Handicap Index. Folia Phoniatr Logop 2012; 64: 20–25

[7] Rosen CA, Lee AS, Osborne J, Zullo T, Murry T. Development and validation of the Voice Handicap Index-10. Laryngoscope 2004; 114: 1549–1556

[8] Rosen CA, Murry T. Voice Handicap Index in singers. J Voice 2000; 14: 370–377

[9] Rosen CA, Murry T, Zinn A, Zullo T, Sonbolian M. Voice Handicap Index change following treatment of voice disorders. J Voice 2000; 14: 619–623

[10] Branski RC, Cukier-Blaj S, Pusic A et al. Measuring quality of life in dysphonic patients: a systematic review of content development in patient-reported outcomes measures. J Voice 2010; 24: 193–198
[11] Cohen SM, Dupont WD, Courey MS. Quality-of-life impact of non-neoplastic voice disorders: a meta-analysis. Ann Otol Rhinol Laryngol 2006; 115: 128–134
[12] Belafsky PC, Postma GN, Koufman JA. Validity and reliability of the Reflux Symptom Index (RSI). J Voice 2002; 16: 274–277
[13] Ramig LO, Gray S, Baker K et al. The aging voice: a review, treatment data and familial and genetic perspectives. Folia Phoniatr Logop 2001; 53: 252–265
[14] Woo P, Casper J, Colton R, Brewer D. Dysphonia in the aging: physiology versus disease. Laryngoscope 1992; 102: 139–144
[15] Davis CB, Davis ML. The effects of premenstrual syndrome (PMS) on the female singer. J Voice 1993; 7: 337–353
[16] Dejonckere PH. Pathogenesis of voice disorders in childhood. Acta Otorhinolaryngol Belg 1984; 38: 307–314
[17] Hirano M. Clinical Examination of Voice. New York, NY: Springer-Verlag; 1981
[18] Lovetri J, Lesh S, Woo P. Preliminary study on the ability of trained singers to control the intrinsic and extrinsic laryngeal musculature. J Voice 1999; 13: 219–226
[19] Morrison MD, Rammage LA. Muscle misuse voice disorders: description and classification. Acta Otolaryngol 1993; 113: 428–434
[20] Morrison M. Pattern recognition in muscle misuse voice disorders: how I do it. J Voice 1997; 11: 108–114
[21] Angsuwarangsee T, Morrison M. Extrinsic laryngeal muscular tension in patients with voice disorders. J Voice 2002; 16: 333–343
[22] Hulshoff AC, Dikkers FG. De stilstaande stemband Ned Tijdschr Geneeskd 1998; 142: 1897–1901
[23] Roy N, Ford CN, Bless DM. Muscle tension dysphonia and spasmodic dysphonia: the role of manual laryngeal tension reduction in diagnosis and management. Ann Otol Rhinol Laryngol 1996; 105: 851–856
[24] Aronson AE. Clinical Voice Disorders. New York, NY: Thieme-Stratton,1980
[25] Mace SE. Blunt laryngotracheal trauma. Ann Emerg Med 1986; 15: 836–842
[26] , sshiki N, Ohkawa M, Goto M. Stiffness of the vocal cord in dysphonia—its assessment and treatment. Acta Otolaryngol Suppl 1984; 419 supplement: 167–174
[27] Eller R, Ginsburg M, Lurie D, Heman-Ackah Y, Lyons K, Sataloff R. Flexible laryngoscopy: a comparison of fiber optic and distal chip technologies. Part 1: vocal fold masses. J Voice 2008; 22: 746–750
[28] Eller R, Ginsburg M, Lurie D, Heman-Ackah Y, Lyons K, Sataloff R. Flexible laryngoscopy: a comparison of fiber optic and distal chip technologies. Part 2: laryngopharyngeal reflux. J Voice 2009; 23: 389–395
[29] Nospes S, Kuhr K, Napiontek U, Keilmann A. Stroboskopi-Befunde: Flexible CCD-Videostroboskopie und klassiche Lupenstroboskopie im Vergleich. Laryngorhinootologie 2011; 90: 218–223
[30] Sato K, Umeno H, Nakashima T. Stroboscopic observation of vocal fold vibration with the videoendoscope. Ann Otol Rhinol Laryngol 2003; 112: 965–970
[31] Kawaida M, Fukuda H, Kohno N. Electronic videoendoscopic laryngostroboscopy. ORL J Otorhinolaryngol Relat Spec 2004; 66: 267–274
[32] Remacle M. The contribution of videostroboscopy in daily ENT practice. Acta Otorhinolaryngol Belg 1996; 50: 265–281
[33] Schade G, Müller F. Hochgeschwindigkeitsglottographische. Diagnostik in der Laryngologie HNO 2005; 53: 1085–1086, 1088–1091
[34] Yiu EM, Kong J, Fong R, Chan KM. A preliminary study of a quantitative analysis method for high speed laryngoscopic images. Int J Speech-Language Pathol 2010; 12: 520–528
[35] Koufman JA, Radomski TA, Joharji GM, Russell GB, Pillsbury DC. Laryngeal biomechanics of the singing voice. Otolaryngol Head Neck Surg 1996; 115: 527–537
[36] Yanagisawa E, Estill J, Mambrino L, Talkin D. Supraglottic contributions to pitch raising. Videoendoscopic study with spectroanalysis. Ann Otol Rhinol Laryngol 1991; 100: 19–30
[37] Belafsky PC, Postma GN, Reulbach TR, Holland BW, Koufman JA. Muscle tension dysphonia as a sign of underlying glottal insufficiency. Otolaryngol Head Neck Surg 2002; 127: 448–451
[38] Behrman A. Common practices of voice therapists in the evaluation of patients. J Voice 2005; 19: 454–469
[39] Koufman JA, Amin MR, Panetti M. Prevalence of reflux in 113 consecutive patients with laryngeal and voice disorders. Otolaryngol Head Neck Surg 2000; 123: 385–388
[40] Dursun G, Sataloff RT, Spiegel JR, Mandel S, Heuer RJ, Rosen DC. Superior laryngeal nerve paresis and paralysis. J Voice 1996; 10: 206–211
[41] Fleischer S, Schade G, Hess MM. Office-based laryngoscopic observations of recurrent laryngeal nerve paresis and paralysis. Ann Otol Rhinol Laryngol 2005; 114: 488–493
[42] Woo P, Colton R, Casper J et al. Diagnostic value of stroboscopic examination in hoarse patients. J Voice 1991; 5: 231–238
[43] Casiano RR, Zaveri V, Lundy DS. Efficacy of videostroboscopy in the diagnosis of voice disorders. Otolaryngol Head Neck Surg 1992; 107: 95–100
[44] Wendler J. Stroboscopy. J Voice 1992; 6: 149–154
[45] Bootle C, McGlashan J, Robinson F. Larynx synchronised stroboscopy—a new tool for outcome measures in the voice clinic. Int J Lang Commun Disord 1998; 33 Suppl: 298–303
[46] Hartnick CJ, Zeitels SM. Pediatric video laryngo-stroboscopy. Int J Pediatr Otorhinolaryngol 2005; 69: 215–219
[47] Elias ME, Sataloff RT, Rosen DC, Heuer RJ, Spiegel JR. Normal strobovideolaryngoscopy: variability in healthy singers. J Voice 1997; 11: 104–107
[48] Schönharl E. Die Stroboskopie in der Praktischen Laryngologie. Stuttgart, Germany: Georg Thieme Verlag; 1960
[49] Colton R, Casper J, Brewer D, Woo P, Bless DM. Stroboscopic evaluation of the larynx. Paper presented at: American Speech-Language-Hearing Association Annual Convention; November 22–25, 1991; Atlanta, GA
[50] Bless DM, Brandenburg JH. Stroboscopic evaluation of functional voice disorders. Paper presented at: Middle Section of the Triological Society; January 22–24,1983; Madison, WI
[51] Ellis SF, Pollak AC, Hanson DG, Jiang JJ. Videolaryngoscopic evaluation of laryngeal intubation injury: incidence and predictive factors. Otolaryngol Head Neck Surg 1996; 114: 729–731
[52] Schutte HK, Svec JG, Sram F. First results of clinical application of videokymography. Laryngoscope 1998; 108: 1206–1210
[53] Deliyski DD, Petrushev PP, Bonilha HS, Gerlach TT, Martin-Harris B, Hillman RE. Clinical implementation of laryngeal high-speed videoendoscopy: challenges and evolution. Folia Phoniatr Logop 2008; 60: 33–44
[54] Safak MA, Göçmen H, Korkmaz H, Kiliç R. Computerized tomographic alignment of Silastic implant in type 1 thyroplasty. Am J Otolaryngol 2000; 21: 179–183
[55] De Cock M, Van Laer C, Vanwambeke K, Salgado R. Chondrosarcoma of the larynx: a report of two cases and a review of the literature. B-ENT 2006; 2: 21–26
[56] Schroeder U, Motzko M, Wittekindt C, Eckel HE. Hoarseness after laryngeal blunt trauma: a differential diagnosis between an injury to the external branch of the superior laryngeal nerve and an arytenoid subluxation. A case report and literature review. Eur Arch Otorhinolaryngol 2003; 260: 304–307
[57] Avrahami E, Frishman E, Spierer I, Englender M, Katz R. CT of minor intubation trauma with clinical correlations. Eur J Radiol 1995; 20: 68–71
[58] Brazeau-Lamontagne L, Charlin B, Levesque RY, Lussier A. Cricoarytenoiditis: CT assessment in rheumatoid arthritis. Radiology 1986; 158: 463–466
[59] Mafee MF, Schild JA, Valvassori GE, Capek V. Computed tomography of the larynx: correlation with anatomic and pathologic studies in cases of laryngeal carcinoma. Radiology 1983; 147: 123–128
[60] Sulica L, Blitzer A. Electromyography and the immobile vocal fold. Otolaryngol Clin North Am 2004; 37: 59–74
[61] Carding PN, Wilson JA, MacKenzie K, Deary IJ. Measuring voice outcomes: state of the science review. J Laryngol Otol 2009; 123: 823–829
[62] Wheeler KM, Collins SP, Sapienza CM. The relationship between VHI scores and specific acoustic measures of mildly disordered voice production. J Voice 2006; 20: 308–317
[63] Rodríguez-Parra MJ, Adrián JA, Casado JC. Voice therapy used to test a basic protocol for multidimensional assessment of dysphonia. J Voice 2009; 23: 304–318
[64] Hernando M, Cobeta I, Lara A, García F, Gamboa FJ. Vocal pathologies of difficult diagnosis. J Voice 2008; 22: 607–610
[65] Burns JA, Hillman RE, Stadelman-Cohen T, Zeitels SM. Phonomicrosurgical treatment of intracordal vocal-fold cysts in singers. Laryngoscope 2009; 119: 419–422
[66] Johns MM. Update on the etiology, diagnosis, and treatment of vocal fold nodules, polyps, and cysts. Curr Opin Otolaryngol Head Neck Surg 2003; 11: 456–461

4 Evaluation and Examination of the Patient with Dysphagia

Pavan S. Mallur and Jo Shapiro

Swallowing is a complex, multistaged process that has both a voluntary and an involuntary component. Cortical and brainstem functions combine with sensory afferent input and efferent activity to coordinate a temporally precise neuromuscular sequence. The end result is a specific sequence of muscle activation and relaxation, leading to the cardinal events of the oropharyngeal swallow: velopharyngeal closure, base of tongue retraction, pharyngeal constrictor contraction, hyolaryngeal elevation, and pharyngoesophageal sphincter (PES) opening (▶ Fig. 4.1). Akin to the engineering tenet that the ability for mechanical failure is proportional to the number of moving parts, during the course of the swallow there are multiple points of potential failure. Detailed knowledge of the swallowing mechanism, along with a differential diagnosis specific to the location of the suspected deficit, allows selection of the appropriate diagnostic workup. Diagnostic testing may yield functional, structural, or physiologic data, contributing information of variable relevance in evaluating individual disease processes.

Ultimately, the goal of the dysphagia evaluation is to correlate symptoms with the diagnostic workup, to establish a diagnosis, and to apply the clinical information in executing a rational therapeutic plan.

4.1 History

The patient with swallowing difficulties may present with an isolated complaint and limited medical history or with multiple symptoms and medical comorbidities; an adequate history will detail complaints related to each phase of swallowing and assess the patient for known and undiagnosed disease processes associated with dysphagia. Swallow-specific history delineates severity of symptoms and helps to localize suspected deficits to the oral, oropharyngeal, or esophageal phases. This initial screening guides the selection of appropriate diagnostic tests, as not all options for workup yield relevant or optimal clinical information. A careful medical history that goes beyond swallow-specific symptoms will inform the physician of potential structural, neurologic, or neuromuscular etiologies.

In an effort to standardize outcome measures, many advocate initial screening with patient questionnaires specific to dysphagia. To this end, several quantifiable, statistically validated scales have been developed that incorporate questions about symptoms and quality of life. The M.D. Anderson Dysphagia Inventory (MDADI), developed for the head and neck cancer population, surveys emotional, functional, and physical aspects of a patient's swallow to establish a score of 0 (low functioning) to 100 (high functioning).[1] Similarly, the SWAL-QOL tool is a 44-item survey that assesses 10 quality-of-life concepts and correlates symptom severity with the calculated numeric scale.[2] The Eating Assessment Tool (EAT-10) has been developed recently to provide an instrument that is rapidly administered and easily scored, facilitating use in clinical practice.[3] Although not specific to dysphagia, the Reflux Symptom Index (RSI) documents perceived severity of laryngopharyngeal reflux symptoms, often comorbid in patients with dysphagia.[4] The scales are a useful adjunct in clinical dysphagia evaluation, providing a quantified outcome for symptom severity; the utility lies in standardization of outcome measures, comparison with normative values, and use in longitudinal assessments to determine treatment efficacy.

The initial history should first clarify whether there is any odynophagia, as this raises concerns for other issues, such as neoplasia or infection. Next should be an attempt to localize symptoms to the oral, oropharyngeal, and/or esophageal phases of swallowing. Though not absolute, symptoms occurring before initiation of the swallow suggest oral-phase deficits, symptoms during or immediately after the swallow suggest oropharyngeal deficits, and symptoms occurring several seconds after the swallow suggest esophageal phase dysphagia. With regard to symptom type, difficulty initiating swallow, cough during or immediately after the swallow, nasal regurgitation, and increased effort or repeated swallows suggest oropharyngeal dysphagia. Localization of symptoms to the upper throat similarly may suggest an oropharyngeal etiology; however, this symptom may be referred from a primary esophageal abnormality. Conversely, symptoms felt in the retrosternal area more reliably suggest esophageal causes and rarely, if ever, point to an oropharyngeal deficit. Beyond this, manometric investigation has shown that perceived localization of esophageal abnormalities correlates poorly with manometric abnormalities, especially with respect to proximal or midesophageal symptoms.[5] Pointing to the importance of history in the dysphagia evaluation, there is evidence that suggests that a careful history can localize the phase of abnormal swallowing in up to 85% of patients.[6]

Although often overlooked, initial history should include assessments of oral-preparatory and oral-phase symptoms. An integral portion of bolus preparation includes adequate lubrication with saliva; complaints of dry mouth can be related to a variety of disorders, including medication-induced, systemic rheumatologic disease, or postradiation xerostomia. Preparation and initial propulsion of the food bolus toward the oropharynx require adequate control of labial, buccal, intrinsic tongue, and mastication musculature, and normally last 1 to 1.5 seconds. Recent evidence suggests the voluntary oral phase is controlled by the primary sensorimotor cortex and premotor cortex and is coordinated via the cerebellum.[7] Prolonged time for oral phase, difficulty coordinating tongue movements, premature coughing while chewing, and difficulty chewing harder foods may be signs of a neurologic disease process, such as stroke,[8,9] or neuromuscular etiology, such as Parkinson disease, amyotrophic lateral sclerosis (ALS), or myasthenia gravis.[10,11] Additionally, complaints of physical tongue tethering with odynophagia may reveal structural abnormalities, such as a carcinoma of the oral cavity.

A history of abnormal pharyngeal phase of swallowing may indicate multiple complaints. Afferent input triggers this phase

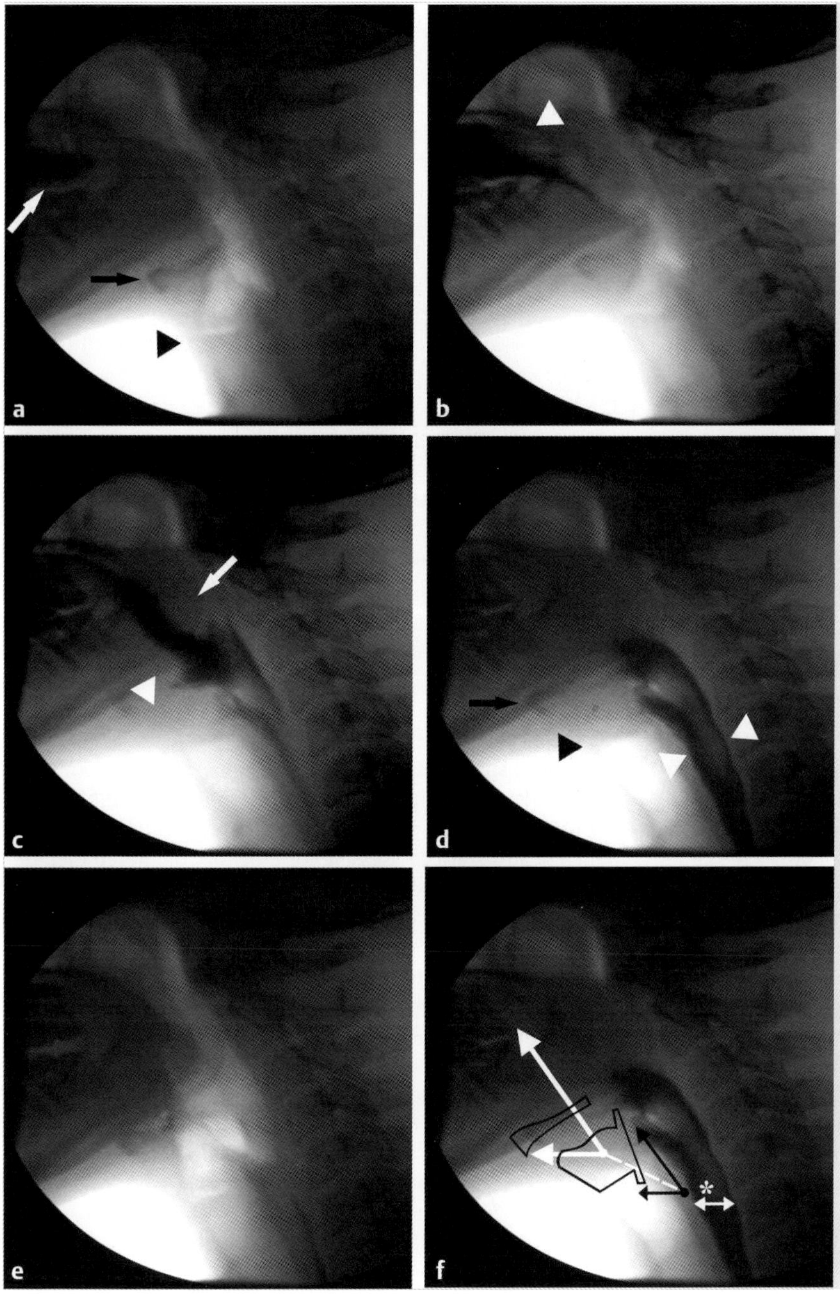

Fig. 4.1 Videofluoroscopy of the normal swallow mechanism. (**a**) Oral preparatory phase with bolus (*white arrow*) held in the oral cavity and normal resting position of hyoid bone (*black arrow*) and thyroid cartilage (*black arrowhead*). (**b**) Initiation of the pharyngeal phase of swallow with velopharyngeal closure (*white arrowhead*). (**c**) Initial propulsion of the bolus through the oropharynx with base of tongue retraction (*white arrowhead*) and superior pharyngeal constrictor contraction (*white arrow*). (**d**) Hyolaryngeal elevation with hyoid (*black arrow*) and thyroid cartilages (*black arrowhead*) anteriorly and superiorly displaced. Note concomitant opening of the pharyngoesophageal sphincter (*white arrowheads*). (**e**) Closure of the pharyngoesophageal sphincter and initiation of esophageal phase of swallow. (**f**) Directional pull of suprahyoid musculature (*white arrows*) elevating the hyolaryngeal complex. Resultant force vector (*black arrows*), along with cricopharyngeal relaxation (*asterisk*), contributes to PES opening (*white double-headed arrow*).

via the glossopharyngeal nerve (cranial nerve [CN] IX) in the oropharynx and internal branch of the superior laryngeal nerve (CN X) in the supraglottic larynx.[12] It has classically been suggested that the internal branch of the superior laryngeal nerve is only present as an accessory input not involved in normal swallowing, though more recent literature places more import on this afferent pathway.[13] The pharyngeal phase is mediated primarily by the lower brainstem, though conscious modulation may occur through descending cortical pathways via the primary sensorimotor cortex.[14,15] Inability to initiate swallow may signal sensory or central neurologic deficiencies along this pathway (▶ Fig. 4.2). Nasal regurgitation during the swallow, with associated hypernasal speech and without structural defects of the soft palate, indicates decreased or absent vagus (CN X) or lower motor neuron innervation. Alternatively, there may be a structural abnormality of the soft palate, either congenital, as seen in cleft palate, postsurgical, as seen in soft palate resection or uvulopalatopharyngoplasty; or postradiation fibrosis, as seen in nasopharyngeal or oropharyngeal carcinoma. Complaints of inefficient swallow, such as bolus sticking in the upper throat or need for repeated swallows, can be related to reduced base of tongue or pharyngeal strength, or may be secondary to outflow obstruction from cricopharyngeal dysfunction, reduced hyolaryngeal elevation, or mechanical obstruction. Typically, this can be localized with greater accuracy than esophageal obstruction, and the onset is during or immediately after the swallow. Difficulty with solids may suggest mechanical obstruction; difficulty with both liquids and solids implies a neurologic or neuromuscular etiology. That said, neuromuscular disorders causing dysphagia due to diffuse pharyngeal

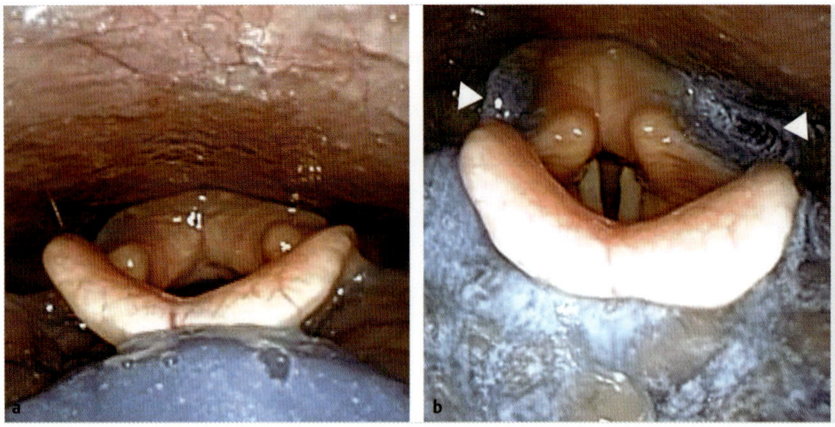

Fig. 4.2 Flexible fiberoptic evaluation of swallow (FEES) demonstrating absent initiation of pharyngeal swallow. (**a**) Pudding-consistency bolus at vallecula/base of tongue level with no trigger of pharyngeal swallow. (**b**) Passive, premature spillage of nectar-thickened liquid bolus into vallecula and piriform sinuses (arrowheads) with failure to trigger pharyngeal-phase swallow.

muscle weakness typically first present with difficulty in solid bolus propulsion.

If there is a history suggestive of bolus propulsion difficulties, it is helpful to elucidate how the patient handles this symptom. Maneuvers range from briefly waiting for the bolus to pass spontaneously to requiring volitional pharyngeal regurgitation to remove the bolus. Such distinctions help to both determine the severity of the dysphagia as well as to localize the region and sometimes the etiology of the symptom. For example, with a lower esophageal obstruction such as a Schatzki ring, the impacted bolus requires forceful regurgitation; attempting to use multiple liquid swallows to pass the bolus merely results in the liquids "backing up" against the impacted solid. On the other hand, solid boluses lodged in a pharyngeal diverticulum will typically be spontaneously regurgitated sometime after a meal.

A history for dysphagia should always note signs and symptoms of aspiration and consider the temporal relation to oropharyngeal swallow. Aspiration occurring before the initiation of the oropharyngeal swallow, for example, while chewing, indicates premature spillage from the oral cavity. Premature transport of solids into the vallecula occurs through active stage II transport, and of liquids into the hypopharynx through a gravity-dependent process in healthy individuals, and is increased in the elderly and with mixed-consistency food consumption.[16,17] However, when control of oral cavity musculature, soft palate movement, or laryngeal sensation is impaired, as seen in stroke patients or postradiation treatment for head and neck cancer, premature spillage may result in aspiration.[18,19] Primary aspiration occurring during the oropharyngeal phase occurs with reduced or absent laryngeal aditus closure or frank glottic incompetence. The former may occur with large anterior cervical spine osteophytes; although this is thought to be secondary to reduced epiglottic inversion from mechanical obstruction, it is controversial.[20] Glottic incompetence is well recognized in unilateral vocal fold immobility/paralysis. This may be increased with high vagal lesions due to reduced laryngeal sensation from superior laryngeal nerve and/or reduced pharyngeal contraction from pharyngeal constrictor paralysis, respectively.[21] The notion that aspiration secondary to high vagal lesions is due to increased propensity for lateral vocal fold position is not substantiated by the available literature.[22,23] Though anecdotally seen with glottic incompetence from vocal fold scar, severe vocal fold atrophy, or vocal fold hypomobility/paresis, aspiration in these entities has not been well studied and may be exacerbated by other factors predisposing to dysphagia. Secondary aspiration occurring after the oropharyngeal swallow results from bolus retention at the level of the vallecula or hypopharynx, or from retrograde transport of esophageal contents into the laryngopharynx. A host of disease processes can contribute to this, and features may include reduced tongue base or pharyngeal strength, mechanically impeded pharyngeal outflow, PES dysfunction, laryngopharyngeal reflux, mechanical esophageal stasis or dysmotility, or an incompetent lower esophageal sphincter.

One final point that should not be ignored in the history of the patient with dysphagia is the overall assessment of the patient's health status. Assessing for a history of altered diet, dehydration, weight loss, or failure to thrive helps delineate the severity of dysphagia. Awareness of global weakness, dysarthria, ptosis, or subtle mental status changes can prompt investigation for neuromuscular or neurologic disease processes. Concomitant medical comorbidities, such as cardiopulmonary disease or overall deconditioning, often will change a patient's tolerance of aspiration, and may prompt more urgent workup and treatment.

4.2 Physical Examination

The physical examination of the patient with dysphagia begins with a complete head and neck examination with a CN assessment. Initial survey should begin with a general assessment of the patient's communication ability, assessing for dysarthria, dysphonia, or hypernasal speech suggestive of poor oral motor control, underlying glottic incompetence, or velopharyngeal insufficiency, respectively. The remainder of the head and neck examination should be directed at identifying abnormal anatomy or frank pathological lesions that may affect swallowing, such as abnormal or missing dentition, physical lesions tethering the tongue, or neck masses or fibrosis reducing hyolaryngeal elevation. The presence of a nasogastric tube for nutrition should be noted, though this does not independently increase risk for dysphagia or aspiration.[24] Examination of the CNs will alert the clinician to deficits in oral motor control, pharyngeal sensitivity, or larger neurologic or neuromuscular processes.

The physical examination for patients with dysphagia is often formalized with the clinical evaluation of swallowing, a functional and structural screening for dysphagia performed without instrumentation or radiographic imaging. Most often performed by speech-language-swallowing pathologists, the exam has portions that overlap the general physical exam. Though it has existed through various iterations, the exam typically consists of an oromotor evaluation and noninstrumented laryngeal evaluation and may include an oral bolus trial to grossly assess swallow. The oromotor evaluation assesses jaw movement, labial movement and oral competence, tongue motion, strength, and sensitivity, and soft palate elevation. This may include testing for the presence or strength of an oropharyngeal gag reflex. In addition, the oromotor evaluation can assess for adequate mental status, ability to follow commands, and suitability for oral trials. The laryngeal evaluation assesses for presence of tracheotomy tube, voice quality, projection, mean phonatory time, and strength of volitional cough. Oral bolus trials, when safe, consist of various volume trials of water, and assess for oral clearing, cough before, during, or after the swallow, palpation for laryngeal elevation, presence of "wet" sounding cough or gurgling, and optimal patient position for swallowing. A history of aspiration, respiratory compromise, "wet" dysphonia, decreased mental status, excessive pooling of secretions, or absent volitional cough should preclude an oral bolus trial.

Though the clinical evaluation of swallowing is useful conceptually, in practice it has variable execution. A systematic review of several trials reports sensitivity ranging from 42% to 92%, and specificity from 59% to 91%, as a predictor of aspiration.[25] Much effort has been made to isolate factors predictive of aspiration in specific patient populations. Palatal asymmetry, incomplete oral clearance, and impaired pharyngeal response with gurgling or cough have been purported to be independent predictors of aspiration, as measured by the gold standard of videofluoroscopy.[26] Absent gag reflex, dysarthria, and abnormal volitional cough have also been suggested as independent predictors of aspiration.[27] Addition of cervical auscultation may increase the sensitivity and specificity of clinical evaluation of swallowing in detecting aspiration.[28] Some have suggested that adding pulse oximetry to larger bolus trials increases sensitivity for aspiration detection to 100%.[29]

A point should be made regarding tracheotomy and its role in dysphagia. Though classically it has been surmised that tracheotomy placement tethers the larynx and prevents hyolaryngeal excursion, recent evidence suggests that hyoid and laryngeal elevation remains normal after tracheotomy placement and decannulation.[30,31] Additionally, removal of a tracheotomy tube does not seem to appreciably alter laryngeal kinematics or expedite return to oral intake.[31,32] It is likely the comorbid conditions, such as overall debilitation, deconditioning, trauma, stroke, and respiratory compromise, predispose patients with tracheotomy to aspiration and pneumonia, rather than the tracheotomy itself.

As part of the physical examination, flexible laryngoscopy with or without stroboscopy should be considered in patients with suspected glottic incompetence. Classically, hoarse or breathy voice, a decrease in mean phonatory time, decreased volume, decreased projection, vocal fatigue, and increased pitch all suggest glottic incompetence to varying extents. It is estimated that aspiration occurs in 44% of patients with unilateral vocal fold immobility and in 57% with bilateral immobility.[33] Though it has not been studied extensively, subtle causes of glottic incompetence, such as vocal fold atrophy or hypomobility, may contribute to dysphagia in patients with comorbid neurologic or neuromuscular disorders. Animal models inducing unilateral vocal fold paralysis confirm that glottic closing pressures are impaired during swallow and that they improve after medialization.[34,35] It is unknown if these data are applicable to vocal fold hypomobility or atrophy, though it is reasonable to surmise that improved glottic competence with these entities may improve pharyngeal pressure during swallow. Regardless, modern materials and techniques allow for restoration of glottic competence on a temporary or trial basis with minimal risk for complication.[36,37] Because of this, videostroboscopy, the gold standard for diagnosis of glottic insufficiency, should be considered in patients with complex dysphagia.

4.3 Differential Diagnosis

The differential diagnosis for dysphagia is extensive, with a wide array of pathophysiologic processes responsible for dysfunctional swallowing. Particular features of pathologic swallowing may be common across multiple diagnoses. Despite this, it is important to search for a definitive cause, as further workup and management may vary considerably. For the purposes of categorization, causes of oropharyngeal dysphagia can be divided into four main categories: structural, neuromuscular, neurologic, and psychological disorders.

4.3.1 Structural Causes

Zenker Diverticulum

Zenker diverticulum is a evagination of the hypopharyngeal mucosa, typically through the Killian triangle, bordered superiorly by the inferior pharyngeal constrictor and inferiorly by the cricopharyngeus muscle. The pathophysiology of a Zenker diverticulum may result from cricopharyngeal (CP) dysfunction; persistent pharyngeal contraction against a closed or incompletely opened PES increases pressures proximally, exploiting the anatomical weakness in the hypopharyngeal wall (▶ Fig. 4.3). The exact nature of CP dysfunction, however, is debated; incomplete or delayed CP relaxation, premature return to tonic contraction before swallow is complete, and poor coordination of pharyngeal contractions and CP relaxation have all been proposed.[38] Some postulate that the anatomical weakness between the lower border of the inferior constrictor and the upper border of the CP may be solely responsible for diverticulum formation, regardless of CP status.

Zenker diverticula present most commonly in men between the ages of 60 and 70. Symptoms include those of CP dysfunction, such as solid boluses sticking in the throat, as well as regurgitation of undigested food after the meal and halitosis. Chronic cough occurs in 30% to 40%.[39] Aspiration and weight loss may occur in severe cases. The association with laryngopharyngeal reflux, as diagnosed by dual-channel pH probe, is suggested to be as high as 72%.[40] This is disputed, however; therefore, symptoms consistent with gastroesophageal reflux disease (GERD) or laryngopharyngeal reflux (LPR) should not be relied upon for diagnosis. Physical examination findings are few, although they may include an audible "gurgling" sound on swallowing or signs of malnutrition.

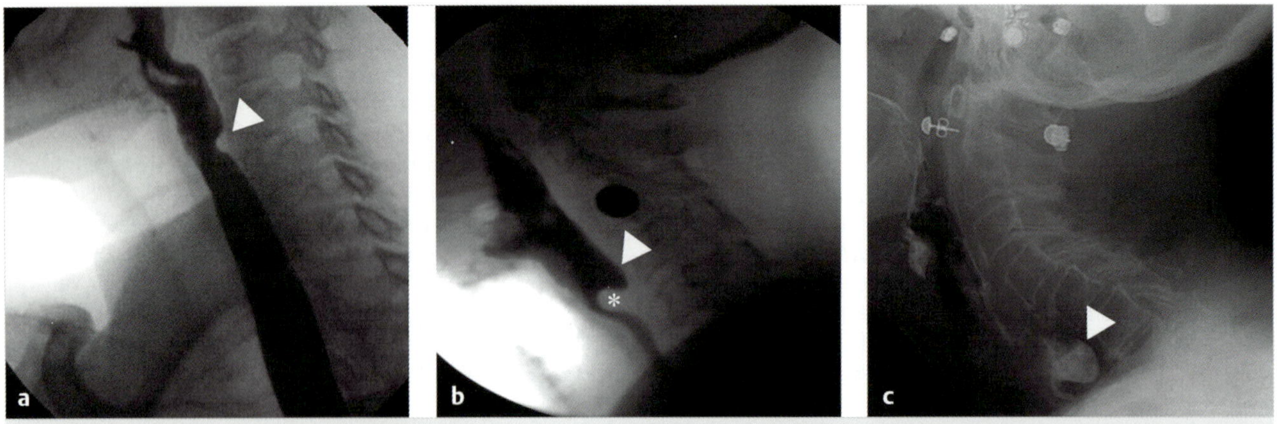

Fig. 4.3 Videofluoroscopy demonstrating spectrum of cricopharyngeal dysfunction with Zenker diverticulum. (a) Prominent posterior cricopharyngeal "bar" (*arrowhead*) with incomplete pharyngoesophageal sphincter opening. (b) Prominent cricopharyngeus (*asterisk*) with small hypopharyngeal diverticulum (*arrowhead*). (c) Larger hypopharyngeal diverticulum with posterior base (*arrowhead*).

Diagnosis is made with a barium esophagram, revealing a hypopharyngeal pouch, usually protruding posteriorly and to the left. Size varies greatly, as does the degree of reflux from the diverticulum. A lateral view is necessary to visualize the PES. Recent evidence suggests that pharyngeal dilation, as evidenced by an increased pharyngeal constriction ratio, also is visible on videofluoroscopy.[41]

Hypopharyngeal Stricture

Stricture of the hypopharynx most commonly results after treatment of head and neck carcinoma; it has been described after concurrent chemotherapy and radiation, endoscopic resection, and open resection with reconstruction. Though rare, it also may occur in Plummer-Vinson syndrome, with web formation in the postcricoid region, or in cicatricial pemphigoid. Symptoms may include varying degrees of bolus obstruction. Diagnosis is made on videofluoroscopy, typically showing narrowing or obliteration of one or both piriforms, or narrowing to complete obstruction at the cricopharyngeal level.

Pharyngocele

Lateral pharyngeal diverticula, or pharyngoceles, are rare acquired diverticula of the piriform sinus. They are presumed to be caused by increased pharyngeal pressures exploiting the muscular weakness between the middle and inferior pharyngeal constrictors. Most are unilateral and range from 1 to 2 cm in size. Symptoms of dysphagia, regurgitation, or pain may occur. Physical exam findings are rare, but may include neck mass. Diagnosis is made by barium swallow or videofluoroscopy, showing a typically round outpouching in the base of the piriform sinus.[42]

Osteophytes

Anterior cervical spine osteophytes occur in age-related degenerative skeletal disease, in the setting of previous trauma, or in the rarely encountered diffuse skeletal idiopathic hyperostosis. Severe dysphagia from anterior cervical spine osteophytes requiring surgical osteophytectomy is relatively infrequent, and outcomes are uncertain.[43] Workup typically includes videofluoroscopy with lateral views, which best reveal osteophyte impingement of the laryngopharynx or upper esophagus and obstruction of bolus. Manometry may reveal increased intrabolus pressures across the osteophyte, which some purport predict improved functional outcomes after surgical intervention.[44]

Head and Neck Cancer

All head and neck malignancies have the potential to cause varying degrees of dysphagia. Poor oral control, odynophagia, difficulty with passage of solid foods, aspiration, need for altered diet, failure to thrive, and weight loss are well described in both pre- and posttreatment cancer patients. A nononcologic workup of dysphagia should include clinical examination of swallowing, and, when indicated, videofluoroscopy or functional endoscopic evaluation of swallowing. Predictors for severe dysphagia or feeding tube dependence include oropharyngeal, laryngeal, and hypopharyngeal sites, pretreatment feeding tube dependence, and higher T stage.[45,46,47] Comparison of the effects of therapy on functional outcomes is controversial, though emerging evidence suggests that newer technology, such as transoral robotic laser resections, have better functional outcomes than open surgical techniques.[45,46] Posttreatment videofluoroscopy may vary considerably, though it is suggested that concurrent chemoradiation therapy for various sites may lead to decreased PES opening and aspiration in up to 30% of patients.[46]

4.3.2 Neurologic Causes

Laryngopharyngeal Paralysis and Paresis

Laryngopharyngeal paralysis is aberrant muscular contraction that may result from a primary neurologic or CN insult. It may occur from a deficit in CNs X or XII, or less commonly from a deficit in CN IX.

Symptoms of laryngopharyngeal paralysis often include poor bolus propulsion and aspiration. The pathophysiologic correlate is dependent on the specific lower CN deficit and may include decreased tongue base retraction (CN XII) and pharyngeal contraction (CN X), as well as reduced contraction of the suprahyoid musculature (CNs IX and XII). Though a variety of disorders may cause laryngopharyngeal paralysis, one of the most recognized is recurrent laryngeal nerve paralysis in isolation, or as part of a higher vagal nerve paralysis. Certain neurologic, neuromuscular, neoplastic, or autoimmune disorders may involve more than one nerve in combination.

The most practical and widely used diagnostic workup for laryngopharyngeal paralysis is videofluoroscopy; recent quantification of metrics on this examination has revealed increased pharyngeal transit times, decreased pharyngeal contraction, and reduced hyolaryngeal excursion.[48] Electromyographic study of hypoglossal, recurrent, and superior laryngeal nerves is often utilized to confirm neurologic or neuromuscular deficits and may provide prognostic information. These studies provide valuable physiologic information; however, they do not yield information on functional status. Currently, high-resolution pharyngeal manometry is the gold standard for functional diagnosis of laryngopharyngeal paralysis. Despite this, it is not widely available and requires considerable experience and expertise for interpretation. It also may be subject to inherent variation. Studies comparing pharyngeal constriction ratio on videofluoroscopy to high-resolution pharyngeal manometry have supported the use of the metric as a valid surrogate for pharyngeal strength.[50,51]

Stroke

Acute cerebrovascular ischemia, particularly involving the vertebrobasilar system or posterior inferior cerebellar arteries, may cause varying degrees of dysphagia. Most commonly, delayed triggering of swallow is responsible for premature spillage into the oropharynx; when combined with the commonly found sensory deficits of the laryngopharynx, it may lead to aspiration. Early clinical assessment of swallow may prompt further assessment, though the modality has variable sensitivity and specificity and is poor in detecting silent aspiration.[52] Videofluoroscopy remains the gold standard for workup and may detect penetration and aspiration in up to 42.8% and 26.5% of patients, respectively.[53] Increase in swallow initiation time, increase in pharyngeal transit time, decrease in laryngeal closure duration, and decrease in cricopharyngeal opening may all be found; however, the former two in combination may be more predictive of aspiration.[54] The estimated incidence of acute stroke-associated pneumonia is 7% and is associated with increased 30-day and 1-year mortality.[55] Because of this, videofluoroscopy, with a higher sensitivity to detect aspiration, is preferred over flexible endoscopic evaluation of swallowing.

4.3.3 Neuromuscular Causes

Parkinson Disease

Parkinson disease (PD) is a progressive disorder caused by abnormalities in the dopamine transmitting cells of the basal ganglia. Characteristic global symptoms include bradykinesia, resting tremor, postural instability, and "cogwheel" muscle rigidity. Mild cognitive impairment may also accompany the other symptoms. There is a high prevalence of oral-phase dysphagia, with repetitive tongue pumping anteriorly to posteriorly, residue in the lateral and anterior sulci, premature spillage, and piecemeal deglutition. Increased pharyngeal transit time and decreased PES opening are also common features. Aspiration may occur in up to 50% of PD patients with reported dysphagia.[56] Although only 30% of PD patients report subjective dysphagia, objective studies show abnormalities in up to 80%.[57] Overall increase in total swallowing time is likened to the global bradykinesia seen in this patient population. With the high risk for aspiration, videofluoroscopy remains the workup of choice.

Amyotrophic Lateral Sclerosis

Amyotrophic lateral sclerosis (ALS), or motor neuron disease, is a progressive disorder of upper and lower motor neurons. Though it may affect any body segment, bulbar and pseudobulbar paralysis are responsible for the dysphagia prevalent in this population. Early signs are predominantly oral-phase deficits, with anterior and posterior tongue exhibiting abnormal movements.[58] Late-stage dysphagia includes poor bolus control in the oral cavity and decreased pharyngeal contraction, though PES opening appears preserved.[59] Aspiration may occur in up to 60% of patients.[60] Videofluoroscopy is most widely utilized to diagnose dysphagia, though use of videofluoromanometry may give physiologic correlates for assessing therapeutic maneuvers.[60]

Multiple Sclerosis

Multiple sclerosis (MS) is an axonal demyelinating disorder that may produce relapsing or progressive sensory or motor deficits. In patients with mild to moderate disease severity, approximately 30% will have some form of dysphagia, with up to 7% experiencing frank aspiration.[61] Delayed onset of pharyngeal swallow, delayed and prolonged laryngeal elevation, and pharyngeal constrictor dysmotility are the predominant findings.[62] Videofluoroscopy or flexible endoscopic evaluation of swallowing may be used to evaluate swallow when indicated.

Myasthenia Gravis

Myasthenia gravis (MG) is a neuromuscular disorder caused by an autoimmune antibody blockade of postsynaptic acetylcholine receptors leading to muscle weakness characterized by early fatigability. Abnormal bolus transport to the oropharynx, pharyngeal constriction, laryngeal elevation, and PES opening are common features and may worsen toward the end of a meal as the patient fatigues. Aspiration may occur in approximately 30% of patients.[63]

Oculopharyngeal Muscular Dystrophy

Oculopharyngeal muscular dystrophy (OPMD) is a variably inherited disorder of the *PABPN1* gene that results in ptosis and dysphagia. Onset is typically after 45 years of age. Early symptoms include subjectively increased time spent in eating and avoidance of dry foods; this corresponds to decreased oral strength, intraoral swallow pressure, and swallow capacity, and increased swallow time.[64] Additionally, aspiration and pneumonia may be a concern in these patients. Pharyngeal pressures detected by manometry corroborate findings of decreased pharyngeal propulsion and PES dysfunction seen commonly on videofluoroscopy or FEES in these patients.[65,66] Additionally, esophageal manometry may demonstrate abnormal esophageal contractions and decreased lower esophageal sphincter relaxation, the presence of which may alter treatment with CP myotomy.[67] Despite the presence of esophageal dysmotility and lower esophageal sphincter dysfunction, patients with OPMD may obtain moderate benefit from cricopharyngeal myotomy for a duration of 1 to 2 years.

Inclusion Body Myositis

Spontaneous inclusion body myositis is an idiopathic inflammatory disorder of skeletal muscle, with histology and inflammatory cytokine expression suggesting both inflammatory fibrosis as well as overall muscle degeneration.[68] Simultaneous videofluoroscopy and manometry suggest the dysphagia is secondary to delayed initiation of swallow, decreased hyolaryngeal excursion, and decreased pharyngeal propulsion. Poor PES opening is a common feature in this disorder, thought to be related to poor hyolaryngeal elevation[69] Abnormalities in manometry are found even in patients without complaints of dysphagia, suggesting the utility of this modality in detecting an early subclinical course.[70] Biopsy of the cricopharyngeus muscle confirms histologic diagnosis.

Inflammatory Myopathies

The inflammatory myopathies are a group of disorders involving skeletal muscle and connective tissue. They include polymyositis, dermatomyositis, and the previously mentioned inclusion body myositis. Prevalence of dysphagia in the group of disorders is estimated at 8%, with 21% of patients exhibiting dysphagia as the presenting symptom. Patients most commonly describe food sticking, particularly solids, such as steak and dry foods, as well as cough with swallowing. Videofluoroscopy reveals pharyngeal stasis and decreased tongue base retraction in the majority of patients, with decreased PES opening and laryngeal elevation in about half of the patients.[71] Electromyographic studies are often normal, without evidence of myopathy. Biopsy confirms the diagnosis with histopathological correlates and absence of inclusion bodies.[72]

Cricopharyngeal Dysfunction

Cricopharyngeal dysfunction results in poor opening of the PES. Opening of the PES involves multiple factors, including cricopharyngeal compliance, hyolaryngeal elevation, pharyngeal driving forces, neurally mediated cricopharyngeal relaxation, and proper coordination of the muscle functions. Symptoms include difficulties with solid-food propulsion requiring multiple liquid swallows to propel the bolus. Aspiration may result from bolus retention above the PES. This is frequently present in myopathic diseases, such as oculopharyngeal muscular dystrophy, inclusion body myositis, polymyositis, and inflammatory myopathy. Diagnostic workup most commonly includes videofluoroscopy, though findings of pharyngeal stasis, incomplete or uncoordinated PES opening, and horizontal, posteriorly based "cricopharyngeal bar" or prominence are nonspecific. Indeed, the presence of a cricopharyngeal bar does not readily correlate with dysphagia symptoms and is seen in approximately 30% of nondysphagic patients. Additionally, only a small percentage of manometrically confirmed failure of PES relaxation will have a cricopharyngeal bar on radiographic examination.[51]

4.3.4 Psychogenic Causes

Psychogenic swallowing disorders, sometimes referred to as phagophobia, involve a functional dysphagia, often secondary to an apprehension of swallowing. Although classically attributed to eating disorders, the entity may be more akin to a somatization disorder, with marked anxiety and psychological distress surrounding eating.[73] Patients will invariably have normal physical examination, videofluoroscopy, and barium esophagram findings.[74] Surface electromyography (EMG) has been proposed as a screening mechanism for this disorder; however, this is not widely in use clinically. Prominent accessory neck muscle tension during observed swallow is a notable feature.[75]

4.4 Diagnostic Testing

4.4.1 Videofluoroscopy

Videofluoroscopy is the mainstay of workup of oropharyngeal dysphagia, and in many cases it is the first and only diagnostic study of choice. It is also called *modified barium swallow*, which distinguishes this test from a standard barium esophagram with small quantities of barium ingested through varying consistencies and primary oropharyngeal fluoroscopy. The test examines oral transit time, pharyngeal transit time, presence of residue in the pharyngeal recesses or postcricoid area, hyolaryngeal excursion, presence of penetration, presence and timing of aspiration, timing and degree of PES opening, cervical esophageal peristalsis, and presence of structural lesions. An examiner also assesses the change of the aforementioned parameters with varying consistencies. One of the most helpful aspects of the study is the ability to assess whether swallowing maneuvers, such as head tilt or supraglottic swallow, will ameliorate the dysphagia.

Indications for videofluoroscopy include a suspected oropharyngeal dysphagia, especially aspiration, abnormal clinical assessment of swallowing, and suspected PES dysfunction. It is considered the gold standard for detecting aspiration and is more sensitive than flexible endoscopic evaluation of swallowing.[76] Videofluoroscopy is less sensitive in estimating severity of pharyngeal residue, a risk factor for aspiration.[77] Additionally, videofluoroscopy with attention to esophageal pathology is limited to a sensitivity of approximately 60%.[78]

4.4.2 Barium Swallow

A standard barium swallow differs from videofluoroscopy in that it uses videoradiography in conjunction with large boluses (200–300 mL) of barium and often includes a supine posture. The resulting esophageal distension allows detection of structural abnormalities, esophageal dysmotility, and gastroesophageal reflux.

There are several indications for a standard barium swallow. It should be performed for suspected anatomical or structural abnormalities of the pharynx and esophagus, such as webs, diverticula, strictures, and Schatzki rings. It is standard as an initial test for suspected esophageal carcinoma and is considered equivalent to esophagoscopy, though inferior to positron emission tomography with 2-deoxy-2-[fluorine-18]fluoro-D-glucose integrated with computed tomography (^{18}F-FDG PET/CT) for detecting synchronous esophageal neoplasms in newly diagnosed head and neck cancer.[79,80] It may be used to screen for esophageal dysmotility and lower esophageal sphincter abnormalities, though high-resolution manometry gives more physiologic information on esophageal contractile properties and bolus transport and more accurately predicts surgical outcomes.[81] Standard barium swallow does not definitively diagnose laryngopharyngeal reflux or gastroesophageal reflux; a 24-hour pH probe/impedance study measures acid and nonacid reflux and is considered the gold standard over a standard esophagram.[82,83] Additionally, mucosal abnormalities, such as esophagitis, are more accurately diagnosed with standard endoscopy and biopsy.

4.4.3 Flexible Endoscopic Evaluation of Swallowing

Flexible endoscopic evaluation of swallowing (FEES) uses flexible laryngoscopy to directly visualize the laryngopharynx before and after the pharyngeal phase of swallowing. Boluses of varying consistencies are dyed with food coloring for assisted visualization. Indications are similar to that for videofluoroscopy. The strength of FEES lies in the ability to directly assess glottic competence, toleration of own secretions/saliva, and presence of vallecular/pharyngeal stasis. If vocal fold immobility or tongue base/pharyngeal constrictor weakness is considered, FEES may be an appropriate examination. The principal drawbacks include inability to assess swallow during pharyngeal contraction, decreased direct visualization of aspiration, and inability to visualize PES function. There is some evidence that FEES may be more sensitive for pharyngeal stasis and may overestimate aspiration.[76,77] If aspiration during the swallow or PES dysfunction is suspected, FEES should be deferred in favor of videofluoroscopy. Its drawbacks limit the clinical utility of FEES, though when videofluoroscopy is not readily available, it is a reasonable diagnostic modality.

4.4.4 Flexible Endoscopic Evaluation of Swallowing with Sensory Testing

Flexible endoscopic evaluation of swallowing with sensory testing (FEEST) combines standard FEES with sensory testing of the laryngopharynx. The test uses a channeled flexible laryngoscope to deliver pulsed air and to visualize the elicited laryngeal adductor reflex. Unilateral or bilateral sensory deficits are described as severe, moderate, or mild, based on the pressure of air (delivered from 0 to 10 mm Hg) required to elicit the reflex.[84] Flexible endoscopic evaluation of swallowing with sensory testing is purported to prognosticate penetration and aspiration by directly observing the brainstem-mediated airway-protection response. The procedure has been shown to be safe and carries limited risk for laryngospasm or airway compromise.[85] Clinically, FEEST may be particularly useful for workup of dysphagia associated with chronic neurologic disease, where sensory deficits figure prominently.[85] Though normative data exist, some question the physiologic validity and applicability of FEEST exams. This, combined with the need for specialized equipment and training, has limited the clinical use of FEEST over videofluoroscopy.

4.4.5 Transnasal Esophagoscopy

Recent advances in distal charge-coupled device imaging have established transnasal esophagoscopy (TNE) as a viable modality for the evaluation of dysphagia. The procedure is performed in the office with only topical anesthetic of the nasal cavity and oropharynx. Insufflation or voluntary swallow allows examination of the esophageal lumen; the former combined with retroflexion of the scope in the stomach allows for complete evaluation of the gastroesophageal junction. Working channels provide ports for biopsy. A formal position statement from the American Bronchoesophagological Association lists the diagnostic indications for TNE as follows: suspected structural cause of dysphagia, esophageal screening in patients with longstanding LPR or GERD, evaluation of abnormalities seen on barium swallow, surveillance and biopsy for Barrett esophagus, and screening for synchronous primary neoplasms of the esophagus in newly diagnosed head and neck cancer (▶ Fig. 4.4).[86] Abnormal findings may occur in up to 50% of patients; those most frequently encountered are esophagitis, Barrett esophagus, and hiatal hernia.[87,88] The procedure is safe, carries minimal risk for complications, and requires no general anesthesia or conscious sedation, making it an ideal screening tool.[87,88] Functional evaluation of esophageal swallow, akin to FEES examination, has been reported as comparable to manometry and fluoroscopy and additionally may be more sensitive for mucosal abnormalities. At this time, TNE as an evaluation of functional esophageal dysphagia remains experimental.[89] Additionally, dysphagia stemming from eosinophilic esophagitis (EoE) may be clinically indistinguishable from GERD; TNE with biopsy of the midesophagus may definitively confirm this.[90]

4.4.6 High-Resolution Manometry

High-resolution manometry (HRM) utilizes closely spaced, circumferential pressure transducers and computer algorithm analysis to generate an intraluminal pressure topograph of esophageal position versus time during a swallow. This has been a significant advancement over traditional manometry (▶ Fig. 4.5). It provides physiologic information of PES resting, relaxation, and closure pressures, as well as esophageal body contraction velocity, amplitude and integrity, dynamics, and intrabolus pressures. It is useful for assessing lower esophageal sphincter (LES) function as well.[91] It is considered the gold standard for diagnosis of nonobstructive esophageal motility disorders. High-resolution manometry has improved classification of esophageal peristalsis, gastroesophageal junction (GEJ) abnormalities (such as hiatal hernia), and LES relaxation: data from HRM studies has established a new classification for achalasia that accurately predicts outcome of LES myotomy.[92] It also aids in diagnosis of surgical failures with Nissen fundoplication for GERD.[93] The utility of HRM is increasingly recognized: Data suggest it is more sensitive than videofluoroscopy for diagnosis

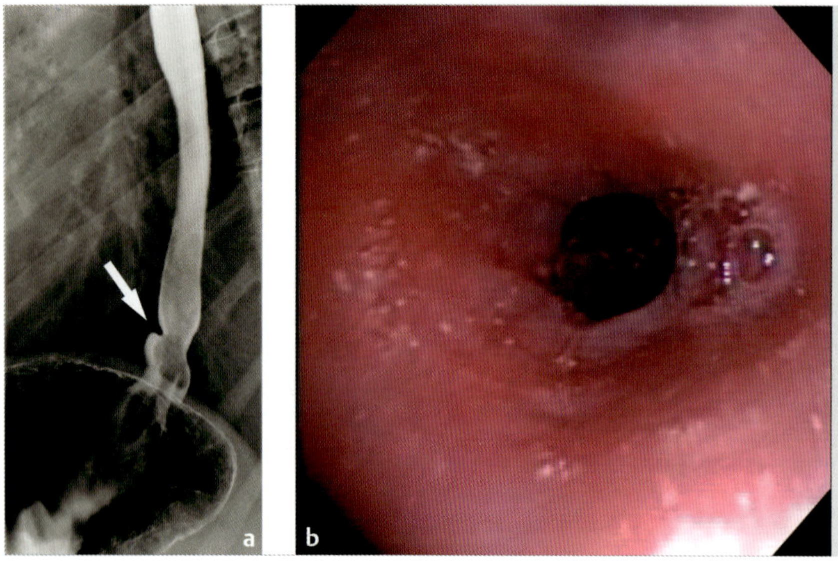

Fig. 4.4 Radiologic and endoscopic imaging of Schatzki ring. (**a**) Barium esophagram showing distal narrowing (*white arrow*) just above the gastroesophageal junction. (**b**) In-office transnasal esophagoscopy confirming intraluminal narrowing without mucosal lesions.

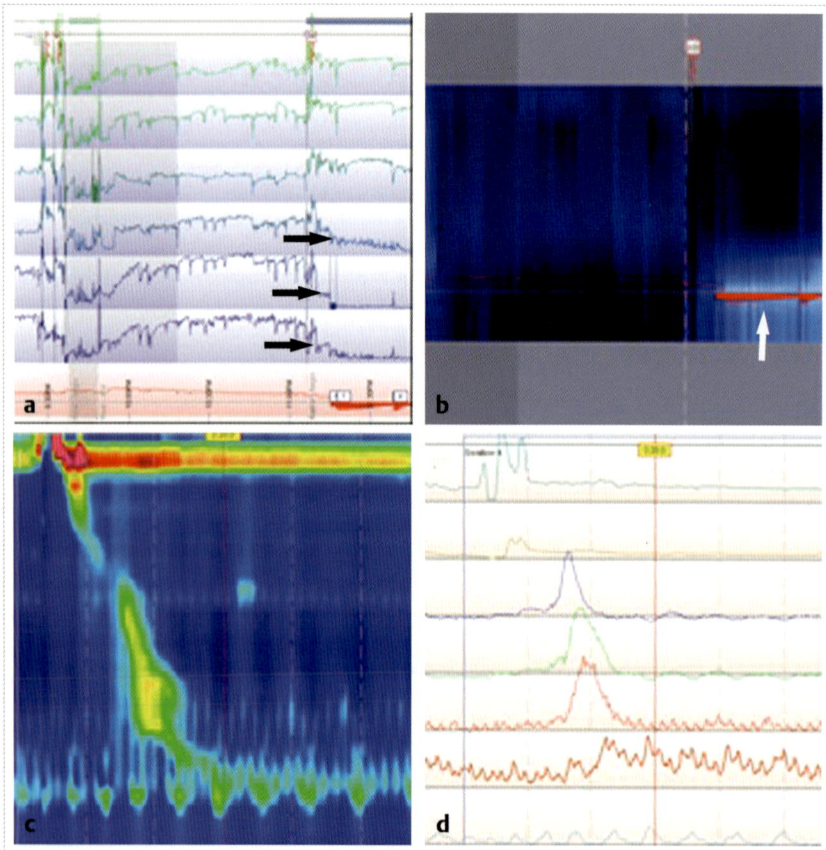

Fig. 4.5 pH/Impedence and manometric evaluation of the esophagus. (**a**) Impedence study showing retrograde propulsion of bolus (*black arrows*) to midesophagus. (**b**) pH confirming acid reflux with pH event below 4 (*arrow*). (**c**) Normal high-resolution manometry compared to (**d**) conventional manometry.

of PES dysfunction in patients with globus sensation.[94,95] In high-volume centers, it is considered the gold standard for diagnosis of PES dysfunction, though it is not widely utilized as yet. At this time, HRM of the hypopharynx, though primarily investigational, is considered promising for diagnosis of pharyngeal weakness.[96,97] Indeed, the ability to glean quantifiable physiologic information that may portend prognosis for intervention has fueled enthusiasm.

4.4.7 Multichannel Intraluminal Impedance and pH Testing

Intraluminal impedance-pH (MII-pH) testing is a more recently developed technology that improves on traditional pH testing by detecting nonacid and acid reflux, distinguishing anterograde from retrograde transport, and detecting gas, liquid, or mixed refluxate.

Catheters with electrodes sense resistance in electrical activity in concert with adjacently placed pH probes, which detect acidic reflux. Adding impedance measurements to the standard 24-hour pH probe dramatically increases sensitivity to nonacid/weakly acidic reflux, and also increases symptom correlation.[98,99] Though the pathophysiologic significance of nonacid reflux is not established, preliminary evidence points to damaging and potentially carcinogenic effect of pepsin on the laryngeal structures.[100,101] A recent modification of impedance testing involves placing probes in the hypopharynx; preliminary data suggest that one episode of laryngopharyngeal reflux in a 24-hour period is abnormal.[102] Indications for MII-pH testing include persistent GERD or LPR symptoms despite acid suppression therapy and preoperative documentation prior to surgical intervention for reflux. Currently, it is considered the gold standard for diagnosis of GERD or LPR.

4.4.8 Cricopharyngeal Electromyography

Electromyography is a potentially useful modality for suspected cricopharyngeal dysfunction. Classically, the cricopharyngeus produces tonic firing on EMG examination, with bursts preceding and following the transient cessation of activity during the swallow. Cricopharyngeal electromyography (CP-EMG) can differentiate peripheral neuropathy (polyphasic waveforms, increased amplitude, and decreased recruitment), myopathy (decreased amplitudes and shorter duration), and central causes of dysphagia (typically normal motor unit potential).[103] Lack of tonic signal cessation during the swallow corresponds to CP dysfunction. However, abnormalities in hyolaryngeal elevation may be more predictive of abnormal PES opening than CP-EMG alone, which may predict response to CP botox treatment.[104] Cricopharyngeal electromyography may be useful for diagnosis of CP dysfunction in relation to recurrent/superior laryngeal nerve paresis, postviral vagal neuropathy, central neurologic disorders, or myopathy.[103,104,105] Importantly, this may prompt treatment with botox or myotomy in the case of vagal paresis, or help guide surgical expectations in the case of myopathy.

4.5 Conclusion

Dysphagia is a complex entity with symptoms that may be induced by a wide variety of pathophysiologic processes. Initial history and physical examination specific to dysphagia may or not be diagnostic, but will often guide further workup. As the range of diagnostic testing increases, results provided by each yield functional, structural, and/or physiologic information of varying clinical significance. The onus is on the clinician to select a workup appropriate to the suspected diagnosis and location of abnormal swallow, as each test has specific diagnostic abilities. Detailed knowledge of disorders and diagnostic testing available facilitates diagnosis, prevents ordering of superfluous and sometimes expensive testing, and, most importantly, guides treatment planning.

References

[1] Chen AY, Frankowski R, Bishop-Leone J et al. The development and validation of a dysphagia-specific quality-of-life questionnaire for patients with head and neck cancer: the M. D. Anderson Dysphagia Inventory. Arch Otolaryngol Head Neck Surg 2001; 127: 870–876

[2] McHorney CA, Robbins J, Lomax K et al. The SWAL-QOL and SWAL-CARE outcomes tool for oropharyngeal dysphagia in adults: III. Documentation of reliability and validity. Dysphagia 2002; 17: 97–114

[3] Belafsky PC, Mouadeb DA, Rees CJ et al. Validity and reliability of the Eating Assessment Tool (EAT-10). Ann Otol Rhinol Laryngol 2008; 117: 919–924

[4] Belafsky PC, Postma GN, Koufman JA. Validity and reliability of the Reflux Symptom Index (RSI). J Voice 2002; 16: 274–277

[5] Roeder BE, Murray JA, Dierkhising RA. Patient localization of esophageal dysphagia. Dig Dis Sci 2004; 49: 697–701

[6] Spieker MR. Evaluating dysphagia. Am Fam Physician 2000; 61: 3639–3648

[7] Malandraki GA, Sutton BP, Perlman AL, Karampinos DC, Conway C. Neural activation of swallowing and swallowing-related tasks in healthy young adults: an attempt to separate the components of deglutition. Hum Brain Mapp 2009; 30: 3209–3226

[8] Hirota N, Konaka K, Ono T et al. Reduced tongue pressure against the hard palate on the paralyzed side during swallowing predicts dysphagia in patients with acute stroke. Stroke 2010; 41: 2982–2984

[9] Kim IS, Han TR. Influence of mastication and salivation on swallowing in stroke patients. Arch Phys Med Rehabil 2005; 86: 1986–1990

[10] Briani C, Marcon M, Ermani M et al. Radiological evidence of subclinical dysphagia in motor neuron disease. J Neurol 1998; 245: 211–216

[11] Willig TN, Paulus J, Lacau Saint Guily J, Béon C, Navarro J. Swallowing problems in neuromuscular disorders. Arch Phys Med Rehabil 1994; 75: 1175–1181

[12] Kitagawa J, Shingai T, Takahashi Y, Yamada Y. Pharyngeal branch of the glossopharyngeal nerve plays a major role in reflex swallowing from the pharynx. Am J Physiol Regul Integr Comp Physiol 2002; 282: R1324–R1327

[13] Jafari S, Prince RA, Kim DY, Paydarfar D. Sensory regulation of swallowing and airway protection: a role for the internal superior laryngeal nerve in humans. J Physiol 2003; 550: 287–304

[14] Steele CM, Miller AJ. Sensory input pathways and mechanisms in swallowing: a review. Dysphagia 2010; 25: 323–333

[15] Verin E, Michou E, Leroi AM, Hamdy S, Marie JP. "Virtual" lesioning of the human oropharyngeal motor cortex: a videofluoroscopic study. Arch Phys Med Rehabil 2012; 93: 1987–1990[epub ahead of print]

[16] Saitoh E, Shibata S, Matsuo K, Baba M, Fujii W, Palmer JB. Chewing and food consistency: effects on bolus transport and swallow initiation. Dysphagia 2007; 22: 100–107

[17] Robbins J, Hamilton JW, Lof GL, Kempster GB. Oropharyngeal swallowing in normal adults of different ages. Gastroenterology 1992; 103: 823–829

[18] Kang SH, Kim DK, Seo KM, Seo JH. Usefulness of videofluoroscopic swallow study with mixed consistency food for patients with stroke or other brain injuries. J Korean Med Sci 2011; 26: 425–430

[19] Logemann JA, Rademaker AW, Pauloski BR et al. Site of disease and treatment protocol as correlates of swallowing function in patients with head and neck cancer treated with chemoradiation. Head Neck 2006; 28: 64–73

[20] Seidler TO, Pèrez Alvarez JC, Wonneberger K, Hacki T. Dysphagia caused by ventral osteophytes of the cervical spine: clinical and radiographic findings. Eur Arch Otorhinolaryngol 2009; 266: 285–291

[21] Périé S, Coiffier L, Laccourreye L, Hazebroucq V, Chaussade S, St Guily JL. Swallowing disorders in paralysis of the lower cranial nerves: a functional analysis. Ann Otol Rhinol Laryngol 1999; 108: 606–611

[22] Woodson GE. Configuration of the glottis in laryngeal paralysis. I: Clinical study. Laryngoscope 1993; 103: 1227–1234

[23] Woodson GE. Configuration of the glottis in laryngeal paralysis. II: Animal experiments. Laryngoscope 1993; 103: 1235–1241

[24] Leder SB, Suiter DM. Effect of nasogastric tubes on incidence of aspiration. Arch Phys Med Rehabil 2008; 89: 648–651

[25] Ramsey DJ, Smithard DG, Kalra L. Early assessments of dysphagia and aspiration risk in acute stroke patients. Stroke 2003; 34: 1252–1257

[26] Mann G, Hankey GJ. Initial clinical and demographic predictors of swallowing impairment following acute stroke. Dysphagia 2001; 16: 208–215

[27] Leder SB, Espinosa JF. Aspiration risk after acute stroke: comparison of clinical examination and fiberoptic endoscopic evaluation of swallowing. Dysphagia 2002; 17: 214–218

[28] Borr C, Hielscher-Fastabend M, Lücking A. Reliability and validity of cervical auscultation. Dysphagia 2007; 22: 225–234
[29] Lim SH, Lieu PK, Phua SY et al. Accuracy of bedside clinical methods compared with fiberoptic endoscopic examination of swallowing (FEES) in determining the risk of aspiration in acute stroke patients. Dysphagia 2001; 16: 1–6
[30] Terk AR, Leder SB, Burrell MI. Hyoid bone and laryngeal movement dependent upon presence of a tracheotomy tube. Dysphagia 2007; 22: 89–93
[31] Leder SB, Joe JK, Ross DA, Coelho DH, Mendes J. Presence of a tracheotomy tube and aspiration status in early, postsurgical head and neck cancer patients. Head Neck 2005; 27: 757–761
[32] Kang JY, Choi KH, Yun GJ, Kim MY, Ryu JS. Does removal of tracheostomy affect dysphagia? A kinematic analysis. Dysphagia 2012; 27: 498–503
[33] Leder SB, Ross DA. Incidence of vocal fold immobility in patients with dysphagia. Dysphagia 2005; 20: 163–167, discussion 168–169
[34] Iwanaga Y, Maeyama T, Umezaki T, Shin T. Intracordal injection increases glottic closing force in recurrent laryngeal nerve paralysis. Otolaryngol Head Neck Surg 1992; 107: 451–456
[35] Sasaki CT, Hundal JS, Eberhardt PR, Riley JT, Ross DA. Glottic closing force: impact of thyroplasty on vocal cord paralysis in a pig model. Ann Otol Rhinol Laryngol 2004; 113: 93–96
[36] Mallur PS, Morrison MP, Postma GN, Amin MR, Rosen CA. Safety and efficacy of carboxymethylcellulose in the treatment of glottic insufficiency. Laryngoscope 2012; 122: 322–326
[37] Song PC, Sung CK, Franco RA. Voice outcomes after endoscopic injection laryngoplasty with hyaluronic acid stabilized gel. Laryngoscope 2010; 120 Suppl 4: S199
[38] Veenker EA, Andersen PE, Cohen JI. Cricopharyngeal spasm and Zenker's diverticulum. Head Neck 2003; 25: 681–694
[39] Ferreira LE, Simmons DT, Baron TH. Zenker's diverticula: pathophysiology, clinical presentation, and flexible endoscopic management. Dis Esophagus 2008; 21: 1–8
[40] Morales-Divo C, Jecker P, Lippert B, Mann WJ. [Extraesophageal reflux in patients suffering from Zenker's diverticulum] HNO 2007; 55: 546–550
[41] Belafsky PC, Rees CJ, Allen J, Leonard RJ. Pharyngeal dilation in cricopharyngeus muscle dysfunction and Zenker diverticulum. Laryngoscope 2010; 120: 889–894
[42] Porcaro-Salles JM, Arantes Soares JM, Sousa AA, Meyer G, Sá Santos MH. Lateral pharyngeal diverticulum: a report of 3 cases. Ear Nose Throat J 2011; 90: 489–492
[43] Carlson ML, Archibald DJ, Graner DE, Kasperbauer JL. Surgical management of dysphagia and airway obstruction in patients with prominent ventral cervical osteophytes. Dysphagia 2011; 26: 34–40
[44] Ozgursoy OB, Salassa JR, Reimer R, Wharen RE, Deen HG. Anterior cervical osteophyte dysphagia: manofluorographic and functional outcomes after surgery. Head Neck 2010; 32: 588–593
[45] Iseli TA, Kulbersh BD, Iseli CE, Carroll WR, Rosenthal EL, Magnuson JS. Functional outcomes after transoral robotic surgery for head and neck cancer. Otolaryngol Head Neck Surg 2009; 141: 166–171
[46] Sinclair CF, McColloch NL, Carroll WR, Rosenthal EL, Desmond RA, Magnuson JS. Patient-perceived and objective functional outcomes following transoral robotic surgery for early oropharyngeal carcinoma. Arch Otolaryngol Head Neck Surg 2011; 137: 1112–1116
[47] Agarwal J, Palwe V, Dutta D et al. Objective assessment of swallowing function after definitive concurrent (chemo)radiotherapy in patients with head and neck cancer. Dysphagia 2011; 26: 399–406
[48] Bleier BS, Levine MS, Mick R et al. Dysphagia after chemoradiation: analysis by modified barium swallow. Ann Otol Rhinol Laryngol 2007; 116: 837–841
[49] Domer A, Leonard R, Belafsky PC. The association between unilateral vocal fold immobility and swallowing function. Paper presented at: International Association for Phonomicrosurgeons; November 2–5, 2011; San Francisco, CA
[50] Leonard R, Belafsky PC, Rees CJ. Relationship between fluoroscopic and manometric measures of pharyngeal constriction: the pharyngeal constriction ratio. Ann Otol Rhinol Laryngol 2006; 115: 897–901
[51] Leonard R, Rees CJ, Belafsky P, Allen J. Fluoroscopic surrogate for pharyngeal strength: the pharyngeal constriction ratio (PCR). Dysphagia 2011; 26: 13–17
[52] Ramsey DJ, Smithard DG, Kalra L. Early assessments of dysphagia and aspiration risk in acute stroke patients. Stroke 2003; 34: 1252–1257
[53] Falsetti P, Acciai C, Palilla R et al. Oropharyngeal dysphagia after stroke: incidence, diagnosis, and clinical predictors in patients admitted to a neurorehabilitation unit. J Stroke Cerebrovasc Dis 2009; 18: 329–335
[54] Power ML, Hamdy S, Goulermas JY, Tyrrell PJ, Turnbull I, Thompson DG. Predicting aspiration after hemispheric stroke from timing measures of oropharyngeal bolus flow and laryngeal closure. Dysphagia 2009; 24: 257–264
[55] Finlayson O, Kapral M, Hall R, Asllani E, Selchen D, Saposnik G Canadian Stroke NetworkStroke Outcome Research Canada (SORCan) Working Group. Risk factors, inpatient care, and outcomes of pneumonia after ischemic stroke. Neurology 2011; 77: 1338–1345
[56] Nagaya M, Kachi T, Yamada T, Igata A. Videofluorographic study of swallowing in Parkinson's disease. Dysphagia 1998; 13: 95–100
[57] Kalf JG, de Swart BJ, Bloem BR, Munneke M. Prevalence of oropharyngeal dysphagia in Parkinson's disease: a meta-analysis. Parkinsonism Relat Disord 2012; 18: 311–315
[58] Kawai S, Tsukuda M, Mochimatsu I et al. A study of the early stage of dysphagia in amyotrophic lateral sclerosis. Dysphagia 2003; 18: 1–8
[59] Higo R, Tayama N, Nito T. Longitudinal analysis of progression of dysphagia in amyotrophic lateral sclerosis. Auris Nasus Larynx 2004; 31: 247–254
[60] Solazzo A, Del Vecchio L, Reginelli A et al. Search for compensation postures with videofluoromanometric investigation in dysphagic patients affected by amyotrophic lateral sclerosis. Radiol Med (Torino) 2011; 116: 1083–1094
[61] Poorjavad M, Derakhshandeh F, Etemadifar M, Soleymani B, Minagar A, Maghzi AH. Oropharyngeal dysphagia in multiple sclerosis. Mult Scler 2010; 16: 362–365
[62] Abraham SS, Yun PT. Laryngopharyngeal dysmotility in multiple sclerosis. Dysphagia 2002; 17: 69–74
[63] Higo R, Nito T, Tayama N. Videofluoroscopic assessment of swallowing function in patients with myasthenia gravis. J Neurol Sci 2005; 231: 45–48
[64] Palmer PM, Neel AT, Sprouls G, Morrison L. Swallow characteristics in patients with oculopharyngeal muscular dystrophy. J Speech Lang Hear Res 2010; 53: 1567–1578
[65] Périé S, Eymard B, Laccourreye L, Chaussade S, Fardeau M, Lacau St Guily J. Dysphagia in oculopharyngeal muscular dystrophy: a series of 22 French cases. Neuromuscul Disord 1997; 7 Suppl 1: S96–S99
[66] Coiffier L, Périé S, Laforêt P, Eymard B, St Guily JL. Long-term results of cricopharyngeal myotomy in oculopharyngeal muscular dystrophy. Otolaryngol Head Neck Surg 2006; 135: 218–222
[67] Castell JA, Castell DO, Duranceau CA, Topart P. Manometric characteristics of the pharynx, upper esophageal sphincter, esophagus, and lower esophageal sphincter in patients with oculopharyngeal muscular dystrophy. Dysphagia 1995; 10: 22–26
[68] Greenberg SA. Inclusion body myositis. Curr Opin Rheumatol 2011; 23: 574–578
[69] Langdon PC, Mulcahy K, Shepherd KL, Low VH, Mastaglia FL. Pharyngeal dysphagia in inflammatory muscle diseases resulting from impaired suprahyoid musculature. Dysphagia 2012; 27: 408–417
[70] Murata KY, Kouda K, Tajima F, Kondo T. A dysphagia study in patients with sporadic inclusion body myositis (s-IBM). Neurol Sci 2012; 33: 765–770
[71] Oh TH, Brumfield KA, Hoskin TL, Stolp KA, Murray JA, Bassford JR. Dysphagia in inflammatory myopathy: clinical characteristics, treatment strategies, and outcome in 62 patients. Mayo Clin Proc 2007; 82: 441–447
[72] Shapiro J, Martin S, DeGirolami U, Goyal R. Inflammatory myopathy causing pharyngeal dysphagia: a new entity. Ann Otol Rhinol Laryngol 1996; 105: 331–335
[73] Barofsky I, Fontaine KR. Do psychogenic dysphagia patients have an eating disorder? Dysphagia 1998; 13: 24–27
[74] Shapiro J, Franko DL, Gagne A. Phagophobia: a form of psychogenic dysphagia. A new entity. Ann Otol Rhinol Laryngol 1997; 106: 286–290
[75] Vaiman M, Shoval G, Gavriel H. The electrodiagnostic examination of psychogenic swallowing disorders. Eur Arch Otorhinolaryngol 2008; 265: 663–668
[76] Kelly AM, Drinnan MJ, Leslie P. Assessing penetration and aspiration: how do videofluoroscopy and fiberoptic endoscopic evaluation of swallowing compare? Laryngoscope 2007; 117: 1723–1727
[77] Kelly AM, Leslie P, Beale T, Payten C, Drinnan MJ. Fibreoptic endoscopic evaluation of swallowing and videofluoroscopy: does examination type influence perception of pharyngeal residue severity? Clin Otolaryngol 2006; 31: 425–432
[78] Allen JE, White C, Leonard R, Belafsky PC. Comparison of esophageal screen findings on videofluoroscopy with full esophagram results. Head Neck 2012; 34: 264–269
[79] Parker JT, Hill JH. Panendoscopy in screening for synchronous primary malignancies. Laryngoscope 1988; 98: 147–149
[80] Haerle SK, Strobel K, Hany TF, Sidler D, Stoeckli SJ. (18)F-FDG-PET/CT versus panendoscopy for the detection of synchronous second primary tumors in

patients with head and neck squamous cell carcinoma. Head Neck 2010; 32: 319–325

[81] Pandolfino JE, Sifrim D. Evaluation of esophageal contractile propagation using esophageal pressure topography. Neurogastroenterol Motil 2012; 24 Suppl 1: 20–26

[82] Kawamura O, Aslam M, Rittmann T, Hofmann C, Shaker R. Physical and pH properties of gastroesophagopharyngeal refluxate: a 24-hour simultaneous ambulatory impedance and pH monitoring study. Am J Gastroenterol 2004; 99: 1000–1010

[83] Kawamura O, Bajaj S, Aslam M, Hofmann C, Rittmann T, Shaker R. Impedance signature of pharyngeal gaseous reflux. Eur J Gastroenterol Hepatol 2007; 19: 65–71

[84] Aviv JE, Kim T, Sacco RL et al. FEESST: a new bedside endoscopic test of the motor and sensory components of swallowing. Ann Otol Rhinol Laryngol 1998; 107: 378–387

[85] Aviv JE, Murry T, Zschommler A, Cohen M, Gartner C. Flexible endoscopic evaluation of swallowing with sensory testing: patient characteristics and analysis of safety in 1,340 consecutive examinations. Ann Otol Rhinol Laryngol 2005; 114: 173–176

[86] Amin MR, Postma GN, Setzen M, Koufman JA. Transnasal esophagoscopy: a position statement from the American Bronchoesophagological Association (ABEA). Otolaryngol Head Neck Surg 2008; 138: 411–414

[87] Postma GN, Cohen JT, Belafsky PC et al. Transnasal esophagoscopy: revisited (over 700 consecutive cases). Laryngoscope 2005; 115: 321–323

[88] Peery AF, Hoppo T, Garman KS et al. Barrett's Esophagus Risk Consortium. Feasibility, safety, acceptability, and yield of office-based, screening transnasal esophagoscopy (with video). Gastrointest Endosc 2012; 75: 945–953, e2

[89] Belafsky PC, Rees CJ. Functional oesophagoscopy: endoscopic evaluation of the oesophageal phase of deglutition. J Laryngol Otol 2009; 123: 1031–1034

[90] Karkos PD, Srivastava R, Kaptanis S, Vaughan C. Eosinophilic esophagitis for the otolaryngologist. Int J Otolaryngol 2012; 2012: 181402

[91] Rice TW, Shay SS. A primer of high-resolution esophageal manometry. Semin Thorac Cardiovasc Surg 2011; 23: 181–190

[92] Pandolfino JE, Kwiatek MA, Nealis T, Bulsiewicz W, Post J, Kahrilas PJ. Achalasia: a new clinically relevant classification by high-resolution manometry. Gastroenterology 2008; 135: 1526–1533

[93] Tatum RP, Soares RV, Figueredo E, Oelschlager BK, Pellegrini CA. High-resolution manometry in evaluation of factors responsible for fundoplication failure. J Am Coll Surg 2010; 210: 611–617, 617–619

[94] Kwiatek MA, Mirza F, Kahrilas PJ, Pandolfino JE. Hyperdynamic upper esophageal sphincter pressure: a manometric observation in patients reporting globus sensation. Am J Gastroenterol 2009; 104: 289–298

[95] Ghosh SK, Pandolfino JE, Zhang Q, Jarosz A, Kahrilas PJ. Deglutitive upper esophageal sphincter relaxation: a study of 75 volunteer subjects using solid-state high-resolution manometry. Am J Physiol Gastrointest Liver Physiol 2006; 291: G525–G531

[96] Mielens JD, Hoffman MR, Ciucci MR, Jiang JJ, McCulloch TM. Automated analysis of pharyngeal pressure data obtained with high-resolution manometry. Dysphagia 2011; 26: 3–12

[97] Takasaki K, Umeki H, Enatsu K et al. Investigation of pharyngeal swallowing function using high-resolution manometry. Laryngoscope 2008; 118: 1729–1732

[98] Hila A, Agrawal A, Castell DO. Combined multichannel intraluminal impedance and pH esophageal testing compared to pH alone for diagnosing both acid and weakly acidic gastroesophageal reflux. Clin Gastroenterol Hepatol 2007; 5: 172–177

[99] Bredenoord AJ, Weusten BL, Timmer R, Conchillo JM, Smout AJ. Addition of esophageal impedance monitoring to pH monitoring increases the yield of symptom association analysis in patients off PPI therapy. Am J Gastroenterol 2006; 101: 453–459

[100] Bulmer DM, Ali MS, Brownlee IA, Dettmar PW, Pearson JP. Laryngeal mucosa: its susceptibility to damage by acid and pepsin. Laryngoscope 2010; 120: 777–782

[101] Johnston N, Yan JC, Hoekzema CR et al. Pepsin promotes proliferation of laryngeal and pharyngeal epithelial cells. Laryngoscope 2012; 122: 1317–1325

[102] Hoppo T, Sanz AF, Nason KS et al. How much pharyngeal exposure is "normal"? Normative data for laryngopharyngeal reflux events using hypopharyngeal multichannel intraluminal impedance (HMII). J Gastrointest Surg 2012; 16: 16–24, discussion 24–25

[103] Shemirani NL, Halum SL, Merati AL, Toohill RJ, Jaradeh S. Cricopharyngeal electromyography: patterns of injury based on etiology. Otolaryngol Head Neck Surg 2007; 137: 792–797

[104] Alfonsi E, Merlo IM, Ponzio M et al. An electrophysiological approach to the diagnosis of neurogenic dysphagia: implications for botulinum toxin treatment. J Neurol Neurosurg Psychiatry 2010; 81: 54–60

[105] Halum SL, Shemirani NL, Merati AL, Jaradeh S, Toohill RJ. Electromyography findings of the cricopharyngeus in association with ipsilateral pharyngeal and laryngeal muscles. Ann Otol Rhinol Laryngol 2006; 115: 312–316

5 Laryngeal Inflammation

Craig Berzofsky and Michael Jay Pitman

Laryngitis is a common term that is often misused by patients and physicians to describe symptoms like hoarseness, throat discomfort, or pain in the throat area. In fact, laryngitis refers only to inflammation of the larynx, which may be caused by a wide spectrum of disorders. Distinguishing the etiology in patients who often have nonspecific throat complaints and nonspecific physical exam findings can be extremely challenging. This chapter explores the causes of laryngitis.

5.1 History and Physical

Laryngitis due to myriad etiologies manifests a similar appearance on laryngoscopy. Therefore, the patient history is vital to obtaining the correct diagnosis and administration of an effective treatment. The most common presenting complaint in patients with laryngeal inflammation is dysphonia. Dysphonia has many different manifestations. The general term may indicate a raspy voice or it can convey vocal breaks, decreased projection, a narrowed range, vocal fatigue or strain, a weak breathy voice, or even aphonia. Whatever the voice quality, patients usually complain of persistent hoarseness that doesn't resolve spontaneously.

Depending on the severity of the inflammation and the edema present, patients may complain of dyspnea. Evaluation for airway compromise is imperative. In patients with respiratory symptoms, differing between laryngeal and pulmonary disease can be challenging. ▶ Table 5.1 provides a comparison between these two causes of dyspnea.

Patients may also complain of dysphagia or odynophagia, depending on how localized or diffuse the inflammation is. Finally, there are often associated laryngeal complaints, such as cough, throat clearing, increased phlegm, and pain. Discussion with the patient should include the time course of the complaints overall and in relation to each other.

Duration of symptoms and determination of sudden versus prolonged onset are essential in determining the ultimate etiology and treatment. Laryngitis is considered chronic if it persists longer than 3 weeks. The differential diagnosis and treatment may differ for acute and chronic laryngitis. The causes of acute laryngitis and chronic laryngitis that are listed below show the differential diagnosis. Qualification of the symptoms and their trajectory is of utmost importance. For example, are they waxing and waning, improving, stable, or progressive?

Table 5.1 History and physical examination findings differentiating laryngeal and pulmonary dyspnea

	Laryngeal	Pulmonary
History of present illness	Dysphonia Dysphagia Cough	Cough Hemoptysis Chest pain
Past medical history	Autoimmune	Autoimmune Chronic obstructive pulmonary disease Emphysema
Physical exam	Stridor	Wheezing Crackles

5.1.1 Causes of Acute Laryngitis

- Infectious
  - Bacterial
  - Viral
  - Fungal
- Noxious chemicals
- Angioedema
- Vocal trauma
- Allergy
- Irritants

5.1.2 Causes of Chronic Laryngitis

- Infectious
  - Bacterial
  - Viral
  - Mycobacterial
  - Spirochetal
  - Fungal
- Allergy
- Laryngopharyngeal reflux
- Smoking
- Radiation
- Vocal abuse
- Environmental irritants

The onset of symptoms is often accompanied by other factors that may aid in directing the physician to the appropriate diagnosis, for example, a preceding upper respiratory infection, unusual voice demands either in business or socially, a new medication, transfer to a new environment with aerosolized irritants or allergens, change in diet, or extreme background noise.

Beyond qualifying the symptoms specific to laryngitis, aspects of the review of systems should focus on the other regions of the head and neck. General upper respiratory tract complaints, including nasal and aural congestion, fever, increased nasal discharge, and sinus pain, can indicate an acute infectious etiology. Patients may also complain of chronic postnasal drip from allergic rhinitis or chronic sinusitis, which can cause laryngeal inflammation. Symptoms of laryngopharyngeal reflux should be elicited, such as globus pharyngeus, throat clearing, coughing, or increased glottal mucus. Additional symptoms of gastroesophageal reflux disease (GERD), including indigestion, heartburn, and sour taste, may support a reflux etiology for laryngeal inflammation. It should, however, be noted that less than 50% of patients with laryngopharyngeal reflux have heartburn.[1] In addition, many of the symptoms of laryngopharyngeal reflux are nonspecific and could arise from any laryngeal irritant.

Symptoms of dysarthria, paresthesias, arthritis, rashes, and night sweats may indicate neurologic, autoimmune, or immunosuppressive disease processes. It is not unusual for a systemic disease to present initially with dysphonia.[2,3,4,5,6]

A review of the patient's medical and surgical history should consider the effects of comorbidities and their treatments, which may also result in laryngitis either directly or indirectly. Autoimmune disorders, pulmonary disease, diabetes, hypertension, and chronic sinusitis are just a few. Head and neck cancer patients who have been treated with radiation therapy are at risk for developing chronic laryngitis.

Medications can impact the larynx. Side effects like dehydration and mucosal drying, which occur with diuretics and antihistamines, can lead to viscous, nonprotective mucus and laryngeal inflammation. Patients with asthma and chronic lung disease may use a corticosteroid inhaler, which will predispose them to fungal laryngitis and chronic vocal fold atrophy, both of which can result in dysphonia. An angiotensin-converting enzyme inhibitor can lead to a chronic dry cough with traumatic inflammation. It is important to note that although angiotensin receptor blockers were developed to decrease this side effect, they too can cause a cough.[7]

Social history will elucidate causes of laryngeal inflammation, particularly those associated with vocal demands and poor vocal hygiene. A patient's occupation and specific daily tasks may suggest vocal abuse, as well as indicate the severity of the impact of the laryngitis, provide a timeline as to how quickly the patient needs the laryngitis to resolve, and how aggressively it needs to be treated. Particular attention should be paid to the overall voice demand and if there are isolated times of extreme demand, such as business conferences or lecturing. The acoustic parameters and availability of a microphone in these situations should be elucidated. Finally, the amount of telephone use is critical. Of special concern is multitasking with holding the handset between the shoulder and ear, resulting in a strained posture, or using a speakerphone, which encourages the patient to overproject the voice, increasing vocal strain and trauma. Social vocal abuse is also common, as seen with loquacious personalities or in patients who attend events with significant background noise.

Tobacco and alcohol use raises concern for malignancy in the differential diagnosis. In addition, smoking directly irritates the vocal folds, predisposing them to inflammation.[8] Alcohol is a diuretic and produces mucosal drying. It is also generally consumed in loud environments and has a disinhibiting effect. Together, these effects increase the risk of laryngeal inflammation secondary to vocal abuse. Patients should be questioned about their toxin or irritant exposure at work or in hobbies. Personal protective equipment may be required in specific work environments. Travel history and current geography are important, as certain fungal infections exist only in specific climates.

A complete otolaryngologic examination is important for patients with laryngitis, as what may seem to be unrelated elements of the examination may help elucidate the underlying etiology and help in the diagnosis and treatment. An assessment of the patient's general appearance may reveal discomfort due to dyspnea or pain, or a toxic appearance due to an infectious etiology. Vital signs should be reviewed, with particular attention to temperature and oxygen saturation, as these may influence the urgency of your treatment decision. A systematic examination should be performed, with visualization of the larynx last. Physical exam findings and their probable causes are seen in ▶ Table 5.2.

Table 5.2 Physical examination findings and possible causes

Site	Finding	Possible causes
Otologic	Purulent otitis	Acute infectious
	Serous otitis	Autoimmune Allergies
	Retraction of tympanic membrane	Allergies
Rhinologic	Sinus tenderness	Acute infectious
	Turbinate hypertrophy	Allergies
	Mucosal edema	Allergies Infectious
	Nasal crusting	Autoimmune
	Clear rhinorhea	Allergies Autoimmune
	Purulent rhinorrhea	Acute infectious
Oral cavity	Tonsillar erythema/exudates	Acute infectious
	Pharyngeal cobblestoning	Allergies
	Bullae	Autoimmune
	Fungal debris	Infectious
Cervical	Adenopathy	Infectious Autoimmune Neoplastic

Laryngologic assessment can be performed with a mirror, flexible fiberoptic laryngoscope, or rigid endoscope. More recently, flexible distal chip digital endoscopes are available that afford images with excellent resolution via a typical transnasal approach. For optimal examination and details of the mucosal wave and phonatory glottal closure, videostroboscopy should be utilized, although it is generally not necessary in the setting of acute laryngitis. For patients with chronic laryngitis that is unresponsive to treatment and with a relatively benign laryngeal exam, stroboscopy may be of significant added benefit.[9] On examination, physicians should note erythema, edema, masses, ulcerations, and exudates in the hypopharynx and larynx. Attention should be paid in particular to the location, color, and morphology of the lesions as well as any abnormality in vocal fold motion. Specific findings associated with diagnoses are discussed in the next section, along with corresponding treatment.

5.2 Diagnosis and Treatment

With the information from the history and physical examination, the cause of laryngitis can usually be elicited. The laryngologic manifestations that are specific to each diagnosis are discussed in this section, as well as the requirement for further testing if necessary. As discussed previously, the differential diagnosis can be divided into acute infectious or chronic infectious, inflammatory, traumatic, autoimmune, or neoplastic categories. The diagnosis and treatment of autoimmune and neoplastic processes are discussed in depth in chapters on systemic diseases and malignancy, respectively.

The fundamental treatment for laryngeal inflammation is conservative behavioral management. Patients are placed on voice rest depending on the degree of inflammation and need for rapid recovery. There is no scientific evidence supporting total voice rest or the appropriate duration of voice rest. The authors recommend only short durations of complete voice rest if prescribed, lasting no more than 3 days. Modified voice use with moderation of time and volume are then recommended. Confidential voice is recommended. This is normal voicing, but at a volume appropriate in a library-type environment. Whispering is absolutely discouraged as it instills poor vocal techniques. Proper vocal hygiene is stressed. This includes hydration and humidification, an antireflux diet, and decreasing coughing and throat clearing. Also, patients are encouraged to pace their voice use throughout the day instead of compacting it to "get the voice use over with." For those with heavy phone use, a headset is recommended to reduce neck tension and the overprojection common with speakerphones.

Future vocal demands on the patient must be elucidated in order to determine how aggressive treatment needs to be. Clearly, a performing vocal artist or trial lawyer with a pending engagement will require different treatment than a retired person living alone with a low voice demand.

Generally, laryngeal inflammation is multifactorial and corresponding treatment is appropriate. If an inciting or contributing factor is identified, then treatment should be aimed at its curative management. This includes nasal steroids for allergic rhinitis, proton pump inhibitor (PPI) for reflux, mucolytics for increased mucus, and cough suppressants for chronic cough. If PPIs are to be prescribed, twice daily dosing is more effective, eliminates the possibility of underdosing the patient, does not add significant morbidity compared to daily dosing when used for less than one year, and allows for step-down therapy after the symptoms have improved.[10] When a cough suppressant is necessary, tramadol has been shown to be more effective than codeine and is well tolerated as it is tapered up to an effective dose.[11] Antihistamines should be avoided if possible, as their drying effect can exacerbate the laryngitis. This must be balanced with the morbidity of the allergies themselves and lack of response to nasal steroids.

If a medication is causing dehydration or an allergen is identified, then avoidance of the substance can help in resolution of the laryngeal inflammation. If a chronic cough is the inciting factor and an ACE inhibitor or angiotensin receptor blocker is the suspected etiology, a 6-week washout period is an acceptable trial to rule out a medication side effect.

5.3 Infectious Laryngitis

Infectious causes of laryngitis can be broken down into acute and chronic. ▶ Table 5.3 is a summary of the most common causative organisms for each microbiological category.

Table 5.3 Common organisms in acute and chronic infectious laryngitis

Organism	Acute	Chronic
Viral	Parainfluenza Influenza Herpes simplex	
Bacterial	*Moraxella catarrhalis* *Haemophilus influenzae* *Streptococcus pneumoniae* *Staphylococcus aureus*	*Klebsiella pneumoniae*
Fungal	*Candida albicans*	*Candida albicans* *Blastomyces dermatitidis* *Histoplasma capsulatum* *Coccidiodes immitis* *Cryptococcus neoformans*
Mycobacterial		*Mycobacterium tuberculosis* *Mycobacterium leprae*
Spirochetal		*Treponema pallidum*

5.3.1 Acute Infectious Laryngitis

Viral Infection

Viruses are the most common cause of laryngitis. Typically, patients have a concurrent upper respiratory tract infection and associated symptoms. Examination reveals erythema and edema of vocal folds, as seen in ▶ Fig. 5.1. If severe, the vocal fold edges may be irregular, and exudate could be present. The most common pathogens for this entity are parainfluenza or influenza virus. Herpes simplex virus infection can cause severe injury, with tissue necrosis affecting the vocal folds as well as the supraglottis and pharynx.[12]

Acute viral laryngitis is usually self-limited and treated with conservative management, as discussed above. If the inflammation is severe and or the patient desires a more rapid recovery, injectable dexamethasone or oral corticosteroids have been shown to reduce symptoms in the first 24 hours in comparison to placebo.[13]

Bacterial Infection

True bacterial laryngitis is rare. The most common pathogens are thought to be normal respiratory pathogens, such as *Moraxella catarrhalis*, *Haemophilus influenzae*, and *Streptococcus pneumoniae*. Some physicians consider purulence in the larynx a sign of bacterial infection. The laryngeal inflammation is severe, often with sloughing of the mucosa, and is not self-limiting. Bacterial laryngitis can be confirmed with sputum culture, although treatment is usually empiric with broad-spectrum oral antibiotics if the inflammation is unusually severe or symptoms become chronic. Recently, reports of methicillin-resistant *Staphylococcus aureus* (MRSA) laryngitis have been increasing.[14]

Acute bacterial laryngitis should be treated in a similar manner to acute viral laryngitis. A Cochrane review analyzed two studies using erythromycin and penicillin V for bacterial laryngitis. There was no significant difference in recovery of the patients compared with conservative management.[15]

Fungal Infection

Acute laryngitis with candidiasis most commonly occurs in immunocompromised patients and patients using inhaled corticosteroids.[16] The onset usually occurs over 24 to 48 hours and the dysphonia can be severe. ▶ Fig. 5.2 shows

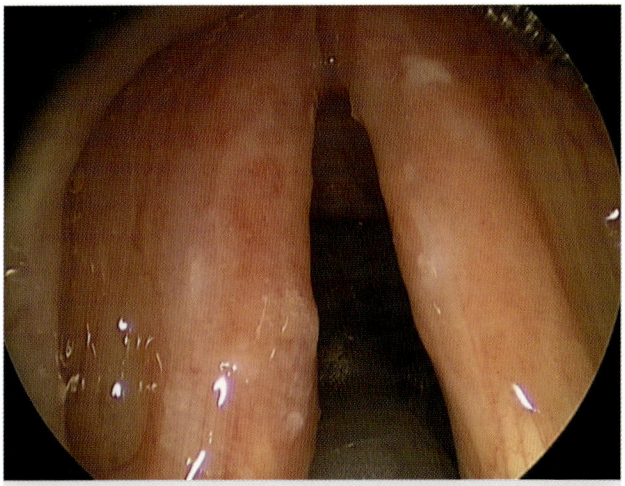

Fig. 5.1 Imaging of acute laryngitis. Note the irregular contours of the vocal fold edge, with edema and thickening of epithelium.

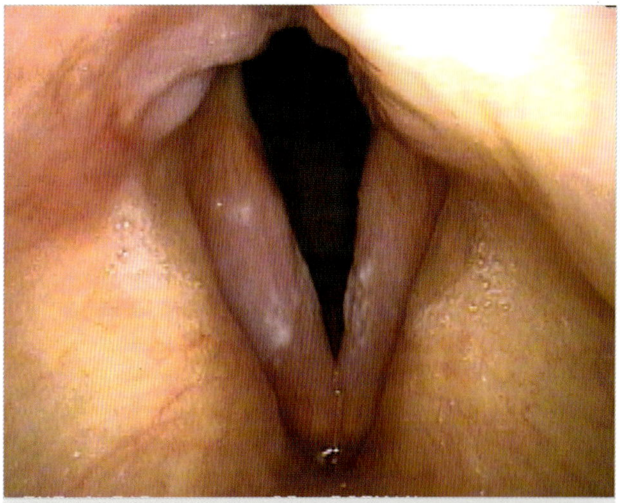

Fig. 5.2 Imaging of fungal laryngitis. Not the typical white plaques on a bed of erythema and edema. The vocal fold edges appear irregular.

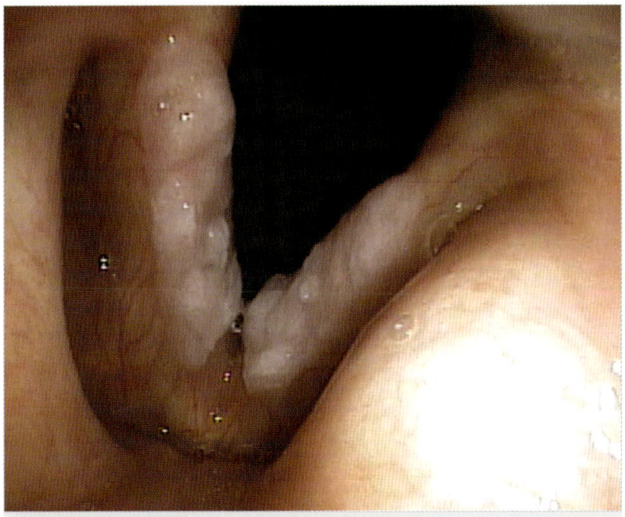

Fig. 5.3 Imaging of exophytic fungal laryngitis lesion resembling carcinoma, although the bilateral lesions in this picture make carcinoma unlikely.

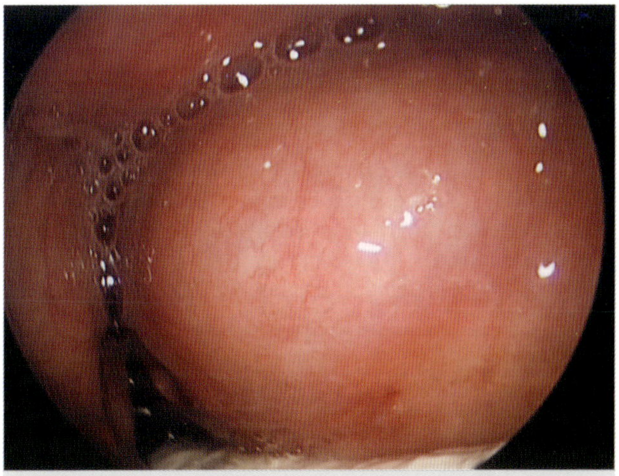

Fig. 5.4 Imaging of the granulomatous stage of *Klebsiella rhinoscleromatis* infection. Note large mucosalized lesion on left supraglottis.

typical bilateral white plaques on a bed of severe erythema. The vocal folds are edematous, with irregular vocal fold edges. Progression of disease can lead to exophytic lesions that resemble carcinoma (▶ Fig. 5.3). If lesions persist despite treatment with antifungal medication, biopsy and fungal stain should be performed to confirm the diagnosis and rule out malignancy, which may present with similar symptoms and appearance.[16]

Fungal laryngitis is treated with oral fluconazole for 2 to 6 weeks. If possible, steroid inhalers should be discontinued. A longer duration is often necessary in patients whose pulmonary disease is so severe that steroid inhaler use cannot be suspended. In these cases, inhalers should be changed to those with less propensity to cause laryngeal fungal infections, such as budesonide or ciclesonide.

5.3.2 Chronic Infectious Laryngitis

Bacterial Infection

Although chronic bacterial laryngitis is rare, *Klebsiella rhinoscleromatis* is a noted cause of severe chronic laryngitis. Although uncommon in the United States, this is seen in patients living in or traveling from the Middle East, Latin America, and Eastern Europe. The disease has a catarrhal, granulomatous, and fibrotic stage. The stages present as purulent rhinorrhea, mucosal granulomas, and synechia with stenosis, respectively. A typical mucosal granuloma can mimic a neoplasm as seen in ▶ Fig. 5.4. Approximately 50% of cases involve the larynx, which can cause life-threatening airway stenosis and obstruction. Diagnosis is made by biopsy and histologic diagnosis depending on the stage of disease. Histology shows Mikulicz cells, which are foamy macrophages. The bacteria are best visualized with Gram or Warthin-Starry stain.[17]

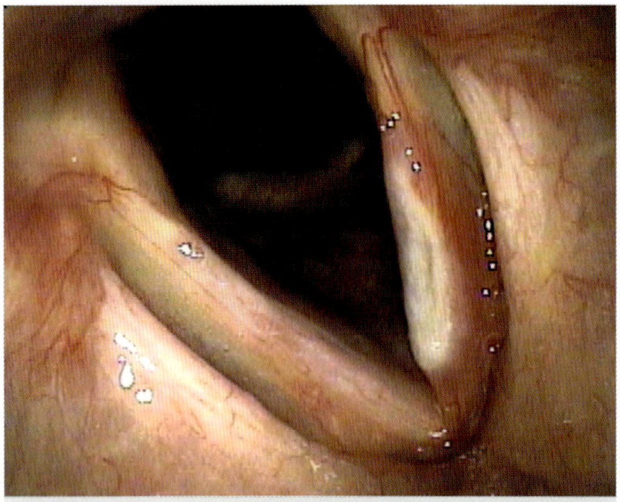

Fig. 5.5 Imaging of vocal fold ulceration. Note the ulcer with associated localized erythema or edema.

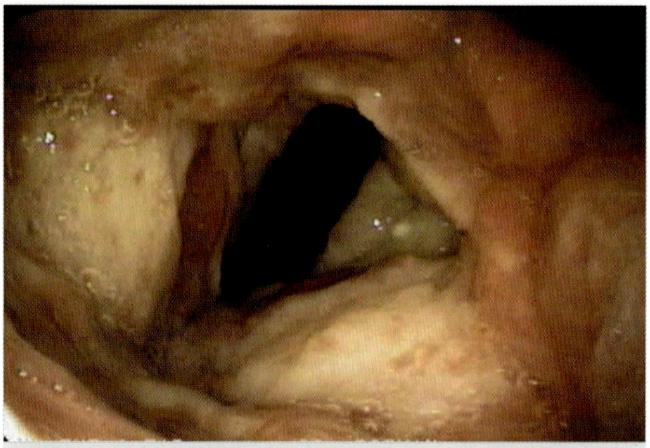

Fig. 5.6 Imaging of *Mycobacterium tuberculosis* in a young female presenting with hoarseness. The diffuse exophytic lesions extend through the entire larynx from epiglottis to glottis, although there is no posterior glottic involvement.

If a chronic bacterial infection is suspected, a culture should be obtained and further treatment based on the causative organism's culture and susceptibilities. An in-office culture can be obtained under topical anesthesia using a brush or can be performed in the operating room via direct laryngoscopy. Rhinoscleroma can be treated with long-term antibiotics depending on the stage of disease. During the catarrhal stage, long-term tetracycline or fluoroquinolones can be used. More advanced cases are treated surgically to secure the airway, along with long-term antibiotics. In a recent review, radiotherapy was used with surgery and antibiotics for cases of relapse.[17]

Viral Laryngitis

Although chronic viral laryngitis is unusual, complications from the acute event may persist. Idiopathic ulcerative laryngitis occurs following upper respiratory tract infection with cough. Patients have midmembranous ulcerative lesions lasting longer than 6 weeks despite various treatments, such as PPI, corticosteroids, antibiotics, and antifungals. Biopsies and cultures reveal only chronic inflammation. The lesion may be purely ulcerative or may be accompanied by exophytic inflammatory tissue (▶ Fig. 5.5). A questionable association with herpes virus is considered, but no evidence exists.[18] The ulcers may take as long as 3 months to resolve with conservative management. Depending on the severity of the resulting fibrosis, permanent dysphonia may occur.

Mycobacterial Infection

Laryngeal *Mycobacterium tuberculosis* infection occurs due to hematogenous or lymphatic spread and from ciliary kinesia of the trachea. The former is consistent with an increased incidence of posterior glottis involvement. A recent review showed 80% involvement of the true vocal fold and 38.5% involvement of posterior commissure and false fold.[19] The infection presents as ulcerative, nodular, or exudative lesions, which can be mistaken for malignancy (▶ Fig. 5.6). Diagnosis is made by PPD, chest x-ray, histology, and culture for acid-fast bacilli.

Mycobacterium leprae is transmitted by aerosolized droplets and occurs mostly in India and Brazil, where the disease is endemic. The erythematous and nodular lesions occur mostly in the epiglottis tip and vocal folds. Complications from the ulceration and scarring can lead to laryngeal stenosis and airway compromise. Diagnosis is confirmed with nasal smears or laryngeal biopsies containing bacilli.[20]

Mycobacterial infections are treated with surgery for relief of stenosis and antibiotic therapy specific for the disease. Tuberculosis is treated with typical tuberculosis four-drug therapy. Culture and sensitivity testing should be performed on biopsy specimens due to the high rate of multiple drug resistant strains of mycobacteria. *Mycobacterium leprae* is treated with dapsone or a combination of dapsone with rifampin. Treatment is continued for 1 to 2 years until negative biopsy specimens are obtained.[19]

Spirochetal Infection

The main spirochete is *Treponema pallidum* and laryngeal involvement occurs with secondary and tertiary syphilis. This causes hyperemia and maculopapular rash or diffuse nodular gummas, respectively. Diagnosis is confirmed with serological testing and pathologic examination of biopsy specimens. Syphilitic infections are treated with penicillin G as the drug of choice. If severe perichondritis or laryngeal stenosis occurs, then surgery or tracheotomy may be required for airway protection.[21]

Fungal Infection

Numerous fungi cause laryngeal infections. The most common pathogens are *Candida albicans, Blastomyces dermatitidis, Histoplasma capsulatum, Coccidioides immitis*, and *Cryptococcus neoformans*. Although *Candida albicans* usually presents as an acute infection, if left untreated it can become chronic and result in irreversible vocal fold fibrosis.

In the United States, blastomycosis occurs mostly in the southeast. The fungus enters through the lungs and spreads hematogenously. Laryngeal lesions are granular, exophytic masses with possible ulcerations. Diagnosis is made by biopsy revealing granulomatous suppurative lesions and fungal stains evidencing budding yeast and septate branching hyphae.[22]

Histoplasmosis is endemic to the Ohio and Mississippi Valley regions of the United States. It is usually a self-limited pulmonary infection except in immunocompromised patients. On examination, the lesions present as painful mucosal ulcers. The infection is lethal and most patients never survive to obtain examination by an otolaryngologist. Biopsy and fungal stains confirm the diagnosis, showing oval yeast and septate branching hyphae.

Coccidioidomycosis is endemic in the southwestern United States and northern Mexico. The infection occurs from spore inhalation and normally affects the lungs. Sputum inoculation or secondary infection can affect the larynx. The lesions are characterized as granulation tissue with ulceration. Diagnosis is by biopsy with histology and fungal stains showing yeast spherules and septate branching hyphae.[23]

Cryptococcosis is acquired by inhalation of spores in bird feces. The infection can be neurotropic and can be life threatening in immunocompromised patients. Diagnosis is confirmed by biopsy and fungal stains showing budding yeast, especially with India Ink and mucocarmine stains due to the encapsulated nature of fungus.[24]

Blastomycosis, histoplasmosis, coccidioidomycosis, and cryptococcosis are treated with intravenous amphotericin B or oral ketoconazole or itroconazole.[21]

5.4 Nonspecific Inflammatory Causes

An inflammation of the larynx can occur secondary to laryngopharyngeal reflux, smoking, allergies, environmental irritants, and radiation. Laryngopharyngeal reflux is often a cause of chronic laryngitis and is discussed in detail in a separate chapter. The diagnosis of laryngopharyngeal reflux has increased precipitously over the last 12 years.[25] Care should be taken not to overdiagnose reflux at the cost of increasing patient morbidity by a misdiagnosis or delay of effective treatment.

Smoking, witheither first-hand or second-hand inhalation of chemicals or particles, can cause irritation and inflammation of the larynx. This is usually a diagnosis of exclusion and is obtained from a proper history.

The role of environmental allergies in laryngitis is unclear.[26] Allergic laryngitis has been proposed in the literature as a primary cause of laryngeal inflammation. It is likely caused by systemic inflammatory mediators rather than by the aspiration of postnasal drip. Allergic rhinitis may also cause laryngeal inflammation secondary to throat clearing in response to increased and tenacious throat mucus.

Angioedema presents as watery edema of laryngeal tissue. It is usually due to anaphylactic reaction and is associated with oral cavity or pharyngeal edema. A common cause of acquired angioedema is a reaction to ACE inhibitors.[27] Angioedema can also be hereditary, in C1 esterase deficiency. Angioedema secondary to ACE inhibitors is not associated with dosage and duration of usage. Hereditary angioedema usually presents with a familial history and abdominal discomfort due to associated intestinal inflammation.

5.5 Radiation Laryngitis

Laryngitis is an acknowledged complication of radiation that may present at the time of treatment or years later. In the acute setting, the entire larynx may become edematous and erythematous in reaction to radiation exposure. Over time, the true vocal folds may become stiff and fibrotic. Destruction of the ventricular salivary glands results in persistent dryness and laryngitis sicca. Relief of symptoms is often difficult to attain for patients who experience chronic radiation laryngitis. Treatment is generally supportive, including hydration and gargles. Saliva stimulants, such as pilocarpine, may be helpful.

5.6 Vocal Overuse and Misuse

Laryngeal inflammation secondary to phonotrauma can occur from chronic vocal abuse or an acute event. The former occurs more often in occupations that require high voice demand, such as waiters and schoolteachers. Traumatic laryngitis does not necessarily require obvious vocally abusive behaviors, but it may be due to chronic inefficient vocal use, especially in the face of poor vocal hygiene or other mediators of vocal fold inflammation. It can also occur with coughing and chronic throat clearing.

The maximal force of vocal fold adduction causes friction, thermal damage, and mucosal breakdown.[28] An acute event can result from persistent elevation of the voice over background noise, or from yelling, shouting, or singing. If the vocal change is abrupt, it may be due to a vocal hemorrhage. In this case, laryngeal examination reveals vocal fold edema, erythema, and pooling of blood in the superficial lamina propria. There may also be herniation of the basement membrane, with formation of a hemorrhagic polyp.

▸ Fig. 5.7 demonstrates a hemorrhage in the superficial lamina propria of a professional singer. This usually resolves without long-term consequences unless it is associated with a polyp. ▸ Fig. 5.8 shows the same vocal fold as in ▸ Fig. 5.7, one month after the acute injury. Complete resolution of the hemorrhage from the superficial lamina propria is seen, with persistence of

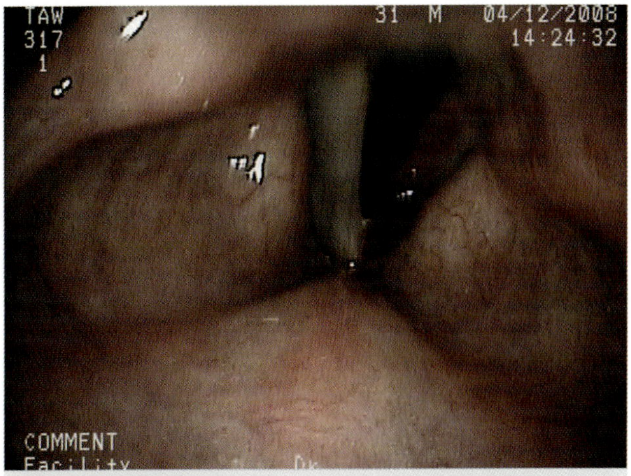

Fig. 5.7 Imaging of acute hemorrhage of left vocal fold. The subepithelial pooling of blood is noted. The inciting lesion, which is either polyp, ectasia, or varix, is noted at the junction of the anterior one third and posterior two thirds of the vocal fold.

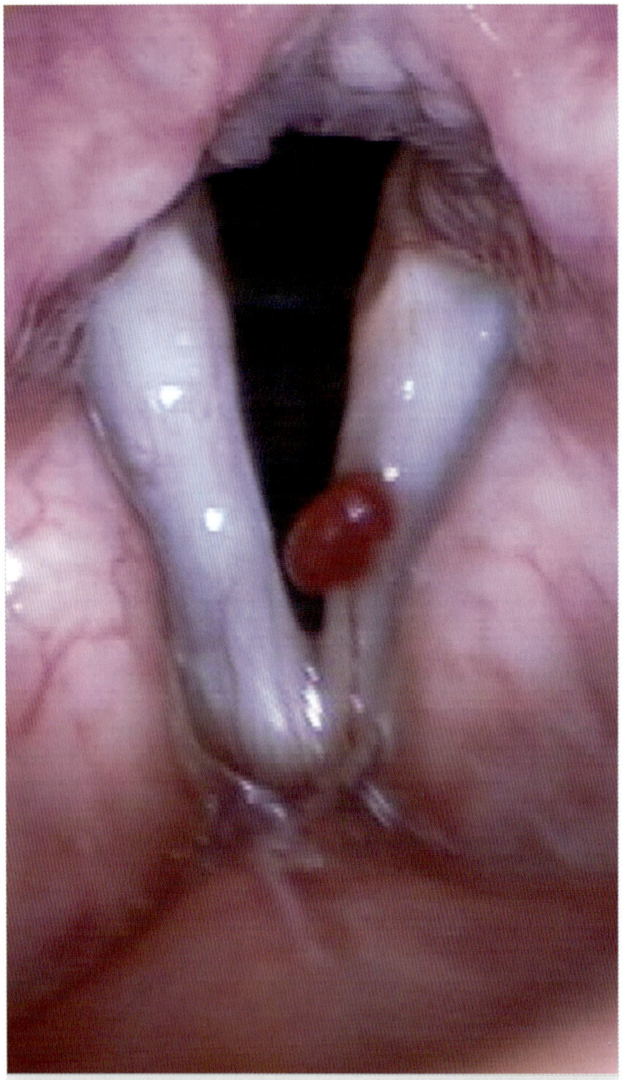

Fig. 5.8 Hemorrhagic polyp with associated dilated vessel.

the hemorrhagic polyp. As is usually the case, this polyp necessitated surgical removed for vocal restoration. Prolonged vocal trauma and inflammation can result in the formation of benign lesions of the vocal fold: nodules, polyps, and cysts. These are discussed in detail in the chapter on benign vocal fold lesions.

5.7 Failures

The disease entities above are usually self-limited or responsive to medication. Although certain etiologies, such as idiopathic ulcerative laryngitis, require many months of treatment, while leprosy requires years of treatment, the ultimate response is resolution of disease. Permanent sequelae may include vocal fold scarring resulting in adynamic segments on stroboscopy and the concordant dysphonia. Although this is rare, it does occur and can be severe. If the signs of laryngitis do not resolve after appropriate management, biopsy should be considered if it has not already been obtained. Many inflammatory lesions resemble carcinoma and this diagnosis should be ruled out before continuing with treatment beyond the expected time.

5.8 Key Points

- Acute laryngitis is usually viral and self-limiting. Supportive care and good vocal hygiene are the fundamental treatment.
- Many chronic inflammatory lesions can resemble carcinoma. If they are unresponsive to therapy, a biopsy should be considered.
- Bacterial causes of chronic laryngitis are rare, but cases caused by MRSA are now occurring more frequently.
- Laryngeal inflammation is usually multifactorial. All the contributing causes should be identified and addressed for optimal therapy.
- Although laryngopharyngeal reflux is a common cause of laryngeal inflammation, it is only one of many causes. Care should be taken not to overdiagnose laryngopharyngeal reflux, with the risk of missing the correct diagnosis and increasing patient morbidity.
- Both ACE inhibitors and angiotensin receptor blockers can cause a chronic cough leading to laryngeal inflammation.

References

[1] Koufman JA. Laryngopharyngeal reflux is different from classic gastroesophageal reflux disease. Ear Nose Throat J 2002; 81 Suppl 2: 7–9

[2] Mayerhoff RM, Pitman MJ. Atypical and disparate presentations of laryngeal sarcoidosis. Ann Otol Rhinol Laryngol 2010; 119: 667–671

[3] Chen A, Garrett CG. Otolaryngologic presentations of amyotrophic lateral sclerosis. Otolaryngol Head Neck Surg 2005; 132: 500–504

[4] Burroughs EI, Aronson AE, Duffy JR, Kyle RA. Speech disorders in systemic amyloidosis. Br J Disord Commun 1991; 26: 201–206

[5] Sanz L, Sistiaga JA, Lara AJ, Cuende E, García-Alcántara F, Rivera T. The prevalence of dysphonia, its association with immunomediated diseases and correlation with biochemical markers. J Voice 2012; 26: 148–153

[6] Simo R, Hartley C, Malik T, Wilson GE, Taylor PH, Mandal BK. Primary non-Hodgkin's lymphoma of the larynx in an AIDS patient. J Laryngol Otol 1998; 112: 77–80

[7] Lacourciére Y Telmisartan Cough Study Group. The incidence of cough: a comparison of lisinopril, placebo and telmisartan, a novel angiotensin II antagonist. Int J Clin Pract 1999; 53: 99–103

[8] Mouadeb DA, Belafsky PC, Birchall M, Hood C, Konia T, Pinkerton KE. The effects of allergens and tobacco smoke on the laryngeal mucosa of guinea pigs. Otolaryngol Head Neck Surg 2009; 140: 493–497

[9] Sataloff RT, Spiegel JR, Hawkshaw MJ. Strobovideolaryngoscopy: results and clinical value. Ann Otol Rhinol Laryngol 1991; 100: 725–727

[10] Park W, Hicks DM, Khandwala F et al. Laryngopharyngeal reflux: prospective cohort study evaluating optimal dose of proton-pump inhibitor therapy and pretherapy predictors of response. Laryngoscope 2005; 115: 1230–1238

[11] Louly PG, Medeiros-Souza P, Santos-Neto L. N-of-1 double-blind, randomized controlled trial of tramadol to treat chronic cough. Clin Ther 2009; 31: 1007–1013

[12] Vrabec JT, Molina CP, West B. Herpes simplex viral laryngitis. Ann Otol Rhinol Laryngol 2000; 109: 611–614

[13] Super DM, Cartelli NA, Brooks LJ, Lembo RM, Kumar ML. A prospective randomized double-blind study to evaluate the effect of dexamethasone in acute laryngotracheitis. J Pediatr 1989; 115: 323–329

[14] Liakos T, Kaye K, Rubin AD. Methicillin-resistant Staphylococcus aureus laryngitis. Ann Otol Rhinol Laryngol 2010; 119: 590–593

[15] Reveiz L, Cardona AF, Ospina EG. Antibiotics for acute laryngitis in adults. Cochrane Database Syst Rev 2005: CD004783

[16] Wong KK, Pace-Asciak P, Wu B, Morrison MD. Laryngeal candidiasis in the outpatient setting. J Otolaryngol Head Neck Surg 2009; 38: 624–627

[17] Zhong Q, Guo W, Chen X et al. Rhinoscleroma: a retrospective study of pathologic and clinical features. J Otolaryngol Head Neck Surg 2011; 40: 167–174

[18] Simpson CB, Sulica L, Postma GN et al. Idiopathic ulcerative laryngitis. Laryngoscope 2011; 121: 1023–1026

[19] Wang CC, Lin CC, Wang CP, Liu SA, Jiang RS. Laryngeal tuberculosis: a review of 26 cases. Otolaryngol Head Neck Surg 2007; 137: 582–588

[20] Soni NK. Leprosy of the larynx. J Laryngol Otol 1992; 106: 518–520

[21] Tulunay OE. Laryngitis—diagnosis and management. Otolaryngol Clin North Am 2008; 41: 437–451, ix

[22] Hanson JM, Spector G, El-Mofty SK. Laryngeal blastomycosis: a commonly missed diagnosis. Report of two cases and review of the literature. Ann Otol Rhinol Laryngol 2000; 109: 281–286

[23] Boyle JO, Coulthard SW, Mandel RM. Laryngeal involvement in disseminated coccidioidomycosis. Arch Otolaryngol Head Neck Surg 1991; 117: 433–438

[24] Reese MC, Colclasure JB. Cryptococcosis of the larynx. Arch Otolaryngol 1975; 101: 698–701

[25] Altman KW, Prufer N, Vaezi MF. A review of clinical practice guidelines for reflux disease: toward creating a clinical protocol for the otolaryngologist. Laryngoscope 2011; 121: 717–723

[26] Roth DF, Ferguson BJ. Vocal allergy: recent advances in understanding the role of allergy in dysphonia. Curr Opin Otolaryngol Head Neck Surg 2010; 18: 176–181

[27] Tai S, Mascaro M, Goldstein NA. Angioedema: a review of 367 episodes presenting to three tertiary care hospitals. Ann Otol Rhinol Laryngol 2010; 119: 836–841

[28] Dworkin JP. Laryngitis: types, causes, and treatments. Otolaryngol Clin North Am 2008; 41: 419–436, ix

6 Laryngopharyngeal Reflux

Ashli O'Rourke and Gregory N. Postma

Laryngopharyngeal reflux (LPR) is often suspected in patients presenting with otolaryngologic complaints. It is due to the retrograde flow of gastric contents into the laryngopharynx. The refluxate is highly injurious to laryngeal epithelium, which lacks the defense mechanisms of the esophageal lining, rendering it more susceptible to acid-induced injury.[1,2] However, not all symptoms attributed to LPR may be associated with direct acid contact with the upper aerodigestive tract epithelium. Some symptoms, such as cough or bronchospasm, are thought to be related to esophagovagal reflexes, triggered by abrupt esophageal distention.

The true prevalence of LPR is unknown, but it is thought to affect between 20 to 30% of patients with laryngologic symptoms. Given the high likelihood that the otolaryngologist will encounter LPR in practice, it is important to be able to clinically diagnose and treat this common problem. It must be understood, however, that other disorders can mimic the symptoms of LPR and overdiagnosis should be avoided. In this chapter, we address the diagnosis of LPR as well as the current guidelines for treatment.

6.1 History

Patients with LPR commonly complain of hoarseness, sore throat, excessive mucus production, throat clearing, cough, globus sensation, and/or dysphagia (▶ Table 6.1).[1,3,4,5,6] To better define the complaints encountered in LPR patients, several symptom indices have been created. The Reflux Symptom Index (RSI) subjectively quantifies the symptoms of LPR and is one of the most widely utilized (▶ Table 6.2).[4] The RSI is a validated, self-administered nine-item questionnaire in which patients are asked to rank symptoms from 0 (no problem) to 5 (severe problem) that have affected them within the past month. In untreated LPR patients, Belafsky et al[4] demonstrated that the RSI was elevated (RSI = 21.2) in comparison to healthy controls (RSI = 11.6). An RSI greater than 13 is considered abnormal and may be indicative of LPR. It is important to interpret the RSI results in the appropriate patient context, as many symptoms that are seemingly suggestive of LPR can be found in the absence of reflux or in other disease processes, such as allergy, rhinosinusitis, or mass lesions of the larynx.[5]

Table 6.1 Otolaryngologic symptoms and associations with laryngopharyngeal reflux

Symptoms	Associations
Dysphonia	Rhinosinusitis
Globus (foreign body) sensation	Otitis media
Chronic cough	Laryngospasm
Soreness or burning in throat	Granuloma
Throat clearing	Airway stenosis
Excessive mucus production	Leukoplakia
Dysphagia	Lingual tonsil hypertrophy
	Obstructive sleep apnea
	Laryngeal carcinoma

In obtaining a patient history, one should attempt to distinguish LPR from gastroesophageal reflux (GER), which is considered a different disease entity. The clinician should also entertain the possibility of coexistent LPR and GER contributing to an individual patient's symptom complex. Laryngopharyngeal reflux is associated with brief episodic reflux with rapid esophageal clearance and occurs primarily in the upright position (mostly during daytime hours). Alternatively, gastroesophageal reflux disease (GERD) is more often associated with supine position, nocturnal regurgitation, and slower clearance of esophageal acid. However, both are associated with transient lower esophageal sphincter relaxations (TLESR) and studies have shown the same prevalence of hiatal hernia and distorted morphology of gastroesophageal junction in the two entities.[7,8,9]

The etiologies of both GERD and LPR are multifactorial and differ in esophageal sphincter function, esophageal versus laryngeal sensitivity, response to treatment, and refluxate exposure times.[10] Although up to 50 acid-exposure events per day in the esophagus can be considered physiologic, two to three episodes of acid exposure to the laryngeal mucosa in the same period are considered abnormal and capable of producing LPR symptoms.[11,12] Keep in mind as well that some extraesophageal symptoms may not be related to direct acid exposure. These symptoms, such as cough or bronchospasm, may be attributable to vagally mediated reflex pathways triggered by the presence of acid within the distal esophagus.[13,14,15] Lastly, weakly acidic or basic refluxate has been shown to be injurious to laryngeal mucosa and may cause LPR signs or symptoms.

Table 6.2 Reflux Symptom Index

Within the last MONTH, how did the following problem affect you?	0 = no problem 5 = severe problem
1. Hoarseness or a problem with your voice	0 1 2 3 4 5
2. Clearing your throat	0 1 2 3 4 5
3. Excess throat mucus or postnasal drip	0 1 2 3 4 5
4. Difficulty swallowing food, liquids, or pills	0 1 2 3 4 5
5. Coughing after you ate or after lying down	0 1 2 3 4 5
6. Breathing difficulties or choking episodes	0 1 2 3 4 5
7. Troublesome or annoying cough	0 1 2 3 4 5
8. Sensations of something sticking in your throat or a lump in your throat	0 1 2 3 4 5
9. Heartburn, chest pain, indigestion, or stomach acid coming up	0 1 2 3 4 5

Source: Used with permission from Belafsky P, Postma G, Koufman J. Validity and reliability of the Reflux Symptom Index (RSI). Journal of Voice 2002; 16 (2):274–277.

The symptom complexes of GERD and LPR differ.[16] GERD is associated with more "classic" symptoms, such as regurgitation or heartburn, which can occur in up to 83% of GERD patients, whereas only 23% of LPR patients have this complaint.[1] Conversely, the majority of patients with LPR have more "atypical" symptoms. For example, 87% of patients with LPR report frequent throat clearing, while only 3% of GERD patients experience this symptom.[3]

6.2 Physical Examination

Many of the symptoms described above may occur in patients without LPR and so diagnosis should not be made based on symptoms alone and must be supplemented with physical examination. Laryngoscopy, either by rigid or flexible examination, is required in addition to a thorough head and neck examination. This is especially true in the patient who presents with dysphonia or airway concerns.

Common laryngoscopic findings of LPR include laryngeal edema, pseudosulcus formation, erythema, posterior commissure hypertrophy, granuloma formation, and/or excessive endolaryngeal mucus.[1,17,18,19,20,21,22] However, these findings in isolation are not proof of reflux-induced laryngeal injury.

Many authors have found posterior laryngeal abnormalities, such as vocal process erythema or posterior commissure hypertrophy, to be associated with LPR.[19,20,21] Ulualp et al[19] found posterior laryngeal abnormalities in 75% of patients with positive pharyngeal pH probe testing. However, Hill et al[22] found no change in posterior commissure hypertrophy in 17 patients with prolonged control of their LPR symptoms. The authors therefore concluded that this finding was not a reliable indicator of active LPR disease.

Diffuse infraglottic edema can create laryngeal pseudosulcus, which is the appearance of a linear indentation of the medial edge of the vocal fold extending from the anterior commissure to the posterior glottis. This is a common laryngeal finding in patients with LPR due the high prevalence of edema, which can be seen in up to 70 to 90% of these patients.[18,23] However, the sensitivity and specificity of this finding are 70% and 77%, respectively, so although suggestive of LPR, it can also be seen in other disorders.[23] Pseudosulcus should not be confused with sulcus vocalis, which is not related to LPR and is caused by loss of the superficial lamina propria with adherence of the overlying epithelium to the deeper underlying vocal ligament.

It cannot be stressed enough that laryngoscopic findings should be considered in the context of the patient's entire disease presentation, because no single laryngoscopic finding is pathognomonic for LPR. In fact, several investigators have demonstrated isolated findings traditionally associated with laryngopharyngeal acid exposure in healthy volunteers.[24,25] To better quantify the constellation of changes of the laryngopharynx that can be seen in LPR, Belafsky et al[17] developed the Reflux Finding Score (RFS). This is a validated, physician-completed scale that documents signs suggestive of reflux laryngitis (▶ Table 6.3).[17] It allows the physician to rank the presence and/or severity of eight common LPR-related laryngoscopic findings, with total scores ranging from 0 (least severe) to 26 (most severe). A score greater than 7, in the appropriate clinical setting, is suggestive of LPR. [17]

6.3 Differential Diagnosis

Reflux-related mucosal inflammation of the laryngopharynx results in symptoms that can be found in many other disease states. These include gastroesophageal reflux disease, chronic rhinosinusitis, allergy, asthma, paradoxical vocal fold motion disorder, muscle tension dysphonia, and mass lesions of the larynx.[5,26,27,28]

6.4 Diagnosis

Although the RSI and RFS are helpful in suggesting the diagnosis, they are not adequate alone to definitively diagnose LPR. Possible further investigations include empiric proton pump inhibitor (PPI) trial, radiography, esophageal manometry, esophagoscopy, and pH and pH-impedance probe testing. In addition, there are some newer technologies being investigated, such as tissue biopsies for the gastric enzyme pepsin. The clinician may have difficulty in knowing where to start. In patients without life-threatening signs or symptoms, it is reasonable to begin with a trial of acid-suppressive medication.

Table 6.3 Reflux Finding Score

Laryngeal finding	Points
Subglottic edema	Absent (0), present (2)
Ventricular obliteration	Partial (2), complete (4)
Erythema/hyperemia	Arytenoids only (2), diffuse (4)
Vocal fold edema	Mild (1), moderate (2), severe (3), polypoid (4)
Diffuse laryngeal edema	Mild (1), moderate (2), severe (3), obstructing (4)
Posterior commissure hypertrophy	Mild (1), moderate (2), severe (3), obstructing (4)
Granuloma/granulation tissue	Absent (0), present (2)
Thick endolaryngeal mucous	Absent (0), present (2)

Source: Used with permission from Belafsky P, Postma G, Koufman J. The validity and reliability of the Reflux Finding Score (RFS). Laryngoscope 2001; 111:1313–1317.

6.4.1 Empiric Medical Therapy

A review of the literature regarding the utility of empiric PPI therapy for the diagnosis of LPR reveals mixed results. In 2003, Bilgen et al[29] attempted to validate empiric antacid therapy as a diagnostic test for LPR. Subjects with RSI and RFS scores suggestive of LPR were placed on lansoprazole 30 mg twice daily for two months followed by 4 months of lansoprazole 15 mg daily. The authors found a significant reduction in RSI and RFS at every 2-month interval during follow-up.[29] However, the same patients who responded to empiric therapy had no difference in proximal reflux events on pH testing as compared to healthy controls. The authors concluded that response to PPI therapy does not necessarily diagnose those with LPR as compared to the gold standard of dual pH-probe testing.

Park et al[30] investigated the optimal dose of PPI in an empiric trial and found at least a 50% reduction in symptoms in 50% of patients after 2 months of twice-daily PPI therapy as compared to a 28% reduction of symptoms in the same number of patients with once-daily therapy. There was no benefit in the addition of histamine-2 (H_2) receptor antagonist therapy. Additionally, they found at least a 50% reduction in symptoms in more than 70% of patients after 4 months of twice-daily PPI therapy.[30] They concluded that acid suppression with twice-daily PPI therapy is warranted for empiric therapy in patients with LPR. However, Qadeer et al[31] completed a meta-analysis of randomized controlled trials utilizing the same outcome of greater than 50% reduction in symptoms. They found no significant difference between placebo and PPI therapy.[31]

Regardless of conflicting studies, most clinicians prescribe a trial of PPI therapy as an initial step in the diagnosis and treatment of individuals suspected to have LPR. The clinician must be aware, however, that if aggressive acid suppression alone does not adequately control symptoms, further investigation, such as pH testing, should be undertaken.

6.4.2 Dual pH-Probe Testing

The gold standard for the objective diagnosis of LPR is dual pH-probe (esophageal and hypopharyngeal) 24-hour monitoring. In dual pH-probe monitoring, a catheter probe is placed through the naris and positioned so that one pH sensor is 1 centimeter (cm) above the upper esophageal sphincter (UES) and a second pH sensor is located 5 cm above the lower esophageal sphincter (LES). This placement requires either prior endoscopy with accurate measurements for location of the sphincters (recorded in cm from the nostril) or manometry (preferred method). Unfortunately, placement of the proximal probe in the pharynx may lead to drying of the probe and false-positive results.[32] This can be improved by placing the proximal probe less than 2 cm above the UES.[33]

It is difficult to ascertain exactly how much pharyngeal acid exposure is pathologic. The literature suggests that both the number of acidic events as well as the percent acid-exposure time are helpful in distinguishing LPR patients from normal individuals.[33] Hypopharyngeal pH testing has the best positive predictive value when performed in patients with laryngoscopic signs suggestive of LPR. Ulualp et al, in two separate studies, found a significantly higher number of pharyngeal acid reflux events in patients with posterior laryngeal signs of LPR versus controls.[19,34] Oelschlager et al[35] found that control subjects had both significantly lower RFS (2.1 vs. 9.6) and pharyngeal acid exposure events (0.2 vs. 3.4) when compared to patients suspected to have LPR. In addition, they identified a subset of patients with RFS > 7 and positive pharyngeal acid events who were twice as likely to respond to acid suppression as patients with negative pH testing and RFS < 7.[35]

6.4.3 Multichannel Intraluminal Impedance-pH Monitoring

Impedance is the measure of electrical resistance, in volts, to the passage of current in a circuit. Esophageal impedance monitoring measures changes in esophageal intraluminal impedance. It utilizes pairs of closely spaced cylindrical metal rings connected in circuit along the probe length. As boluses pass by the catheter, changes in impedance are recorded (▶ Fig. 6.1). Fluid boluses change impedance by "connecting the circuit" and decreasing resistance (and therefore impedance) between electrodes. A liquid reflux event is defined as a sequential retrograde drop in impedance by 50% from baseline across at least two consecutive sensors.

Multichannel intraluminal impedance-pH (MII-pH) probe testing has several benefits over pH probe testing alone. First, MII-pH monitoring can detect acidic, weakly acidic, weakly alkaline, and/or alkaline episodes of reflux, whereas traditional pH monitoring only records events with pH less than 4 or 5. Second, the proximal progress and direction of flow (anterograde vs. retrograde) of an event can be assessed. Lastly,

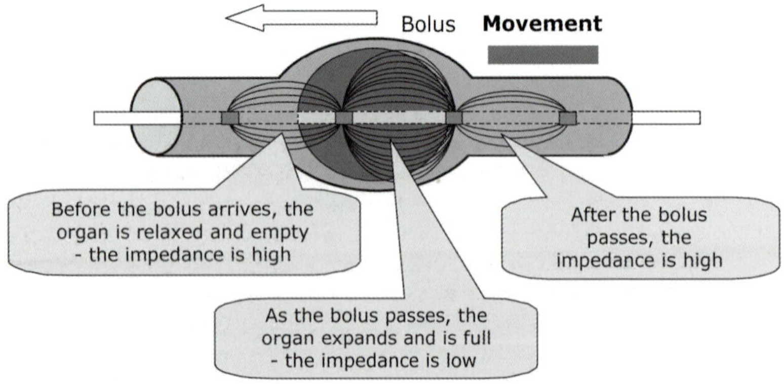

Fig. 6.1 Multichannel esophageal intraluminal impedance testing. (Used with permission from Wise JL, Murray JA. Utilising multichannel intraluminal impedance for diagnosing GERD: a review. Diseases of the Esophagus 2007; 20: 83–88.)

impedance can give information regarding whether a reflux event was gas, liquid, or a mixed bolus.

Impedance testing can be very sensitive. Aslam et al[36] revealed that impedance can consistently detect pharyngeal reflux events as small as 0.1 mL. However, this minute amount of reflux may not be abnormal.

Hoppo et al[12] compared the amount of pharyngeal reflux exposure between patients with LPR symptoms and normal individuals on and off PPI therapy using MII-pH monitoring. A total of 9.3% (55/590) of reflux events in patients with LPR symptoms reached the hypopharynx. In contrast, 0.14% (1/705) of events in control patients off PPI and 0.74% (4/542) of events in controls on PPI were LPR events. Given these results, the authors concluded that one or more pharyngeal reflux events during 24-hour MII-pH testing is abnormal in patients with LPR symptoms and pharyngeal acid exposure is a rare event in asymptomatic patients.[12] These findings warrant further investigation.

6.4.4 Oropharyngeal pH Monitoring

The ResTech pH probe device (Respiratory Technology Corp, San Diego, CA), was created in an attempt to minimize the invasiveness of pharyngeal pH testing, thereby creating a more comfortable evaluation as well as detecting both acidic and weakly acidic extraesophageal reflux.[37] Unlike previous pH probes, it is designed for the detection of oropharyngeal reflux alone. The ResTech device is inserted through the naris and is positioned behind the soft palate to detect aerosolized refluxate in the oropharynx. Studies directly comparing dual pH-probe monitoring with the ResTech device have shown 90% sensitivity and 80% specificity in correlating pharyngeal pH drops with more distal esophageal events as well as the presence of esophagitis.[38] Chheda et al[39] found a high correlation between oropharyngeal events detected with the ResTech device and hypopharyngeal and esophageal events identified by traditional pH dual probe testing. However, Weiner et al[38] found that hypopharyngeal events on traditional dual probe testing did not correlate well with acidic events detected by the ResTech probe, with the latter being more sensitive.

The normative data for oropharyngeal testing are somewhat controversial. Sun et al[37] suggested using a threshold of upright pH of less than 5 in patients with LPR symptoms. Others have suggested that a 10% decrease in pH from the individual's baseline may be a more accurate assessment of abnormal pharyngeal pH values.[38]

6.4.5 Radiography and Esophageal Manometry

Although useful in the evaluation of dysphagia, barium swallow (also called an esophagram at some institutions) and esophageal manometry do not greatly contribute to the evaluation of LPR. A barium swallow may reveal dysmotility, esophageal reflux, or complications associated with GER (stricture, webs, etc.). However, GER may be stimulated by provocative measures during a barium swallow and may signal LES incompetence. Esophageal dysmotility seen on manometry may predispose a patient to reflux. However, on their own, neither radiography nor manometry is adequate to diagnose LPR, and they should be considered ancillary investigations.

6.4.6 Esophagoscopy

Esophagoscopy, either by unsedated transnasal esophagoscopy (TNE) or conventional sedated esophagoscopy, should be completed in cases of chronic LPR to screen for esophageal disease. Reports have shown a wide range in the incidence of esophagitis in LPR patients, between 10 and 55%, but these studies vary in their criterion for the diagnosis of LPR (i.e., symptom complex, laryngoscopic findings, or pH testing).[40,41,42,43,44,45] Koufman et al[46] found esophagitis during TNE in 12% (7/58) of LPR patients with abnormal pharyngeal pH studies. In a study of 405 consecutive patients with otolaryngologic complaints, Poelmans et al[47] found erosive esophagitis in 212 (52.3%) of patients. Metaplastic changes, such as Barrett esophagus, have also been identified in patients with predominantly extraesophageal symptoms. Perry et al discovered Barrett esophagus in 15.6% of patients with LPR, while Koufman et al found a lower prevalence of 7% in a similar study population.[9,46] Interestingly, isolated LPR symptoms, especially chronic cough, were the presenting complaints in 30% of patients eventually found to have esophageal adenocarcinoma in a retrospective review by Reavis et al in 2004.[48] Esophageal screening should be completed after 2 to 3 weeks of PPI therapy to decrease the incidence of minor esophagitis.

6.4.7 Future Investigations

Some groups have focused on the detection of refluxate components in the upper aerodigestive tract as an alternative to pH testing for LPR diagnosis. Many of these investigations stem from evidence that mucosal injury is due not only to acidic pH, but also to the active components of refluxate, such as pepsin or bile acids in weakly acidic or basic duodenal refluxate.

Pepsin is a proteolytic enzyme that is secreted by the gastric chief cells as inactive pepsinogen. Pepsinogen is cleaved at pH 5 to form the active enzyme pepsin. Gastric pepsin is a good marker for reflux because it is only present in gastric secretions and is not produced by other organs. Several authors have found higher levels of pepsin in the laryngopharyngeal mucosa of patients with LPR as compared to controls.[49,50] Blumin and Johnston[51] also detected pepsin in the subglottic mucosa of 13 of 22 (59%) patients with idiopathic subglottic stenosis. Other investigators have shown an increase in the concentration of pepsin in the sputum of LPR patients.[52,53,54] Furthermore, Wassenaar et al[54] demonstrated a decrease in pepsin levels detected in the sputum samples of patients following surgical fundoplication.

Lastly, exhaled breath condensate (EBC) pH detection is a relatively new and potentially valuable noninvasive methodology that can be used to detect airway acidification. Exhaled breath condensate is produced from the airway lining fluid that is aerosolized by turbulent airflow and/or the opening of distal airways.[55] The pH of EBC can be measured and the acidification of the pharynx and upper aerodigestive tract is detectable with EBC analysis.[55] The most common EBC collection device in the United States is the R-Tube (Respiratory Research Inc, Austin, TX) collection system. Exhaled breath condensate is collected by having a patient breath into a small portable tube equipped with a one-way valve. Children as young as 4 years of age have been able to use this device. Although some studies have shown an association between acidic EBC pH values and cough, the ability of EBC pH to accurately detect LPR is still unknown.[55]

6.5 Treatment

The appropriate level of treatment for LPR is largely dependent upon the severity of disease as well as the impact of LPR on a specific patient's lifestyle or occupation. Although a trial of conservative measures (e.g., diet modifications) may be sufficient initial management of mild LPR in the casual voice user, LPR in the professional singer could be career threatening and necessitates more aggressive intervention. Postma et al[56] described LPR as minor, major, or life-threatening based on the severity of patient symptoms, laryngoscopic findings, and impact on occupation (see box "Characteristics of life-threatening laryngopharyngeal reflux"). Minor LPR is characterized by symptoms, such as globus or throat clearing, which may be annoying but do not greatly impact social or professional life. Mild laryngeal edema may be noted on laryngeal examination. Major LPR, however, does have significant impact on social or occupational function.[56] This category may include patients with persistent hoarseness that impairs the ability to perform critical vocal tasks at work or nonobstructing granulomas. Life-threatening LPR includes patients with airway compromise, significant respiratory symptoms, dysplasia, and/or laryngeal carcinoma.[56] Intuitively, the more severe the category, the more aggressive the clinician should be in treating the patient's LPR. Patients with life-threatening LPR should undergo more rigorous diagnostic work-up and require close follow-up during treatment.

Characteristics of life-threatening laryngopharyngeal reflux

Airway obstruction
- Glottic stenosis
- Subglottic stenosis
- Laryngeal webbing
- Laryngospasm
- Severe paradoxical vocal fold movement disorder

Respiratory symptoms
- Reactive airway disease
- Asthma
- Pneumonitis

Histologic changes
- Dysplasia
- Carcinoma

6.5.1 Behavioral and Dietary Modifications

Behavioral and dietary modifications have been shown to improve LPR, at least in the short term.[57] These modifications can be used either alone (in patients with minor LPR) or in conjunction with other treatment modalities. Behavioral modifications are aimed primarily at decreasing the incidence of GERD and thus LPR (see box, "Behavioral modifications for the treatment of laryngopharyngeal reflux (p.52)"). Patients should avoid foods that result in symptoms as well as those known to weaken the LES or promote acid production (see box "Dietary modifications for the treatment of laryngopharyngeal reflux (p.52)").

Behavioral modifications for the treatment of laryngopharyngeal reflux

- Weight loss
- Avoidance of "trigger" foods
- Smoking cessation
- Eat smaller meals
- Limit alcohol consumption
- Avoid eating before lying down
- Elevate head of bed

Dietary restrictions for the treatment of laryngopharyngeal reflux

Diet restrictions
- Caffeine
- Chocolate
- Peppermint
- Fatty foods
- Acidic foods (citrus fruits, tomatoes, jams/jellies, barbecue sauce, most salad dressings)
- Spicy foods (hot mustards, curry, hot peppers)
- Carbonated beverages
- Red wine

6.5.2 Medical Therapy

Laryngopharyngeal reflux typically requires more aggressive and prolonged treatment than GERD and often does not respond to over-the-counter antacid medications, such as H_2 receptor antagonists or buffer agents.[30,58] Proton pump inhibitors directly target the production of acid by irreversibly blocking the hydrogen/potassium adenosine triphosphatase (H^+-K^+ ATPase) enzyme system. The targeting of this terminal step in acid production and the resistance to tachyphalaxis seen with H_2 receptor antagonists make PPIs potent antacid medications. Patients should be instructed to take PPIs approximately 30 minutes prior to mealtimes to ensure peak serum drug levels at the time of maximum H^+-K^+ ATPase stimulation. This is an important point to stress to patients; in a recent analysis in a tertiary laryngology office, nearly half of patients were found to be taking their PPI medication in a suboptimal manner.[59]

The controversy regarding appropriate dosing of PPIs was discussed earlier in this chapter. Review of this literature advocates treatment with twice-daily PPI (e.g., omeprazole 20 mg twice daily or lansoprazole 30 mg twice daily) for at least 2 months before consideration of more aggressive therapy. The reality of insurance reimbursement for PPI therapy, however, may require a failed trial of once-daily therapy. Therefore a practical approach is a trial of once-daily PPI dosing with education about behavior and diet modifications in patients without alarming symptoms and mild signs of LPR on endoscopy. If symptoms do not resolve in 2 months, then dosing should be increased to twice daily. For patients with severe LPR associated with airway stenosis, recurrent granulomas, leukoplakia, or laryngospasm, treatment should begin with twice-daily PPI dosing.

Patients should be followed at 2- to 3-month intervals and treatment response evaluated with the RSI and RFS. It has been found that LPR symptoms respond more rapidly to PPI therapy than resolution of findings on endoscopy, which can take up to 6 months.[60] Once symptoms are controlled and there is documentation of endoscopic improvement, attempts should be made to wean the patient off of PPI therapy while maintaining behavioral and diet modifications. However, many patients are not able to be completely weaned from therapy without symptom recurrence.[58] Bove and Rosen[58] suggested an RSI < 6 and RFS < 10 on two consecutive examinations as an appropriate benchmark to begin PPI tapering. If symptoms return, patients are replaced on the previous dosing that results in symptom control. After tapering to once-daily dosing, patients should begin every-other-day dosing before discontinuing use. Current practice recommends this gradual tapering of PPIs to prevent rebound reflux symptoms, although the literature supporting this is conflicting.[61] However, in a randomized, double-blind, placebo-controlled trial, Reimer et al[62] demonstrated that the abrupt discontinuation after 8 weeks of PPI therapy produced reflux symptoms in 44% (26/59) of healthy volunteers.

As stated before, patients who do not fully respond to empiric PPI therapy should undergo further diagnostic evaluation and the possibility that the diagnosis is something other than LPR must be entertained. In addition, some believe that changing to a different PPI may provide better symptom control in some patients. This is based on heritable differences in cytochrome P450 mediated metabolism of PPIs.[63,64,65] A different PPI should be considered only after increased dosing of the initial PPI has failed to control symptoms. Unfortunately, some LPR patients are refractory to appropriate trials of PPI therapy.[30] This may be due to the fact that while PPI therapy may decrease the acidity of refluxate, it does not reduce the number or duration of reflux events.[66] Weakly acidic reflux injury is difficult to treat with antacid therapy. Alternative therapeutic agents aimed at decreasing transient lower esophageal relaxations, such as baclofen, atropine, cholecystokinin receptor antagonists, morphine, and nitric oxide synthase inhibitors, have been limited by their side-effect profiles.[67,68] Therefore, severe weakly acidic reflux may be best treated surgically.

Lastly, patients should be appropriately treated for comorbid conditions that may contribute to increased reflux. For example, a patient with gastroparesis may also benefit from promotility agents.

6.5.3 Surgical Management

Patients failing maximum medical therapy may be candidates for surgical intervention. Surgery may also be considered for younger patients (less than 40 years old) who would require long-term medical therapy for LPR control.[56] Fundoplication is the primary surgery performed, although there are some newer procedures being investigated to mechanically improve LES tone. In a fundoplication procedure, the upper portion of the stomach (fundus) is wrapped around the lower end of the esophagus. This corrects hiatus hernia and reinforces closure of the LES. Originally introduced by Rudolph Nissen in 1956, the procedure has since undergone many modifications and is now commonly performed laparoscopically. A benefit of fundoplication is that instead of treating just the acidity of refluxate, it decreases all reflux so that exposure to the nonacid components of refluxate can be controlled.

Although early reports suggested that fundoplication is effective in nearly 100% of patients, some have questioned the efficacy of surgery in improving LPR symptoms.[1,69,70] So et al[69] reported that surgical fundoplication was more efficacious in relieving typical GER symptoms (e.g., heartburn) versus atypical LPR symptoms. Swoger et al,[70] in a small prospective case-controlled study, found that only one out of 10 (10%) LPR patients who had failed PPI therapy had improvement of their symptoms after surgical fundoplication. However, most of the evidence appears to support fundoplication in LPR refractory to aggressive antacid therapy.[71,72,73,74,75] Westcott et al[71] found an 84% improvement in 41 patients' RSI scores after a mean follow-up time of 14 months. Rakita et al[74] reported a 67% to 82% improvement in extraesophageal symptoms in 322 patients who underwent fundoplication for moderate to severe LPR. The primary benefit appears to come from the reduction of pharyngeal acidic events, with subsequent improvement in laryngoscopic findings.[73,76] However, structural laryngeal findings, such as vocal fold scar, granuloma, subglottic stenosis, or carcinoma, are not likely to improve after fundoplication alone.[71]

Preoperative MII-pH testing and its prediction of fundoplication success in treating weakly acidic reflux are promising. Mainie et al[75] found good improvement in symptoms for patients whose preoperative symptoms coincided with reflux on MII-pH testing. Del Genio et al[77] also found symptom improvement in patients with negative pH, but positive impedance events after fundoplication.

6.6 What to Do When Treatment Fails

Medical treatment failure can be addressed with surgical intervention, as described above. However, any patient who is not responding to treatment as expected requires a thorough examination, including laryngoscopy, esophagoscopy, esophageal manometry, and/or barium swallow. The clinician should be vigilant for gastric complaints, such as early satiety, dyspepsia, and abdominal pain, which necessitate appropriate referral to a gastroenterologist for sedated esophagogastroduodenoscopy. A different diagnosis, other than LPR or GER, must be considered for any patient failing to respond to appropriate treatment.

6.7 Key Points

- Laryngopharyngeal reflux is common in patients with laryngologic complaints.
- The symptoms of LPR may be caused by direct acid contact with the upper aerodigestive tract epithelium or may be related to esophagovagal reflexes, triggered by esophageal distention.

- Weakly acidic or basic refluxate can be injurious to laryngeal mucosa and may cause LPR signs or symptoms.
- While obtaining a patient history, one should attempt to distinguish LPR from GER, which is considered a different disease entity.
- Common laryngoscopic findings of LPR include laryngeal edema, pseudosulcus formation, erythema, posterior commissure hypertrophy, granuloma formation, and/or excessive endolaryngeal mucus.
- The appropriate level of treatment for LPR is largely dependent upon the severity of disease as well as the impact of LPR on specific patients' lifestyle or occupation.
- The otolaryngologist must formulate an appropriate differential diagnosis for patients with symptoms suggestive of LPR, as there are many other disease processes that share the same symptoms. Particular care should be taken to avoid overdiagnosis as well as overtreatment of mild acid reflux.

References

[1] Koufman JA. The otolaryngologic manifestations of gastroesophageal reflux disease (GERD): a clinical investigation of 225 patients using ambulatory 24-hour pH monitoring and an experimental investigation of the role of acid and pepsin in the development of laryngeal injury. Laryngoscope 1991; 101 Suppl 53: 1–78

[2] Johnston N, Bulmer D, Gill GA et al. Cell biology of laryngeal epithelial defenses in health and disease: further studies. Ann Otol Rhinol Laryngol 2003; 112: 481–491

[3] Book DT, Rhee JS, Toohill RJ, Smith TL. Perspectives in laryngopharyngeal reflux: an international survey. Laryngoscope 2002; 112: 1399–1406

[4] Belafsky PC, Postma GN, Koufman JA. Validity and reliability of the Reflux Symptom Index (RSI). J Voice 2002; 16: 274–277

[5] Ford CN. Evaluation and management of laryngopharyngeal reflux. JAMA 2005; 294: 1534–1540

[6] Ahmed TF, Khandwala F, Abelson TI et al. Chronic laryngitis associated with gastroesophageal reflux: prospective assessment of differences in practice patterns between gastroenterologists and ENT physicians. Am J Gastroenterol 2006; 101: 470–478

[7] Dodds WJ, Dent J, Hogan WJ et al. Mechanisms of gastroesophageal reflux in patients with reflux esophagitis. N Engl J Med 1982; 307: 1547–1552

[8] Schoeman MN, Tippett MD, Akkermans LMA, Dent J, Holloway RH. Mechanisms of gastroesophageal reflux in ambulant healthy human subjects. Gastroenterology 1995; 108: 83–91

[9] Perry KA, Enestvedt CK, Lorenzo CS et al. The integrity of esophagogastric junction anatomy in patients with isolated laryngopharyngeal reflux symptoms. J Gastrointest Surg 2008; 12: 1880–1887

[10] Groome M, Cotton JP, Borland M, McLeod S, Johnston DA, Dillon JF. Prevalence of laryngopharyngeal reflux in a population with gastroesophageal reflux. Laryngoscope 2007; 117: 1424–1428

[11] Postma GN, Tomek MS, Belafsky PC, Koufman JA. Esophageal motor function in laryngopharyngeal reflux is superior to that in classic gastroesophageal reflux disease. Ann Otol Rhinol Laryngol 2001; 110: 1114–1116

[12] Hoppo T, Sanz AF, Nason KS et al. How much pharyngeal exposure is "normal"? Normative data for laryngopharyngeal reflux events using hypopharyngeal multichannel intraluminal impedance (HMII). J Gastrointest Surg 2012; 16: 16–24, discussion 24–25

[13] Wright RA, Miller SA, Corsello BF. Acid-induced esophagobronchial-cardiac reflexes in humans. Gastroenterology 1990; 99: 71–73

[14] Shaker R, Dodds WJ, Ren J, Hogan WJ, Arndorfer RC. Esophagoglottal closure reflex: a mechanism of airway protection. Gastroenterology 1992; 102: 857–861

[15] Schan CA, Harding SM, Haile JM, Bradley LA, Richter JE. Gastroesophageal reflux-induced bronchoconstriction. An intraesophageal acid infusion study using state-of-the-art technology. Chest 1994; 106: 731–737

[16] Koufman JA. Laryngopharyngeal reflux is different from classic gastroesophageal reflux disease. Ear Nose Throat J 2002; 81 Suppl 2: 7–9

[17] Belafsky PC, Postma GN, Koufman JA. The validity and reliability of the Reflux Finding Ccore (RFS). Laryngoscope 2001; 111: 1313–1317

[18] Hickson C, Simpson CB, Falcon R. Laryngeal pseudosulcus as a predictor of laryngopharyngeal reflux. Laryngoscope 2001; 111: 1742–1745

[19] Ulualp SO, Toohill RJ, Hoffmann R, Shaker R. Pharyngeal pH monitoring in patients with posterior laryngitis. Otolaryngol Head Neck Surg 1999; 120: 672–677

[20] Ylitalo R, Lindestad PA, Ramel S. Symptoms, laryngeal findings, and 24-hour pH monitoring in patients with suspected gastroesophago-pharyngeal reflux. Laryngoscope 2001; 111: 1735–1741

[21] Qadeer MA, Swoger J, Milstein C et al. Correlation between symptoms and laryngeal signs in laryngopharyngeal reflux. Laryngoscope 2005; 115: 1947–1952

[22] Hill RK, Simpson CB, Velazquez R, Larson N. Pachydermia is not diagnostic of active laryngopharyngeal reflux disease. Laryngoscope 2004; 114: 1557–1561

[23] Belafsky PC, Postma GN, Koufman JA. The association between laryngeal pseudosulcus and laryngopharyngeal reflux. Otolaryngol Head Neck Surg 2002; 126: 649–652

[24] Hicks DM, Ours TM, Abelson TI, Vaezi MF, Richter JE. The prevalence of hypopharynx findings associated with gastroesophageal reflux in normal volunteers. J Voice 2002; 16: 564–579

[25] Milstein CF, Charbel S, Hicks DM, Abelson TI, Richter JE, Vaezi MF. Prevalence of laryngeal irritation signs associated with reflux in asymptomatic volunteers: impact of endoscopic technique (rigid vs. flexible laryngoscope). Laryngoscope 2005; 115: 2256–2261

[26] Vaezi MF, Qadeer MA, Lopez R, Colabianchi N. Laryngeal cancer and gastroesophageal reflux disease: a case-control study. Am J Med 2006; 119: 768–776

[27] Richter JE. Extraesophageal presentations of gastroesophageal reflux disease. Semin Gastrointest Dis 1997; 8: 75–89

[28] el-Serag HB, Sonnenberg A. Comorbid occurrence of laryngeal or pulmonary disease with esophagitis in United States military veterans. Gastroenterology 1997; 113: 755–760

[29] Bilgen C, Ogüt F, Kesimli-Dinç H, Kirazli T, Bor S. The comparison of an empiric proton pump inhibitor trial vs 24-hour double-probe Ph monitoring in laryngopharyngeal reflux. J Laryngol Otol 2003; 117: 386–390

[30] Park W, Hicks DM, Khandwala F et al. Laryngopharyngeal reflux: prospective cohort study evaluating optimal dose of proton-pump inhibitor therapy and pretherapy predictors of response. Laryngoscope 2005; 115: 1230–1238

[31] Qadeer MA, Phillips CO, Lopez AR et al. Proton pump inhibitor therapy for suspected GERD-related chronic laryngitis: a meta-analysis of randomized controlled trials. Am J Gastroenterol 2006; 101: 2646–2654

[32] Sermon F, Vanden Brande S, Roosens B, Mana F, Deron P, Urbain D. Is ambulatory 24-h dual-probe pH monitoring useful in suspected ENT manifestations of GERD? Dig Liver Dis 2004; 36: 105–110

[33] Merati AL, Lim HJ, Ulualp SO, Toohill RJ. Meta-analysis of upper probe measurements in normal subjects and patients with laryngopharyngeal reflux. Ann Otol Rhinol Laryngol 2005; 114: 177–182

[34] Ulualp SO, Toohill RJ, Shaker R. Pharyngeal acid reflux in patients with single and multiple otolaryngologic disorders. Otolaryngol Head Neck Surg 1999; 121: 725–730

[35] Oelschlager BK, Eubanks TR, Maronian N et al. Laryngoscopy and pharyngeal pH are complementary in the diagnosis of gastroesophageal-laryngeal reflux. J Gastrointest Surg 2002; 6: 189–194

[36] Aslam M, Bajaj S, Easterling C et al. Performance and optimal technique for pharyngeal impedance recording: a simulated pharyngeal reflux study. Am J Gastroenterol 2007; 102: 33–39

[37] Sun G, Muddana S, Slaughter JC et al. A new pH catheter for laryngopharyngeal reflux: Normal values. Laryngoscope 2009; 119: 1639–1643

[38] Wiener GJ, Tsukashima R, Kelly C et al. Oropharyngeal pH monitoring for the detection of liquid and aerosolized supraesophageal gastric reflux. J Voice 2009; 23: 498–504

[39] Chheda NN, Seybt MW, Schade RR, Postma GN. Normal values for pharyngeal pH monitoring. Ann Otol Rhinol Laryngol 2009; 118: 166–171

[40] Wiener GJ, Copper JB, Richter JE et al. Is hoarseness an atypical manifestation of gastroesophageal reflux (GER)? An ambulatory 24-hour pH study. Gastroenterol 1986; 90: A1691

[41] Ossakow SJ, Elta G, Colturi T, Bogdasarian R, Nostrant TT. Esophageal reflux and dysmotility as the basis for persistent cervical symptoms. Ann Otol Rhinol Laryngol 1987; 96: 387–392

[42] Batch AJ. Globus pharyngeus. J Laryngol Otol 1988; 102: 152–158

[43] McNally PR, Maydonovitch CL, Prosek RA, Collette RP, Wong RK. Evaluation of gastroesophageal reflux as a cause of idiopathic hoarseness. Dig Dis Sci 1989; 34: 1900–1904

[44] Ness J, Sontag S, Schnell T. Prevalence of gastroesophageal reflux (GER) in consecutive patients with hoarseness. Gastroenterol 1992; 102: A134

[45] Tauber S, Gross M, Issing WJ. Association of laryngopharyngeal symptoms with gastroesophageal reflux disease. Laryngoscope 2002; 112: 879–886

[46] Koufman JA, Belafsky PC, Bach KK, Daniel E, Postma GN. Prevalence of esophagitis in patients with pH-documented laryngopharyngeal reflux. Laryngoscope 2002; 112: 1606–1609

[47] Poelmans J, Feenstra L, Demedts I, Rutgeerts P, Tack J. The yield of upper gastrointestinal endoscopy in patients with suspected reflux-related chronic ear, nose, and throat symptoms. Am J Gastroenterol 2004; 99: 1419–1426

[48] Reavis KM, Morris CD, Gopal DV, Hunter JG, Jobe BA. Laryngopharyngeal reflux symptoms better predict the presence of esophageal adenocarcinoma than typical gastroesophageal reflux symptoms. Ann Surg 2004; 239: 849–856, discussion 856–858

[49] Johnston N, Knight J, Dettmar PW, Lively MO, Koufman J. Pepsin and carbonic anhydrase isoenzyme III as diagnostic markers for laryngopharyngeal reflux disease. Laryngoscope 2004; 114: 2129–2134

[50] Jiang A, Liang M, Su Z et al. Immunohistochemical detection of pepsin in laryngeal mucosa for diagnosing laryngopharyngeal reflux. Laryngoscope 2011; 121: 1426–1430

[51] Blumin JH, Johnston N. Evidence of extraesophageal reflux in idiopathic subglottic stenosis. Laryngoscope 2011; 121: 1266–1273

[52] Knight J, Lively MO, Johnston N, Dettmar PW, Koufman JA. Sensitive pepsin immunoassay for detection of laryngopharyngeal reflux. Laryngoscope 2005; 115: 1473–1478

[53] Wang L, Liu X, Liu YL et al. Correlation of pepsin-measured laryngopharyngeal reflux disease with symptoms and signs. Otolaryngol Head Neck Surg 2010; 143: 765–771

[54] Wassenaar E, Johnston N, Merati A et al. Pepsin detection in patients with laryngopharyngeal reflux before and after fundoplication. Surg Endosc 2011; 25: 3870–3876

[55] Hunt JF, Yu Y, Burns J et al. Identification of acid reflux cough using serial assays of exhaled breath condensate pH. Cough 2006; 2: 3

[56] Postma GN, Johnson LF, Koufman JA. Treatment of laryngopharyngeal reflux. Ear Nose Throat J 2002; 81 Suppl 2: 24–26

[57] Steward DL, Wilson KM, Kelly DH et al. Proton pump inhibitor therapy for chronic laryngo-pharyngitis: a randomized placebo-control trial. Otolaryngol Head Neck Surg 2004; 131: 342–350

[58] Bove MJ, Rosen C. Diagnosis and management of laryngopharyngeal reflux disease. Curr Opin Otolaryngol Head Neck Surg 2006; 14: 116–123

[59] Chheda NN, Postma GN. Patient compliance with proton pump inhibitor therapy in an otolaryngology practice. Ann Otol Rhinol Laryngol 2008; 117: 670–672

[60] Belafsky PC, Postma GN, Koufman JA. Laryngopharyngeal reflux symptoms improve before changes in physical findings. Laryngoscope 2001; 111: 979–981

[61] Hunfeld NG, Geus WP, Kuipers EJ. Systematic review: Rebound acid hypersecretion after therapy with proton pump inhibitors. Aliment Pharmacol Ther 2007; 25: 39–46

[62] Reimer C, Søndergaard B, Hilsted L, Bytzer P. Proton-pump inhibitor therapy induces acid-related symptoms in healthy volunteers after withdrawal of therapy. Gastroenterology 2009; 137: 80–87, e1

[63] Furuta T, Shirai N, Sugimoto M, Ohashi K, Ishizaki T. Pharmacogenomics of proton pump inhibitors. Pharmacogenomics 2004; 5: 181–202

[64] Fock KM, Ang TL, Bee LC, Lee EJ. Proton pump inhibitors: do differences in pharmacokinetics translate into differences in clinical outcomes? Clin Pharmacokinet 2008; 47: 1–6

[65] Sugimoto M, Furuta T, Shirai N, Ikuma M, Hishida A, Ishizaki T. Initial 48-hour acid inhibition by intravenous infusion of omeprazole, famotidine, or both in relation to cytochrome P450 2C19 genotype status. Clin Pharmacol Ther 2006; 80: 539–548

[66] Tamhankar AP, Peters JH, Portale G et al. Omeprazole does not reduce gastroesophageal reflux: new insights using multichannel intraluminal impedance technology. J Gastrointest Surg 2004; 8: 890–897, discussion 897–898

[67] Koek GH, Sifrim D, Lerut T, Janssens J, Tack J. Effect of the GABA(B) agonist baclofen in patients with symptoms and duodeno-gastro-oesophageal reflux refractory to proton pump inhibitors. Gut 2003; 52: 1397–1402

[68] Vela MF, Tutuian R, Katz PO, Castell DO. Baclofen decreases acid and non-acid post-prandial gastro-oesophageal reflux measured by combined multichannel intraluminal impedance and pH. Aliment Pharmacol Ther 2003; 17: 243–251

[69] So JB, Zeitels SM, Rattner DW. Outcomes of atypical symptoms attributed to gastroesophageal reflux treated by laparoscopic fundoplication. Surgery 1998; 124: 28–32

[70] Swoger J, Ponsky J, Hicks DM et al. Surgical fundoplication in laryngopharyngeal reflux unresponsive to aggressive acid suppression: a controlled study. Clin Gastroenterol Hepatol 2006; 4: 433–441

[71] Westcott CJ, Hopkins MB, Bach K, Postma GN, Belafsky PC, Koufman JA. Fundoplication for laryngopharyngeal reflux disease. J Am Coll Surg 2004; 199: 23–30

[72] Del Genio G, Rossetti G, Brusciano L et al. Laparoscopic Nissen-Rossetti fundoplication is effective to control gastro-oesophageal and pharyngeal reflux detected using 24-hour oesophageal impedance and pH monitoring (MII-pH). Acta Otorhinolaryngol Ital 2006; 26: 287–292

[73] Ogut F, Ersin S, Engin EZ et al. The effect of laparoscopic Nissen fundoplication on laryngeal findings and voice quality. Surg Endosc 2007; 21: 549–554

[74] Rakita S, Villadolid D, Thomas A et al. Laparoscopic Nissen fundoplication offers high patient satisfaction with relief of extraesophageal symptoms of gastroesophageal reflux disease. Am Surg 2006; 72: 207–212

[75] Mainie I, Tutuian R, Agrawal A, Adams D, Castell DO. Combined multichannel intraluminal impedance-pH monitoring to select patients with persistent gastro-oesophageal reflux for laparoscopic Nissen fundoplication. Br J Surg 2006; 93: 1483–1487

[76] Oelschlager BK, Eubanks TR, Oleynikov D, Pope C, Pellegrini CA. Symptomatic and physiologic outcomes after operative treatment for extraesophageal reflux. Surg Endosc 2002; 16: 1032–1036

[77] del Genio G, Tolone S, del Genio F et al. Prospective assessment of patient selection for antireflux surgery by combined multichannel intraluminal impedance pH monitoring. J Gastrointest Surg 2008; 12: 1491–1496

[78] Wise JL, Murray JA. Utilising multichannel intraluminal impedance for diagnosing GERD: a review. Dis Esophagus 2007; 20: 83–88

7 Benign Lesions of the Vocal Folds

Steven M. Zeitels

The management of benign mucosal lesions of the vocal folds was initiated soon after the widespread adoption of mirror laryngoscopy and the origin of laryngology in the mid-19th century.[1,2,3] The introduction of topical cocaine anesthesia[4] in the latter part of that century promoted the development of diagnostic and therapeutic laryngoscopic methods.[5] We experienced a range of surgical innovations in the 20th century that allowed for enhanced precision in surgery of the phonatory mucosa. They included a suspension device,[6] which supported bimanual dissection; the surgical microscope,[7] enabling magnification; general endotracheal anesthesia[8] and laser technology.[9] In the latter part of the 20th century, von Leden[10,11] and Hirano[12,13] championed the integration of physiological principles of glottal sound production into innovative achievements in diagnostic and therapeutic laryngology that were facilitated by laryngeal stroboscopy.[14]

The general otolaryngologist today encounters issues similar to those that 19th century clinicians faced. Typically, a patient presents with voice deficits and is seeking an explanation and/or assistance. The otolaryngologist, prior to designing a plan for restoration of vocal function, will undertake imaging of the vocal folds. Given the relatively low cost and ease of office endoscopy and photo documentation, all patients with voice deficits should undergo office laryngoscopy (flexible and/or telescopic). Stroboscopy should be performed if available. Otherwise, patients should be referred for this evaluation either by a laryngologist or speech-language pathologist if there is persistent hoarseness beyond several weeks. Laryngeal stroboscopy provides the only diagnostic strategy to fully analyze deficits of phonatory mucosal vibration. Except in extreme circumstances of technology unavailability, it is advisable that patients have a stroboscopic assessment prior to undergoing any type of voice-enhancing procedure.

Phonatory epithelium is a delicate membrane that encapsulates the tissues underlying it and reflects the viscoelastic properties, rheology, and vibration characteristics of the subepithelial soft tissues. Optimal laryngeal sound production requires apposition of the vocal fold edges, which are driven into entrained oscillation by the sustained subglottal aerodynamic pressure from the tracheo-bronchial tree. Lesions along the rima glottidis impair entrained oscillation by creating stiffness in the diseased vocal fold and by preventing smooth vocal-edge closure. These factors result in an aerodynamically inefficient glottal valve. Based on the individual circumstances, initial management may include voice rest, voice activity modification, and voice therapy, as well as adjustments in diet and/or medications.

If there is a mass, such as a polyp, cyst, or large fibrovascular nodules, phonomicrosurgery is likely to be the ultimate solution. Phonomicrosurgical procedures are designed to improve aerodynamic efficiency and vocal quality by creating a smooth vocal-fold edge that is not excavated with epithelium that is pliable.[15] The surgical intervention is usually elective and is seldom urgent, and, ultimately, detailed discussions about the operation should be reserved for the surgeon who will perform the procedure.

Given the fact that a majority of benign lesions that result in hoarseness will eventually require surgery to achieve resolution, it is important for the general otolaryngologist to have an overarching understanding of current techniques. All patients considering surgery must be warned that it is possible for the voice to be worse after the surgery. Therefore, the surgeon must have an accurate and realistic assessment of his or her microphonosurgical skills and available equipment. Twenty years ago, most general otolaryngologists performed microsurgery for benign vocal fold lesions. Given the innovations in these procedures, however, and the increasing amount of fellowship-trained laryngologists, consideration of referral to subspecialists is warranted. Patients should also understand that it is very common to identify more pathology during microlaryngoscopy than can be appreciated by videostroboscopy. With the use of telescopes, examination in the operating room provides significantly greater magnification as well as the ability to examine surfaces that are tangential and/or obscured in the clinic exam.

7.1 Polyps

Vocal fold polyps (▶ Fig. 7.1) present in a spectrum of sizes, shapes, and tissue composition. They are typically the result of trauma to the superficial lamina propria (SLP), and most frequently, the microvasculature. Polyps are commonly found in the middle portion of the musculomembranous region because the aerodynamically induced shearing and collision forces on the SLP are greatest in this region. The lesions may be sessile or pedunculated and they may also be vascular, fibrotic, or mixoid. They are often accompanied by aberrant varices and ectasias.

There is great variation in the magnitude of involvement and replacement of the SLP by these lesions. This critical information is initially assessed by stroboscopy in the clinic, as well as by palpation under anesthesia with high-magnification observation. Frequently, a smaller traumatic fibrovascular lesion will be noted on the opposing surface of the contralateral vocal fold. It can be difficult to determine whether the collision trauma from the polyp induced the smaller lesion or whether there were bilateral lesions in which one grew larger. This differentiation is only of academic interest because both lesions should typically be resected if there is palpable tissue alteration.

A 532-nm-pulsed KTP (potassium titanyl phosphate) laser[16] can effectively photocoagulate associated varices, ectasias, and feeding vessels. When resecting polyps, an epithelial cordotomy adjacent to the lesion provides definitive information about the nature of the involvement of the normal SLP and is the initial step in the resection of the lesion. Because the epithelium overlying a sessile polyp is typically normal, all or a portion of it is usually preserved to facilitate rapid healing.[17] Essentially, sessile polyps are being managed similarly to subepithelial cysts. Pedunculated polyps are often amputated by means of retraction and resection with microscissors.

Subepithelial infusion of saline and epinephrine[18,19,20] enhances the precision of the resection of most of these lesions. The infusion places the normal mucosa on tension, which facilitates the epithelial cordotomy. The infusion also increases the depth of the SLP and exaggerates the discrepancy of the normal SLP from the fibrovascular polyp tissue. These factors enhance

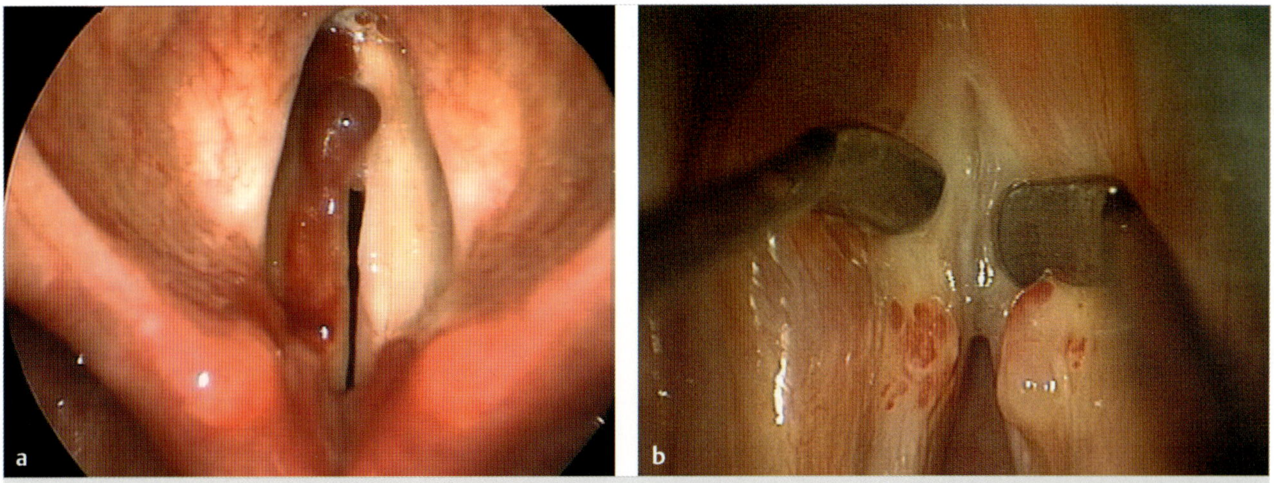

Fig. 7.1 A 50-year-old man, who had sustained severe phonotrauma for many years. (**a**) Office telescopic examination revealed a large polyp of the left vocal fold as well as an acute hemorrhage. (**b**) Microlaryngeal examination one month later revealed large fibrovascular nodules once the sessile polyp was retracted. There were multiple varices and ectasias in both vocal folds.

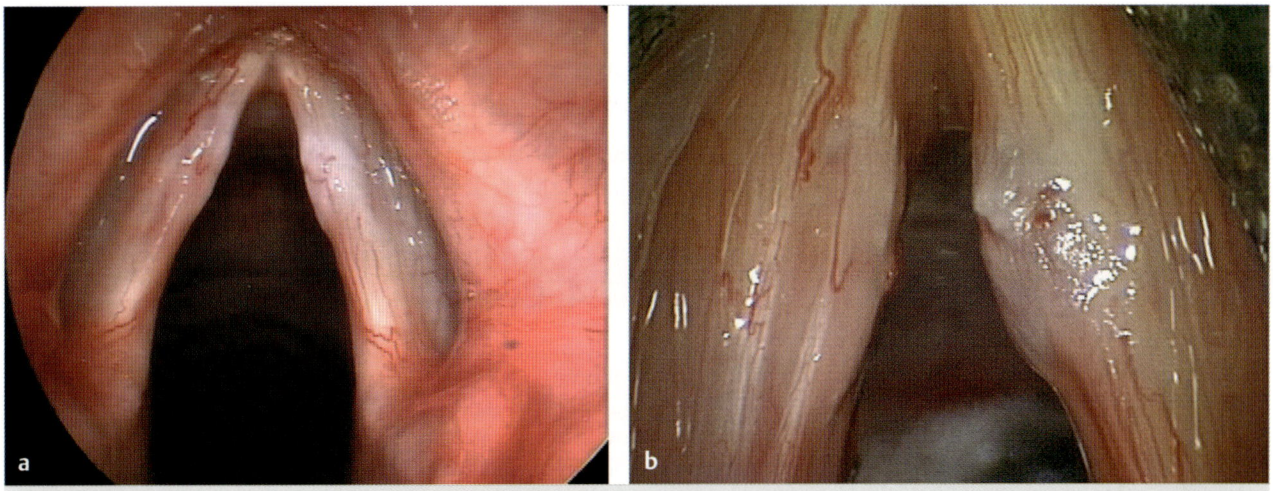

Fig. 7.2 A 25-year-old woman, who is an outgoing aspiring musical-theater performer. (**a**) Office telescopic examination revealed bilateral sessile fibrovascular nodules. (**b**) Microlaryngeal examination revealed large fibrovascular nodules, a sulcus deformity of the left vocal fold, and multiple ectasias and varices.

maximal preservation of normal SLP during the dissection. The epinephrine in the solution as well as the hydrostatic pressure within the Reinke compartment improves hemostasis, which is critical when working at high magnification.

As stated earlier, sessile lesions are ideally removed by means of an epithelial microflap and subepithelial resection of the polyp contents.[16,17,20] Pedunculated lesions with a narrow pedicle are optimally resected by retraction and amputation. The surgeon will need to individualize the resection approach based on pathological presentation. Care should be taken to palpate the component of the polyp that is in the SLP so that it is adequately excised.

7.2 Fibrovascular Nodules

Vocal fold nodules (▶ Fig. 7.2) may present visually and acoustically in a varied manner. There are divergent opinions as to the value of phonomicrosurgical intervention. It is likely that the different opinions about the efficacy of surgical intervention are based (in part) on confusion in the literature as to what constitutes vocal nodules. Remarkably, the most common phonomicrosurgical lesions that we encounter for resection in vocalists are nodules; they are most commonly found in opera singers.[20] There is little disagreement that these lesions are the result of vocal abuse or inappropriate vocal use. Therefore, irrespective of the decision to excise vocal nodules, virtually all of these individuals will benefit from vocal therapy.

Strobovideolaryngoscopy is critical when assessing nodules. High-pitch assessment is necessary to analyze the mechanical effect that fibrovascular nodules have on vocal fold vibration.[20] The nodules may be even better defined if the high-frequency phonatory task is also done with low subglottal pressures so that the patient becomes diplophonic or aphonic with an aperiodic mucosal wave or the acoustic signal ceases. In this setting, stretching the vocal fold physiologically thins any residual SLP that is left under the fibrovascular nodule so that the voice becomes disordered. This type of evaluation also exhibits evidence that surface nodular excrescences frequently have significant unrecognized involvement of the SLP that might not be clinically suspected during stroboscopic examination at a normal pitch frequency. This iceberg effect is found intraoperatively when an epithelial cordotomy is performed.

In most cases, it is advantageous to employ surgery as secondary management. The philosophy regarding surgical intervention is highly individualized to patients and surgeons as well as associated involved professionals, such a speech-language pathologists and voice teachers, who spend the greatest amount of time with the patient. An initial trial of vocal therapy should reduce hyperfunctional behavior and reduce the generalized edema of the SLP that typically accompanies these lesions. Even if the nodules do not resolve and disappear visually, the patient may be satisfied with the quality and stamina of his or her voice such that surgical intervention is not necessary. If the patient desires further improvement, and clear nodules are seen, phonomicrosurgical excision may further enhance vocal quality. The prior vocal therapy will benefit the patient during the postoperative rehabilitative process to prevent injury and recurrence.

The philosophy that "nodules should not be resected despite their continued presence after adequate vocal rehabilitation" arose from unsatisfactory surgical outcomes. In many cases, the trauma induced by the procedure was more deleterious to vocal fold vibration than the lesion itself. This is especially true when the CO_2 laser is used injudiciously and/or small nodules are avulsed or stripped.

Similar to the aforementioned techniques for excising vocal polyps, fibrovascular nodules are optimally removed by means of a subepithelial resection.[20] However, this is technically challenging and is limited by suboptimal hand instrumentation. Cold instruments provide improved precision considering the small size of these lesions and the need for palpation during the procedure. The subepithelial infusion technique must be used selectively. Some nodules that are less well defined visually and by palpation may become obscured by the infusion-induced distension of the SLP.

7.3 Varices and Ectasias

Varices and ectasias (▸ Fig. 7.1 and ▸ Fig. 7.2) of the vocal folds are the result of microvascular trauma within the SLP. The majority of patients with a history of recurrent vocal hemorrhage who require phonomicrosurgical intervention are female vocalists. Many patients will undergo resection of these vascular malformations while the surgeon is excising separate vocal fold pathology, which was the indication for the surgery. Lesions were most frequently noted on the superior surface of the middle musculomembranous vocal fold, which has been termed the *striking zone*. In the 1990s, these lesions were treated by cold-instrument dissection.[21] The 532-nm-pulsed KTP laser has become the treatment of choice because optimal selective photoangiolysis can be achieved with minimal collateral heat to the surrounding SLP.[16]

These superior-surface lesions are generally situated where the lateral extent of mucosal wave excursion would reverse direction. This suggests that these vascular injuries are the result of a deceleration force similar to a whiplash injury. It is believed that the inertial force of the mucosal wave of the SLP and the intralumenal blood of the microvasculature are restricted by the elastic recoil of the tissues and the overlying epithelium. This leads to subepithelial vascular trauma, which is easily visible through the normal translucent epithelium. The cushioning effect of the SLP prevents vessel rupture deeper within the Reinke compartment. The superficial location of the vascular malformations just under the basement membrane facilitates surgical accessibility without significant trauma to the underlying SLP.

If a pulsed angiolytic laser is not available, vascular lesions can be resected by means of cold instruments and multiple epithelial cordotomies. The approach is analogous to a vein stripping of the superficial venous system from the lower extremity to redistribute the aberrant vascularity. It is advantageous to redistribute the susceptible central vascular malformations of the vocal folds out of the striking zone, where they were much more likely to hemorrhage.

Cold-instrument resection is highly successful in preventing recurrent hemorrhage, and despite multiple epithelial cordotomies, there is no postoperative deterioration in vocal function or mucosal wave pliability.[21] This is true even when (1) many incisions are made on the medial vocal fold surface, and (2) virtually all of the patients are singers. Also, patients heal more slowly after CO_2 laser ablation than after cold-instrument resection.

7.4 Cysts

Subepithelial cysts[20,22] (▸ Fig. 7.3) arise in the SLP and present in a variety of sizes. They may be attached to the vocal ligament and/or the epithelial basement membrane. Small cysts may also be freely suspended within the SLP. Small cysts may be confused with nodules if visual examination is performed without stroboscopy, as stroboscopy can help delineate the differences among benign vocal fold lesions. Stroboscopic examination typically reveals a characteristic asymmetric disordered oscillation of the mucosa because of the well-circumscribed stiffness in the area of the cyst. If the cyst protrudes from the medial surface of the glottal edge, a nodule may be observed on the contralateral vocal fold. Asymmetric spheroid masses on the medial surface of the vocal fold should alert the clinician that there may be a cyst on one side.

Most subepithelial cysts probably arise from obstructed ducts within the SLP. They may contain mucus or may be composed of an epithelial rest (similar to a cholesteatoma). On occasion, small ovoid subepithelial masses that are thought preoperatively to be cysts within the SLP are found at microlaryngoscopy to be fibrous masses. These masses are usually firmer to palpation and may be the result an old microvascular injury or a rheumatoid lesion. The subepithelial infusion technique[18,19] is extremely helpful during the phonomicrosurgical resection of well-defined cysts and firm masses within the SLP.

Masses within the SLP should be resected with cold instruments with few exceptions.[20,23] It is not uncommon for the cyst to rupture, especially toward the end of the dissection, while

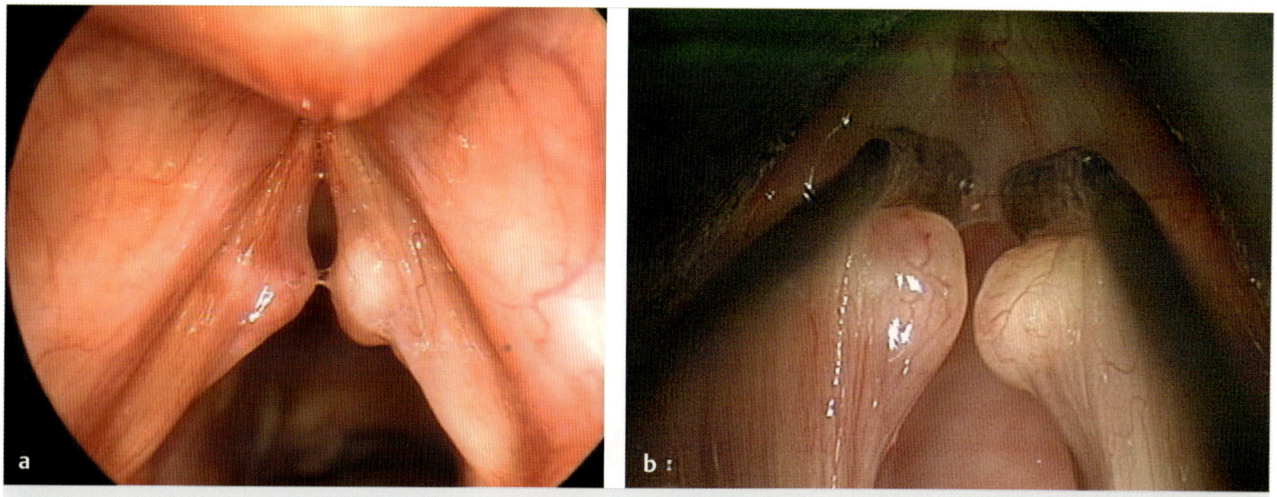

Fig. 7.3 A 42-year-old woman who has been hoarse since childhood and has been overusing her voice throughout her life. (**a**) Office telescopic examination revealed bilateral cysts that were likely congenital. (**b**) Microlaryngeal examination further illustrates the lesions. Curved dissectors are positioned at the anterior commissure to retract the vocal fold soft tissue.

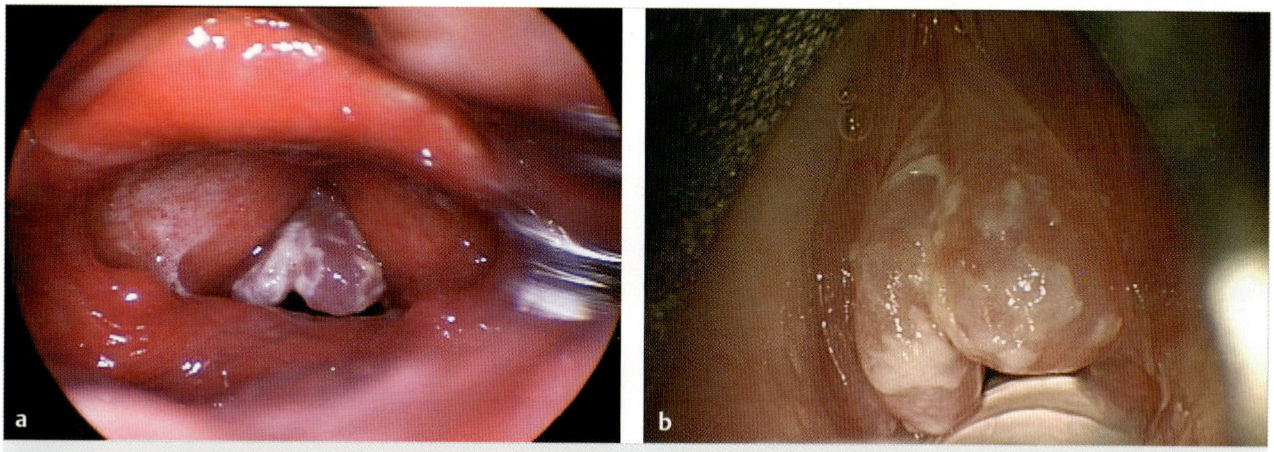

Fig. 7.4 A 52-year-old woman whose conversational voice frequency is ~90 Hz. She is a two-pack-per-day smoker, is obese, and is very talkative. (**a**) Office telescopic examination revealed asymmetric polypoid corditis (Reinke's edema) with diffuse keratosis with dysplasia. (**b**) Microlaryngeal examination illustrates the lesions in more detail.

the surgeon is grasping the fragile wall for retraction. The surgeon must be careful to retrieve the entirety of the cyst wall without undo trauma to the underlying normal SLP. Great care should be taken to minimally disturb any normal SLP and epithelium. This approach will optimize postoperative mucosal-wave oscillation and vocal quality. Although the wave usually improves, it does not typically return to normal if the cyst has already replaced a substantial amount of normal SLP, which will not regenerate. The need for extremely fine, delicate, tangential dissection precludes effective use of the CO_2 laser or other continuous-wave lasers.

7.5 Polypoid Corditis/Reinke's Edema

Polypoid corditis (▸ Fig. 7.4) presents as extensive swelling of the SLP (Reinke's space). The swelling is usually situated on the superior surface of the musculomembranous vocal fold.[24] This entity is another manifestation of vocal-fold pathology that is of multifactoral genesis. The patients typically smoke extensively, have laryngopharyngeal reflux, and demonstrate vocal hyperfunction. The swelling probably occurs from the increased aerodynamic pressures that drive vocal-fold mucosal oscillation in a general environment of glottal mucositis, which is secondary to smoking and reflux. The swelling is typically bilateral, but often asymmetric in volume. Often keratosis with dysplasia is observed.

Individuals with polypoid corditis describe gradual onset of a rough and abnormally low-pitched voice (females: < 130 Hz, males: < 110 Hz) because the mass-loaded folds oscillate at an inordinately low frequency. Women present more frequently than men and undergo phonomicrosurgical management more frequently because of the greater discrepancy from their normal fundamental frequency (180–230 Hz).

Airway symptoms are unusual if the arytenoids abduct normally because the edema is confined to the anterior glottal aperture. Epithelial pliability and mucosal-wave characteristics vary greatly between patients and are dependent on the viscoelasticity of the pathological SLP. Some individuals have hyperdynamic pliable waves and others, who have sustained severe phonotrauma, demonstrate poor pliability and mass motion of the epithelium and pathological SLP. When the edema is extensive, it can potentially obscure an occult malignancy.

Treatment of Reinke's edema begins with elimination of predisposing risk factors. Patients should discontinue smoking, have their reflux controlled, and should undergo preoperative vocal therapy. Systemic or topical steroids are not routinely used to treat Reink'se edema. Patients should be advised that if they continue to smoke, the problem will not resolve without surgery and will likely recur subsequent to surgical resection. Furthermore, extensive edema may prevent the identification of an early malignancy in the office so that some individuals will undergo earlier microlaryngoscopic intervention if keratosis is noted.

Surgery has been the mainstay of treatment for Reinke's edema. Vocal-fold stripping was designed as a one-handed, unmagnified treatment for Reinke's edema by means of a monocular laryngoscope.[25,26] Unfortunately, this procedure is imprecise; frequently, excessive SLP and epithelium are removed. This can result in a prolonged period of healing, and often, stiff scarred vocal folds. Although the vocal folds appear normal on a mirror or fiberoptic exam, stroboscopy reveals loss of epithelial pliability and lack of vibration.

A number of years ago, Hirano[27] described a more precise technique, which involves incising the epithelium and elevating the mucosa as a flap. Then the gelatinous matrix within the SLP is reduced, followed by redraping the flap and trimming the excess mucosa. A microscissor is used for the initial incision unless there is prominent subepithelial vascular injection, in which case a KTP laser can be advantageous. The gelatinous hypertrophied SLP should then be carefully contoured and reduced to a more normal volume. This can be done by suctioning or by direct removal. Great care must be taken not to overreduce the SLP, which results in an inordinately stiff vocal system. The vocal ligament should never be visualized directly. Overreduction of the SLP can result in a severely strained, harsh voice because these individuals already employ high subglottal pressures to drive their floppy mass-loaded folds. Vocally, it is preferable to leave a larger fold than to create a visually pleasing smaller fold.

Once the SLP has been reduced, the epithelium is redraped and trimmed appropriately. There are varied opinions about whether both vocal folds should be worked on simultaneously. Exuberant resection of epithelium and SLP anteromedially may leave two opposed raw surfaces at the anterior commissure, which can lead to web formation. If the incisions and dissection are confined to the superior surface of the vocal folds, bilateral procedures are not associated with complications.[24]

Microflap cytoreduction avoids removing excessive amounts of mucosa, and healing time is therefore shortened. If leukoplakia/keratosis or other suspicious process involves the mucosa, that tissue should also be removed for pathologic examination. This may cause a defect that will lengthen the healing time. After an initial period of vocal rest (~10 days), patients should receive vocal therapy and should be monitored closely. Preventing recurrence is dependent on modification of the predisposing factors, especially smoking.

Control of the medical factors along with surgical resection will usually elevate the fundamental frequency of female patients to approximately 150 Hz, which is commensurate with the normal fundamental frequency for female smokers.[24] Patients should also undergo a course of voice therapy postoperatively because the biomechanics of glottal sound production have been radically altered and patients have become accustomed to phonating with excessive subglottal pressure.

7.6 Summary

Laryngeal and voice problems are universal throughout the world, irrespective of age, gender, or social stratification; benign vocal-edge lesions are the most common problem. These benign phonatory lesions are commonly encountered in a general otolaryngology practice. However, microlaryngeal surgical interventions have evolved into a subspecialty because of extensive recent innovations and the increasing importance of the human voice in communication-based societies. It behooves general otolaryngologists to have access to stroboscopic equipment and to familiarize themselves with state-of-the-art techniques to optimally manage phonatory disorders.

References

[1] Garcia M. Observations on the human voice. Proc R Soc Lond 1855; 7: 397–410

[2] Mackenzie M. The Use of the Laryngoscope in Diseases of the Throat with an Appendix on Rhinoscopy. London: J & A Churchill; 1865

[3] Elsberg L. Laryngoscopal Surgery Illustrated in the Treatment of Morbid Growths within the Larynx. Philadelphia, PA: Collins; 1866

[4] Jelinek E. Das cocain als anastheticum und analgeticum fur den pharynx und larynx. Wien Med Wochenschr 1884; 45: 1334–1337, 1364–1367

[5] Kirstein A. Autoscopy of the larynx and trachea (direct examination without mirror). Philadelphia: F.A. Davis; 1897

[6] Killian G. Die Schwebelaryngoskopie. Archiv Fur Laryngologie Und Rhinologie 1912; 26: 277–317

[7] Scalco AN, Shipman WF, Tabb HG. Microscopic suspension laryngoscopy. Ann Otol Rhinol Laryngol 1960; 69: 1134–1138

[8] Elsberg CA. Clinical experiences with intratracheal insufflation [Meltzer], with remarks upon the value of the method for thoracic surgery. Ann Surg 1910; 52: 23–29

[9] Jako GJ, Kleinsasser O. Endolaryngeal micro-diagnosis and microsurgery. Paper presented at: The Annual Meeting of the American Medical Association; June 26–30, 1966; Chicago, IL

[10] von Leden H, Moore P, Timcke R. Laryngeal vibrations: measurements of the glottic wave: part III. the pathological larynx. Arch Otolaryngol 1960; 71: 16–35

[11] Von Leden H. Laryngeal physiology. Cinematographic observations. J Laryngol Otol 1960; 74: 705–712

[12] Hirano M, Koike Y, Von Leden H. Maximum phonation time and air usage during phonation. Clinical study. Folia Phoniatr (Basel) 1968; 20: 185–201

[13] Hirano M. Phonosurgery: Basic and clinical investigations. Otologia (Fukuoka) 1975; 21: 239–442

[14] Von Leden H. The electronic synchron-stroboscope. Its value for the practicing laryngologist. Trans Am Laryngol Assoc 1961; 82: 200–214

[15] Zeitels SM, Healy GB. Laryngology and phonosurgery. N Engl J Med 2003; 349: 882–892

[16] Zeitels SM, Akst LM, Bums JA, Hillman RE, Broadhurst MS, Anderson RR. Pulsed angiolytic laser treatment of ectasias and varices in singers. Ann Otol Rhinol Laryngol 2006; 115: 571–580

[17] Hochman II, Zeitels SM. Phonomicrosurgical management of vocal fold polyps: the subepithelial microflap resection technique. J Voice 2000; 14: 112–118

[18] Zeitels SM, Vaughan CW. A submucosal true vocal fold infusion needle. Otolaryngol Head Neck Surg 1991; 105: 478–479

[19] Kass ES, Hillman RE, Zeitels SM. Vocal fold submucosal infusion technique in phonomicrosurgery. Ann Otol Rhinol Laryngol 1996; 105: 341–347

[20] Zeitels SM, Hillman RE, Desloge RB, Mauri M, Doyle PB. Phonomicrosurgery in singers and performing artists: treatment outcomes, management theories, and future directions. Ann Otol Rhinol Laryngol Suppl 2002; 190: 21–40

[21] Hochman I, Sataloff RT, Hillman RE, Zeitels SM. Ectasias and varices of the vocal fold: clearing the striking zone. Ann Otol Rhinol Laryngol 1999; 108: 10–16

[22] Burns JA, Hillman RE, Stadelman-Cohen T, Zeitels SM. Phonomicrosurgical treatment of intracordal vocal-fold cysts in singers. Laryngoscope 2009; 119: 419–422

[23] Zeitels SM. Laser versus cold instruments for microlaryngoscopic surgery. Laryngoscope 1996; 106: 545–552

[24] Zeitels SM, Hillman RE, Bunting GW, Vaughn T. Reinke's edema: phonatory mechanisms and management strategies. Ann Otol Rhinol Laryngol 1997; 106: 533–543

[25] Lore JM. Stripping of the vocal cords. Laryngoscope 1934; 44: 803–816

[26] Lore JM. Stripping of the vocal cords. Arch Otolaryngol 1945; 42: 378–383

[27] Hirano M, Shin T, Morio M, Kasuya T, Kubyashi S. An improvement in surgical treatment for polypoid vocal cord: sucking technique. Otologia (Fukuoka) 1976; 22: 583–589

8 Benign Tumors of the Larynx

Sapna A. Patel and Albert L. Merati

Benign tumors of the larynx include papillomas, rhabdomyomas, lipomas, neural tumors, granular cell tumors, hemangiomas, laryngoceles, and saccular cysts. They may appear in any part of the larynx. As with all bulky masses in the larynx, they present with hoarseness, dyspnea, aspiration, dysphagia, pain, otalgia, and/or hemoptysis. In this chapter, we explore each of these pathologies and their management.

8.1 Recurrent Respiratory Papillomata

Papillomas are the most common benign laryngeal tumor and were first differentiated from other laryngeal masses in the late 19th century.[1] Fecurrent respiratory papillomatosis (RRP) is also the most common neoplasia in the larynx in children.[2] The incidence of RRP is 4.6 per 100,000 children and 1.8 per 100,000 adults.[3,4] This benign disease can be quite frustrating to treat due to its unpredictable nature, tendency to recur and spread, and malignant potential, with a 3 to 7% risk of conversion.[5] Typically, there are two main clinical entities of RRP: adult onset and juvenile onset. Based on its bimodal distribution, juvenile onset usually occurs in children younger than 5 years and adult onset usually occurs between 20 to 40 years of age.[6] Although the concepts of adult and juvenile onset are descriptive of the age of onset and give a strong indication of clinical behavior, these characterizations are not always clinically predictive or helpful.

There is great variability in the presentation and clinical course of RRP, making management difficult. It can afflict patients as young as one day old and has been reported in patients as old as 84 years. Of the two clinically recognized entities of RRP, juvenile onset is thought to be the more aggressive. Much of this is outlined in the pediatric laryngology chapter in this volume (see Chapter 21). The earlier the presentation, the more likely it is to require several surgical interventions and the greater likelihood of needing a tracheotomy, due to a greater severity/more aggressive form of the disease and a smaller caliber airway.[7,8,9,10] One study noted that children diagnosed before 3 years of age are 3.6 times more likely to require greater than four surgical procedures per year and are 2 times as likely to have involvement of multiple sites.[3] Usually, in adults, the disease is clinically less aggressive, often with localized or solitary lesions. However, adult-onset disease can present as aggressively as juvenile onset. Another important distinction between the two forms is that juvenile-onset disease is almost twice as likely (30%) of having extralaryngeal spread, compared to the adult form (16%).[3]

Among all benign laryngeal tumors, RRP is the only one with an infectious etiology, the human papilloma virus (HPV). This small nonenveloped DNA virus has over 100 identifiable strains. The two most commonly implicated strains in laryngeal growths are HPV 6 and 11.[11] The latter is linked to a more aggressive form of RRP, one that presents earlier, requires more frequent surgical intervention, is more likely to have extralaryngeal involvement, and thus more often requires a tracheotomy. Long-term results with a 20-year follow-up support this and have also noted a higher incidence of malignant transformation and mortality with HPV type 11.[9,12]

Aside from the strain of HPV, variable outcomes seen with RRP could be linked to one's immune status or acquired factors. Malignant transformation of HPV 6 strain has been noted, with an increased incidence in those previously exposed to radiation. Other potential oncogenic cofactors include smoking, immunologic disturbance, and viral coinfection.[12] Stern et al[13] assessed the role of immune response and noted a significantly decreased CD4/CD8 ratio and lymphocyte response in afflicted children compared to age-matched controls, but the temporal sequence is unclear.

The human papilloma virus has long been known to infect the anogenital tract of both males and females and is considered to be the most commonly sexually transmitted infection. Infected women vertically transmit the virus to their child through their birth canal, thus leading to the theory that children born vaginally in primigravid females with HPV infection are more likely to manifest RRP. Primigravid women tend to experience a prolonged second stage of labor, which increases potential contact time. Kashima et al[14] suggested that newly acquired genital HPV lesions are more likely to shed virus than long-standing lesions. Despite this theory, there are documented reports of RRP manifesting in those born via caesarean section, suggesting a potential for perinatal transfer.[9] The actual incidence of RRP is quite low in comparison with the high prevalence of HPV infection. This suggests a multifactorial nature of transmission, in which one must also take into account patient immunity, length/volume of viral status, local trauma, etc. The course and severity of RRP vary with the strain of virus, which holds true during pregnancy. Disease progression is more likely among pregnant women with HPV type 11, particularly with involvement of lung tissue, rapid growth of papillomas, and more frequent recurrence.[15] Regardless of the stage of disease or the strain of the virus, patients are able to have healthy children.

As with any space-occupying lesion of the larynx, symptomatology is highly variable and depends on the size and location of the lesion. The usual presenting sign is hoarseness and voice changes, but less commonly, one can present with acute respiratory distress due to airway obstruction. In children, the diagnosis is often delayed because voice changes go uninvestigated. Furthermore, other commonly presenting symptoms, such as stridor, result in misdiagnosis as asthma, croup, or other respiratory pathologies. This can lead to a delay in diagnosis on average of 1 year.[16,17] One should obtain information about the age of onset, progression of symptoms, and pertinent medical history regarding previous trauma, surgeries, and infections; as well as perinatal history if obtainable. Slow, progressive dysphonia in a child younger than 5 years should merit further evaluation.

The physical examination should focus on an assessment of the respiratory status and oxygenation. Auscultation with a stethoscope can help localize the tumor based on the type of stridor and breathing patterns. Altering the patient's position usually results in changes in stridor, which can help rule out diagnoses like laryngomalacia. If the patient is clinically stable, a flexible endoscopic examination should be performed to allow for direct visualization of the upper aerodigestive tract. If examination is limited, which often occurs in young children, further evaluation under anesthesia with direct laryngoscopy is advised. This would also allow for histopathologic confirmation of the diagnosis. Visualization of the full extent of the tumor is essential for careful surveillance to monitor progression. Most pediatric patients require general anesthesia owing to their smaller airway and cooperation issues.[6]

On gross examination, the tumors are generally exophytic, but they can also be sessile and velvety (▶ Fig. 8.1); the latter is more common among the adult population. They can be pink to white in color. On microscopic examination, papillomas contain nonkeratinized stratified squamous epithelium surrounding a core of fibrous stroma. There is often abnormal cellular differentiation with some degree of atypia. Usually these occur in juxtaposing areas of squamous and ciliated epithelium. The most common sites include the limen vestibuli, the nasopharyngeal surface of the soft palate, the laryngeal surface of the epiglottis, the ventricle, the undersurface of the vocal folds, the carina, and the bronchial spurs. In decreasing order of involvement, extralaryngeal lesions are found in the oral cavity, trachea, and bronchi.

After identification and diagnosis of the papillomas, proper documentation of the findings is crucial to monitor disease progression. There is no uniformly accepted staging system, but numerous systems have been proposed. One designed by Derkay et al[18] allows for both subjective and objective assessment, combining both functional parameters and evaluation of the full extent of the disease at one or more subsites.

Counseling is of utmost importance for patients and their family. Recurrent respiratory papillomatosis inflicts a heavy emotional burden and require repeated surgeries, and its economic cost is high, estimated at $150 million annually.[3] Furthermore, it can affect the quality of life. One study reported that severely affected patients had lower scores in all dimensions of the SF-36, with greater differences compared to controls in the domains of pain, physical limitation, and energy/vitality.[19]

There should be emphasis on the clinical course and prognosis of RRP, both of which are highly variable. For juvenile-onset RRP, lifetime surgical treatments range from 2 to 179, with significantly more surgeries noted among those diagnosed less than 4 years of age. The mean number of surgical procedures for children per year is 4.4. Current age, rather than age at diagnosis, dictates surgical frequency, as smaller airways require more regular intervention to maintain patency. Children with disease of the upper airway, specifically superior to the larynx, tend to be older and manage disease better.[2] Despite this, the disease is unpredictable, thus frequent office visits and endoscopic exams are required. Patients and/or their families should be educated about signs of disease progression and what requires clinical evaluation sooner, rather than later. Most importantly, there should be particular emphasis on the lack of any single effective curative modality.

Treatment ranges from simple observation to surgical debulking. In some cases, there are no options for management due to the extent of spread within the pulmonary parenchyma. Overall goals of therapy include eradicating gross disease, maintaining the airway, improving the voice quality, minimizing or preventing spread of disease, and decreasing the number of surgical debridements, all while avoiding secondary complications like stenosis. There are multiple ways to surgically remove these tumors, including laser excision, the microdebrider, and the cold knife technique—each has its own advantages and disadvantages. It is important to realize that surgery removes the visible warty growth, but the HPV genome remains in normal-appearing tissue.[20]

Overall, surgical management is very practitioner-dependent regarding type of anesthesia, technique, frequency of biopsy, and whether any imaging is obtained. Some prefer jet ventilation, noting that driving jet pressures approximate those

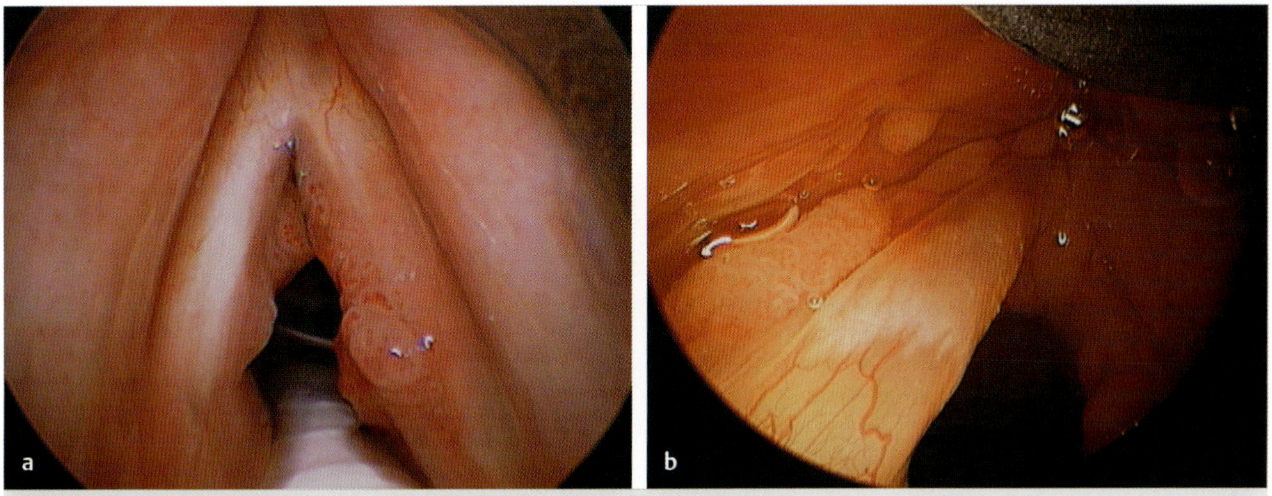

Fig. 8.1 (a) Recurrent respiratory papillomatosis (RRP) on the left vocal fold and in the recess of the left ventricle of a 44-year-old male smoker. The 70-degree telescope allows excellent visualization of the lateral aspects of the ventricles. Also note that this patient has both low-lying (superficial spreading) RRP on the membranous vocal fold and more exophytic papillomata elsewhere. (b) Recurrent respiratory papillomatosis in the anterior commissure area in a 56-year-old man with adult persistence of juvenile-onset RRP. This is a zero-degree operative image demonstrating scarring, anterior webbing (iatrogenic), and scattered RRP.

created during normal respiration, and thus cause no increased harm. An alternative technique is apneic ventilation, which requires repeated insertion and removal of the endotracheal tube. However, this raises concern for possible tracheal seeding of the papilloma. A recent American Society of Pediatric Otolaryngology (ASPO) survey commented on anesthesia management during laryngeal papilloma surgery: 47 (63.5%) preferred spontaneous or apneic ventilation techniques, while 18 (24.3%) preferred jet ventilation.[21]

There is also much debate on how often to perform a biopsy. In the same survey, about one third of respondents obtain a repeat biopsy of the papilloma at every surgery. This is presumably due to concern about the progression from squamous papilloma to papilloma with atypia or possibly to full malignant conversion. In contrast, about half of respondents only perform a repeat biopsy if there has been a change in the growth pattern. The remaining group performs a yearly biopsy or uses some other criteria to dictate whether a biopsy is warranted.[21]

Surgical methods have changed with advances in technology and time. The oldest method utilized for primary surgical excision was cold steel technique, but with newer technologies, it has lost popularity. Many still prefer it, as it avoids potential thermal heat transfer and thus minimizes scarring and damage to healthy surrounding tissue. Unfortunately, one runs the risk of increased blood loss and the potential for losing fragments into the lower airway, resulting in possible seeding.

Laser excision allows for greater precision, thereby limiting secondary damage to the vocal cords and scarring, while also maximizing hemostasis. Furthermore, with a laser, one can employ a defocused mode for debulking by vaporization, and then switch to a focused beam in areas that require precision cutting. Principles of laser surgery must be applied, specifically constant awareness and adjustment of the laser power output, spot size, and duration of exposure to papillomas. One should have constant awareness of the line of demarcation between normal and abnormal tissues and avoid continuous application to the same area and accumulation of char. There should be constant suction/removal of char to avoid overheating tissue, continuous microscopic visual and palpable inspection of both diseased and normal tissue with appropriate instruments, and awareness of the location and extent of disease involvement, especially important functional areas, such as the true vocal cords, false vocal folds, and arytenoid cartilages.

Many different lasers are employed for the management of RRP, including carbon dioxide (CO_2), pulse-dyed laser (PDL), neodymium-doped yttrium aluminium garnet (Nd-YAG), and potassium titanyl phosphate (KTP). The CO_2 laser first became available for use in 1971.[22] With a wavelength of 10,600 nm, this laser has a high absorption for water that enables a precise superficial vaporization and ablation of papilloma tissue with only minimal bleeding. Furthermore, one can use it in an office setting. The downfall of using CO_2 laser therapy for treatment is the need for multiple surgeries because of the superficial thermal effect. This results in greater risk of complications, such as scarring, webbing, and hoarseness, and has the potential for endotracheal tube ignition.[23]

The PDL is nonablative, targets microvasculature, and takes advantage of the 585-nm wavelength, which is one of the two peaks of chromophore of oxyhemoglobin. It is delivered with flexible fiberoptics, which makes it easy to treat hard-to-reach lesions and safe in the office setting.

Also deliverable via flexible fiberoptics, the KTP laser is at a wavelength of 532 nm, close to the other peak of chromophore of oxyhemoglobin. Burns et al[24] suggested that a KTP laser is better than PDL because its target wavelength is closer to the absorption peak of oxyhemoglobin, and the associated extended pulse width results in better clinical efficacy.

Another type that has been employed is the Nd-YAG laser. Its usage has been linked to a lower rate of recurrence (1 treatment per year for each patient) of RRP compared to treatment with a CO_2 laser. The support for this finding is based on the ability of the Nd-YAG laser to provide deeper coagulation, allowing for the destruction of the basal layer of epithelium, which is the origination of papillomatous lesions. The capability of reaching greater depths should be used with caution, as it can also lead to more deleterious effects, such as damaging vocal cord mobility, scarring, or acute postoperative edema with dyspnea.[23]

The endoscopic microdebrider has also grown in popularity and was noted to be the preferred method among ASPO members. This technique is better for larger lesions that require debulking, and for subglottic or tracheal extension where exposure for laser application may be more limited, but it is less advantageous in troublesome areas that require more precision. Several studies have concluded that the use of a microdebrider leads to a shorter operating time, less expense, decreased pain, minimal collateral laryngeal mucosal damage, less thermal trauma, decreased risk to the operative team, and improved voice quality when compared with the CO_2 laser.[25,26] In comparing the various excisional techniques, Schraff et al[21] noted that the microdebrider and carbon dioxide (CO_2) laser were the preferred means for surgical removal of laryngeal RRP, with 39 (52.7%) preferring the microdebrider and 31 (41.9%) the CO_2 laser.

About 20% of patients require adjuvant medical management.[21] The criteria that most practitioners have used for initiation of this are that the patient has had (1) more than four surgical procedures per year, (2) the presence of distal spread of disease, or (3) rapid regrowth with airway compromise.[21]

The most commonly employed treatment is cidofovir, a nucleotide analog, which has been shown to induce apoptosis in HPV-infected cells. Currently, it is approved by the U.S. Food and Drug Administration only for retinitis caused by cytomegalovirus. Its use has been widely published, but there is great variability in the dosing, interval of treatment, duration of treatment, and number of injections. Intralesional cidofovir use was described in 1995.[27] In an extensive literature review of intralesional use of cidofovir for RRP in both adults and children, direct injection into the site of the papillomata was associated with partial-to-complete regression of papillomata, improvement in voice quality and airway status, and decreased need for surgery.[28,29] The recommended intralesional dose of cidofovir in adults is less than 3 mg/kg.[30]

There has been concern about the risk of laryngeal dysplasia among those who receive intralesional cidofovir, but an extensive review noted that the incidence is similar to the rate of spontaneous malignant transformation, which ranges from 2 to 5%. There is speculation that malignant transformation is increased in the presence of smoking or radiation.[31] Other potential routes of administration are intravenous and via nebulizer.

The former use is uncommon for RRP; based on published literature, it has been limited to those with aggressive disease and extralaryngeal spread. There are reported side effects of alopecia and leukopenia, and based on its use in the treatment of CMV retinitis, other systemic side effects, specifically nephrotoxicity and neutropenia, are possible. Thus, if it is used intravenously, many advocate that the administration of oral probenecid and intravenous hydration before and after each cidofovir dose remains important to minimize the risk of these systemic effects. Giles et al[32] reported the effects of nebulized cidofovir for RRP with pulmonary spread, noting that the lesions responded and diminished in size; the course, however, was complicated by hemoptysis, which resolved when the dose of cidofovir was reduced.

Regardless of the route of administration of cidofovir, the side effects should not be forgotten. They include a cutaneous rash, headache, compromised airway, and disorders of hematologic and chemical parameters in blood, such as neutropenia and elevated liver enzymes, if used systemically; localized injection can lead to local inflammatory response and vocal cord scarring. Most advocate monitoring blood cell counts, kidney function, and liver studies prior to and during treatment with cidofovir.[30]

Interferon therapy was popular in the early 1990s, with 9% of children with RRP receiving the drug.[33] However, its use has now declined to less than 4%. This decrease is likely a combination of its unfavorable side-effect profile, which includes hepatic and renal dysfunction as well as spastic diplegia, rapid recurrence noted after discontinuation of therapy, and overall mixed clinical success, with a 30 to 60% complete response rate.[21,34] The varied success rate may be related to the strain of HPV, as one study noted a better response among cases infected with HPV 6 compared to those infected with HPV 11 or those that were HPV negative.[35] Theories regarding its mechanism of action include its influence on estradiol metabolism, or that it binds to a cell-specific receptor, which leads to a special transcription that makes the cells viral resistant. Alpha-interferon can be administrated intramuscularly, intravenously, or subcutaneously. The dose is increased gradually to a target of 3 MU/m^2 body surface daily for a month, and then reduced to 3 times per week for at least 6 months. The proposed dose for children weighing less than 25 kg is 100 to 200 mg daily.[16]

Due to the microvascularity of RRP, many believe that vascular endothelial growth factor (VEGF) plays a role in the progression; a commonly used inhibitor of VEGF for ophthalmologic neovascular growth is bevacizumab (monoclonal immunoglobulin), and it has been used off label as an adjunct to KTP laser therapy of RRP. Zeitels et al noted that it is safe locally and systemically; they concluded that there was a statistically significant reduction in lesions in those treated with adjuvant bevacizumab.[24]

Photodynamic therapy has also been explored. Hematoporphyrin derivative or HPD had less promising results, but preliminary results with a newer agent, meso-tetra hydroxyphenylchlorin (mTHPC), showed remission after a single treatment in six out of seven patients. For the remaining patient, who had extralaryngeal spread, improvement was noted.[34]

Further research into the molecular pathways of HPV-infected cells led to the discovery of differences in the cyclooxygenase 2 (COX-2) signaling cascade. This suggested a new potential target for treatment. Currently, there is a multiinstitutional study to assess the effects of COX-2 inhibitors in RRP patients—both adults and children.[6]

Other less commonly employed therapies include ribavarin, which was noted to lead to greater intervals between surgeries in a small Minnesota-based study, and cimetidine, which has conflicting results regarding its efficacy.[36] Preventative and therapeutic vaccines are objects of growing interest, especially the quadrivalent HPV vaccine. The vaccine promotes immunity against four of the common strains of HPV, including type 6 and type 11. It is theorized that increased use of the vaccine could result in transplacental transfer of antibodies and thereby prevent or ameliorate the severity of RRP.[34]

For some, disease extent may be so severe that a tracheotomy is necessary. Incidence of tracheotomy ranges from 1.6 to 64%.[37] Some believe that tracheotomy results in spread to the trachea, bronchi, and lungs; others feel that more aggressive disease warrants tracheotomy and the severity of the disease alone would have resulted in extralaryngeal spread.[38,39,40,41] Regardless, most advocate avoidance of a tracheotomy unless it is absolutely necessary.[42] If it is performed, decannulation should be considered as soon as the disease is managed effectively.

All surgical treatments have the potential for complications. These include stenosis, webbing, recurrence, vocal cord scarring, granulation tissue formation, tracheal perforation, tracheo-esophageal fistula, respiratory arrest, bronchitis, pneumonia, pneumothorax, hemorrhage, and death. In a published case series of laser management of RRP, there was a linear relationship between the number of complications and the frequency of laser microlaryngoscopies.[43] Death is a possibility; close to 50% of responding ASPO practices have had at least one patient with RRP die, with 89% of 25 deaths due to direct RRP-related causes, such as progressive pulmonary disease, anesthesia-related complications, or malignant transformation of disease. The remaining three patients died of causes possibly related to RRP. Thirty-one (50.0%) of the 62 practices reported that a patient with RRP had died under their care.[21]

When performing any surgical excision, it is wise to leave minimal amounts of papilloma at sites where irreparable scarring may occur, especially at the anterior commissure and the posterior glottis. Often, patients are placed on antireflux medications to minimize soft tissue inflammation in the post-surgical setting. Regardless of what technique is employed or what postoperative management is followed, the goals of the surgery should be maintained, and one should be open to leaving residual disease behind rather than causing potential damage to the vocal folds.

8.2 Rhabdomyoma

Rhabdomyomas, compared to their malignant counterpart, are very rare, with less than 50 reported cases arising from intrinsic laryngeal musculature.[44] The term *rhabdomyoma* was introduced by Zenker in 1864.[45] The tumors are classified as cardiac and extracardiac; the latter originate from the mesoderm of branchial arches. Extracardiac rhabdomyomas are further classified into fetal, genital, and adult types based on the histologic differentiation of their skeletal muscle components. The fetal type can be cellular or myxoid. Adult and fetal types show no clinical difference when found in the larynx.[44,45,46]

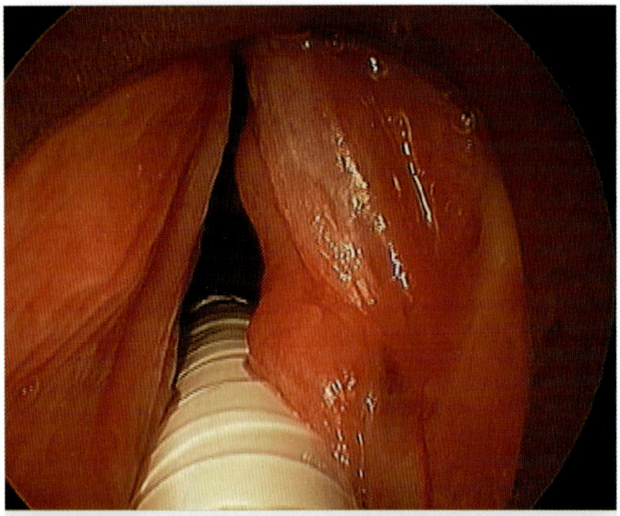

Fig. 8.2 Rhabdomyoma in a 60-year-old male smoker. The lesion is hanging from the right vocal fold; the vocal fold itself is abnormal due to tobacco use and other irritants.

Over 90% of the adult type are found in the head and neck region, particularly the larynx and pharynx.[44] There is a predilection in males, and it is usually diagnosed in the fifth decade, but has been reported in 8- to 85-year-olds. A majority of the lesions are solitary.[47] Currently, there are no reports of malignant transformation of the adult form.[44]

Symptoms at time of presentation, like those of other tumors of the larynx, vary widely based on the size and location of the lesion. They include globus sensation, painless neck mass, dysphagia, dyspnea, dysphonia, cough, and stridor.[48,49] The duration is typically long due to their benign nature. Both computed tomography (CT) and magnetic resonance imaging (MRI) are useful to evaluate the full extent of the tumor and multifocality, if present.[44]

On gross appearance, the tumors are soft, often lobulated, and can be reddish brown or gray (▶ Fig. 8.2). Histologic appearance shows large polygonal or ovoid cells with eosinophilic cytoplasm. According to Liang et al, unlike their malignant counterparts, these lesions have well-circumscribed margins, absence of invasion of surrounding soft tissues, and a submucosal location.[46,48]

Many of the earlier descriptions of rhabdomyomas actually may have been reports of granular cell tumors, which represent the main differential diagnosis.[50] Granular cell tumors are distinguished from rhabdomyomas based on the lack of cross striations and immunohistochemical staining.[51] According to Helliwell et al, granular cell tumors do not stain for desmin or myoglobin like rhabodmyomas.[45,52]

Surgical excision is curative, whether endoscopic or through an open transcervical approach. Recurrence rates up to 40% have been reported, often months to years after excision due to their slow progressive growth.[44] Kapadia et al[53] noted that recurrences are most commonly associated with incomplete excision and have been reported to occur in more than one-third of cases. Follow-up must be long term, as recurrence can occur after as long as 35 years. Tumor recurrence also should alert one to the possibility of rhabdomyosarcoma.[46,53]

8.3 Lipomas

With fewer than 115 cases reported in the medical literature, laryngeal lipomas are another rare entity.[54] Clinically, they do occur more frequently in the pharynx and upper esophagus. They represent 0.1 to 0.6% of all benign laryngeal tumors.[55,56] They usually present in adults during the fourth to fifth decade, and are rarely seen in the pediatric population.[57,58]

Adipose tissue is a natural component in the area of the vestibular fold. Based on their origination, a majority of lipomas arise from the supraglottis, particularly the aryepiglottic folds, epiglottis, and laryngeal vestibule. The tumors can be submucosal or polypoid.[59]

Similar to rhabdomyomas, lipomas are slow-growing tumors that can present with various symptoms due to mass effect, with obstruction and compression on surrounding structures. Symptoms are similar to those seen with other masses of the larynx, and duration is also variable, from months to years.

On examination, the tumors usually appear as solitary, smooth masses, pedunculated or sessile, which are often confused with retention cysts and laryngoceles. If multicentric, they are often associated with syndromes like neurofibromatosis, Gardner syndrome, Launois-Bensaude syndrome, Madelung disease, and Dercum disease.[58] Once there is suspicion of a laryngeal tumor, imaging is often used to determine its true extent, with characteristic findings of a homogenous, low-attenuated tumor with few septations. Magnetic resonance imaging allows for better visualization of the margins, and the adipose composition is well appreciated on T1-weighted images.[54]

The main differential diagnosis of lipoma is its malignant counterpart, liposarcoma.[59] Histologic evaluation is required, as both appear similar on gross examination.[54] Lipomas are well encapsulated and consist of mature adipocytes, which can often exhibit secondary changes, such as hemorrhage, calcification, cyst formation, fat necrosis, and infarction. There can also be other mesenchymal components mixed with the adipocytes, such as mucoid substances in myxlipomas, vasculature in angiolipomas, or fibrous connective tissues, as with fibrolipomas.[59] Liposarcomas, however, tend to be infiltrative and have cytological evidence of atypia, pleomorphism, and lipoblasts.

Surgical removal can be curative if it is complete.[58]This can be performed endoscopically or via an external approach, with the latter reserved for larger tumors. Recurrences have been reported in about 5% of patients.[54] They are more common when the lipoma is associated with generalized lipomatosis, when the mass is not completely removed during a previous surgery, or when the tumor is a well-differentiated liposarcoma incorrectly diagnosed as a benign lipoma.[58,59,60]

8.4 Neural Tumors

Neurogenic tumors of the larynx comprise a wide variety of lesions. A majority of the tumors are neurinomas, which are also known as neurilemommas and Schwannomas. They are clinically and histologically different from neurofibromas.[61,62]

Both neurinomas and neurofibromas originate from Schwann cells, but there are a few key differences between the two lesions. Neurinomas are usually solitary, encapsulated, and rarely undergo malignant sarcomatous change. Neurofibromas, however, are more likely to be multiple and nonencapsulated and to undergo malignant transformation in about 12% of cases.[63] Neurinomas are rarely associated with neurofibromatosis 2, unlike neurofibromas. Histologically, they are different as well, in that neurinomas are attached to or surrounding the nerve, while neurofibromas occur within the sheath.

Laryngeal neurinomas account for 0.1% of all benign tumors. The lesions are more frequently observed in patients between 25 to 50 years and have a slight female preponderance.[63,64] Despite their close proximity to nerves, neural deficits usually are not observed, as they remain extrinsic to the fascicles. Most laryngeal neurinomas are found in the supraglottis, usually involving the A-E folds.[56,65] Based on their typical location, most presume the nerve of origin is the internal branch of the superior laryngeal nerve.[66] There has been report, however, of vocal cord paralysis in the setting of this lesion, suggesting involvement of the recurrent laryngeal nerve.[67] Usually, impaired vocal cord mobility is noted on the affected side, but normal mobility has also been seen.[68,69] The tumors tend to be submucosal. There are two distinct histological types based on the arrangement of the cellular components, Antoni A and Antoni B, with the former having a more organized array. Neurinomas are more likely to become cystic, hemorrhagic, hyalinized, or calcified as they enlarge.[63] Diagnosis with biopsy is often difficult due to the solid capsule. Incomplete resection can lead to rapid regrowth.[70]

Laryngeal neurofibromas commonly involve the aryepiglottic folds and arytenoids, both of which are rich in terminal nerve plexuses.[61] These tumors are round, white lesions that are attached to the neural sheath. Generally, they are unencapsulated, and they tend to be intertwined with the parental nerve fascicles. Histologically, one finds prominent collagen fibers with numerous mast cells. There are three potential patterns: plexiform, diffuse, or a combination of the two. Per Supance et al, women are more likely to be affected than men.[71] Due to the tumor's slow growth, the duration of symptoms can last up to years. Most are solitary and sporadic, but they can be multifocal and up to 50% of cases are associated with von Recklinghausen disease.[72] Imaging is often obtained, with MRI being superior due to its soft tissue characterization. An infiltrative nature is associated with a higher likelihood of recurrence.[73,74] Close follow-up is necessary to monitor for potential malignant transformation, which is often characterized by an increase in size and pain.[61]

Paragangliomas of the larynx are fairly rare; they were first reported in 1955 by Blanchard and Saunders, but since then over a 100 reports have been published in the literature.[75] These benign tumors, usually occur in the fourth to sixth decades of life with a female preponderance.[76] They are slow-growing submucosal lesions that are highly vascularized. Histologically, one finds a combination of chief and sustentacular cells arranged in a Zelballen pattern.

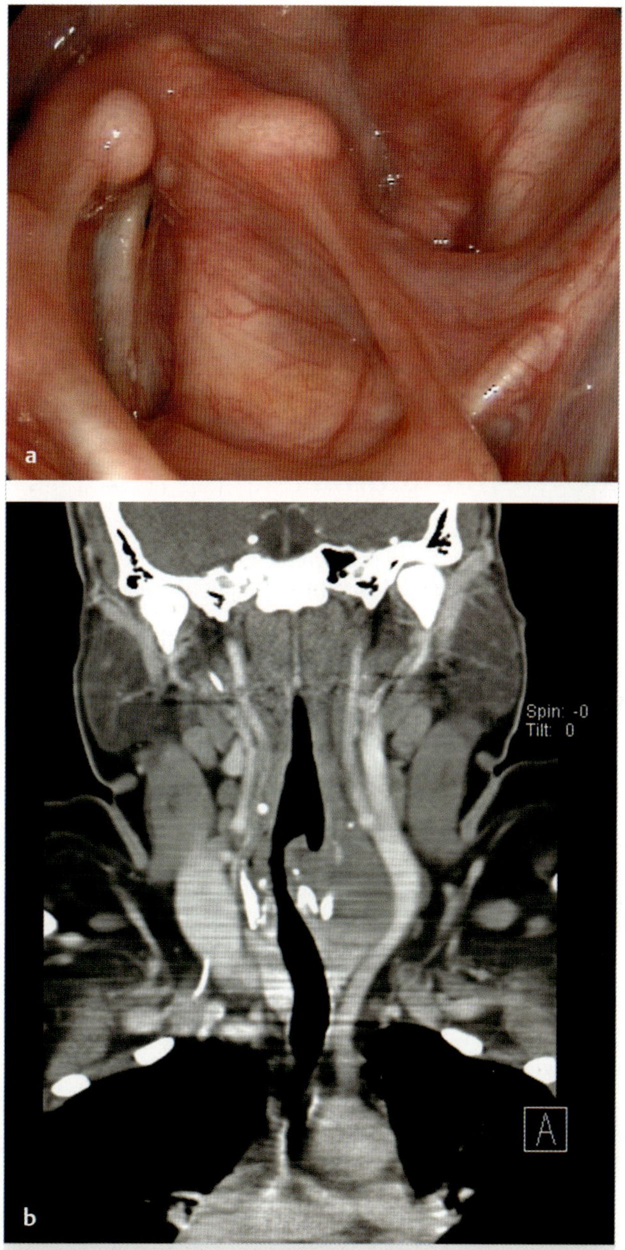

Fig. 8.3 (**a**) Endoscopic exam and (**b**) coronal computed tomography scan of granular cell tumor in the left posterior paraglottic space in a 33-year-old female. This tumor was quite large and extended out to the deep neck, displacing the carotid. It was removed with a partial laryngectomy.

8.5 Granular Cell Tumors

Granular cell tumors have a predilection for females and are most common among the African American population. The typical location in the larynx is the posterior third of the true vocal cords (▶ Fig. 8.3). They are usually solitary lesions, but multiple satellite nodules are seen in up to 15% of cases.[77] Although they usually present between the third and sixth decades of life, these tumors can occur in the pediatric population, where they generally involve the anterior larynx and subglottis.[78]

Initially, many thought that these tumors originated from skeletal muscle, but now most acknowledge that they derive from Schwann cells.[79] Grossly, these are pink firm masses that present, on average, within 7 months of symptoms. They are well-circumscribed, unencapsulated lesions with large polygonal cells that consist of periodic acid-Schiff and Sudan black B positive granules, which represent lysosomes. These tumors stain positive for S-100 and neuron-specific enolase.[80] In at least 50% of cases, the overlying epithelium has pseudo-epitheliomatous hyperplasia.[81,82] This often causes confusion with squamous cell carcinoma, which is the most common differential diagnosis.

Surgical excision is the mainstay for treatment, as these tumors are radioresistant.[79] There are varied rates of recurrence, ranging from 2 to 20%.[78,82,83] Regardless of the true percentage, recurrence is possible. Thus, follow-up with long-term surveillance is recommended, with both clinical examination and MRI.[78] The presence of a positive margin does not guarantee tumor recurrence; so conservative resection is recommended, with repeat excision as needed.[81] Malignancy is present in less than 5% of these tumors and is identified by cellular histology. Suspicion for malignancy arises in masses that are greater than 4 cm, have rapid growth, have recurred, or have infiltrated into surrounding tissue.[78,84]

8.6 Hemangiomas

The first description of hemangiomas was by Mackenzie, but they were not further distinguished into the two common forms, infantile and adult, until 1921. Adult hemangiomas were noted to be sharply demarcated, located in the supraglottis, typically cavernous, and projected or pedunculated, while infantile hemangiomas were in the subglottis, purplish or bluish, capillary, and sessile. The distinction between capillary and cavernous is made histologically based on the caliber of the vascular channels, with the former appearing similar to capillaries while the latter are much larger.

Hemangiomas are self-involuting endothelial cell tumors that can be cutaneous or found within the airway. Infantile laryngeal hemangiomas are one of the most common neoplasms of the infant airway, with females being two times more likely to be affected.[89]They are rarely diagnosed in newborns and 12-month-olds; most will present during the first 6 months of life.

In the past, infantile hemangiomas of the larynx were referred to as *subglottic hemangiomas*. Although most infantile hemangiomas were isolated to the subglottis, 15% percent were diffuse and widespread in their distribution, mirroring the patterns of hemangiomas found on skin. These diffuse lesions, unlike the focal lesions, were usually associated with a segmental hemangioma of the face. The *airway hemangiomas* may therefore be focal, as in isolated subglottic hemangiomas, or they may be segmental, usually transglottic, with possible extension into the trachea, where mucosal staining is seen (▶ Fig. 8.4 and ▶ Fig. 8.5).[90] About 30% of infants with segmental hemangiomas will have associated PHACES (posterior fossa malformations–hemangiomas–arterial anomalies–cardiac defects–eye abnormalities–sternal cleft and supraumbilical raphe syndrome) syndrome and will therefore need to be further investigated for this.[91]

The natural history of hemangiomas includes progressive airway obstruction during the proliferative phase, followed by resolution during the involutive phase.[89] Involution may take many years to complete, but as it takes place in a rapidly expanding airway it will usually relieve airway obstruction symptoms by 18 to 24 months of age.[90] Histologic examination of infantile hemangiomas reveals high rates of mitosis of endothelial cells during the proliferation stage, followed by apoptosis and fibrofatty replacement during involution. The proliferation stage is characterized by increased fibroblast growth factor and increased vascular endothelial growth factor. Involution is characterized by apoptosis, inhibition of angiogenesis, increased amounts of mast cells, and tissue inhibitor metalloproteinase.[88]

Infants usually have a normal voice and normal swallowing, with a croup-like cough and/or biphasic stridor. Due to the gradual onset and nonspecific symptoms, infants are often misdiagnosed with croup or another upper respiratory illness, thus delaying the true diagnosis. Up to 50% of cases will have associated cutaneous hemangiomas, so physical exam findings of cutaneous hemangiomas should raise suspicion for laryngeal hemangioma.[89,93,94] Because the subglottis is the narrowest part of the infant airway, if they are large enough, these lesions can cause airway obstruction and even death. Respiratory distress

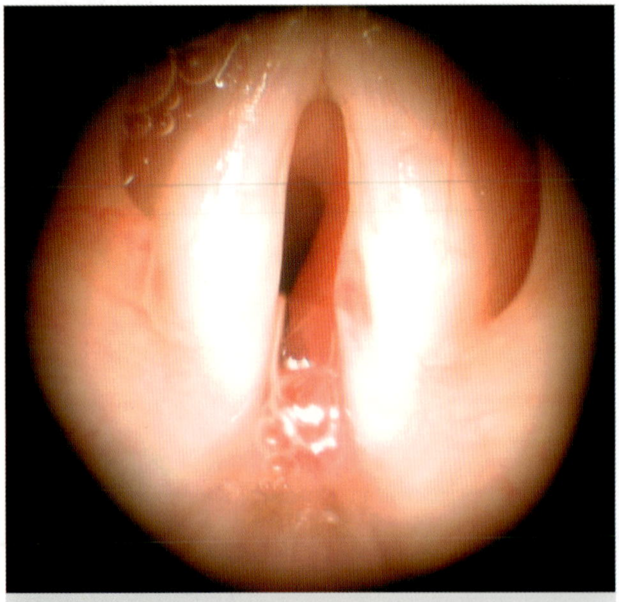

Fig. 8.4 Direct laryngoscopic image of a focal subglottic hemangioma on the right side in an infant.

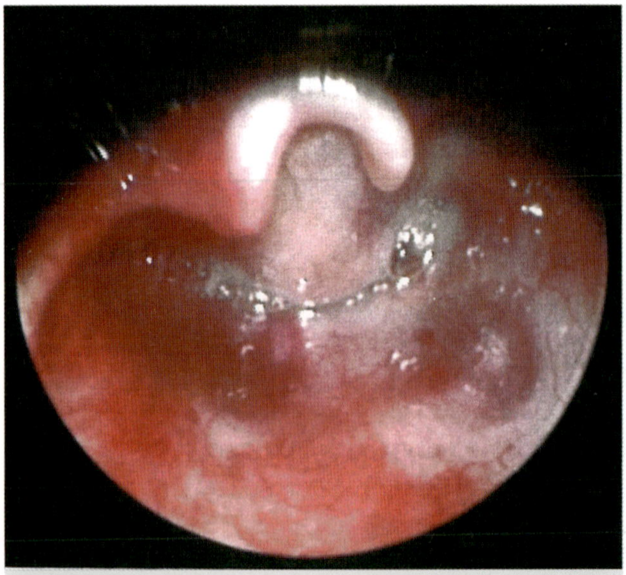

Fig. 8.5 Direct laryngoscopic image of a segmental hemangioma in an infant who also had a segmental facial hemangioma. (Courtesy of Teresa Min-Jung O, MD, and Milton Waner, MD.)

is variable, as it is aggravated by excitement and ameliorated by rest.[92]

If there is suspected a hemangioma based on clinical presentation, further examination is warranted. One must use caution when performing a flexible endoscopic examination to avoid any acute respiratory distress. For infants, examination under general anesthesia using endoscopy is recommended; the infant should be allowed to breathe spontaneously. Diagnosis is based on clinical and endoscopic findings. Focal airway hemangiomas present as a submucosal mass and can be red or blue, depending on the thickness of the overlying mucosa and the degree of vascularity. These lesions are usually unilateral but can be posterior or circumferential; they are rarely found in the anterior subglottis.[89] Segmental airway hemangiomas have, invariably, red staining of the mucosa where the disease is superficial, and the deeper components can be appreciated by their mass effect. Biopsy provides histological confirmation, but it is rarely employed due to the risk of hemorrhage.[92]

For infantile hemangiomas, the goals of treatment are to maintain the airway, to prevent compromise, especially during the proliferative phase, and to minimize long-term sequelae. For cases with less severe symptoms, observation is recommended because many of the lesions will spontaneously involute.[92] Current treatments are aimed at temporarily relieving airway obstruction or transiently decreasing tumor size until normal resolution occurs with spontaneous involution. Preoperative CT angiography is commonly obtained to create a high-resolution three-dimensional image of the lesion that allows for individualized treatment plans. Initial evaluation with direct microlaryngoscopy using laryngeal distending forceps is helpful to accurately identify the true extent of the tumor.[91]

Numerous methods have been used to treat hemangiomas including radiation, cryotherapy, and tracheotomy with observation. Hemangiomas are known to be radioresponsive, but regression may not be appreciated until a year after treatment.[95] Furthermore, response to treatment tends to decrease with increasing age.[96,97] Also, radiation therapy can predispose to other malignancies and is unpredictable with regard to lesion resolution. Therefore, it was abandoned in the 1970s.[88] Cryotherapy was difficult to apply, was unpredictable with respect to tissue depth penetration, and had associated subglottic stenosis, so it has been abandoned as well.[88,98] Tracheotomy with observation was first reported in 1940. It is generally not recommended unless there are multiple lesions located in the glottis or supraglottis, or if there is a contraindication to other therapies.[88]

With technologic advances, laser excision and ablation have become popular. Regardless of what type of laser is used, caution should be employed to avoid burning surrounding structures. In 1970, Simpson et al reported their first treatment of subglottic hemangioma with the CO_2 laser.[99] Usually, multiple treatments are required. This type of laser is more effective for cutting rather than for coagulation due to its wavelength. Random bursts, rather than a continuous mode, are recommended to avoid overheating the tissue. Of note, there is a case series reporting a 20% incidence of subglottic stenosis among those treated with CO_2 laser excision of their subglottic hemangiomas.[89]

The Nd-YAG laser has also been employed for hemangiomas. Its low tissue absorption allows for deeper penetration. This results in treatment of a large tissue volume, which leads to more tissue necrosis compared to other lasers.[100] The KTP laser has been explored as well; it is delivered via fiberoptic fibers, which allows for greater precision. Its downfalls include obscured visibility with blood and debris and loss of depth perception, as one must use monocular vision with this technique.[101] Both the KTP and the Nd-YAG lasers are critiqued for their deeper penetration, resulting in potential thermal damage to the surrounding cartilage, but their preferential absorption of hemoglobin based on their respective wavelengths and their minimal disruption of the overlying mucosa are advantageous in decreasing the risk of scarring and subglottic stenosis, both of which are complications often seen with CO_2 laser therapy.[100,102,103] Regardless of which laser is used, the techniques and success are user dependent, and careful monitoring postoperatively is needed due to increased edema from thermal trauma.

Open surgical excision has been widely reported, with stenosis noted more commonly among bilateral and circumferential lesions. Often, an anterior cricoid split is done to minimize this risk. Also, patients require at least a week-long intubation after excision.[102]

Medical therapy is commonly used, but it is difficult to attribute any success to it because these lesions have a spontaneous involution phase. Steroids were previously popular; they function by blocking estradiol receptors, which stimulate endothelial cell proliferation. Systemic administration of steroids is used infrequently because they have variable effects on airway hemangiomas at the cost of multiple side effects, including growth retardation, Cushing syndrome, and immunodeficiency. If steroids are tried, the recommended dose is 2 to 3 mg/kg/d of prednisone.[88] Results are usually seen after a few weeks of treatment; if no response is noted, the steroid dose should be tapered quickly and other treatment modalities should be explored. Intralesional injection is more effective, but it still has an unpredictable response, ranging from 30 to 60%.[88,102] Treatment is required for at least 6 months before any resolution is noted. For this form of administration, repeated endoscopies under anesthesia are required.

Interferon 2-alpha inhibits endothelial cell migration and angiogenesis. Improvement in the size of the hemangioma is biphasic, with initially rapid diminishment followed by a slower phase. According to Anger et al, abrupt disruption can cause a rebound of symptoms.[104] Subcutaneous injection of interferon alpha has been utilized, as its treatment in cervicofacial and life-threatening hemangiomas has been effective.[88] However, there is a wide range of side effects with interferon therapy. Neurotoxicity, usually in the form of spastic diplegia, is the most severe, and it is noted with prolonged use. It is seen in 5 to 20% of cases.[88] Due to the unacceptable morbidity associated with this medication, interferon 2-alpha use has been abandoned for the treatment of hemangiomas and should only be considered in life-threatening cases where there is no alternative.

The newest therapy to be reported is the use of propranolol, which allows for the avoidance of surgery, decannulation, and tapering off of steroids. In a reported case series, all patients underwent a baseline electrocardiogram and blood-pressure assessment.[105] Since it is a newer therapy, there are many questions yet to be answered, including the ideal dose, how it should be administered, if other beta blockers are effective, what the appropriate length of therapy is, and whether the dose should be tapered. Doses should be given with meals to minimize risk of hypoglycemia. In one of the published case series, six out of the seven patients had resolution of their hemangiomas despite failing systemic steroids, intralesional steroids, and surgery; the remaining patient underwent surgical excision and the lesion turned out to be a pyogenic granuloma.[105]

Adult vascular malformations tend to be more common in men. They rarely progress to the point of respiratory distress.[85] These lesions can occur at any age and are usually found in the glottis or supraglottis. They are commonly cavernous and rarely involute. Unlike infantile hemangiomas, they are much slower to grow, so treatment is often conservative.[106] It is important to rule out any extralaryngeal involvement.[107] Angiography and MRI are useful to confirm the extent of the lesion.[108]

With adult lesions, because most are cavernous, management goals are to reverse or to minimize any functional impairment, pain, hemorrhage, thrombocytopenia, and high-output status. Malignancy should be suspected for lesions that present outside the clinical norm, as development of hemangiosarcoma from a subglottic hemangioma that was excised, yet had multiple recurrences requiring repeat excisions, has been reported in an adult.[106] Treatment methods utilized for infantile hemangiomas can be used for the adult forms if needed, but most can usually be managed conservatively with observation.

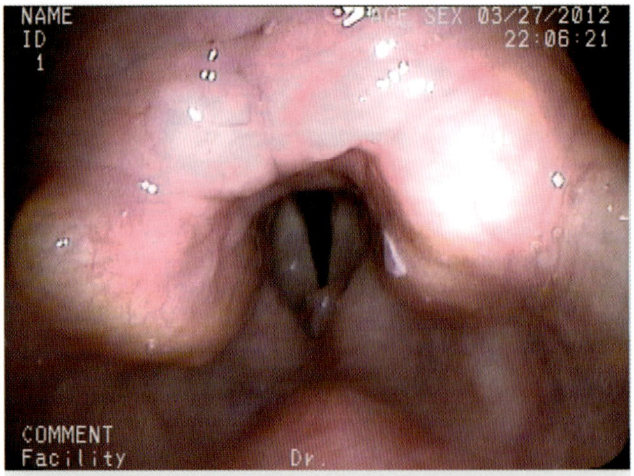

Fig. 8.6 Right anterior saccular cyst in a 56-year-old Hispanic man who presented with hoarseness, but who was otherwise asymptomatic.

8.7 Laryngoceles and Saccular Cysts

During the second month of gestation, the laryngeal ventricle develops as an evagination of mucosa that splits the false vocal folds from the true vocal cords; the apex of this pouch forms the saccule. In adults, the saccule courses posteriorly and superiorly from the anterior ventricle and is lined with pseudostratified ciliated columnar epithelium. The entire saccule is pocketed within a fibrous capsule that is continuous with the true vocal cord. Its medial border is the mucosa of the aryepiglottic fold and the ventricular band, while laterally the thyroepiglottic muscle separates it from the thyroid cartilage. The saccular orifice is normally 0.5 to 1 mm in diameter and acts as a valve to store the mucous secretions of the underlying glands, which are released when the surrounding muscles contract.

Saccular cysts are rare. Holinger et al noted that over a period of 30 years, only 20 cases were diagnosed.[109,110] A saccular cyst is a mucous-filled dilated saccule that is not connected to the laryngeal lumen. It is generally submucosal and covered by the mucosal membrane. There are two commonly accepted types of saccular cysts, lateral and anterior. The former are more common and tend to distend parts or all of the supraglottis (false vocal folds, AE folds, or the ventricle) and sometimes extend up to or through the thyrohyoid membrane. Anterior saccular cysts extend medially into the laryngeal lumen between the true and false vocal folds (▶ Fig. 8.6), often causing distortion of the larynx and making origination difficult to ascertain.

Laryngoceles are air-filled dilated saccules that do connect with the laryngeal lumen; when infected, they are referred to as laryngopyoceles. They can be further divided, based on the size and direction of the extension or dissection, as internal, external, or both internal and external. The internal part extends posterosuperior into the false vocal fold or the AE folds; the external component goes beyond the thyrohyoid membrane, often with palpable swelling in the neck, and can course along the superior laryngeal nerve and vessels. Some have been reported to extend as far as the axillary space or supraclavicular region.[111] Of the three types of laryngoceles, the most common is the combination of both external and internal components, while the least common is an isolated external type. Internal laryngoceles that become infected or a laryngopyocele is often indistinguishable from an infected saccular cyst.[112] According to de Vincentiis, 80 to 90% of laryngoceles occur in men, usually in the fifth and sixth decades.[113] Laryngoceles are less common in children than in adults.[111]

The main difference between the two is that saccular cysts have an isolated lumen that does not contain air. Saccular enlargements that fill or empty with air with coughing or speaking represent intermittent symptoms, implying a patent saccular orifice, and thus should be considered a laryngocele.

These entities should not be confused with ductal cysts, which are common cysts found anywhere in the larynx. Usually, these are less than 1 cm, superficial, lined by ductal type cells, and created by retained mucus that was secreted by submucosal glands. They are 3 times more common than saccular cysts. They must also be distinguished from ventricular prolapse, often seen in those with prolonged intubation, in which the mucosa and submucosa protrude into the laryngeal lumen.

There is a spectrum of theories about formation for saccular cysts and laryngoceles: congenital, congenital defect exacerbated by habitual increased intralaryngeal pressure, or acquired. Congenital lesions occur due to atresia of the orifice. Causes of acquired lesions include trauma, neoplasm, inflammation, and fibrosis. Hobbies or occupations that lead to increased pressure in the laryngeal lumen include singing, glass blowing, playing wind instruments, and chronic coughing.[114]

Patients have varied symptomatology depending on the size and extension, but more often than not, hoarseness is noted due to downward pressure on the vocal cords. Other commonly described symptoms include cough, stridor, sore throat, snoring, and dysphagia. These can be severe enough to cause airway obstruction or death. Often, infants with these cysts cannot cry, have labored breathing, and easily become cyanotic.[115] The presence of a neck mass is suggestive of a lateral saccular cyst or a laryngocele with an external component. Airway compromise due to saccular cyst lesions can be severe; in the series reported by Kristensen and Tveteras, almost 50% of the cases were diagnosed at autopsy, emphasizing the need for early recognition and management.[116] Soft tissue radiographs of the neck show air densities lateral to the thyroid ala or hyoid bone. Computed tomography is useful to distinguish between air- and fluid-filled sacs, and to help diagnose the presence of a mixed laryngocele if present.[112] Endoscopic evaluation is usually the next step. If the sac is not distended with air, the larynx may appear normal, but a Valsalva maneuver can help identify these lesions. Larger cysts can bulge superiorly into the floor of vallecula or laterally into the piriform sinus. Tracheotomy should be used only when absolutely needed.[110]

Treatment varies based on age and has evolved over time. Management of saccular cysts has evolved from needle aspiration and decompression to external excision, with endoscopic techniques favored when applicable. For infants, needle aspiration is usually the initial treatment, and if the condition recurs, repeat aspiration can be pursued or one can unroof the superior extent of the cyst and use forceps to remove any redundant mucosa. In adults, anterior cysts are treated via excision using forceps during laryngoscopy, while lateral lesions are treated with endoscopic marsupialization followed by re-excision if needed.[114]Traditionally, a tracheotomy was always performed, but this is no longer necessary. Frequent recurrence has been associated with aspiration and marsupialization, with rates of 50% and 78% in children and adults, respectively.[114] Recurrence can vary from 2 months after initial excision up to 1.5 years; this wide range suggests the need for more frequent short-term follow-up.[117]

When treated endoscopically, some prefer the use of a laser, as it causes less destruction and trauma than a cold steel technique, and thus decreased postoperative edema and adhesion formation.[118] Endoscopic management is usually reserved to internal laryngoceles and anterior saccular cysts. Larger or recurrent lesions, lateral saccular cysts, and laryngoceles with an external component typically require a transcervical approach for excision, often via a superior laryngofissure. This requires going through the thyrohyoid membrane and rarely involves a thyrotomy. Any specimen that is removed should be sent to pathology to rule out carcinoma.[112]

Acquired saccular disorders have been noted in various conditions. There is a 5% incidence of a simultaneous presence of carcinoma.[119] They have also been noted in those with amyloidosis. The theory is that deposition of amyloid in the laryngeal tissue leads to decreased resilience. There has been much debate about development of these lesions in those who have undergone neck surgery. Previous reports support the rarity of these lesions after surgeries like tracheotomy, partial laryngectomy, and hemithyroidectomy. The authors concluded that previous surgery in the paralaryngeal region may result in a soft spot that interrupts the intralaryngeal pressure from its normal steady-state status, resulting in a one-way valve that predisposes to cyst formation.[119,120,121,122]

A variant of saccular disorders is the oncocytic cyst, which tends to occur around the ventricle in the elderly.[115] Oncocytic cysts comprise 35% of saccular cysts.[114] They are often compared to oncocytomes and Warthin tumors of the parotid. Histologically, the cells are filled with mitochondria and active enzymes. Oncocytic laryngeal cysts tend to recur.[112]

8.8 Conclusion

Benign laryngeal tumors encompass a wide variety of pathologic origins, including epithelial, glandular, vascular, adipose, muscular, and neural. With the exception of papilloma, most of the tumors are rare, especially in comparison to benign mucosal lesions of the larynx. The pathologies cannot be distinguished based upon symptomatology or even laryngoscopy in many cases. Careful functional evaluation and diagnosis with histopathology is necessary to determine an appropriate plan of care.

8.9 Key Points

- The distinction of epithelial from subepithelial disease is important in diagnosis as well as understanding the pathophysiology and treatment of the laryngeal disorder.
- Laryngoscopy with videostroboscopy is critical in the assessment of patients with these lesions.
- Recurrent respiratory papilloma continues to be a dominant issue in contemporary laryngology. Historically, its treatment has involved careful surgical removal of symptomatic lesions. With the advent of the pulsed-dye and KTP lasers, this paradigm has evolved.
- The use of adjunctive medical therapy, intralesionally or systemically, remains controversial in RRP.

References

[1] Smith HG, Healy GB, Vaughan CW, Strong MS. Topical chemotherapy of recurrent respiratory papillomatosis. A preliminary report. Ann Otol Rhinol Laryngol 1980; 89: 472–478

[2] Reeves WC, Ruparelia SS, Swanson KI, Derkay CS, Marcus A, Unger ER. National registry for juvenile-onset recurrent respiratory papillomatosis. Arch Otolaryngol Head Neck Surg 2003; 129: 976–982

[3] Derkay CS. Task force on recurrent respiratory papillomas. A preliminary report. Arch Otolaryngol Head Neck Surg 1995; 121: 1386–1391

[4] Cohn AM, Kos JT, Taber LH, Adam E. Recurring laryngeal papillopa. Am J Otolaryngol 1981; 2: 129–132

[5] Lie ES, Engh V, Boysen M et al. Squamous cell carcinoma of the respiratory tract following laryngeal papillomatosis. Acta Otolaryngol 1994; 114: 209–212

[6] Gallagher TQ, Derkay CS. Recurrent respiratory papillomatosis: update 2008. Curr Opin Otolaryngol Head Neck Surg 2008; 16: 536–542

[7] Leung R, Hawkes M, Campisi P. Severity of juvenile onset recurrent respiratory papillomatosis is not associated with socioeconomic status in a setting of universal health care. Int J Pediatr Otorhinolaryngol 2007; 71: 965–972

[8] Wiatrak BJ. Overview of recurrent respiratory papillomatosis. Curr Opin Otolaryngol Head Neck Surg 2003; 11: 433–441

[9] Wiatrak BJ, Wiatrak DW, Broker TR, Lewis L. Recurrent respiratory papillomatosis: a longitudinal study comparing severity associated with human papilloma viral types 6 and 11 and other risk factors in a large pediatric population. Laryngoscope 2004; 114 Suppl 104: 1–23

[10] Derkay CS, Darrow DH. Recurrent respiratory papillomatosis. Ann Otol Rhinol Laryngol 2006; 115: 1–11

[11] Corbitt G, Zarod AP, Arrand JR, Longson M, Farrington WT. Human papillomavirus (HPV) genotypes associated with laryngeal papilloma. J Clin Pathol 1988; 41: 284–288

[12] Gerein V, Rastorguev E, Gerein J, Draf W, Schirren J. Incidence, age at onset, and potential reasons of malignant transformation in recurrent respiratory papillomatosis patients: 20 years experience. Otolaryngol Head Neck Surg 2005; 132: 392–394

[13] Stern Y, Felipovich A, Cotton RT, Segal K. Immunocompetency in children with recurrent respiratory papillomatosis: prospective study. Ann Otol Rhinol Laryngol 2007; 116: 169–171

[14] Kashima HK, Shah F, Lyles A et al. A comparison of risk factors in juvenile-onset and adult-onset recurrent respiratory papillomatosis. Laryngoscope 1992; 102: 9–13

[15] Gerein V, Soldatski IL, Babkina N, Onufrieva EK, Barysik N, Pfister H. Children and partners of patients with recurrent respiratory papillomatosis have no evidence of the disease during long-term observation. Int J Pediatr Otorhinolaryngol 2006; 70: 2061–2066

[16] Stamataki S, Nikolopoulos TP, Korres S, Felekis D, Tzangaroulakis A, Ferekidis E. Juvenile recurrent respiratory papillomatosis: still a mystery disease with difficult management. Head Neck 2007; 29: 155–162

[17] Armbruster C. Novel treatments for recurrent respiratory papillomatosis. Expert Opin Investig Drugs 2002; 11: 1139–1148

[18] Derkay CS, Malis DJ, Zalzal G, Wiatrak BJ, Kashima HK, Coltrera MD. A staging system for assessing severity of disease and response to therapy in recurrent respiratory papillomatosis. Laryngoscope 1998; 108: 935–937

[19] Hill DS, Akhtar S, Corroll A, Croft CB. Quality of life issues in recurrent respiratory papillomatosis. Clin Otolaryngol Allied Sci 2000; 25: 153–160

[20] Leventhal BG, Kashima HK, Weck PW et al. Randomized surgical adjuvant trial of interferon alfa-n1 in recurrent papillomatosis. Arch Otolaryngol Head Neck Surg 1988; 114: 1163–1169

[21] Schraff S, Derkay CS, Burke B, Lawson L. American Society of Pediatric Otolaryngology members' experience with recurrent respiratory papillomatosis and the use of adjuvant therapy. Arch Otolaryngol Head Neck Surg 2004; 130: 1039–1042

[22] Strong MS, Vaughan CW, Cooperband SR, Healy GB, Clemente MA. Recurrent respiratory papillomatosis: management with the CO2 laser. Ann Otol Rhinol Laryngol 1976; 85: 508–516

[23] Janda P, Leunig A, Sroka R, Betz CS, Rasp G. Preliminary report of endolaryngeal and endotracheal laser surgery of juvenile-onset recurrent respiratory papillomatosis by Nd:YAG laser and a new fiber guidance instrument. Otolaryngol Head Neck Surg 2004; 131: 44–49

[24] Zeitels SM, Barbu AM, Landau-Zemer T et al. Local injection of bevacizumab (Avastin) and angiolytic KTP laser treatment of recurrent respiratory papillomatosis of the vocal folds: a prospective study. Ann Otol Rhinol Laryngol 2011; 120: 627–634

[25] Holler T, Allegro J, Chadha NK et al. Voice outcomes following repeated surgical resection of laryngeal papillomata in children. Otolaryngol Head Neck Surg 2009; 141: 522–526

[26] El-Bitar MA, Zalzal GH. Powered instrumentation in the treatment of recurrent respiratory papillomatosis: an alternative to the carbon dioxide laser. Arch Otolaryngol Head Neck Surg 2002; 128: 425–428

[27] Van Cutsem E, Snoeck R, Van Ranst M et al. Successful treatment of a squamous papilloma of the hypopharynx-esophagus by local injections of (S)-1-(3-hydroxy-2-phosphonylmethoxypropyl)cytosine. J Med Virol 1995; 45: 230–235

[28] Wierzbicka M, Jackowska J, Bartochowska A, Józefiak A, Szyfter W, Kędzia W. Effectiveness of cidofovir intralesional treatment in recurrent respiratory papillomatosis. Eur Arch Otorhinolaryngol 2011; 268: 1305–1311

[29] Shehab N, Sweet BV, Hogikyan ND. Cidofovir for the treatment of recurrent respiratory papillomatosis: a review of the literature. Pharmacotherapy 2005; 25: 977–989

[30] Broekema FI, Dikkers FG. Side-effects of cidofovir in the treatment of recurrent respiratory papillomatosis. Eur Arch Otorhinolaryngol 2008; 265: 871–879

[31] Bauman NM, Smith RJ. Recurrent respiratory papillomatosis. Pediatr Clin North Am 1996; 43: 1385–1401

[32] Giles BL, Seifert B. CR12/339—Nebulized cidofovir for recurrent respiratory papillomatosis: a case report. Paediatr Respir Rev 2006; 7 Suppl 1: S330

[33] Avidano MA, Singleton GT. Adjuvant drug strategies in the treatment of recurrent respiratory papillomatosis. Otolaryngol Head Neck Surg 1995; 112: 197–202

[34] Auborn KJ. Therapy for recurrent respiratory papillomatosis. Antivir Ther 2002; 7: 1–9

[35] Szeps M, Dahlgren L, Aaltonen LM et al. Human papillomavirus, viral load and proliferation rate in recurrent respiratory papillomatosis in response to alpha interferon treatment. J Gen Virol 2005; 86: 1695–1702

[36] McGlennen RC, Adams GL, Lewis CM, Faras AJ, Ostrow RS. Pilot trial of ribavirin for the treatment of laryngeal papillomatosis. Head Neck 1993; 15: 504–512, discussion 512–513

[37] Doyle DJ, Gianoli GJ, Espinola T, Miller RH. Recurrent respiratory papillomatosis: juvenile versus adult forms. Laryngoscope 1994; 104: 523–527

[38] Weiss MD, Kashima HK. Tracheal involvement in laryngeal papillomatosis. Laryngoscope 1983; 93: 45–48

[39] Boston M, Rutter M, Myer CM, Cotton RT. Airway reconstruction in children with recurrent respiratory papillomatosis. Int J Pediatr Otorhinolaryngol 2006; 70: 1097–1101

[40] Blackledge FA, Anand VK. Tracheobronchial extension of recurrent respiratory papillomatosis. Ann Otol Rhinol Laryngol 2000; 109: 812–818

[41] Cole RR, Myer CM, Cotton RT. Tracheotomy in children with recurrent respiratory papillomatosis. Head Neck 1989; 11: 226–230

[42] Derkay CS, Wiatrak B. Recurrent respiratory papillomatosis: a review. Laryngoscope 2008; 118: 1236–1247

[43] Wetmore SJ, Key JM, Suen JY. Complications of laser surgery for laryngeal papillomatosis. Laryngoscope 1985; 95: 798–801

[44] Papaspyrou G, Werner JA, Roessler M, Devaney KO, Rinaldo A, Ferlito A. Adult rhabdomyoma in the parapharyngeal space: report of 2 cases and review of the literature. Am J Otolaryngol 2011; 32: 240–246

[45] Johansen EC, Illum P. Rhabdomyoma of the larynx: a review of the literature with a summary of previously described cases of rhabdomyoma of the larynx and a report of a new case. J Laryngol Otol 1995; 109: 147–153

[46] Brys AK, Sakai O, DeRosa J, Shapshay SM. Rhabdomyoma of the larynx: case report and clinical and pathologic review. Ear Nose Throat J 2005; 84: 437–440

[47] Liess BD, Zitsch RP, Lane R, Bickel JT. Multifocal adult rhabdomyoma: a case report and literature review. Am J Otolaryngol 2005; 26: 214–217

[48] Liang GS, Loevner LA, Kumar P. Laryngeal rhabdomyoma involving the paraglottic space. AJR Am J Roentgenol 2000; 174: 1285–1287

[49] LaBagnara J, Hitchcock E, Spitzer T. Rhabdomyoma of the true vocal fold. J Voice 1999; 13: 289–293

[50] Smith HW. Skeletal muscle rhabdomyoma of the larynx: report of a case. Laryngoscope 1959; 69: 1528–1536

[51] Hamper K, Renninghoff J, Schäfer H. Rhabdomyoma of the larynx recurring after 12 years: immunocytochemistry and differential diagnosis. Arch Otorhinolaryngol 1989; 246: 222–226

[52] Helliwell TR, Sissons MC, Stoney PJ, Ashworth MT. Immunochemistry and electron microscopy of head and neck rhabdomyoma. J Clin Pathol 1988; 41: 1058–1063

[53] Kapadia SB, Meis JM, Frisman DM, Ellis GL, Heffner DK, Hyams VJ. Adult rhabdomyoma of the head and neck: a clinicopathologic and immunophenotypic study. Hum Pathol 1993; 24: 608–617

[54] Durr ML, Agrawal N, Saunders JR, Ha PK. Laryngeal lipoma associated with diffuse lipomatosis: case report and literature review. Ear Nose Throat J 2010; 89: 34–37

[55] Lippert BM, Eggers S, Schlüter E, Rudert H, Werner JA. Lipoma of the larynx. Report of 2 cases and review of the literature. Otolaryngol Pol 2002; 56: 669–674

[56] Jones SR, Myers EN, Barnes L. Benign neoplasms of the larynx. Otolaryngol Clin North Am 1984; 17: 151–178

[57] Dinsdale RC, Manning SC, Brooks DJ, Vuitch F. Myxoid laryngeal lipoma in a juvenile. Otolaryngol Head Neck Surg 1990; 103: 653–657

[58] De Vincentiis M, Greco A, Mascelli A, Soldo P, Zambetti G. Lipoma of the larynx: a case report. Acta Otorhinolaryngol Ital 2010; 30: 58–63

[59] Wenig BM. Lipomas of the larynx and hypopharynx: a review of the literature with the addition of three new cases. J Laryngol Otol 1995; 109: 353–357

[60] Kapur TR. Recurrent lipomata of the larynx and the pharynx with late malignant change. J Laryngol Otol 1968; 82: 761–768

[61] Rahbar R, Litrovnik BG, Vargas SO et al. The biology and management of laryngeal neurofibroma. Arch Otolaryngol Head Neck Surg 2004; 130: 1400–1406

[62] Aponte GE, Vicens EA. Neurogenic tumors of the larynx. Ann Otol Rhinol Laryngol 1955; 64: 319–325

[63] Fini-Storchi I, Frosini P. Laryngeal neurinoma. A case report and review. ORL J Otorhinolaryngol Relat Spec 1997; 59: 182–185

[64] Schaeffer BT, Som PM, Biller HF, Som ML, Arnold LM. Schwannomas of the larynx: review and computed tomographic scan analysis. Head Neck Surg 1986; 8: 469–472

[65] Gooder P, Farrington T. Extracranial neurilemmomata of the head and neck. J Laryngol Otol 1980; 94: 243–249

[66] Nanson EM. Neurilemoma of the larynx: a case study. Head Neck Surg 1978; 1: 69–74

[67] al-Otieschan AT, Mahasin ZZ, Gangopadhyay K, al-Dayel F, Jamshed A. Schwannoma of the larynx: two case reports and review of the literature. J Otolaryngol 1996; 25: 412–415
[68] Ebmeyer J, Reineke U, Gehl HB et al. Schwannoma of the larynx. Head Neck Oncol 2009; 1: 24
[69] Cadoni G, Bucci G, Corina L, Scarano E, Almadori G. Schwannoma of the larynx presenting with difficult swallowing. Otolaryngol Head Neck Surg 2000; 122: 773–774
[70] Rosen FS, Pou AM, Quinn FB. Obstructive supraglottic schwannoma: a case report and review of the literature. Laryngoscope 2002; 112: 997–1002
[71] Supance JS, Quenelle DJ, Crissman J. Endolaryngeal neurofibromas. Otolaryngol Head Neck Surg (1979) 1980; 88: 74–78
[72] Puri R, Berry S, Srivastava G. Solitary neurofibroma of the larynx. Otolaryngol Head Neck Surg 1997; 117: 713–714
[73] Stanley RJ, Scheithauer BW, Weiland LH, Neel HB. Neural and neuroendocrine tumors of the larynx. Ann Otol Rhinol Laryngol 1987; 96: 630–638
[74] Garabédian EN, Ducroz V, Ayache D, Triglia JM. Results of partial laryngectomy for benign neural tumors of the larynx in children. Ann Otol Rhinol Laryngol 1999; 108: 666–671
[75] Lewis JS, Ferlito A, Gnepp DR et al. International Head and Neck Scientific Group. Terminology and classification of neuroendocrine neoplasms of the larynx. Laryngoscope 2011; 121: 1187–1193
[76] Angouridakis N, Goudakos J, Karayannopoulou G, Triaridis S, Nikolaou A, Markou K. Primary neuroendocrine neoplasms of the larynx. A series of 4 cases reported and a review of the literature. Head Neck 2012
[77] Qureshi NA, Tahir M, Carmichael AR. Granular cell tumour of the soft tissues: a case report and literature review. Int Semin Surg Oncol 2006; 3: 21
[78] Sataloff RT, Ressue JC, Portell M et al. Granular cell tumors of the larynx. J Voice 2000; 14: 119–134
[79] Arevalo C, Maly B, Eliashar R, Gross M. Laryngeal granular cell tumor. J Voice 2008; 22: 339–342
[80] Kamal SA, Othman EO. Granular cell tumour of the larynx. J Laryngol Otol 1998; 112: 83–85
[81] White JB, Glade R, Rossi CT, Bielamowicz S. Granular cell tumors of the larynx: diagnosis and management. J Voice 2009; 23: 516–517
[82] Pelucchi S, Amoroso C, Grandi E, Carinci F, Pastore A. Granular cell tumour of the larynx: literature review and case report. J Otolaryngol 2002; 31: 234–235
[83] Conley SF, Milbrath MM, Beste DJ. Pediatric laryngeal granular cell tumor. J Otolaryngol 1992; 21: 450–453
[84] Park JH, Do NY, Cho SI, Choi JY. Granular cell tumor on larynx. Clin Exp Otorhinolaryngol 2010; 3: 52–55
[85] Bridger GP, Nassar VH, Skinner HG. Hemangioma in the adult larynx. Arch Otolaryngol 1970; 92: 493–498
[86] Doermann P, Lunseth J, Segnitz RH. Obstructing subglottic hemangioma of the larynx in infancy; review of the literature and report of a deceptive case. N Engl J Med 1958; 258: 68–71
[87] Mulder JJ, van den Broek P. Surgical treatment of infantile subglottic hemangioma. Int J Pediatr Otorhinolaryngol 1989; 17: 57–63
[88] Rahbar R, Nicollas R, Roger G et al. The biology and management of subglottic hemangioma: past, present, future. Laryngoscope 2004; 114: 1880–1891
[89] Sie KC, McGill T, Healy GB. Subglottic hemangioma: ten years' experience with the carbon dioxide laser. Ann Otol Rhinol Laryngol 1994; 103: 167–172
[90] O TM, Alexander RE, Lando T et al. Segmental hemangiomas of the upper airway. Laryngoscope 2009; 119: 2242–2247
[91] Perkins JA, Duke W, Chen E, Manning S. Emerging concepts in airway infantile hemangioma assessment and management. Otolaryngol Head Neck Surg 2009; 141: 207–212
[92] Choa DI, Smith MC, Evans JN, Bailey CM. Subglottic haemangioma in children. J Laryngol Otol 1986; 100: 447–454
[93] Narcy P, Contencin P, Bobin S, Manac'h Y. Treatment of infantile subglottic hemangioma. A report of 49 cases. Int J Pediatr Otorhinolaryngol 1985; 9: 157–164
[94] Shikhani AH, Jones MM, Marsh BR, Holliday MJ. Infantile subglottic hemangiomas. An update. Ann Otol Rhinol Laryngol 1986; 95: 336–347
[95] Huang CM, Lee KW, Huang CJ. Radiation therapy for life-threatening huge laryngeal hemangioma involving pharynx and parapharyngeal space. Head Neck 2013; 35: E98–E101
[96] Shpitzer T, Noyek AM, Witterick I et al. Noncutaneous cavernous hemangiomas of the head and neck. Am J Otolaryngol 1997; 18: 367–374
[97] Zheng JW, Zhou Q, Yang XJ et al. Treatment guideline for hemangiomas and vascular malformations of the head and neck. Head Neck 2010; 32: 1088–1098
[98] Seikaly H, Cuyler JP. Infantile subglottic hemangioma. J Otolaryngol 1994; 23: 135–137
[99] Simpson GT, Healy GB, McGill T, Strong MS. Benign tumors and lesions of the larynx in children. Surgical excision by CO2 laser. Ann Otol Rhinol Laryngol 1979; 88: 479–485
[100] McCaffrey TV, Cortese DA. Neodymium:YAG laser treatment of subglottic hemangioma. Otolaryngol Head Neck Surg 1986; 94: 382–384
[101] Kacker A, April M, Ward RF. Use of potassium titanyl phosphate (KTP) laser in management of subglottic hemangiomas. Int J Pediatr Otorhinolaryngol 2001; 59: 15–21
[102] Pransky SM, Canto C. Management of subglottic hemangioma. Curr Opin Otolaryngol Head Neck Surg 2004; 12: 509–512
[103] Bitar MA, Moukarbel RV, Zalzal GH. Management of congenital subglottic hemangioma: trends and success over the past 17 years. Otolaryngol Head Neck Surg 2005; 132: 226–231
[104] Anger J, Carneiro RG, Pinus J, Ernesto JM, Faiwichow G. The rebound effect in the treatment of complex hemangioma with interferon alpha 2A. Sao Paulo Med J 1998; 116: 1826–1828
[105] Truong MT, Perkins JA, Messner AH, Chang KW. Propranolol for the treatment of airway hemangiomas: a case series and treatment algorithm. Int J Pediatr Otorhinolaryngol 2010; 74: 1043–1048
[106] McRae RD, Gatland DJ, McNab Jones RF, Khan S. Malignant transformation in a laryngeal hemangioma. Ann Otol Rhinol Laryngol 1990; 99: 562–565
[107] Nishimura T, Takimoto T, Ishikawa S, Ohmura K. Venous haemangioma of the neck and mediastinum. J Laryngol Otol 1991; 105: 386–388
[108] Lucioni M, Marioni G, Della Libera D, Rizzotto G. Adult laryngeal hemangioma CO2 laser excision. A single institution 3-year experience (Vittorio Veneto 2001–2003). Acta Otolaryngol 2006; 126: 621–626
[109] Holinger PH, Brown WT. Congenital webs, cysts, laryngoceles and other anomalies of the larynx. Ann Otol Rhinol Laryngol 1967; 76: 744–752
[110] Suhonen H, Kero PO, Puhakka H, Vilkki P. Saccular cyst of the larynx in infants. Int J Pediatr Otorhinolaryngol 1984; 8: 73–78
[111] Civantos FJ, Holinger LD. Laryngoceles and saccular cysts in infants and children. Arch Otolaryngol Head Neck Surg 1992; 118: 296–300
[112] Myssiorek D, Persky M. Laser endoscopic treatment of laryngoceles and laryngeal cysts. Otolaryngol Head Neck Surg 1989; 100: 538–541
[113] de Vincentiis I, Biserni A. Surgery of the mixed laryngocele. Acta Otolaryngol 1979; 87: 142–151
[114] Holinger LD, Barnes DR, Smid LJ, Holinger PH. Laryngocele and saccular cysts. Ann Otol Rhinol Laryngol 1978; 87: 675–685
[115] Kinnunen I, Klemi P, Grenman R. Saccular laryngeal cysts. Three case studies and review of the literature. ORL J Otorhinolaryngol Relat Spec 2000; 62: 109–111
[116] Kristensen S, Tveterås K. Congenital laryngeal cyst in infancy. A rare cause of life-threatening stridor. ORL J Otorhinolaryngol Relat Spec 1986; 48: 150–155
[117] Young VN, Smith LJ. Saccular cysts: a current review of characteristics and management. Laryngoscope 2012; 122: 595–599
[118] Abramson AL, Zielinski B. Congenital laryngeal saccular cyst of the newborn. Laryngoscope 1984; 94: 1580–1582
[119] Marom T, Roth Y, Cinamon U. Laryngocele: a rare long-term complication following neck surgery? J Voice 2011; 25: 272–274
[120] Upile T, Jerjes W, Sipaul F et al. Laryngocele: a rare complication of surgical tracheostomy. BMC Surg 2006; 6: 14
[121] Naudo P, Laccourreye O, Weinstein G, Jouffre V, Laccourreye H, Brasnu D. Complications and functional outcome after supracricoid partial laryngectomy with cricohyoidoepiglottopexy. Otolaryngol Head Neck Surg 1998; 118: 124–129
[122] Carrat X, François JM, Carles D, Devars F, Traissac L. Laryngomucocele as an unusual late complication of subtotal laryngectomy. Case report. Ann Otol Rhinol Laryngol 1998; 107: 703–707

9 Vocal Fold Immobility

Roger L. Crumley

Any discussion of vocal fold motion impairment must begin with an explanation of certain terms. There is no single term that defines the various vocal fold motion impairments; rather they are truly a mixed bag of disorders. Vocal fold immobility has become a more commonly used term, implying a vocal fold that has neither active abduction nor active adduction; i.e., it is motionless. It is arguably a satisfactory replacement for the older, less accurate term *vocal cord/fold paralysis*, which was previously used in virtually every situation in which the vocal fold did not move properly. With improved recognition of the various disorders that cause vocal fold immobility as well as improved technologies in videostroboscopy and distal chip endoscopes, we now have a much greater knowledge of these disorders, and hence need better nomenclature.

Vocal fold immobility seems simple enough, implying that the vocal fold does not move. However, there is one significant problem with this term. Because the passive mobility test is one of the most important evaluations done in management of patients with vocal fold immobility or motion impairment, usage of the term can create a clinical conundrum. If one uses the term vocal fold immobility (VFI), it implies that the vocal fold does not move. However, in preparing to perform such procedures as thyroplasty, arytenoid adduction, reinnervation, and vocal fold injections it is useful (if not imperative) for the clinician to know whether there is passive mobility of the arytenoid cartilage at the cricoarytenoid joint. Accordingly, the well-known maneuver that is performed during direct laryngoscopy is to gently push the vocal process laterally and to ascertain whether passive mobility of the arytenoid is present or not (passive mobility test). In many, if not most, cases of motion impairment/immobility (VFI), the vocal fold and arytenoids are in fact mobile on the passive mobility test. This creates a scenario in which the patient has VFI and yet the arytenoid has passive mobility, for example, is "mobile."

For this reason, vocal fold motion impairment (VFMI) may be a more accurate term because it implies that even though the vocal fold may be immobile in terms of active movements, it may still have a normal passive mobility test. This term describes VF motion as simply abnormal or impaired. Another term that the author likes almost as much as VFMI is *VF dysmotility*.[1] However, the status of the literature is such that VFI is currently a very common term and the "horse may be out of the barn" in trying to change this terminology to something more accurate. Hence, VFI will be used in this chapter.

With regard to older terminology, vocal fold paralysis and vocal cord paralysis are terms still used in the literature. However, fortunately, they are gradually disappearing. The terms are inaccurate because many patients with VFI or VFMI do not really have true paralysis: rather, the laryngeal muscles are actually innervated, with synkinetic movements or other dysfunctional movements, such that "paralysis" is simply not an accurate or correct term. Paresis is an important currently used term that implies partial motion impairment or partial paralysis and is still useful because it implies that VF movements are present although they are smaller and less dynamic than normal. Paresis frequently coexists with synkinesis. In this chapter, the author uses the terms VFI and VFMI—mostly VFI for brevity.

Laryngeal synkinesis is another term that is frequently useful in explaining clinical VF motion disorders. Synkinesis is generally not present for 2 to 4 months after a recurrent laryngeal nerve (RLN) injury. However, when it appears, it may replace what appears to be true paralysis. Accordingly, an understanding of synkinesis is very important for the otolaryngologist and laryngologist.

In summary, in this chapter, several of these terms are used. This preliminary discussion should enable the reader to understand the subtle differences that may make a very vast difference in treatment and end results.

9.1 Causes of Vocal Fold Immobility

It should be noted that there are a wide variety of recurrent laryngeal nerve disorders, many of which can cause paresis, paralysis, and immobility syndromes. They are covered more extensively later in this chapter.

9.1.1 Nonneurogenic (RLN-Unrelated) Causes of Vocal Fold Immobility

When the entire structure of a vocal fold, including the cartilaginous vocal process and entire membranous vocal fold, is truly motionless, the clinician should consider a very long list of etiologies (and not make the assumption that RLN injury is the cause). The astute clinician will not assume that a patient with a new vocal fold immobility syndrome has a recurrent laryngeal nerve disorder (or idiopathic vocal fold paralysis) unless there is a history of a thyroidectomy, skull base procedure, cervical spine operation, or other operations in the chest, neck, or thorax that might have endangered the integrity of the RLN. The author has seen several instances when such things as vocal cord cancer, amyloidosis, or scar have all produced VF motion impairment, and these important disorders were missed by a clinician who treated the patient as if the problem were vocal fold paralysis or idiopathic vocal fold paralysis. Vocal fold immobility then is a very important finding for the clinician as it may be the first sign of a malignant tumor of the vocal fold, subglottis, paraglottic space, arytenoid cartilage, or cricoarytenoid joint.

Laryngeal scar may tether one vocal fold to the other, producing a relative immobility on one or both sides. These cicatrical bands or other webs may present anteriorly at the anterior commissure, or posteriorly anywhere from the vocal process to the true posterior commissure. The entire arytenoid cartilage medial surface may be tethered by scar to the opposite arytenoid. Indeed the posterior commissural scar that causes an apparent bilateral vocal fold paralysis, or bilateral vocal fold immobility, is one of the more difficult diagnoses for many laryngologists and otolaryngologists to make. Such scarring can follow endotracheal intubation, airway burns, laser burns, or other glottic injuries. If it is confused with true bilateral neurogenic motion impairment/immobility, the correct treatment (lysis/release of the scar with mucosal resurfacing of the denuded margin) may never be achieved. It is important to restress how easy it is for this diagnosis to be missed during direct laryngoscopy if the otolaryngologist is not actively thinking about it, considering it, and looking for it.

9.2 History and Physical Examination

9.2.1 History Taking

Most patients with VFI/VFMI will present with either dysphonia (hoarseness) or some other form of vocal dysfunction. Given that there are several causes of immobility, the history is extremely important and often provides the best clue as to whether the VFI is RLN-related. Accordingly, the following questions are essential components of the vocal/clinical history:

1. How long has your voice been abnormal?
2. Have you had this problem with your voice previous to this occurrence? When?
3. Have you had recent surgery or trauma? (It is important for the otolaryngologist to ask several questions re vocal abuse. Many patients do not understand what it is. Answers should be clarified accordingly.)
4. Smoking history, including exposure to secondary smoke.
5. History of heartburn, gastroesophageal reflux disease (GERD), or other gastrointestinal symptoms?
6. Does anything make the hoarseness worse? Better?
7. Do you have a new home, job, work environment, car? (Are there any major changes in the patient's life recently that might have a bearing on causation?)
8. Do you have trouble being heard in a quiet room, loud room, or car, or on the telephone?
9. What do you use your voice for? (Professional usage, such as singing, public speaking, or office job, or working at home, retired, etc.?)

These nine questions will often move the clinician in the direction of a preliminary diagnosis. It is important to consider all the possibilities in the differential diagnosis. If there has been a recent surgical procedure in the neck or thorax (thyroidectomy, cervical spine exploration, mediastinal exploration, aortic arch procedure, etc.) one would obviously be thinking of RLN-related VFI/VFMI. The most common cervical surgical procedures resulting in VFI/VFMI include thyroidectomy, parathyroidectomy, anterior approach to cervical spine, carotid endarterectomy, open Zenker diverticulectomy and cricopharyngeal myotomy, and vagal nerve stimulators (placed for management of seizure disorders). Thoracic surgical procedures most frequently associated with VFI/VFMI include pneumonectomy, lobotomy, mediastinal procedures, cardiac and aortic procedures, esophagectomy, and other esophageal procedures.[2]

9.2.2 Differential Diagnosis

Vocal fold motion impairment and immobility have a number of causes that can be sorted into recurrent laryngeal nerve-related (neurogenic) disorders and non-RLN-related causes.[3]

The RLN-related causes include vagus or recurrent laryngeal nerve injuries, with synkinesis, paresis, or paralysis. The injury may be at the skull base, the cervical vagus, the thoracic vagus and RLN, or the cervical RLN. If not due to a distinct injury along the course of the vagus nerve or RLN, it may be an idiopathic vocal fold paralysis or secondary to stroke or central nervous system injuries.

Of note, this is not a complete differential diagnosis; the reader is referred to other sources for more comprehensive listing of all the various causes.[2,4]

Non-RLN causes for immobility of the vocal fold include arytenoid fixation, neoplasm (notably squamous cell carcinoma without obvious mucosal ulceration), benign tumors of the vocal fold or paraglottic space, iatrogenic injury from prior surgery, vocal fold scar, webs, synechiae, or prior radiation.

9.2.3 Physical Examination

The otolaryngologist should first examine the patient's ears, nose, nasopharynx, oral cavity, pharynx, and neck. It is important to look assiduously for surgical scars reflecting procedures that the patient may have forgotten about. A careful indirect mirror laryngoscopy should always be performed prior to fiberoptic evaluation and videostroboscopy. The mirror exam yields information regarding the gag reflex (vagus), and tremor and other abnormal muscular movements, as well as vallecular and piriform sinus pooling. In addition, the time-proven mirror laryngeal exam provides a "wider angle" view of the laryngeal vestibule, supraglottic larynx, and glottis when compared with fiberoptic laryngoscopy.

The thyroid prominence, thyroid cartilage, cricoid cartilage, and thyroid gland should be carefully palpated from behind as well as in front. Evaluate any asymmetry of either the thyroid or cricoid cartilages that may exist, as well as lymphadenopathy, thyromegaly, or other abnormal masses in the region. Have the patient swallow and note laryngeal ascent, which should be at least 2 cm or greater. A full cranial nerve examination is advisable, particularly looking for other evidence of cranial nerve weakness, such as palatal movement asymmetries or weakness of the sternocleidomastoid or trapezius muscles.

9.2.4 Videostroboscopy and Flexible Fiberoptic Laryngoscopy

Outpatient endoscopy and videostroboscopy could be considered as additional diagnostic tests, but among laryngologists these techniques are almost routinely performed on all patients presenting with dysphonia or other phonatory disorders. Accordingly, it is appropriate to include them here in the physical examination. Just as a mirror laryngoscopy should be performed in every laryngology patient, the flexible fiberoptic laryngoscope is an indispensable tool (if possible the distal chip version) for all patients with laryngeal disorders. Although the distal chip (DC) scope has higher resolution, it is not essential that every practicing otolaryngologist must purchase a DC fiberscope, insofar as a study by Eller et al revealed that the standard fiberoptic laryngoscope performed as well as the more expensive DC fiberoptic laryngoscope.[5]

Most clinicians feel that the flexible fiberoptic laryngoscope provides the best view of the vocal folds during phonation, inspiration, cough, throat clearing, and all laryngeal functions. The rigid endoscope often provides a good view, but the necessary tongue retraction renders the exam less physiological than the fiberoptic endoscope passed transnasally. The newer DC scopes offer resolution rivaling that of the rigid scopes and are preferred by many. The larynx should be first viewed (and recorded) during quiet respiration, then during "ee-ee" phonation, and then during sniffing to demonstrate abduction. If the clinician or facility has both rigid and fiberoptic laryngoscopes, it is preferable to perform videolaryngoscopy with both rigid and flexible fiberoptic laryngoscopes. The rigid scope is preferred by some, and according to Eller et al may be better than flexible endoscopy for some lesions.[2,5]

Rigid telescopic videolaryngoscopy and videostroboscopy offer the advantage of being relatively quick and easy. The clinician grasps the patient's tongue tip with a 4 × 4 gauze sponge and slides the scope posteriorly along the midline of the tongue until the larynx comes into view. It is helpful to have the patient lean forward from the hips for the best laryngeal exposure. This exam generally requires no anesthesia; hence, it can be done somewhat faster than the flexible transnasal fiberoptic technique. which requires anesthetic spraying of the nose. (It is also helpful to spray the vallecula and epiglottis.)

Following rigid videoendoscopy (with the tongue being grasped and pulled slightly anteriorly), it is advisable to then complete a transnasal fiberoptic exam. This arguably offers a more physiologic view of the larynx, in that the tongue is in its normal position and with normal untethered lingual and palatal mobility. During the flexible portion of the exam, it is useful to stop the advance of the scope as soon as the epiglottic tip is passed to obtain a wide-angle view of the supraglottis, glottis, and laryngeal vestibule. Subsequently, the clinician should pass the scope on into the laryngeal inlet, so that both false and true vocal folds can be viewed during phonation ("eeee-ee"), connected speech, coughing, and inspiratory sniffing. Additionally, remember to pass the fiberscope farther inferiorly and very close to the true VF surface so that mucosal lesions, hypervascularity, and other tiny lesions may be noted. Ask the patient to sniff and then rapidly say "eee-ee" three times in succession. In addition it is often useful to have the patient whistle a short segment of a simple tune, such as "Happy Birthday," while the VF movements are being observed. Whistling is a good test of rapid abduction, adduction, and VF coordination and will allow for detection of dysdiadochokinesis and other movement disorders.[6]

During each portion of the exam, be sure to observe the two sides carefully, comparing one to the other, as well as looking for abnormal "associated" movements. Small jerks or tremors (caused by synkinesis) can often best be detected by watching the corniculate cartilage area atop the arytenoid cartilages. These fine movements may be the best indication that unfavorable synkinesis is at least a part of the etiology of the dysphonia.

If one suspects RLN-related (neurogenic) VFI, it is prudent to observe closely the configuration and position of the ipsilateral arytenoid cartilage. Characteristically in the early phase (before any RLN or other nerve regeneration can occur) the arytenoid will be subluxated medially and slightly anteriorly (▶ Fig. 9.1). This is because the normal vectors pulling posteriorly, inferiorly, and laterally on the vocal process (lateral cricoarytenoid muscle [LCA] and posterior cricoarytenoid muscle [PCA] muscle) are paralyzed and unopposed. Additionally, the vocal ligament attached to the thyroid cartilage anteriorly exerts an anterior pull on the arytenoid, while the partially innervated interartenoid (IA) muscle exerts a medial pull. This combination of vectors results in the arytenoid being malpositioned, as described and shown in ▶ Fig. 9.2, and this results in the vocal process being rotated inferiorly relative to the level of the vocal process on the opposite side.

9.3 Diagnosis

Given that the differential diagnosis of vocal fold immobility includes a variety of non-RLN causes, as well as RLN-related causes (including synkinesis and central disorders, such as strokes and brainstem lesions), it follows that other clinical tests are often used to further elucidate an accurate diagnosis. These tests include:

- Laryngeal electromyography (LEMG)
- Imaging (computed tomography [CT], magnetic resonance imaging [MRI], standard chest x-ray [CXR])
- Speech pathology testing, including acoustic and aerodynamic measurements

The speech pathology tests are helpful not only to identify and quantify the degree of difficulty the patient is having, but also to document the degree of improvement from treatment,

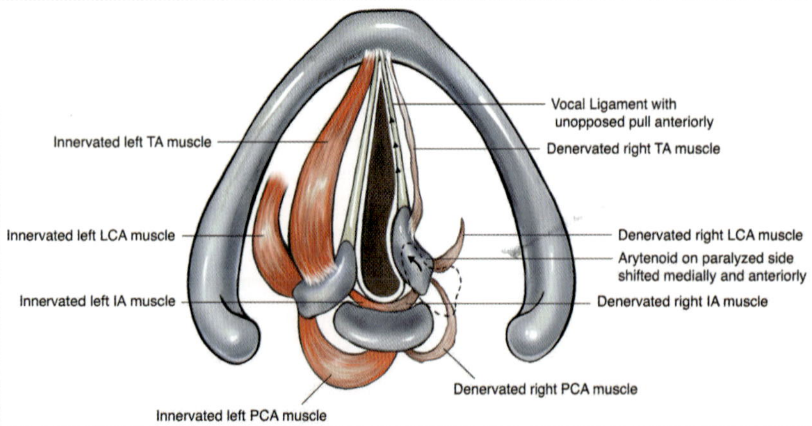

Fig. 9.1 Artist's depiction of a vocal fold following recurrent laryngeal nerve transection with paralysis of ipsilateral thyroarytenoid muscle (TA), lateral cricoarytenoid muscle (LCA), posterior cricoarytenoid muscle (PCA), and interartenoid (IA) muscles, acute phase. Note that the absence of PCA (posteroinferior) and LCA (anteriorly and anteroinferior) forces on the muscular process allows vocal ligament pull anteriorly, and interarytenoid pull medially, to rock the arytenoid medially and anteriorly, which shifts the vocal process and posterior portion of the vocal fold inferiorly.

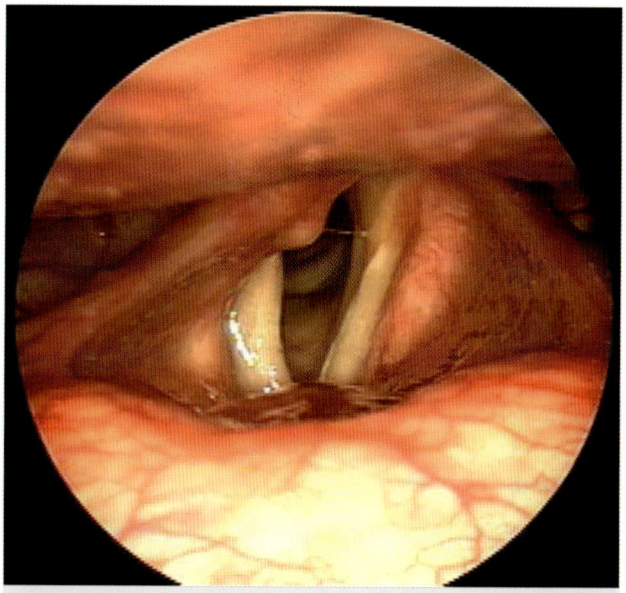

Fig. 9.2 Clinical photograph of patient with acute-phase recurrent laryngeal nerve transection.

once the problem is identified. The tests include, but are not limited to:

- Jitter and shimmer
- Maximum phonation time
- Harmonic to noise ratio

When ordering or performing diagnostic tests, the otolaryngologist should always consider expense and necessity. Routine serologic tests are usually unnecessary and add little or no new clinical information. Panendoscopy (laryngoscopy, bronchoscopy, and esophagoscopy) has been a recommended part of the routine diagnostic workup of all patients with vocal cord paralysis in prior years, but this is no longer necessary, in part due to improvements in imaging technology and resolution.

The history and physical exam will often help ascertain whether a lesion is RLN-related or non-RLN related and should help guide the diagnostic workup. For example, not every VFI patient needs LEMG. The history, comprehensive otolaryngologic exam, and videostroboscopy should give a strong indication of whether an RLN lesion is causative. For example, if a 38-year-old woman had undergone a thyroidectomy 6 weeks earlier and immediately noted the onset of hoarseness, and the surgical operative note confirmed there was difficulty in dissecting the RLN ipsilateral to the immobile VF, then there would be little reason for imaging studies to be done. Acoustic and aerodynamic testing by a speech-language pathologist, however, would help document and quantify the degree of speech difficulty and dysphonia. LEMG could provide some evidence as to the degree of RLN injury sustained, and yet many would argue that it would do little to influence the management of the patient.

Because a large percentage of VFI patients will have paralysis, paresis, or synkinesis, it is important to pursue the diagnostic workup consistent with the history. As mentioned previously, the patient with a recent skull base, cervical, or thoracic surgical procedure and onset of dysphonia immediately postoperatively can be assumed to have an RLN-related cause of immobility. Accordingly, if the physical exam and videostroboscopic findings are consistent with RLN lesion, it is perfectly prudent to pursue treatment of the immobility with an appropriate modality, such as VF injection, medialization, arytenoid adduction, or reinnervation, depending on timing and clinical details, as discussed below. Conversely, a 60-year-old male smoker might be seen with a 2-month history of hoarseness/dysphonia. Mirror indirect laryngoscopy and videostroboscopy could both show VF immobility, with no visible VF mass or ulceration. In this instance, it would be important to obtain a CT or MRI scan of the larynx, and also to obtain a biopsy at an early juncture. In this patient, LEMG is unnecessary unless the imaging and biopsy are both negative for tumor.

Accordingly, it requires considerable insight, forethought, and judgment to order the appropriate tests for each case of VFI.

9.3.1 Laryngeal Electromyography

The scope of this chapter does not allow a full or extensive discussion of LEMG. However, a brief explanation of the role of this technique in diagnostic testing and follow-up in patients with VFI is appropriate. For further information, see Chapter 11 and the references cited here.[1,7,8,9]

Much has been learned about EMG evaluation of the larynx in the past 20 years; yet it is not necessary nor useful in every case of VFI. The most important information that may be derived from LEMG is whether the immobile VF has viable muscle fibers (e.g., is not "electrically silent" when the electrode is placed) and clarification of the status of innervation or reinnervation (e.g., normal potentials with phonation seen with paresis and sometimes synkinesis vs. nascent or polyphasic potentials seen during the reinnervation process vs. fibrillation potentials seen as a result of muscle denervation). Serial LEMG exams may measure and illustrate the course of RLN recovery and the return of muscle innervation, and/or development of synkinesis. After a significant RLN injury, such as complete transection, one expects the laryngeal muscles to demonstrate electrical silence immediately and during the first 14 days following injury. After that initial postinjury period, one should hear/see fibrillation potentials demonstrative of the expected muscle denervation. Beyond this initial time frame, depending on whether the RLN was repaired or is otherwise capable of regeneration, LEMG should demonstrate early nascent potentials as regenerating axons arrive back at their laryngeal motor end plates, and these potentials will grow in volume as increasing numbers of axons regenerate through the lesion and back to the laryngeal intrinsic muscles.

9.3.2 Imaging

Imaging will be useful in many if not most cases of VFI/VFMI. There are several specific instances when scans should be ordered, and a standard CXR should be routine in the diagnostic workup.

Chest X-Ray

A CXR has long been an important part of the workup of vocal cord paralysis, or in RLN-related VFI. Particularly with left-sided VFI without known RLN injury, the otolaryngologist should view and interpret the CXR even if the radiologist submits a normal report. Check carefully the aortic arch area, the mediastinum, and the rest of the course of the RLN in its ascending pathway to the larynx.

Computerized Tomography Scan

If the history and/or exam suggest an RLN-related cause (and if this cause is not obvious or apparent, such as immediately following thyroidectomy or anterior approach to C-spine) the entire course of the RLN should be imaged. This entails CT of the skull base for the jugular foramen area, CT of the neck for the entire cervical course of the vagus nerve and RLN, and chest CT to include the aortic arch and mediastinum as far as the aorticopulmonary window (for left-sided VFI), or subclavian artery (brachiocephalic artery) (for right-sided VFI).[10,11]

A CT scan of the larynx will sometimes provide additional information about the configuration and positioning of the arytenoid cartilages and vocal folds and should be requested at the time of ordering a neck CT.[10] Metastatic mediastinal masses in particular are imaged much more accurately with CT than with CXR.[12] Magnetic resonance imaging has been recommended when high vagal lesions are suspected in the area of the skull base, or even intracranially, because small lesions can be missed in this area.[13] Otherwise, most clinicians and investigators prefer CT to MRI for the workup of VFI. It is important to recognize the various RLN lesions caused by mediastinal disease. A partial list of these and other causes was recently enumerated by Paquette et al as follows:[12]

Vascular and Cardiac Causes of Vocal Fold Immobility

- Aortic dissection
- Pseudoaneurysm
- Left atrial enlargement
- Congenital heart disease
- Pulmonary artery enlargement
- Pulmonary embolism

Neoplastic Causes

- Bronchogenic carcinoma
- Lymphoma
- Esophageal carcinoma
- Neurogenic tumors (paraganglioma, schwannoma)
- Thyroid carcinoma
- Thymic malignancy
- Nodal metastasis
- Retrosternal goiter

Surgical and Iatrogenic Causes

- Cardiac surgery or median sternotomy (valve repair, coronary artery bypass graft)
- Patent ductus arteriosus ligation or embolization
- Left pneumonectomy or lobectomy
- Mediastinoscopy
- Radical esophagectomy
- Tracheal resection
- Thymectomy
- Central venous line catheterization (more commonly right RLN)
- Anterior approach to cervical spine
- Carotid endarterectomy
- External radiation therapy

Inflammatory Causes

- Sarcoidosis
- Silicosis
- Fibrosing mediastinitis

Infiltrative Causes

- Amyloidosis

Infectious Causes

- Tuberculosis
- Histoplasmosis
- Coccidioidomycosis
- Bacterial abscess
- Mycotic infection
- Aortic pseudoaneurysm

Traumatic Causes

- Endotracheal intubation
- Deceleration injuries
- Penetrating injuries

In addition, the author has seen two patients with unilateral immobility from RLN paralysis secondary to cardiac radiofrequency ablation for atrial fibrillation. However, a PubMed search did not show this as documented in the literature yet.

In summary, imaging is generally best performed using standard CXR and CT techniques, being careful to image all regions of the ipsilateral RLN.[13]

9.4 Treatment

Treatment for patients with VFI/VFMI must be directed toward the primary causation of the VFMI. As there are many RLN-unrelated (nonneurologic) causes, and many of them are covered in other chapters of this book, the following discussion focuses on management of the RLN-related causes, primarily paralysis, paresis, and synkinesis. Obviously, the clinician is always dealing with two vocal folds; accordingly, the status of both right and left individual VFs is vitally important to laryngeal function, and particularly to phonatory quality and airway. Most of the following discussion about management of RLN-related VFI assumes that the contralateral VF is functioning normally in both abduction and adduction; we discuss therapeutic options for the patient with unilateral VFI secondary to an RLN lesion. It should be pointed out also that there is necessary overlap between this section and Chapter 17. Furthermore, this discussion assumes that the clinician has performed the diagnostic workup outlined above and has concluded that an RLN lesion is the only cause for the unilateral VFI (otherwise, the non-RLN lesion —tumor, scar, etc.—causing the immobility should be treated appropriately).

9.4.1 Treatment of Unilateral Vocal Fold Immobility (RLN-Related, Neurogenic)

The management of RLN-related VFI/VFMI should always be determined by a careful analysis of the neurophysiologic status of the immobile VF. That is to say, that it is important for the otolaryngologist to understand the exact state of paresis, synkinesis, or full paralysis that exists in the VF. In addition, the timing of treatment is vitally important because the neurophysiologic status of the VF will most probably be changing for at least the first 9 months after onset, if not a full year. Accordingly, this is where EMG may be helpful in deciding a treatment plan. The flow diagram in ▶ Fig. 9.3 provides an overview of the diagnosis and treatment paradigms for VFI.

Early Treatment (First 4 to 6 Weeks)

Patients who suffer an acute RLN injury—traumatic, postsurgical (thyroidectomy, cardiothoracic procedure, anterior approach to C-spine, etc.) or idiopathic—should ideally be seen as soon after the injury as possible. With acute full paralysis (as from RLN transection) the vocal fold will be immediately flaccid and immobile. Aspiration very possibly will be an early comorbidity and is almost certain if the nerve injury is high vagal, or if the superior laryngeal nerve is otherwise damaged. These patients may need an acute injection of Radiesse Voice (Merz Aesthetics, San Mateo, CA), CyMetra (Lifecell Corp, Branchburg, NJ), fat, or other injectable [such as Gelfoam paste (Pfizer, Inc., New York, NY)] to move the flaccid VF toward the midline and provide for glottic closure in swallowing as well as phonation. My

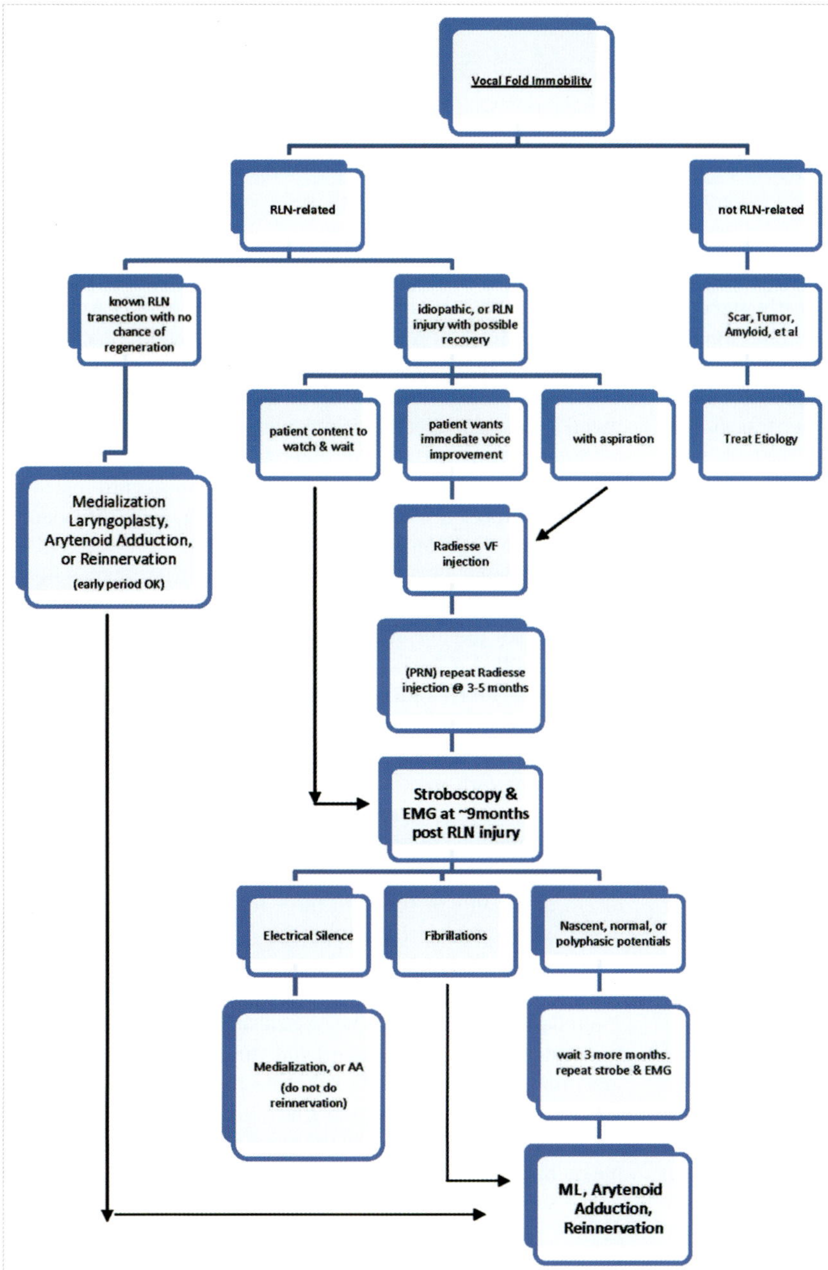

Fig. 9.3 Treatment flow diagram for vocal fold immobility. (VF, vocal fold; AA, arytenoid adduction, EMG, electromyography; PRN, as needed; RLN, recurrent laryngeal nerve; ML, medicalization laryngoplasty)

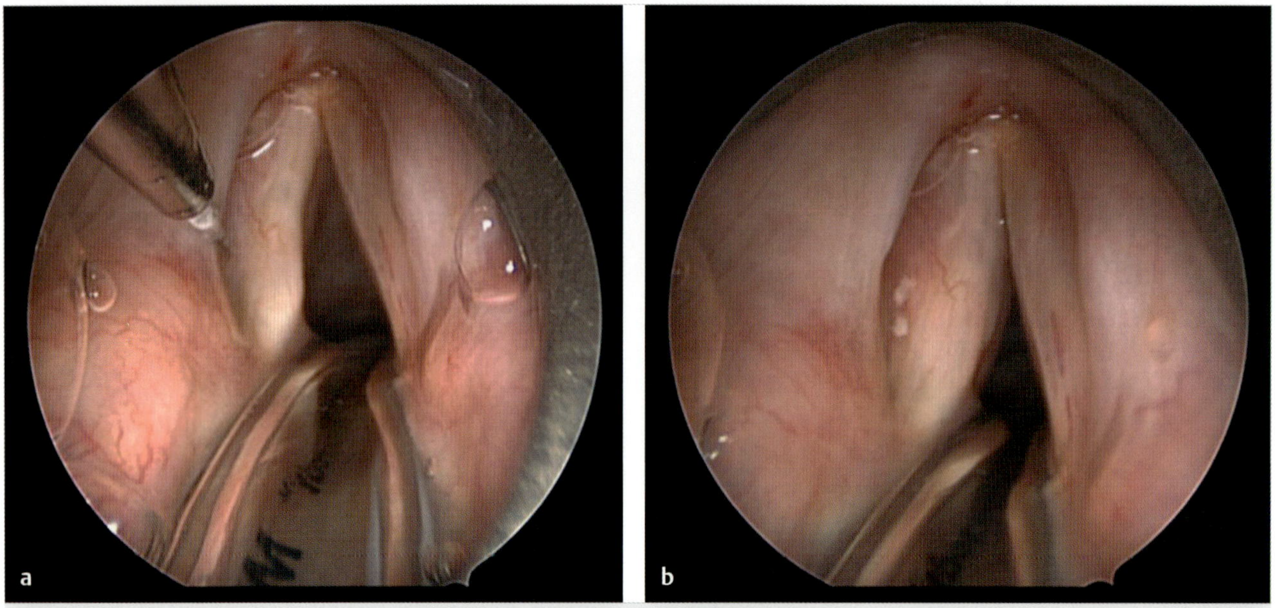

Fig. 9.4 (**a**) Needle positioned posteriorly for injection into lateral aspect of middle third of the vocal fold (VF). (Note that many surgeons believe that a second injection immediately lateral to the vocal process may move the vocal process medially, improving overall result.) (**b**) Medialized VF following injection of ~0.8 cc Radiesse Voice (Merz Aesthetics, San Mateo, CA).

preference in this scenario is Radiesse (generally, Radiesse Voice is better than Radiesse Voice Gel because the gel is usually too short-acting for these patients' needs). This early injection (often soon after the patient is first seen, in the initial week or weeks after RLN injury) is often done in the office, clinic, or voice lab setting with the patient in the sitting position, using transnasal fiberoptic videolaryngoscopy and either transoral or transcutaneous delivery of the Radiesse Voice. As the half-life of Radiesse Voice may be short (only 2–3 months in some patients), the injection can be repeated as necessary while awaiting possible RLN recovery. In an occasional patient, injection may have to be performed in the operating room via direct laryngoscopy. Other temporary injections have been described with various collagen-based compounds[14] or micronized human dermis (CyMetra).[15,16]

At this stage following RLN injury, it is generally imprudent to perform a permanent procedure, such as arytenoid adduction or ansa cervicalis-RLN anastomosis, unless it is absolutely certain that the RLN was completely transected and has no chance for significant return. In that scenario (such as when the RLN was purposefully removed for thyroid or other malignancy, the vagus nerve was resected for a schwannoma, or the RLN was transected and not repaired in an aortic arch procedure), any and all treatment can be considered appropriate, including medialization, arytenoid adduction, or laryngeal reinnervation.

Some patients with RLN injuries have dysphonia but no dysphagia or aspiration when first seen by the otolaryngologist or laryngologist. In those instances, management of the dysphonia should be guided by a discussion with the patient regarding his or her vocal needs, the degree of dysphonia that exists, and the prognosis in the short/intermediate time frame. If the cause is deemed to be "idiopathic VF paralysis" (which increasingly appears to be a herpetic viral neuritis[17,18]) then it is reasonable to pursue a conservative (expectant) course because many will undergo partial or full recovery. It is possible in such cases that the dysphonia will resolve in a matter of weeks, or 2 to 3 months, without treatment. Accordingly, if the patient can tolerate the phonatory difficulty in the short term, it is acceptable to offer no surgical treatment and simply have the patient return every 2 to 4 weeks to track the anticipated return of function. During this initial period, the otolaryngologist can recommend a course of speech therapy with a knowledgeable speech pathologist/clinician. On the other hand, if the patient wants and needs an immediate return of voice, a vocal cord injection may be performed in the office/clinic setting, or in the operating room via direct laryngoscopy (▶ Fig. 9.4).

For such injections, the author frequently uses flexible fiberoptic videolaryngoscopy for monitoring and a transcutaneous technique for the injection of Radiesse Voice. The technique has been described elsewhere but can be easily performed with a 22-gauge, 1.5-inch, or 2.0-inch needle, which can be introduced in several ways.

Through the upper midline of the cricothyroid membrane, angled superiorly and laterally such that it can be seen via the video laryngoscope to pass under and then into the lateral aspect of the middle third of the lateralized vocal fold. As much as 0.4 cc can be placed in two locations (avoiding the most anterior cm of the VF), or 0.3 cc in three locations or more. Usually 1.0 cc is adequate, although there is no reason why additional material cannot be injected if adequate medialization is not achieved.

Similarly, the needle can be passed slightly lateral to the midline and angled slightly upward and laterally. This technique allows the needle to pass directly into the substance of the VF without a needle puncture in the mucosa of the VF, but it is slightly less accurate because the exact puncture site is not visible on the video screen.

The suprathyroid technique is best performed with a 2-inch needle. (Some surgeons prefer a 25-gauge needle, but the Radiesse Voice is more easily passed through the larger 22- or

23-gauge needle. In addition, slightly heating the Radiesse Voice to at least body temperature improves ease of injectability.) The needle should be bent approximately 75 degrees, introduced immediately over the thyroid notch, and downward. The advantage of this technique is that the needle is now visible above the VF, but it may be slightly more difficult to control the exact anteroposterior orientation of the injection. A second advantage of this technique is that there is no calcification encountered with it, as opposed to the frequent calcifications found in the cricothyroid membrane and the lower portions of the thyroid cartilage with the first two techniques.

A fourth, oral technique is preferred by some. The manufacturer of Radiesse Voice provides a long needle that can be bent to the proper curvature to introduce through the mouth, the oropharynx, posterior to the epiglottis, and directly into the superior surface of the true vocal cord. Again, the Radiesse Voice can be placed primarily in the lateral aspect of the middle third of the lateralized immobile VF, with a slightly smaller amount posteriorly, just lateral to the vocal process, and a smaller amount just anterior to the first portion. It is worth repeating that injection of the anterior third of the VF is to be avoided as it will lead to poor phonatory/vocal results.

Intermediate Period (6 Weeks to 9 Months)

Following the early period, some patients begin to compensate slightly with the contralateral VF. As mentioned previously, if the degree of injury and the amount of recovery are not clearly established (which is the norm in many cases), the patient and the otolaryngologist should wait approximately 9 months for recovery to occur. During this first 9 months after the onset of neurogenic immobility, the RLN may or may not regenerate to the point of partial or complete VF recovery. In such patients, a full paralysis with VF lateralization and flaccidity may transition into a VF paresis with improved positioning, a balance of abductive and adductive forces with favorable synkinesis and good voice, other synkinetic outcomes with jerkiness or other VF incoordination (and poor voice), or remain lateralized, paramedian, or otherwise suboptimal for achieving satisfactory phonatory voice. During this period, frequent (every 2 months) videostroboscopic exams are useful to document changes in arytenoid position, vocal process position, and VF position.

During this period, the clinician needs to remain supportive of patient and remind them that a more permanent surgical solution may await them at the 9- to 12-month mark following RLN injury. (medialization laryngoplasty with or without arytenoid adduction, VF fat injection, or laryngeal reinnervation with or without arytenoid adduction). Voice therapy may be useful; many patients will learn tips on how to use their weakened vocal instrument more efficiently during this recovery period. Some otolaryngologists feel that it is acceptable to perform medialization (Isshiki 1) laryngoplasty in either the early or the intermediate period, insofar as the technique is theoretically reversible (by simply removing the implant). In this regard, it is a technically easier surgical task to remove a Silastic implant than a Gore-Tex (W.L. Gore & Associates, Elkton, MD) implant. In addition, some laryngeal surgeons feel that medialization laryngoplasty changes the VF and the paraglottic space; hence, even if the implant is removed, the procedure is not completely reversible. On the other hand, there are some patients in whom VF movements have been recovered following RLN injury; the laryngoplasty implants have been left in situ with no airway or phonatory defect noted.

Late Period (9 Months after RLN Injury and Later)

After 9 months have elapsed following RLN injury, there will be little or no significant additional nerve regeneration and recovery. For known injuries of the cervical vagus nerve, aortic arch injuries, or mediastinal lesions, it is conjectural that one should wait one full year before undertaking permanent treatment. However, it is known that the more proximal the nerve injury (e.g., thorax, cervical vagus, or high cervical vagus and skull base), the less chance that nerve regeneration and recovery will occur. Therefore, in general, a 9-month waiting period is adequate. By that time, the extent of nerve regeneration and quantity and quality of VF movements restored will be readily apparent. Accordingly, a permanent treatment for the patient's VF immobility can be discussed and implemented.

At this juncture, the modified 10-point Vocal Handicap Index (VHI) should be administered and recorded. Again, laryngeal videostroboscopy should be done and compared with previous exams. It is important to note whether the arytenoid has returned to its normal symmetrical position with respect to the other arytenoid. If not, it is likely that the vocal process is inferior to the normal side at rest, and possibly is pushed superior to the normal side by subglottal air pressure during phonation. It is important also to note carefully any accessory movements of the arytenoid during the exam. These are often best noted by observing the corniculate cartilage area atop the arytenoid mound. Look for slight twitching or jerky movements, especially if accompanied by dysphonia. Also look for unintended abductive movements during phonation, or adductive movements during attempted inspiration, both evidence of unfavorable laryngeal synkinesis.

It is important to be aware of the various possibilities for VF movements that may result from misdirected RLN regeneration and VF synkinesis. This author has attempted to classify some of these possibilities into four types of laryngeal synkinesis.[19,20]

Type I, the only favorable type, results in excellent arytenoid and VF position, with no inappropriate movements. Although there will be little or no observable VF movement (abduction or adduction) upon phonation or inspiration, the resting muscle tone and balance of abductive and adductive forces allow the VF to entrain properly with the normal opposite side. In such cases the voice can be excellent or even normal, depending on the patient's age, pulmonary status, and the health and vitality of the contralateral VF.

The other three types of laryngeal synkinesis are associated with poor phonatory quality and/or airway compromise. Type II is a VF that has flawed twitching, jerky, or other aberrant movements, particularly during attempted phonation, such that the arytenoid cartilage, vocal process, and attached VF are moving in an uncoordinated manner during phonation. The voice may be good during the onset of phonation but is generally unreliable, with breaks and other abnormalities during prolonged vowels. Treatment is either short term with botox injections to the TA or lateral LCA, or longer term with RLN transection and anastomosis with the ansa cervicalis. The latter reinnervation procedure quiets the unintended movements and usually improves the voice rather markedly.

Type III synkinesis results in VF movements medially (adduction) during inspiration. These may be subtle—hence compatibility with VFI. A videostroboscopic exam will document adductive movements during sniff testing, while the other VF abducts appropriately. Some of these patients will have presented to the clinician with a complaint of airway distress, especially upon climbing stairs or other exertion. Typically, the symptom is not present during the first 3 to 4 months of the RLN-related immobility because it does not appear until the former PCA muscle/abductive (inspiratory-firing) nerve fibers have regenerated far enough to reinnervate TA, LCA, or IA abductor muscle fibers. Treatment of type III synkinesis is by botox injections to the LCA and/or TA muscles or by ansa-RLN anastomosis.

Type IV seems to be the least common of the four types and describes the VF that abducts during attempted phonation. This is caused by aberrant and faulty reinnervation of portions of the abductor PCA muscle by formerly phonatory nerve fibers (axons), which previously innervated the TA, IA, or LCA muscle. The fibers then produce PCA contraction during phonation, which abducts the vocal process and pulls the VF away from the adducting other side during attempted phonation. Treatment is either botox injection to the offending PCA muscle or ansa-RLN anastomosis.

Most frequently in RLN-related (neurogenic) VF immobility or paresis at 9 months (or later) following RLN injury, the VF presents somewhat lateral to its most optimal position, with little or no abductive or adductive movement, and with minimal obvious synkinetic movements of type II, III, or IV. With attempted phonation during stroboscopy, the examiner will note significant air escape and poor glottal closure and VF entrainment. What is needed for improved phonation is for the involved VF to be moved medially. In this most common clinical scenario, the patient can be treated by medialization laryngoplasty with or without arytenoid adduction (see Chapter 17), VF injection, or ansa-RLN reinnervation with or without arytenoid adduction.

9.4.2 Medialization Laryngoplasty

The most frequently used of the treatment options is medialization laryngoplasty (ML), described in Chapter 17. The author has treated virtually all neurogenic VFI patients with either ML or reinnervation. Others have combined the techniques and have described success.[15,21] After the appropriate interval (9–12 months) has elapsed to allow for physiological regeneration and recovery, it is appropriate to proceed with ML. Many authors have described the technique, which is usually performed under local anesthesia with sedation. Phonatory improvement is usually immediate (see Chapter 17).[22,23,24]

9.4.3 Lipoinjection

Injection laryngoplasty techniques and materials are discussed earlier in this chapter. Some phonosurgeons use fat injection as a permanent method for treating unilateral VFI.[25,26] This has not realized universal acceptance because the persistence of the injected fat has proven to be variable. However, it is a technique that warrants further research and review. The fat is harvested from the abdominal wall under sterile conditions using standard liposuction technique. Subsequently, the fat is rinsed with saline and then treated with insulin to stabilize cell membranes and promote fat survival. It is then injected via an appropriate injector (Brunings syringe, Storz, St. Louis, MO; or Lipoinjector, Instrumentarium, Montreal, Canada).[27] Producing a convez VF edge by overinjection is necessary because a variable amount of the injected fat is either absorbed or undergoes necrosis.

9.4.4 Laryngeal Reinnervation

Another treatment option for RLN-related VFI involves reinnervating the paralyzed or paretic intrinsic muscles with a different nerve. As noted above, the most common nerve is the ansa cervicalis, although use of the hypoglossal nerve has been described.[17,18] Reinnervation is not as commonly performed as is ML, but it does offer some advantages in certain patients.[28] I prefer to use reinnervation in younger patients, those who use their voices professionally (singers, public speakers, etc.), and those in whom it is highly probable that both RLN and ansa cervicalis can be surgically identified. ▶ Table 9.1 shows the advantages and disadvantages of reinnervation when compared to ML.

My technique for laryngeal reinnervation is a simple three-suture nerve anastomosis of the largest ansa cervicalis branch or branches to the distal stump of the RLN (▶ Fig. 9.5).[30] (Paniello has also described using the hypoglossal nerve as a reinnervation source[31]; others have used the ansa cervicalis by utilizing the neuromuscular pedicle concept popularized by Tucker.[32]) Our series currently numbers just over 100 patients, although Zheng reported a much larger series of 237 cases recently using essentially the same technique.[33] The procedure consists of three stages:

1. Identifying the ansa cervicalis (and dissecting one, two, or three branches distally) (▶ Fig. 9.6a)

Table 9.1 Ansa reinnervation (vs. medialization laryngoplasty)

Advantages	Disadvantages
1. Phonatory improvement usually permanent 2. No alteration of VF, arytenoid, or other parts of larynx (no implants) 3. Replaces what is missing (muscle tone in intrinsic muscles) 4. Permanent reinnervation of intrinsic muscles (a "babysitter" if, in the future, a new procedure evolves that can evoke physiological movements—abduction and adduction) 5. Produces physiological arytenoid adduction and puts vocal process at physiologically normal inferiosuperior level	1. Usually requires general anesthesia 2. Actual reinnervation (and return of phonation) occurs 3–4 months postop (requiring temporary injection usually) 3. Not possible if distal recurrent laryngeal nerve or ansa unavailable (contralateral ansa can be used)[29] 4. Not advisable in elderly or diabetic patients

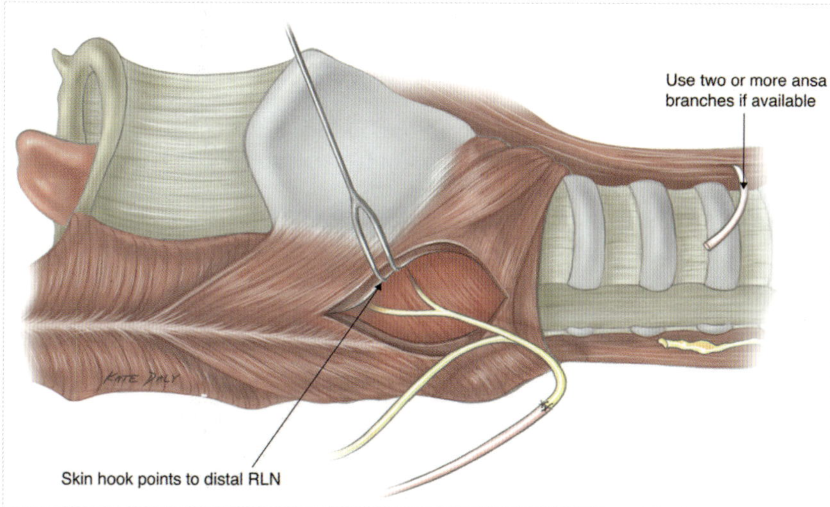

Fig. 9.5 Illustration of ansa cervicalis–recurrent laryngeal nerve (RLN) anastomosis. Ansa to strap muscles has been transected and turned medially. Recurrent laryngeal nerve has been transected distal to nerve injury, and distal RLN has been sutured to ansa cervicalis.

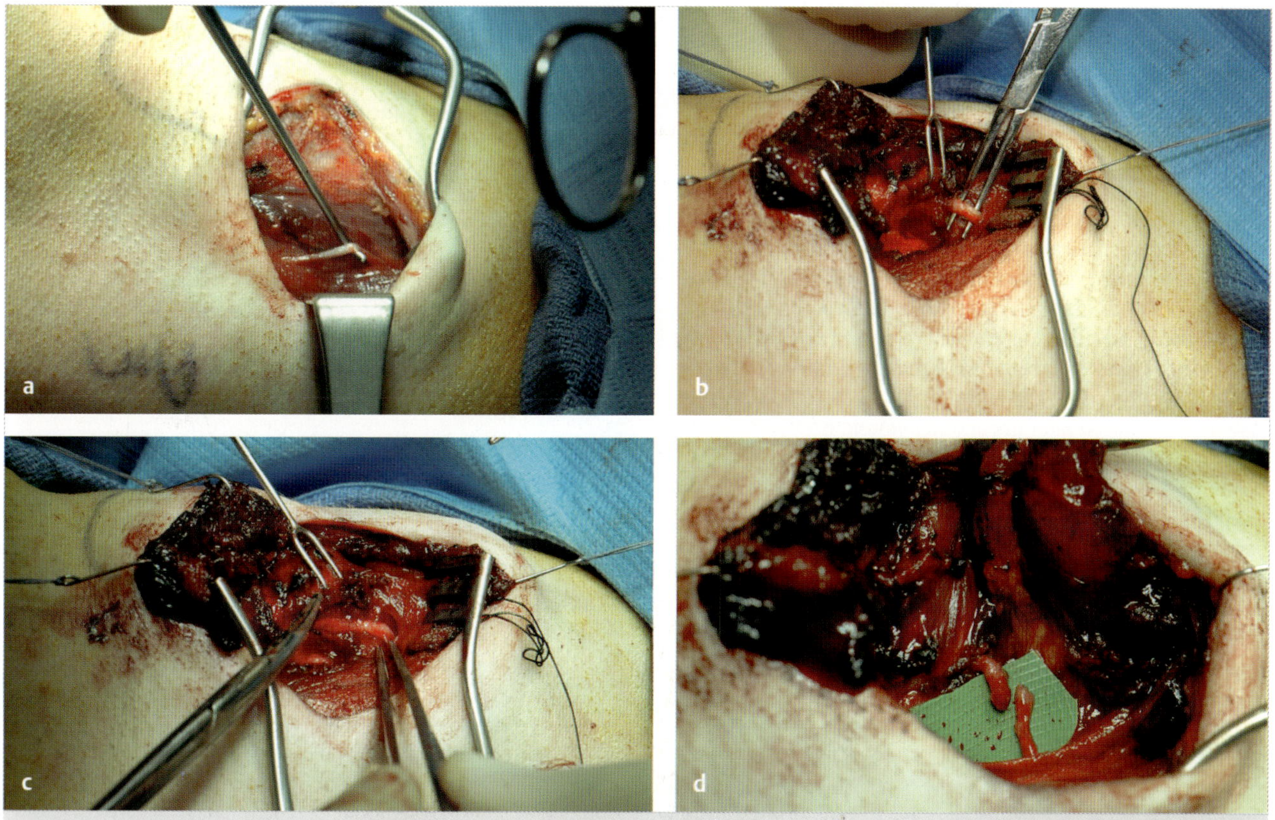

Fig. 9.6 (**a**) The right ansa cervicalis is identified and dissected distally to its entry point into the strap muscles. The largest of the ansa's branches, or preferably two largest branches, should be identified, dissected, and prepared for anastomosis. (**b**) The right recurrent laryngeal nerve (RLN) is identified. Notice how careful placement of the double-prong skin hook at the most inferior point of the right thyroid ala points directly to the RLN, which is 3 to 5 mm below the hook, and deep to the cricopharyngeus muscle. (**c**) Further dissection of the RLN confirms and clarifies the usefulness of the hook as an anatomic indicator. The RLN is ready for transection and suture. The ansa is out of view, lower to the right with a silk suture looped around it. (**d**) The nerves have been transected and positioned against microsurgical background material for anastomosis.

2. Identifying the RLN near the larynx (▶ Fig. 9.6b,c)
3. Suturing as many ansa branches as will reach to the RLN's distal stump using simple epineural sutures of 8–0 or 9–0 nylon (▶ Fig. 9.6d)

Operative details. The ansa cervicalis is identified overlying the internal jugular vein. The largest and most electrically stimulable branch should be used (usually this is the branch to the sternohyoid muscle), but if possible use each and every ansa branch that is long enough to reach the RLN's suture site. The nerve stimulator is often helpful in finding and identifying which branch(es) are the most active.

RLN identification. Because it is optimal for the anastomosis to be performed distally, the RLN is identified just below the cricothyroid joint. Place a double-prong skin hook on the lowest portion of the thyroid ala, just above the cricoid, and rotate the thyroid cartilage anteriorly and toward the opposite side. The lower hook of the double hook will point at the RLN, which will be found 3 to 4 mm from the end of the hook and immediately deep to the cricopharyngeus muscle. Essentially a cricopharyngeal myotomy is performed, then the RLN is found using a McCabe nerve dissector (Pilling/Teleflex, Durham, NC), and then the RLN dissected inferiorly, deep to the thyroid gland. In most cases, a nerve stimulator may be used and is often helpful in identifying the RLN. We have found it useful to use the RLN integrity monitor system, including an endotracheal tube with EMG electrodes (NIM, Medtronic, Minneapolis, MN),[34] insofar as it often saves time in locating the RLN in this distal location. In most cases, the distal RLN is electrically excitable, despite the clinical status of neurogenic VFI (due to laryngeal synkinesis). If possible, dissect the RLN 1.5 to 2.0 cm inferiorly so as to leave enough nerve length available to turn the distal stump laterally for anastomosis to the ansa. Sometimes it is helpful to transect the strap muscles and/or to mobilize the superior pole of the thyroid gland, to facilitate exposure of the RLN as well as to facilitate exposure of the ansa-RLN anastomosis site.

Microsurgical background material is then placed, the transected nerve ends (ansa branch or branches) severed distally, and the RLN ends are then placed near one another on the colored background material. We usually use an operating microscope for the nerve anastomosis, although if 8–0 nylon is used, 2.5 or 3.0 × surgical loupes will suffice. Usually a half-inch Penrose drain is placed laterally and the wound is closed in layers, including the strap muscles if they were transected.

After wound closure, an operating laryngoscope is then placed, and an ipsilateral Radiesse Voice or Cymetra injection is performed via direct laryngoscopy (for short-term phonatory enhancement during the 3-month + period until the reinnervating nerve fibers reach the laryngeal muscles).

At approximately 2.5 months postoperatively, videolaryngoscopy will reveal the arytenoid cartilage to be moving toward a more normal and symmetrical position, from its common abnormal VFI location of anteriomedial subluxation. This also means that the vocal process and VF have moved higher and are now at approximately the same inferiosuperior level as the contralateral vocal process. When this arytenoid repositioning is noted, it is usually not more than 2 weeks later that the patient reports that the phonatory voice has markedly improved. Anecdotally, sometimes patients report that this occurs overnight, or over a 24-hour period.

9.5 Treatment Failure

Considering that the main symptom of RLN-related VFI is hoarseness, dysphonia, poor voice quality, and/or diplophonia, the goal of treatment is to restore the most normal phonatory voice possible. Treatment failure then is defined as poor vocal quality following completion of one of the described treatments (VF injection laryngoplasty, Isshiki I ML, arytenoid adduction, or reinnervation). Following reinnervation, one should wait 9 months before making the assumption that the reinnervation failed. Objective assessments of voice to ascertain success or failure would entail such parameters as jitter, shimmer, maximum phonation time (MPT), harmonics/noise ratio, as well as a subjective VHI-10.

If the vocal quality and results of the above parameters are such that the laryngologist and the patient both feel further improvement is necessary and feasible, then an additional intervention should be discussed. The selection of a procedure depends on what is deemed to be responsible for the resultant dysphonia. Some examples follow.

Postoperative dysphonia causes and possible resolutions

Fat Injection

- Overinjection → Laser or cup-forcep removal[29]
- Underinjection, or loss of fat → Reinject fat, Radiesse Voice®, Cymetra®, or do medialization laryngoplasty

Medialization Laryngoplasty

- Implant malposition → Surgically replace implant
- Implant too small, too large → Surgically replace implant

Arytenoid Adduction

- Arytenoid too medial → Revise adduction suture
- Arytenoid not adducted enough → Revise adduction suture, medialization laryngoplasty
- Vocal process inferior or superior → Revise adduction suture

Reinnervation

- Poor phonatory quality → Medialization laryngoplasty → Injection
- Posterior glottal gap → Arytenoid adduction

9.6 Key Points

- VFI can be confusing if the important passive mobility test reveals normal arytenoid mobility (VF motion impairment or "dysmotility" may be more accurate).
- It is critical to rule out all RLN-unrelated causes of VFI prior to undertaking treatment of neurogenic (RLN-related) causes because the unrelated ones include VF cancer, scar, and infiltrative lesions, such as amyloidosis, etc.
- A careful history is often the key to identifying the etiology of VFI and may also yield important information regarding whether it is necessary to wait the usual 9 to 12 months to allow for RLN recovery and contralateral VF compensation.
- Whenever feasible, perform both rigid and fiberoptic videolaryngoscopy and videostroboscopy.
- Consider the entire course of the RLN's fibers from brainstem through the skull base, cervical vagus, thorax, mediastinum, and cervical RLN when assessing neurogenic VFI.

- Obtain CXR in all cases of VFI, and use CT in cases when the cause is not readily apparent. Remember to obtain CT images of the larynx in addition to imaging the course of the RLN.
- Use LEMG for determining the extent and quality of existing innervation in the laryngeal muscles, for tracking RLN regeneration during the intermediate period, and for assessing whether full regeneration has occurred at the 9-month mark following RLN injury.
- Remember that combinations of paresis and synkinesis may explain certain VF configurations and behaviors as well as treatment failures of ML or VF injections; understand how synkinetic reinnervation may influence these movements.
- Unless an RLN resection or transection (without repair) is known, wait at least 9 months to allow for normal RLN regeneration before performing permanent neurogenic VFI surgical treatment.
- During the course of management, the otolaryngologist should remain supportive and recommend voice therapy (and sometimes psychological counseling) during any interval in which it may be deemed helpful. Many patients are emotionally devastated by VFI dysphonia.

References

[1] Hillel A, Robinson L. Diagnostic electromyography for unilateral vocal fold dysmotility. In: Sulica L, Blitzer A, eds. Vocal Fold Paralysis. New York, NY: Springer; 2006: 63–73

[2] Sulica L, Cultrara A, Blitzer A. Vocal fold paralysis: causes, outcomes, and clinical aspects. In: Sulica L, Blitzer A, eds. Vocal Fold Paralysis. New York, NY: Springer; 2006: 38–48

[3] Simpson CB, Fleming DJ. Medical and vocal history in the evaluation of dysphonia. Otolaryngol Clin North Am 2000; 33: 719–730

[4] Titche LL. Causes of recurrent laryngeal nerve paralysis. Arch Otolaryngol 1976; 102: 259–261

[5] Eller R, Ginsburg M, Lurie D, Heman-Ackah Y, Lyons K, Sataloff R. Flexible laryngoscopy: a comparison of fiber optic and distal chip technologies. Part 1: vocal fold masses. J Voice 2008; 22: 746–750

[6] Warner T, Bressman S. Laryngeal dystonia. In: Clinical Diagnosis and Management of Dystonia. London: Informa Healthcare; 2007: 113–115

[7] Meyer TK, Hillel AD. Is laryngeal electromyography useful in the diagnosis and management of vocal fold paresis/paralysis? Laryngoscope 2011; 121: 234–235

[8] Blitzer A, Crumley RL, Dailey SH et al. Recommendations of the neurolaryngology study group on laryngeal electromyography. Otolaryngol Head Neck Surg 2009; 140: 782–793

[9] Maronian NC, Robinson L, Waugh P, Hillel AD. A new electromyographic definition of laryngeal synkinesis. Ann Otol Rhinol Laryngol 2004; 113: 877–886

[10] Benninger MS, Crumley RL, Ford CN et al. Evaluation and treatment of the unilateral paralyzed vocal fold. Otolaryngol Head Neck Surg 1994; 111: 497–508

[11] Paquette CM, Manos DC, Psooy BJ. Unilateral vocal cord paralysis: a review of CT findings, mediastinal causes, and the course of the recurrent laryngeal nerves. Radiographics 2012; 32: 721–740

[12] Glazer HS, Aronberg DJ, Lee JK, Sagel SS. Extralaryngeal causes of vocal cord paralysis: CT evaluation. AJR Am J Roentgenol 1983; 141: 527–531

[13] Koufman JA, Postma GN, Whang CS et al. Diagnostic laryngeal electromyography: the Wake Forest experience 1995–1999. Otolaryngol Head Neck Surg 2001; 124: 603–606

[14] Ford CN, Martin DW, Warner TF. Injectable collagen in laryngeal rehabilitation. Laryngoscope 1984; 94: 513–518

[15] Pearl AW, Woo P, Ostrowski R, Mojica J, Mandell DL, Costantino P. A preliminary report on micronized AlloDerm injection laryngoplasty. Laryngoscope 2002; 112: 990–996

[16] Courey MS. Homologous collagen substances for vocal fold augmentation. Laryngoscope 2001; 111: 747–758

[17] Bhattacharyya N, Kotz T, Shapiro J. Dysphagia and aspiration with unilateral vocal cord immobility: incidence, characterization, and response to surgical treatment. Ann Otol Rhinol Laryngol 2002; 111: 672–679

[18] Amin MR, Koufman JA. Vagal neuropathy after upper respiratory infection: a viral etiology? Am J Otolaryngol 2001; 22: 251–256

[19] Crumley RL. Laryngeal synkinesis: its significance to the laryngologist. Ann Otol Rhinol Laryngol 1989; 98: 87–92

[20] Crumley RL. Laryngeal synkinesis revisited. Ann Otol Rhinol Laryngol 2000; 109: 365–371

[21] Chhetri DK, Gerratt BR, Kreiman J, Berke GS. Combined arytenoid adduction and laryngeal reinnervation in the treatment of vocal fold paralysis. Laryngoscope 1999; 109: 1928–1936

[22] Koufman JA. Laryngoplasty for vocal cord medialization: an alternative to Teflon. Laryngoscope 1986; 96: 726–731

[23] Netterville JL, Stone RE, Luken ES, Civantos FJ, Ossoff RH. Silastic medialization and arytenoid adduction: the Vanderbilt experience. A review of 116 phonosurgical procedures. Ann Otol Rhinol Laryngol 1993; 102: 413–424

[24] McCulloch TM, Hoffman HT. Medialization laryngoplasty with expanded polytetrafluoroethylene. Surgical technique and preliminary results. Ann Otol Rhinol Laryngol 1998; 107: 427–432

[25] Mikaelian DO, Lowry LD, Sataloff RT. Lipoinjection for unilateral vocal cord paralysis. Laryngoscope 1991; 101: 465–468

[26] Brandenburg JH, Kirkham W, Koschkee D. Vocal cord augmentation with autogenous fat. Laryngoscope 1992; 102: 495–500

[27] Rosen C. Autologus fat for vocal fold injection. In: Sulica L, Blitzer A, eds. Vocal Fold Paralysis. New York, NY: Springer; 2006: 105–110

[28] Paniello RC, Edgar JD, Kallogjeri D, Piccirillo JF. Medialization versus reinnervation for unilateral vocal fold paralysis: a multicenter randomized clinical trial. Laryngoscope 2011; 121: 2172–2179

[29] Wang W, Chen S, Chen D et al. Contralateral ansa cervicalis-to-recurrent laryngeal nerve anastomosis for unilateral vocal fold paralysis: a long-term outcome analysis of 56 cases. Laryngoscope 2011; 121: 1027–1034

[30] Crumley RL, Izdebski K. Voice quality following laryngeal reinnervation by ansa hypoglossi transfer. Laryngoscope 1986; 96: 611–616

[31] Paniello RC, West SE, Lee P. Laryngeal reinnervation with the hypoglossal nerve. I. Physiology, histochemistry, electromyography, and retrograde labeling in a canine model. Ann Otol Rhinol Laryngol 2001; 110: 532–542

[32] Tucker HM. Long-term preservation of voice improvement following surgical medialization and reinnervation for unilateral vocal fold paralysis. J Voice 1999; 13: 251–256

[33] Wang W, Chen D, Chen S et al. Laryngeal reinnervation using ansa cervicalis for thyroid surgery-related unilateral vocal fold paralysis: a long-term outcome analysis of 237 cases. PLoS ONE 2011; 6: e19128

[34] Randolph G. Surgical anatomy of the recurrent laryngeal nerve. In: Surgery of the Thyroid and Parathyroid Glands. Philadelphia, PA: Elsevier; 2003: 316

10 Laryngeal Stenosis

Chandra M. Ivey

Laryngeal stenosis is an uncommon problem that may be difficult to diagnose and treat. This chapter explores the etiologies, work-up and techniques for intervention in the various forms of this disease.

10.1 History and Physical Examination

10.1.1 The Normal Airway

The normal airway starts at the nares and oral cavity and ends in the mainstem bronchi. It includes the nasopharynx, oropharynx, larynx, and trachea. The larynx is further subdivided into the supraglottis, glottis, and subglottis. This system is designed to provide an adequate airflow from the environment to the lungs and to maintain normal minute ventilation while allowing for special functions like airway protection, cough, voice, and deglutition. Any change to the airway may compromise these abilities. One of the most important considerations for the maintenance of ventilation is size and location of the narrowest segment of the airway. In the pediatric population, the narrowest point is at the cricoid cartilage in the subglottis. As the laryngeal framework grows, the narrowest segment becomes the vocal folds at the level of the glottis. Changes at either of these structures have the potential to narrow the airway. Narrowing may cause turbulence and contribute to inefficient coordination of respiration, speaking, and swallowing. This, combined with the Bernouli effect, can produce stridor. Airway size has become even more important during general anesthesia and endotracheal intubation. Although pediatric airway size is often estimated using the formula $4 + (\text{AGE} \times ¼)$ to determine proper endotracheal tube size, there is no standard way to estimate the airway size in the adult population due to the common practice of using cuffed endotracheal tubes. In situations when an endotracheal tube is improperly sized, when prolonged intubation is required, when an intubated patient has significant inflammation of the larynx, or when there is persistent movement of the endotracheal tube in the airway, there is potential for trauma, subsequent edema, and scarring resulting in airway stenosis.

10.1.2 Patient History

Laryngeal stenosis can be caused by multiple factors that culminate in shortness of breath as the primary symptom. Patients complain of persistent exercise intolerance and/or noisy breathing, often with voice changes. Cough may be present and is often barking in nature. The goal of the history and physical examination is to determine whether the symptoms are due to airway stenosis and to establish the etiology in order to decide on appropriate management. The underlying cause of laryngeal stenosis is often different in adult and pediatric groups. Onset of symptoms may be congenital, insidious in nature, or immediate after trauma or intubation. Worsening of symptoms can be associated with recent weight gain or pregnancy. Patients are often misdiagnosed with asthma and fail to improve with bronchodilators or inhaled steroids. Associated fatigue, arthralgia, rashes, and gastrointestinal symptoms should be investigated. Prior history of prematurity with possible intubation, history of neck irradiation, or family history of autoimmune disease are important factors that can contribute to development of airway problems. Key points of patient history for diagnosis of laryngeal stenosis are summarized in ▶ Table 10.1.

10.1.3 Differential Diagnosis

Although the workup may be standardized, the etiologies and differential diagnoses in pediatric and adult laryngeal stenosis are often variable. Congenital laryngeal pathology should be ruled out in the pediatric population. Laryngomalacia and unilateral vocal fold paralysis are more common than congenital laryngeal stenosis and are easy to diagnose on flexible laryngoscopy. It is possible, particularly in the pediatric population, to have multiple upper airway problems. A positive diagnosis of laryngomalacia, for example, does not fully rule out a concurrent diagnosis of subglottic stenosis. In the acute setting, an airway foreign body, as well as infections like supraglottitis and croup, may present with sudden progressive dyspnea and airway noise and are often handled in an emergent manner. Subglottic stenosis should be suspected and ruled out in children with recurrent croup. Laryngeal stenosis is often misdiagnosed

Table 10.1 Components of the history necessary for determination of laryngeal stenosis

History component	Patient response
Onset	Fast, emergent Slow, progressive
Concurrent symptoms	Cough Dyspnea with speaking Exercise intolerance Pain Stridor
Past medical history	Asthma Autoimmune disease Caustic ingestion Intubations Neck irradiation Pregnancy Prematurity Pulmonary disease Weight gain
Past surgical history	Neck surgery Postsurgical complications Tracheotomy
Social history	Alcohol Chemical exposure Smoking
Family history	Autoimmune disease Genetic disease

as asthma and should be ruled out in cases that are unresponsive to treatment. Asthma tends to cause expiratory wheezing and laryngeal stenosis is often associated with inspiratory stridor; however, both may have cough as a primary symptom.

The adult population is more susceptible to laryngeal trauma from neck injuries due to the lower anatomical location of the larynx. Airway compression from hematoma, bleeding, or laryngeal fracture must be ruled out if there is a history of trauma. Adult patients are more likely to have acute respiratory compromise from angioedema due to the wide use of angiotensin-converting enzyme (ACE) inhibitors in the American population. The symptoms may mimic laryngeal stenosis but must be treated as an airway emergency. Laryngospasm and paradoxical vocal fold motion should be included in the differential for laryngeal stenosis; however, in these cases symptoms are episodic and are differentiated by history. The differential diagnoses for laryngeal stenosis in the pediatric and adult populations are summarized in ▶ Table 10.2.

10.1.4 Physical Examination

A complete physical examination inclusive of neck and pulmonary auscultation is essential in the diagnosis of laryngeal stenosis. Although vital signs are usually normal, occasionally mild tachypnea and tachycardia may be present. Oxygen saturation is usually normal. Assessment of the patient's body positioning and level of distress is important to determine whether acute intervention may be necessary. Patients may be comfortable at rest but need multiple breaths to complete a sentence when speaking, indicating they are unable to take in enough air. Stridor may be present at rest, or it may manifest with speaking or activity. Attention should be paid to presence of suprasternal or supraclavicular retractions with inspiration. Wheezing is typically not present. The head and neck should be examined for radiation changes or scarring from previous neck procedures, such as thyroidectomy or tracheotomy. Often, the head and neck examination is nonlocalizing until laryngoscopy is performed. Supraglottic or glottic masses can be easily visualized by laryngoscopy. Vocal fold motion and glottic aperture are also evaluated on the exam. It is important to note scarring and fibrosis when present, as they can narrow the anterior glottis, as in the case of anterior glottic webbing, or decrease vocal fold abduction with presence of posterior scar band. The immediate subglottis or even trachea can be evaluated by visualizing the airway through the vocal folds on laryngoscopy or performing in-office tracheoscopy. Auscultation of the neck for inspiratory and expiratory stridor can assist with diagnosis. Presence of wheezing, rhonchi, rales, or crackles on lung auscultation may point toward other causes for dyspnea.

Table 10.2 Differential diagnosis of laryngeal stenosis; Xs indicate common diagnoses in the pediatric and adult populations

	Pediatric population	Adult population
Laryngomalacia	X	
Unilateral vocal fold paralysis	X	
Supraglottitis	X	X
Croup	X	
Asthma	X	X
Acute trauma	X	X
Angioedema		X
Neoplasm	X	X
Paradoxical vocal fold motion		X
Foreign body	X	X

10.2 Diagnosis

Pathologic conditions that may cause airway narrowing can also lead to laryngeal stenosis. Because this is truly a condition and not a specific disease, each etiology must be considered and ruled out. It is also important to remember that airway stenosis can involve multiple levels. Some systemic diseases may affect multiple parts of the larynx and affect different patients in different ways. The larynx is subdivided into three anatomical subsites: supraglottis, glottis, and subglottis. Narrowing in these subsites often has separate etiologies, symptoms, and management. Laryngeal stenosis may further be categorized based on infiltrative versus exophytic processes, intrinsic versus extrinsic etiologies, and soft tissue versus cartilaginous involvement. These distinctions assist in decision making for both treatment and operative intervention.

10.2.1 Supraglottic Stenosis

Supraglottic stenosis is defined as narrowing of the larynx above the level of the vocal folds and is depicted in ▶ Fig. 10.1. This is a very rare diagnosis, and may involve the epiglottis, arytenoids, aryepiglottic folds, and false folds. It can be caused by congenital malformations of any of the above structures. Hemangioma formation, although uncommon, may involve these areas and cause airway narrowing. Trauma and scarring can occur as a result of caustic or thermal ingestion, difficult intubation, prior surgery, and neck irradiation. Inflammatory conditions associated with supraglottic stenosis include sarcoidosis, Granulomatosis with polyangitis (GPA, formerly known as Wegener granulomatosis), and other rare autoimmune diseases, such as relapsing polychondritis. Infections, including supraglottitis and tuberculosis, may cause swelling, obstruction, or long-term scarring. There is thought to be a role for laryngopharyngeal reflux in either the etiology or worsening of this condition.[1] Supraglottic stenosis may also be idiopathic.

10.2.2 Glottic Stenosis

Glottic stenosis is defined as narrowing of the airway at the level of the vocal folds. This may be congenital in children, as seen in congenital glottic atresia, congenital bilateral vocal fold paralysis, anterior webbing, or posterior banding of the vocal folds. An example of congenital laryngeal web is depicted in ▶ Fig. 10.2. Cases of severe glottic stenosis may present with inspiratory or biphasic stridor necessitating intubation or

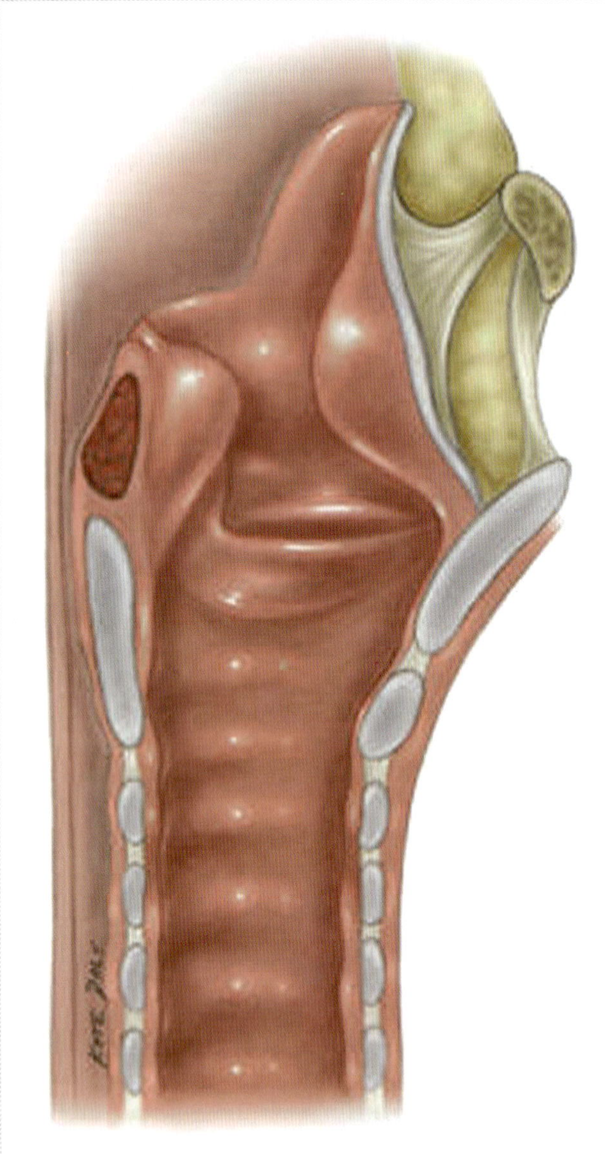

Fig. 10.1 Anatomical location of supraglottic stenosis.

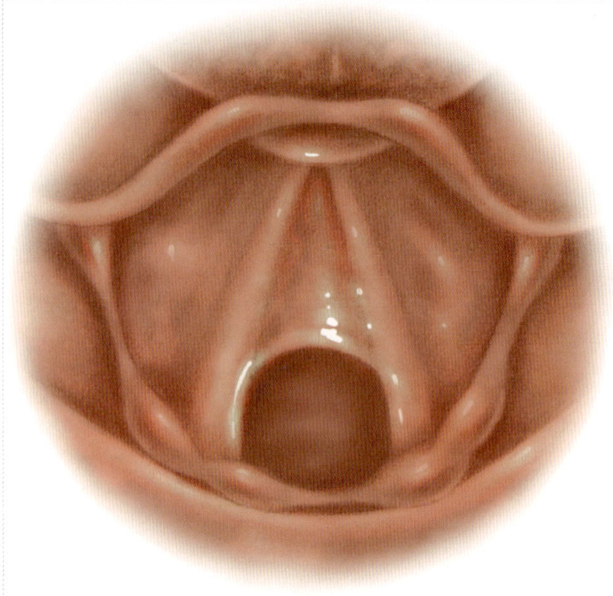

Fig. 10.2 Congenital anterior glottic web resulting in narrowed airway.

tracheotomy placement. Patients with laryngeal neoplastic lesions, such as primary squamous cell carcinoma, recurrent respiratory papillomatosis, and hemangioma can have significant disease causing narrowing at the glottis. These lesions may be more insidious in nature but are often diagnosed due to the presence of voice changes prior to airway obstruction. Traumatic causes, such as difficult intubation, surgery involving the vocal folds, or neck irradiation, can lead to scar tissue formation that narrows the glottis. Bilateral vocal fold paralysis or ankylosis of the cricoarytenoid joints can cause functional stenosis. Severe infections may narrow the glottic inlet; however, they are rarely the cause of scarring and long-term stenosis, with some exceptions, such as tuberculosis, which is known to cause stenosis by granuloma formation. GPA, sarcoidosis, and amyloidosis may affect the glottic aperture by inflammatory and infiltrative changes to the normal tissue.

10.2.3 Subglottic Stenosis

Subglottic stenosis connotes narrowing of the airway below the vocal folds and is illustrated in ▶ Fig. 10.3. Subglottic stenosis can be membranous, cartilaginous, or both, depending on the type of tissue involved at the site of narrowing. Congenital stenosis can affect either tissue type. Soft tissue trauma is the most common cause of scarring and stenosis in patients with a history of prolonged intubation; however, cartilage can be involved as well. Inflammatory or autoimmune diseases tend to cause changes in all tissues and may occur at different sites as a result of the underlying systemic process. If no intrinsic laryngeal lesions are identified, it is important to evaluate for any extrinsic processes causing compressive airway narrowing. Examples include vascular sling, cervical neoplasm, or lymphadenopathy.

Degree of subglottic stenosis has been described based on the percentage of airway obstruction. Myer et al proposed a classification of subglottic stenosis based on measurement of the airway size utilizing endotracheal tubes.[2] Grade I stenosis corresponds to 0 to 50%, Grade II to 51 to 70%, and Grade III to 71 to 99% airway obstruction. Grade IV stenosis indicates no appreciable lumen in the subglottis. This classification system is helpful for the consistent description of subglottic lesions and assists in choices for intervention. This system does not differentiate between cartilaginous and membranous lesions or assess the length of stenosis. A representation of this grading system is displayed in ▶ Fig. 10.4.

Congenital subglottic stenosis is most commonly found in children and has multiple etiologies. Subglottic narrowing may occur as a result of congenital malformation of the cricoid cartilage or excessive subglottic mucosal thickening. Other congenital causes are subglottic cysts, entrapment of the first tracheal cartilage within the cricoid ring, and benign

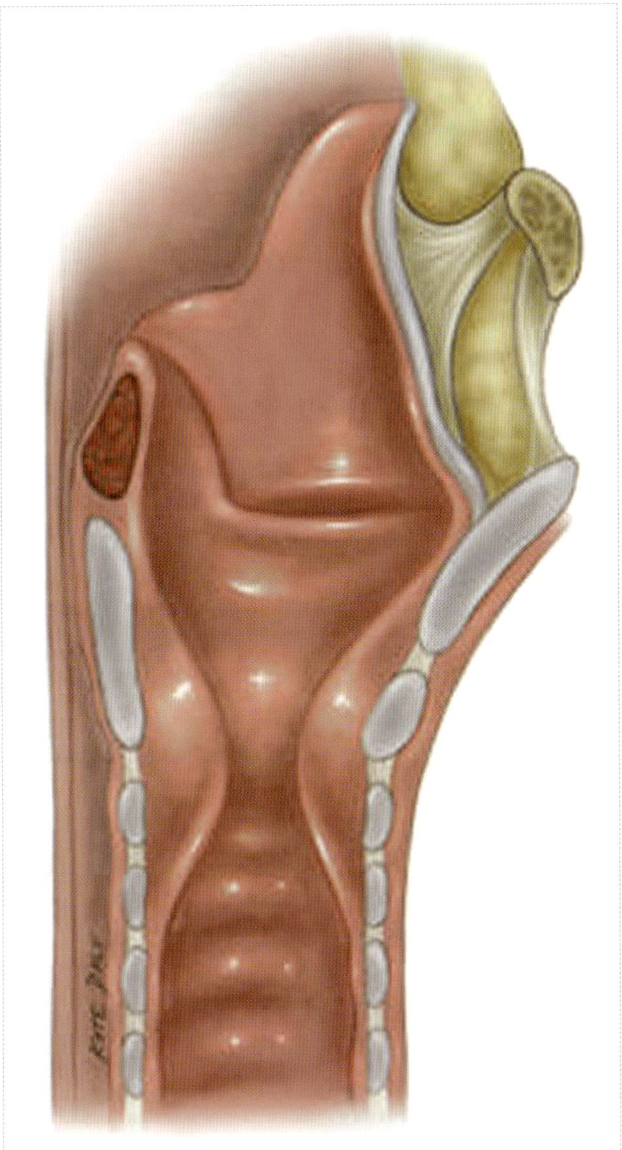

Fig. 10.3 Anatomical location of subglottic stenosis.

neoplastic processes, such as recurrent respiratory papillomatosis or subglottic hemangioma. Neoplastic causes of subglottic stenosis include chondroma, chondrosarcoma, rare primary tumors of the subglottis, and invasion of carcinoma from the hypopharynx or thyroid. Inflammatory conditions, such as acid reflux, have been shown to play a role in subglottic stenosis.[3] Eosinophilic esophagitis has been identified as a coincident, if not a causative, factor of subglottic stenosis.[4] In adults, conditions causing inflammation and infiltration of the subglottic tissue with fibroblasts and multinucleated giant cells can cause stenosis. Association of GPA with subglottic stenoisis has been extensively reported in the literature; however, cases associated with relapsing polychondritis, psoriatic arthritis, and vasculitis have also been described.[5,6] Postradiation fibrosis may also affect the subglottis. Traumatic conditions, including prolonged intubation, high tracheotomy, and prior surgical intervention, can potentially cause narrowing of the subglottic airway. Idiopathic cases, including sarcoid, have been described in the literature.

10.2.4 Further Procedures

Tracheoscopy/Bronchoscopy

After thorough history and physical examination, tracheal evaluation, if deemed safe, can further assist in evaluation of stenosis. Office-performed tracheoscopy can be used postoperatively to ensure that no significant restenosis has occurred. Four percent lidocaine spray through a mucosal atomizer or transtracheal lidocaine injection through the cricothyroid membrane is often adequate to anesthetize the endolarynx for visualization of the subglottis. At times, nebulized lidocaine can assist with this examination. Additional information can be obtained with video-recording equipment where the saved images can be retrospectively evaluated. The grade of subglottic stenosis can be estimated in this fashion. With adequate local anesthesia, the area of stenosis can be carefully traversed to visualize the trachea and carina to evaluate for the presence of multilevel disease. The length of stenosis can be evaluated in this manner. It is important to monitor patients' vital signs and minimize respiratory distress during the procedure. It is imperative to avoid tissue trauma, because in high grades of stenosis this may lead to swelling of the airway and cause an emergency situation. This procedure cannot typically be performed in patients with significant glottic stenosis because their glottic aperture during abduction of the vocal folds will not allow safe passage of the endoscope. If the patient is deemed unstable, or if the grade of stenosis is high, further evaluation in the controlled operating room setting is preferable. ▶ Fig. 10.5 demonstrates an in-office tracheoscopy displaying the glottis, grade II subglottic stenosis, and normal trachea.

Pulmonary Function Testing

A pulmonary function test (PFT) as an adjunct examination can assist in confirming a fixed-airway lesion. Although PFTs are not often available in an otolaryngologist's office, they are common practice for a pulmonologist. The PFT provides information about flow dynamics of the upper and lower airways. Typically, the upper airway is presumed normal, thus the test is used to gain information about the smaller diameter bronchioles when evaluating for asthma or the resistance of the alveolar complexes evaluated in fibrotic states and emphysema. A PFT is sensitive to upper airway changes and can show reproducible findings consistent with upper airway stenosis. Pathologic states with discernable patterns on flow-volume loops are bilateral vocal fold paralysis and fixed stenosis at any level of the trachea, subglottis, or glottis. Unilateral vocal fold paralysis and supraglottic stenosis may also show changes on PFT; however, patterns may be inconsistent. Bilateral vocal fold paralysis typically causes a restricted inspiratory loop without significantly changing the expiratory loop on the PFT. Fixed stenosis causes a restriction in both inspiratory and expiratory loops. Inspiratory and expiratory volumes and flow information may be used to discern functional severity of disease. ▶ Fig. 10.6 demonstrates the common flow-volume loops for upper airway stenosis.

Electromyography Testing

Needle electrode testing of the intrinsic laryngeal musculature is a helpful adjunct when vocal fold immobility is noted. In the

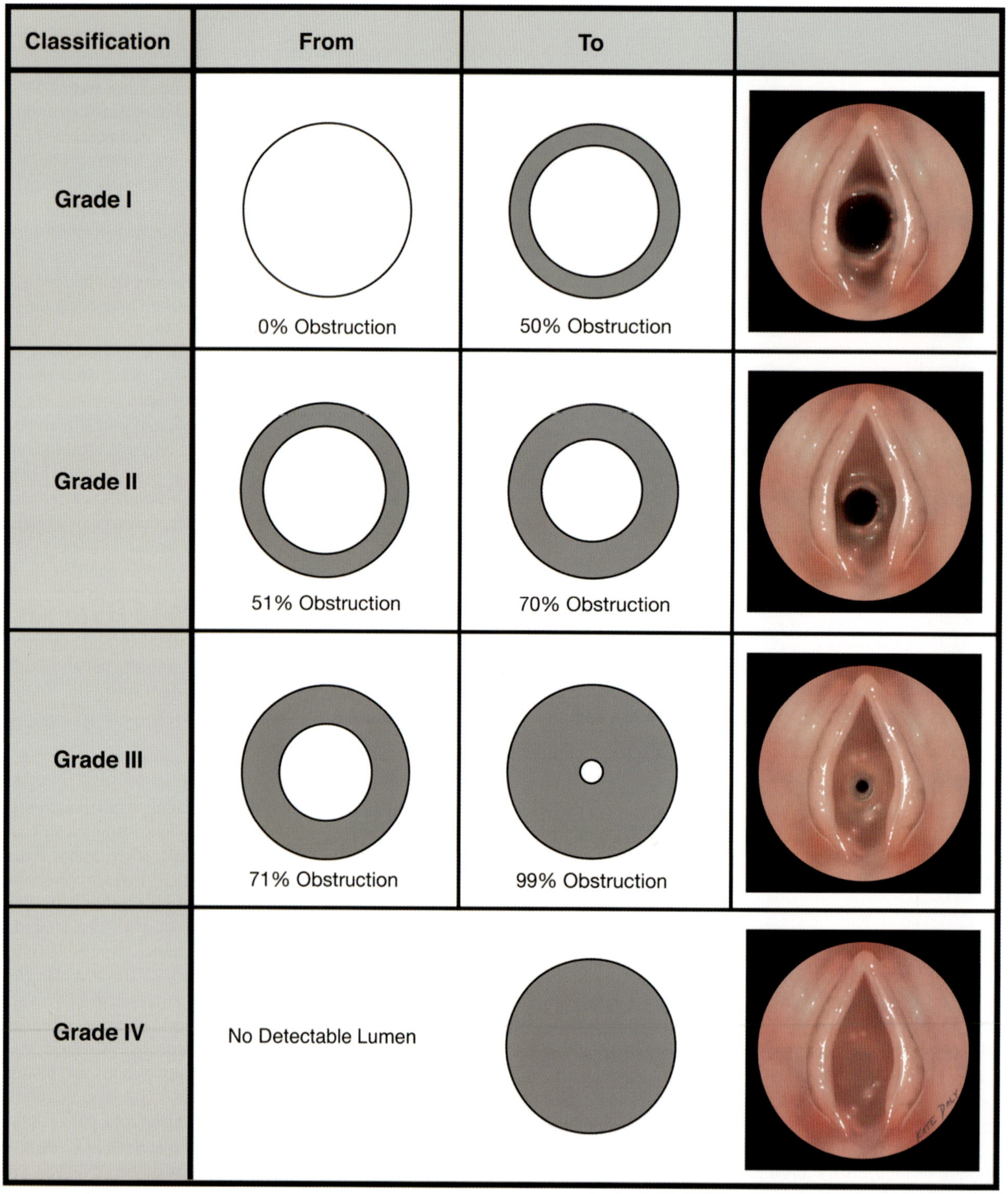

Fig. 10.4 Cotton-Myer subglottic stenosis classification system.

setting of trauma or prolonged intubation, it may be difficult to distinguish between ankylosis of the cricoarytenoid joints and true nerve damage as a cause of immobility. Testing of the thyroarytenoid muscles often assists with differentiation between the two. Electromyography (EMG) would show normal compound action potentials if joint fixation is the cause of stenosis. It is important to recognize that EMG testing for bilateral vocal fold paralysis has potential to cause bleeding or swelling, leading to further compromise of an already narrowed airway.

Imaging

Imaging can assess both intrinsic and extrinsic causes of laryngeal stenosis. Lateral neck x-ray (XR) is a useful screening tool

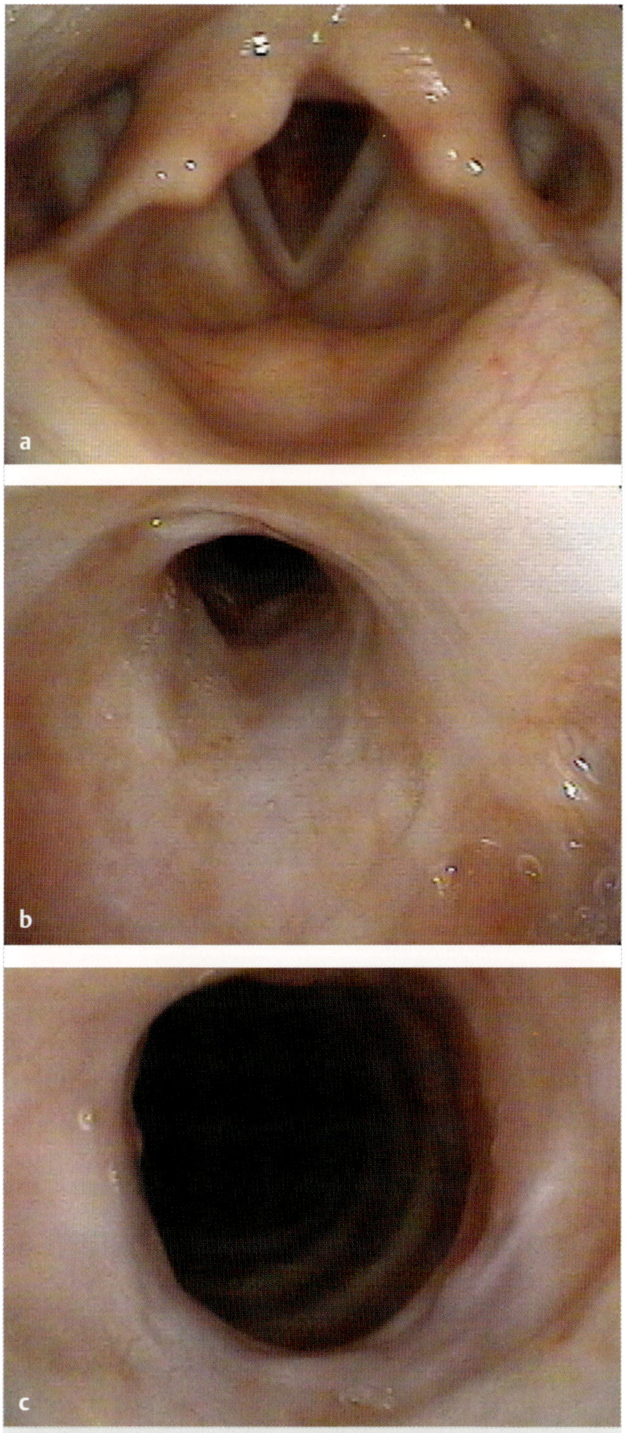

Fig. 10.5 In-office tracheoscopy to evaluate subglottic stenosis. Displayed is (a) the normal appearing glottis, (b) grade II subglottic stenosis, and (c) the distal trachea of normal caliber.

for airway narrowing. It has been used in evaluation of supraglottitis, croup, or more distal airway narrowing and compression. Retropharyngeal swelling causing airway compression is discernible with this imaging modality. X-ray is an easy and quick test and with positive findings may help to focus further evaluation on a more limited region of the airway. X-ray is commonly used in children because it is fast and noninvasive.

Computed tomography (CT) scan gives a significant amount of information about location and type of airway lesion. The study allows serial axial and sagittal sections through the airway to be traced and helps to differentiate between bony/cartilaginous and soft tissue defect as the primary etiology of stenosis. Computed tomography aids with diagnosis and preoperative evaluation of lesions or masses that cause external airway compression. Vascular slings and innominate artery compression are also discernible on CT. Computed tomography scanning is most useful when performed with intravenous contrast. The test takes a moderate amount of time to perform and should not be used in patients deemed unstable. Magnetic resonance imaging (MRI) is becoming more commonly used due to its superior soft tissue definition. This examination takes significantly longer than the alternatives and is often not feasible in children unless they are sedated prior to testing. Imaging modalities like chest XR and CT of the chest help to evaluate for lung disease associate with sarcoidosis and tuberculosis and to recognize other underlying disease processes contributing to laryngeal stenosis.

Laboratory Investigations

Laboratory tests are often normal in patients with laryngeal stenosis. At times, laboratory investigation may help elucidate a cause for dyspnea, such as severe anemia or thyroid abnormality. Most often, testing is aimed toward diagnosing inflammatory or autoimmune disorders that can cause laryngeal stenosis. These tests and associated diagnoses are listed in ▶ Table 10.3.

10.3 Treatment

Treatment of laryngeal stenosis is based on etiology of the narrowing, severity of symptoms and level of involvement. In cases of subglottic cyst or primary neoplasm, immediate surgical treatment may offer definitive management. In cases of systemic inflammatory or autoimmune diseases, medical management of the underlying condition may improve the symptoms of dyspnea without the need for surgical intervention. Emergency cases may necessitate tracheotomy prior to conclusive diagnosis and treatment.

10.3.1 Medical Management

Medical treatment is attempted in any patient with mild symptoms or without a known etiology for stenosis. Patients whose level of disease has not been elucidated are often started on oral steroids as initial management in case the underlying etiology is inflammation or granulation formation.[6] Often this may improve symptoms until the full workup is completed and a decision on management is made. In cases of systemic autoimmune disorder, patients may be maintained on long-term anti-inflammatory treatment to control symptoms because there is no true "cure." Steroid doses may be pulsed to determine effectiveness and are often titrated based on patient response. At times, if a lesion is small or there is only superficial mucosal involvement causing stenosis, inhaled steroids may be considered. Use of postoperative steroids after surgeries that have a high risk for stenosis is not routinely practiced. Steroids may have some utility in patients after difficult or prolonged intubation where the risk of stenosis is higher.

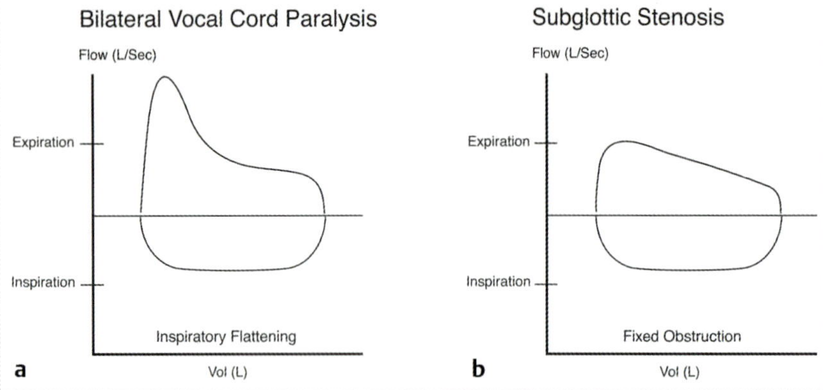

Fig. 10.6 Common flow-volume loops for upper airway stenosis. (**a**) Inspiratory flattening with normal expiratory loop is often encountered with bilateral vocal fold paralysis. (**b**) Flattening of both inspiratory and expiratory loops displays fixed stenosis as encountered with subglottic stenosis.

Table 10.3 Common laboratory tests ordered to assist in determining the etiology of laryngeal stenosis

Laboratory test	Associated diagnosis
Complete blood count with differential	Anemia, leukemia
Complete metabolic panel	Electrolyte abnormality, estimate of calcium, magnesium
Thyroid function studies	Hyperthyroidism
Angiotensin converting enzyme (ACE)	Sarcoidosis
ESR/CRP	Generalized inflammatory factors
ANA/RF	Generalized autoimmune factors
C-ANCA	Generalized vasculitis
P-ANCA	GPA, vasculitis
PPD	Tuberculosis

Abbreviations: ESR, erythrocyte sedimentation rate; CRP, C-reactive protein; ANA, antinuclear antibody; RF, rheumatoid factor; C-ANCA, cytoplasmic antineutrophil cytoplasmic antibodies; P-ANCA, perinuclear antineutrophil cytoplasmic antibodies; PPD, purified protein derivative.

Medical treatment of inflammatory mediators, as in laryngopharyngeal reflux, eosinophilic esophagitis, allergy, and pulmonary disease, is imperative for effective management of stenosis. Failure rates are thought to be increased when these factors are not taken into account. Depending on severity of reflux, treatment may include once or twice daily proton pump inhibitors. A team approach involving otolaryngology, pulmonary medicine, gastroenterology, and possibly rheumatology facilitates comprehensive workup and evaluation of various factors that can contribute to the development of stenosis. There are case studies supporting a role of reflux in the development of subglottic stenosis; some individual reports imply that treatment of reflux-associated inflammation can decrease stenosis and at times eliminate the need for surgical intervention.[3]

Patients who have elements of supraglottic stenosis or bilateral vocal fold paralysis may benefit from noninvasive ventilator support during sleep. Bilevel positive airway pressure (BiPAP) often facilitates air entry into the larynx so that patients can rest more easily. Because expiration is often less compromised, this serves to improve the inspiratory parameters in either patients with borderline disease not warranting surgical intervention or those who do not want surgical intervention. Oxygen supplementation has been used in some cases but does not change the underlying disease process in any way.

Certain lesions causing laryngeal stenosis have medical therapies that have been shown to be very effective. For example, propranolol is now primary therapy for hemangioma prior to surgical intervention unless there is emergent airway obstruction.[7] Use of propranolol has significantly changed the management approach to airway hemangioma and has decreased the need for surgery in many patients. Although treatment for recurrent respiratory papillomatosis continues to be primarily surgical, trials using antiviral therapy with cidofovir and antineoplastic agents like avastin continue to show efficacy in reducing disease burden in some patient populations.[8,9]

Medical treatment is warranted only in mild cases of stenosis. In cases of severe stenosis associated with stridor and dyspnea, surgical intervention is often required. When discussing medical treatment with patients, it is important to discuss that stenosis may continue to progress, and that medical treatment is often a stop-gap measure if stenosis continues to progress. When surgical treatment is recommended and patients opt for medical management instead, it is important to make patients aware that a controlled, but symptomatic disease could quickly progress and lead to an emergency situation. It is also important to discuss the risks of long-term steroid use with any patient who is being treated for autoimmune disease.

10.3.2 Surgical Management

Any surgical intervention should begin with a risk–benefit discussion. Surgical management is typically the most effective treatment for cases of stenosis. It can cause near-immediate improvement in airway size and symptom severity. In many cases, only a few procedures are necessary to permanently improve airway size. Unfortunately, when a patient with a compromised airway is placed under anesthesia, there is always a risk of inability to ventilate and the necessity for emergent airway management, including tracheotomy. The inability to ventilate for any significant amount of time carries the risk of hypoperfusion of the brain and other vital organs, causing ischemic injury or death. Instrumentation of a narrow airway, even for diagnostic purposes, may lead to swelling and airway compromise. Postoperative restenosis is always a risk with some of the common surgical procedures. Some surgical procedures require intubation or short-term tracheotomy placement for stenting purposes.

In many cases of laryngeal stenosis, definitive diagnosis is not achieved prior to an attempt at surgical intervention to improve symptoms. Full intraoperative diagnostic evaluation of the area, including biopsy of the stenotic segment, is recommended. Biopsy may assist in determining etiology regardless of the level of stenosis, and biopsy is often necessary to diagnose GPA, relapsing polychondritis, sarcoidosis, and amyloidosis.

Supraglottic Management

Surgical treatment of supraglottic stenosis is aimed at removing or opening stenotic tissue to allow proper access to the glottis. This is often achieved with some form of supraglottoplasty or supraglottic laryngectomy. Depending on the severity of stenosis, awake tracheotomy may be necessary for airway protection and maintenance during the procedure. A transoral procedure utilizing a carbon dioxide (CO_2) laser is often attempted as a first line of treatment in supraglottic stenosis cases.[10] Management of supraglottic stenosis is tailored to address the areas of significant scarring. Removal of obstructive supraglottic tissue or release of scar is possible with a laser approach.

If transoral access to the supraglottis is not possible, or if laser excision has failed, an open supraglottic laryngectomy technique may be used. The procedure involves removal of tissue from the ventricle superiorly followed by reconstruction, suspending the remainder of the thyroid cartilage from the hyoid and tongue base for airway protection. If scarring of the ventricle is present, this approach may lead to scarring of the glottis, resulting in decreased voice quality.

Glottic Management

Management decisions in cases of glottic stenosis are based on etiology. Bilateral vocal fold paralysis or ankylosis can be managed in a multitude of ways. If voice preservation is desired, tracheotomy continues to be an acceptable treatment for this condition and should always be discussed with patients. When voice preservation is not a high priority, transoral endoscopic unilateral posterior cordotomy combined with partial or total arytenoidectomy can improve the glottic opening. This is often accomplished with use of a CO_2 laser. Proper evaluation prior to definitive treatment is imperative in these cases. A posterior glottic scar band tethering the posterior larynx can appear similar to bilateral ankylosis or paralysis. If noted intraoperatively, release of the scar can improve the glottic opening without significant voice changes. More recently, an endoscopic approach to posterior cartilage grafting has been reported to improve posterior glottic stenosis from bilateral vocal fold paralysis or ankylosis.[11] Anterior glottic stenosis or webbing must be fully evaluated to assess depth and type of lesion. If a web is purely mucosal in nature, microlaryngoscopy with web division and microflap reconstruction of the surface of one vocal fold may improve breathing and offer good voice outcomes. If there is an anterior scarring component to the stenosis, then division the scar tissue with a CO_2 laser is necessary to maximally improve the airway.

If transoral access is not optimal, open surgical management of glottic stenosis is performed through a laryngofissure approach. With this technique, anterior or posterior stenosis can be addressed. For bilateral ankylosis or vocal fold paralysis, posterior cricoid cartilage grafting is possible to widen the posterior glottic aperture. Stent placement at the level of the glottis may be necessary to keep a posterior cartilage graft in place, and the stent is typically removed once mucosal healing has been established. Anterior scar can be removed or divided; a keel is often temporarily placed to prevent repeat scarring or web reformation. If a stent or keel is used, a short-term tracheotomy must be placed for airway management.

Subglottic Management

Subglottic stenosis is amenable to multiple surgical approaches, depending on type of stenosis and length of involvement. A subglottic cyst is commonly found to narrow the infant airway and can be marsupialized using endoscopic technique. If soft tissue stenosis comprises the majority of a lesion, many options are available for increasing the diameter of the subglottis. Carbon dioxide laser division of stenosis, with or without dilation, has been the mainstay of endoscopic treatment for subglottic stenosis. This may be performed with access through a laryngoscope with telescopic visualization, a laryngoscope placed subglottically with microscopic visualization, or through a bronchoscope. Both radial dilation using balloon and classic dilation using laryngeal dilators or endotracheal tubes have been described for enlarging the stenotic region.[12] ▶ Fig. 10.7 displays the

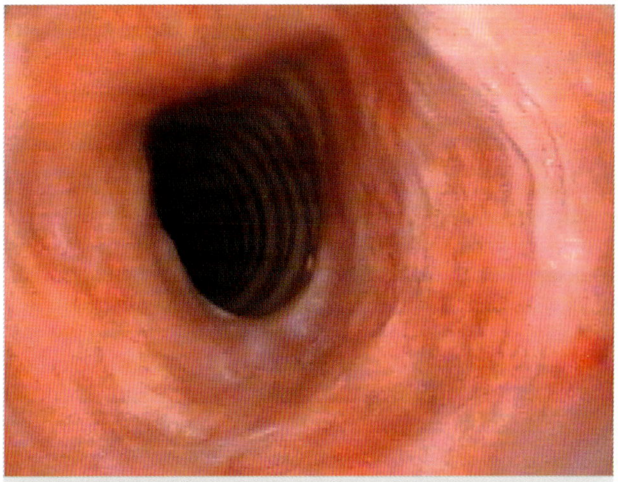

Fig. 10.7 Successful endoscopic management of subglottic stenosis by endoscopic carbon dioxide laser division and balloon dilation. Original stenosis is displayed in ▶ Fig. 10.5. Patient was photographed 3 months after airway intervention.

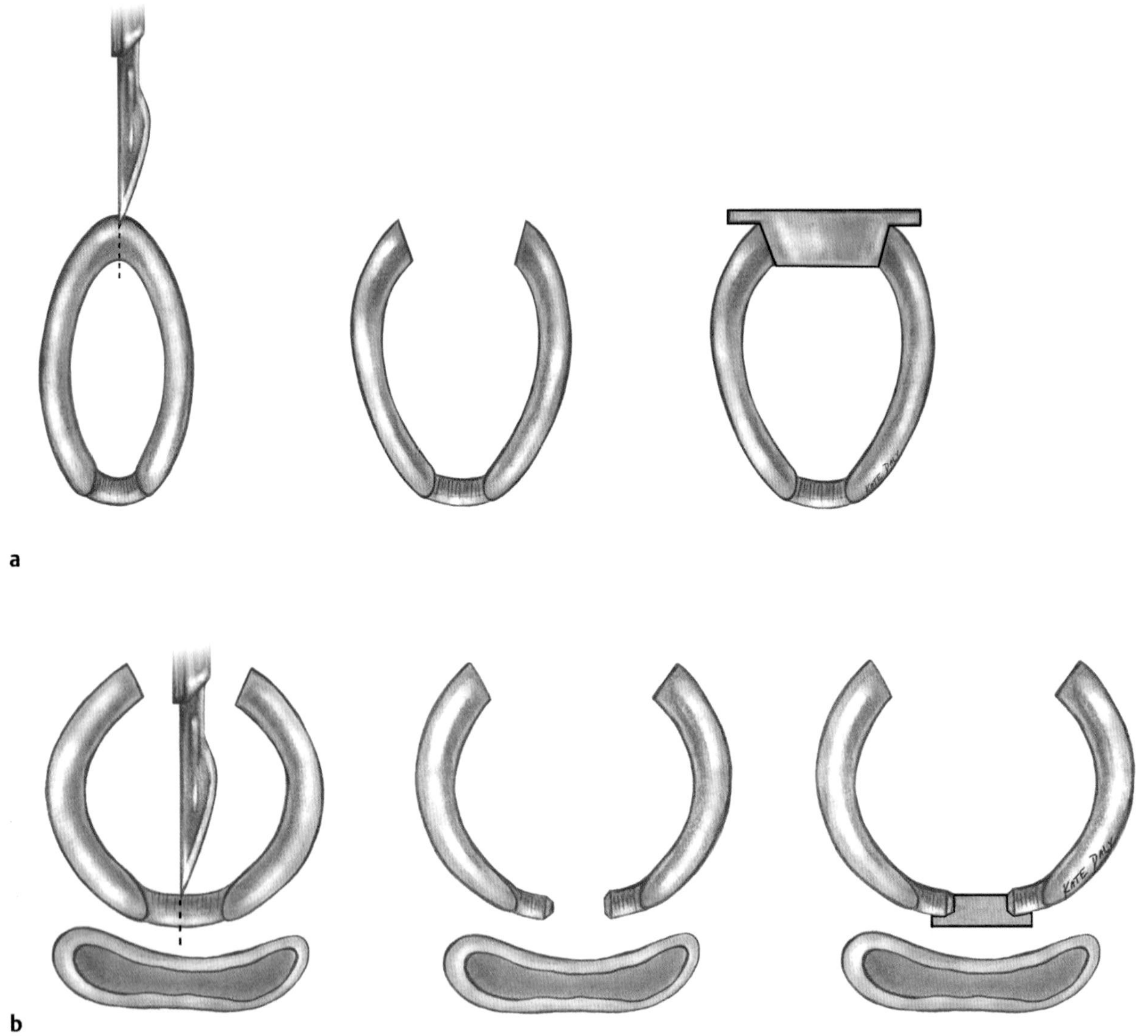

Fig. 10.8 Sketch of laryngotracheoplasty with cartilage grafting to increase luminal diameter in subglottic stenosis. (**a**) Anterior. (**b**) Posterior.

successful result of endoscopic CO_2 laser and balloon dilation of grade II subglottic stenosis originally pictured in ▶ Fig. 10.5. Endoscopic techniques have been used preferentially as initial treatment for grade I and II subglottic stenosis, but some surgeons are finding success even in cases of grade III stenosis. Although useful, endoscopic techniques are less likely to succeed in long-segment stenosis or severe grades of stenosis.

Traditional open procedures for subglottic stenosis are laryngotracheoplasty with cartilage grafting, and cricotracheal resection with reanastomosis. In infants with a narrow cricoid ring, it is possible to perform open or endoscopic anterior cricoid split without grafting to provide a small increase in luminal diameter that may allow for extubation or decannulation. Laryngotracheoplasty with anterior cartilage grafting, or with more severe stenosis, anterior and posterior cartilage grafting, can provide a significant increase in luminal diameter. This is depicted in ▶ Fig. 10.8. Because these techniques require grafts that must be held in a stable position while mucosalization occurs, stenting is often necessary. Placement of an endotracheal tube or an in-dwelling stent that requires tracheotomy for airway patency is commonly used after surgical intervention. Laryngotracheoplasty techniques have traditionally been used in long-segment stenosis or stenosis that involves the glottis as well as the subglottis. In comparison, cricotracheal resection, depicted in ▶ Fig. 10.9, involves single-step excision of the anterior portion of the cricoid cartilage along with the stenotic segment, and reanastomosis by release and pull-up of the healthy distal tracheal segment. This has traditionally been the procedure of choice in high-grade short stenotic segments. This procedure is technically challenging but has been found to have a low morbidity rate and low failure rate with properly chosen patients.[13,14] Major risks for these procedures include graft failure, anastomotic failure, and restenosis. Infection is also a significant risk factor for failure.

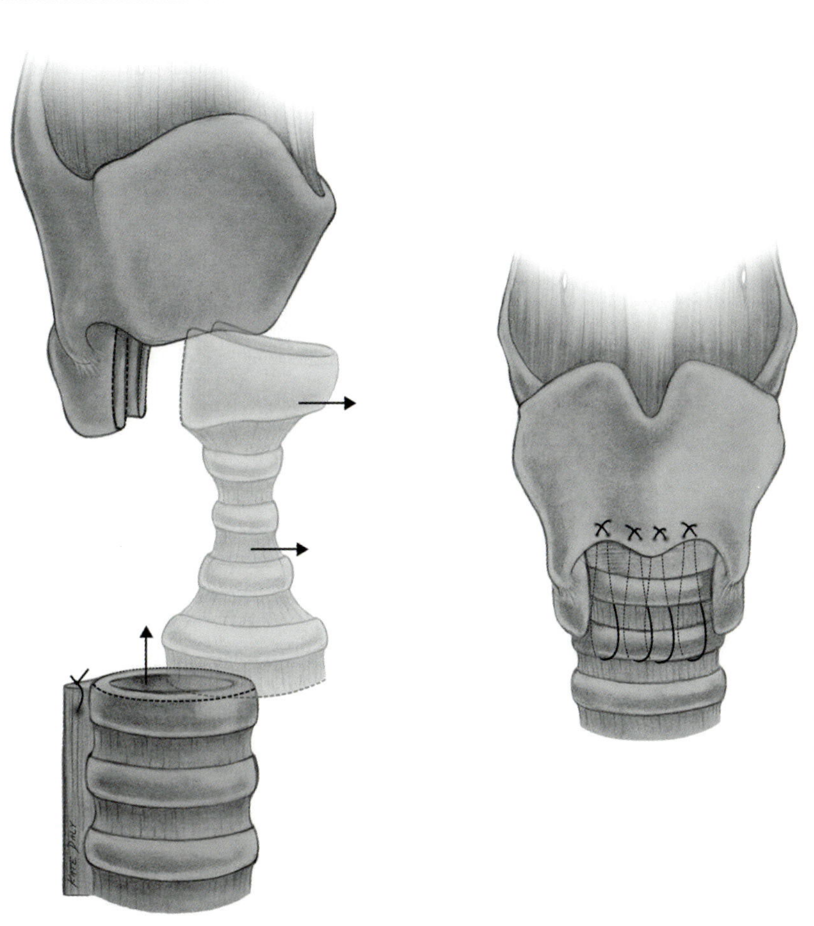

Fig. 10.9 Sketch depiction of a cricotracheal resection to increase luminal diameter in subglottic stenosis.

Repeat endoscopy and revision endoscopic management of postoperative granulation tissue and stenosis is common after any surgical procedure for laryngeal stenosis. Most often this entails endoscopic surveillance and if indicated, dilation and/or laser division of scar. Intralesional steroids as well as mitomycin-C application have been utilized intraoperatively as adjuncts to dilation to improve airway patency during the healing process and to maximize the symptom-free time between procedures.[15] Their use is controversial and varies from institution to institution.

10.3.3 Prognosis

With proper diagnosis and management, many patients with laryngeal stenosis have an improvement in symptoms. Success rate of endoscopic management in properly chosen cases varies from approximately 60 to 100%. [16,17] Studies have shown that endoscopic techniques have high success with mild, short-segment, and intrinsic mucosal abnormalities. Open techniques are usually performed in higher grades of stenosis, stenosis involving longer segments, and in cases that have failed endoscopic techniques. Studies have shown a 63 to 91% success rate over time.[18,19] Patients with underlying systemic diseases are more likely to have prolonged airway difficulty because surgical intervention only helps to improve symptoms and does not cure the underlying condition.

10.4 Treatment Failure

10.4.1 Definition of Failure

As previously established, surgical intervention for laryngeal stenosis has the potential for long-term improvement of symptoms. It is also accepted that the majority of patients will need multiple procedures. Second-stage surgeries or endoscopic dilation after open procedures are common to remove granulation tissue or to dilate the anastomotic site for optimal benefit. Treatment failure is thus not defined as the necessity for further operative intervention, but instead as continued severe symptoms despite the interventions. Some studies use inability to decannulate as indicative of failure.

10.4.2 Next Step

If the original treatment failed to widen the airway for symptom control, the etiology of stenosis and the treatment algorithm should be reassessed. Depending on the areas and severity or restenosis, repeat endoscopic or open surgical interventions are often indicated for patients with supraglottic stenosis. In cases of conservative management of the glottis, revision arytenoidectomy or cordotomy may be necessary. These procedures often carry a risk of poor voice outcome and need to be discussed frankly with patients. If endoscopic methods to manage subglottic stenosis fail, evaluation for open laryngotracheoplasty or cricotracheal resection may be indicated. It must be ensured that a second site of stenosis was not overlooked in the diagnostic workup. If treatment fails due to restenosis after initial improvement, repeat procedures may be indicated. Restenosis often suggests that the inflammatory mediators in the area are not being fully addressed. Adjuvant medical treatments like steroids or mitomycin-C may be considered during repeat procedures. Planned endoscopic re-evaluations can detect scar tissue formation before symptoms become severe. Although not a favorable option, it is important to remember that a tracheotomy can be performed in any of the cases if the patient becomes unstable. In cases of worsening systemic disease, a tracheotomy may be a viable alternative treatment until disease treatment is optimized.

10.4.3 Referral Recommendations

Often patients with laryngeal stenosis will be referred to tertiary care centers for airway management. These institutions have access to equipment that may not be available in a community setting, such as the CO_2 laser and endoscopic instruments. Anesthesiologists and surgeons at these centers tend to be more familiar with difficult airway management, as they generally treat larger numbers of complex patients. Laryngeal stenosis cases often require postoperative intubation for airway stenting and intensive-care unit care. Pediatric centers use a multispecialty team approach to evaluate difficult airway cases in order to make a proper diagnosis and to optimize the outcome. Many adult centers are now implementing the same model to improve adult airway management.

10.5 Key Points

- Dyspnea is the most common symptom and stridor is the most common sign in laryngeal stenosis.
- Flexible laryngoscopy, tracheoscopy, and often operative microlaryngoscopy with bronchoscopy are necessary to fully evaluate laryngeal stenosis.
- Traumatic, scarring, or inflammatory conditions are likely to cause laryngeal stenosis regardless of the level of involvement. Pediatric stenosis may also be from congenital causes.
- Medical management may be indicated when patients have minor stenosis with good exercise tolerance.
- Identification and management of factors that cause airway inflammation, including laryngopharyngeal reflux, will improve treatment outcomes for laryngeal stenosis.
- Supraglottic stenosis may be managed by endoscopic or open partial supraglottic laryngectomy, but restenosis often occurs.
- Unilateral cordotomy with or without arytenoidectomy may treat glottic stenosis caused by vocal fold immobility, but scar tissue or webs may be endoscopically divided.
- Endoscopic laser and/or balloon dilation is often a primary treatment for subglottic stenosis, and laryngotracheoplasty and cricotracheal resection are reserved for more severe cases of stenosis or endoscopic failures.
- Tracheotomy may be necessary, either short term or long term for treatment failures.
- Tertiary care referral may be necessary for patients with laryngeal stenosis.

References

[1] Krishna PD, Malone JP. Isolated adult supraglottic stenosis: surgical treatment and possible etiologies. Am J Otolaryngol 2006; 27: 355–357

[2] Myer CM, O'Connor DM, Cotton RT. Proposed grading system for subglottic stenosis based on endotracheal tube sizes. Ann Otol Rhinol Laryngol 1994; 103: 319–323

[3] Maronian NC, Azadeh H, Waugh P, Hillel A. Association of laryngopharyngeal reflux disease and subglottic stenosis. Ann Otol Rhinol Laryngol 2001; 110: 606–612

[4] Dauer EH, Ponikau JU, Smyrk TC, Murray JA, Thompson DM. Airway manifestations of pediatric eosinophilic esophagitis: a clinical and histopathologic report of an emerging association. Ann Otol Rhinol Laryngol 2006; 115: 507–517

[5] Langford CA, Sneller MC, Hallahan CW et al. Clinical features and therapeutic management of subglottic stenosis in patients with Wegener's granulomatosis. Arthritis Rheum 1996; 39: 1754–1760

[6] Erickson VR, Hwang PH. Wegener's granulomatosis: current trends in diagnosis and management. Curr Opin Otolaryngol Head Neck Surg 2007; 15: 170–176

[7] Fuchsmann C, Quintal MC, Giguere C et al. Propranolol as first-line treatment of head and neck hemangiomas. Arch Otolaryngol Head Neck Surg 2011; 137: 471–478

[8] Donne AJ, Rothera MP, Homer JJ. Scientific and clinical aspects of the use of cidofovir in recurrent respiratory papillomatosis. Int J Pediatr Otorhinolaryngol 2008; 72: 939–944

[9] Zeitels SM, Barbu AM, Landau-Zemer T et al. Local injection of bevacizumab (Avastin) and angiolytic KTP laser treatment of recurrent respiratory papillomatosis of the vocal folds: a prospective study. Ann Otol Rhinol Laryngol 2011; 120: 627–634

[10] Vira D, DeConde A, Chhetri DK. Endoscopic management of supraglottic laryngopharyngeal stenosis. Otolaryngol Head Neck Surg 2012; 146: 611–613

[11] Thakkar K, Gerber ME. Endoscopic posterior costal cartilage graft placement for acute management of pediatric bilateral vocal fold paralysis without tracheostomy. Int J Pediatr Otorhinolaryngol 2008; 72: 1555–1558

[12] Lee KH, Rutter MJ. Role of balloon dilation in the management of adult idiopathic subglottic stenosis. Ann Otol Rhinol Laryngol 2008; 117: 81–84

[13] Grillo HC, Mathisen DJ, Ashiku SK, Wright CD, Wain JC. Successful treatment of idiopathic laryngotracheal stenosis by resection and primary anastomosis. Ann Otol Rhinol Laryngol 2003; 112: 798–800

[14] Yamamoto K, Kojima F, Tomiyama K, Nakamura T, Hayashino Y. Meta-analysis of therapeutic procedures for acquired subglottic stenosis in adults. Ann Thorac Surg 2011; 91: 1747–1753

[15] Simpson CB, James JC. The efficacy of mitomycin-C in the treatment of laryngotracheal stenosis. Laryngoscope 2006; 116: 1923–1925

[16] Quesnel AM, Lee GS, Nuss RC, Volk MS, Jones DT, Rahbar R. Minimally invasive endoscopic management of subglottic stenosis in children: success and failure. Int J Pediatr Otorhinolaryngol 2011; 75: 652–656

[17] Bakthavachalam S, McClay JE. Endoscopic management of subglottic stenosis. Otolaryngol Head Neck Surg 2008; 139: 551–559

[18] Lano CF, Duncavage JA, Reinisch L, Ossoff RH, Courey MS, Netterville JL. Laryngotracheal reconstruction in the adult: a ten year experience. Ann Otol Rhinol Laryngol 1998; 107: 92–97

[19] Ashiku SK, Kuzucu A, Grillo HC et al. Idiopathic laryngotracheal stenosis: effective definitive treatment with laryngotracheal resection. J Thorac Cardiovasc Surg 2004; 127: 99–107

11 Neurologic and Neuromuscular Diseases of the Larynx

Catherine F. Sinclair, Lowell E. Gurey, and Andrew Blitzer

Evolution of the human laryngopharynx has allowed for complex forms of verbal communication; however, its anatomical structure whereby inspired air and ingested food traverse the same space can be perilous in the absence of coordinated motor activity and appropriate response to sensory feedback. The larynx must be open during breathing and tightly closed during swallowing and activities that require positive intrathoracic pressure (e.g., defecation, heavy lifting). It must open just before respiration and close gradually, during exhalation, thereby braking expiratory airflow and influencing the rate of breathing.[1] Sound production (phonation) requires that the vocal folds be appropriately approximated with a three-dimensional shape that imparts favorable glottic aerodynamic features.[1,2,3] Control of vocal fold length and tension is required to produce normal inflections in pitch and tone; in the absence of such control, the voice may be flat and expressionless or distorted by uncontrolled pitch breaks.[1] Resonance of the phonated sound is modulated by motor activity of the pharynx, soft palate, and oral cavity and articulation at the level of the lips, tongue, palate, pharynx, and larynx helps shape the voice into words.[1,2,3] Feedback from a variety of sensory receptors assists with all these functions although the exact sensory feedback loops involved are not well understood.[4,5,6] Neurologic disorders can thus impair aerodigestive tract function by diverse mechanisms including motor weakness, incoordination, or impairment of sensation.[4,5] Such disorders can be difficult to diagnose and require an awareness of the possibility of neural dysfunction, familiarity with the signs and symptoms of such dysfunction, and a systematic examination approach. In this chapter, we will outline an approach to the history and physical examination of patients with a suspected neurologic disorder, use of ancillary tests, and discussion of management options for some of the more frequently encountered neurologic disorders that affect the larynx.

11.1 History and Physical Examination

The standard neurologic examination does not directly address functional activity of the throat and larynx due to their relatively inaccessability. Similarly, the standard otolaryngologic examination will often fail to address many aspects of the standard neurologic assessment. Proper diagnosis and management thus typically requires a team approach involving an otolaryngologist, neurologist, and speech-language pathologist.

11.1.1 History

Neurologic disorders can affect both motor and sensory functions. Movement disorders result from a disorder of motor programming, resulting in either a paucity of movement (akinesia or bradykinesis) or excessive movement (hyperkinesia), or a combination thereof. In addition, sensory functions can be affected either in isolation or in concert with a movement disorder. The type of symptoms and symptom complexes present can help guide further questioning by narrowing the differential diagnosis (▶ Table 11.1). Specific questions for laryngeal pathology include presence of vocal fatigue, pain with speaking, increased effort required for speech, glottal tightness, pitch breaks, tremor, and dysphagia. Age and rapidity of onset plus timing and duration of symptoms should be determined. Symptoms of sudden onset may suggest a vascular or infective cause such as stroke or vocal fold paresis secondary to viral infection. Insidious onset is common in generalized neurologic conditions including Parkinson disease (PD) and multiple sclerosis (MS). Involvement of other body parts and questioning about autonomical functions (e.g., bowel/bladder control, blood pressure) can assist in differentiating localized from generalized processes. Past medical history including history of head trauma, family history, prior treatments (including prior neurologist review), current medications, and symptom improvement with alcohol ingestion (dystonia, essential tremor) should also be elucidated.

11.1.2 Examination

The objectives of the examination are to assess the integrity of the lower cranial nerves and to systematically seek signs of central nervous system (CNS) disorders as outlined below and summarized in ▶ Table 11.2.

11.1.3 General and Voice

Observe the patient's posture, gait, and facial expressions as he walks into and sits in the room, noting presence (or absence) of signs like bradykinesia, dystonic limb or cervical movements, tremor, and facial dyskinesias. Listen to the voice for the symptoms listed in ▶ Table 11.2.

11.1.4 Neurologic

Cranial nerve examination should be done to assess for bulbar or muscular abnormalities (▶ Table 11.2). Check hands for

Table 11.1 Symptoms suggesting neuropathology

Function	Symptom
Speech	Lack of volume Breathiness Instability of pitch or volume Lack of voice inflection Abnormal resonance Dysarthria
Swallowing	Oral incompetence Velopharyngeal incompetence Inability to initiate a swallow Aspiration
Breathing	Fluctuating inspiratory stridor Weak breathy cough "Gurgly" breathing noises

Table 11.2 Clinical examination findings

	Symptoms	Possible diagnostic consideration
General Inspection	Bradykinesia Tremor	PD, MSA PD, ET, dystonia
Voice	Hypophonia Strain / breaks Tremor Articulation	PD, MSA Dystonia, MTD Dystonia, ET, PD Dystonia, bulbar palsy, ALS
Oral cavity	Spontaneous movement • Slow/athetoid • Fasciculations • Spasmodic • Blinking/Jaw thrusting Palate abnormalities • Spontaneous contractions • Decreased elevation with speech • Deviated uvula	Tardive dyskinesia ALS Meige syndrome Palatal myoclonus Bulbar palsy, negative dystonia Vagal dysfunction

Abbreviations: ALS, amyotrophic lateral sclerosis; ET, essential tremor; MSA, multiple system atrophy; MTD, muscle tension dysphonia; PD, Parkinson disease.

tremor with arms outstretched. Eye closure can exacerbate symptoms. Observe for intention tremor during finger-nose pointing.

11.1.5 Oral Cavity

Observe the lips, palate, and tongue for abnormal spontaneous movement (see the box "Clinical uses for laryngeal electromyography and interpretation of findings (p. 98)"). Assess range of motion, strength, and symmetry of the mouth and palate muscles by asking the patient to purse the lips, protrude the tongue and move it from side to side, and open the mouth and say "ah." Assess tongue strength by having the patient push his or her tongue against the buccal mucosa while you palpate the cheek externally.[2] In addition to strength testing, central control of lip and tongue muscles should also be assessed. Rapid repetition of the syllable /Pa/ shows lip function. A healthy person is able to maintain a regular rhythm at a rapid rate. A lower motor neuron lesion decreases the strength of this action. Upper motor neuron involvement decreases the rate at which the patient can repeat the syllable, but regular rhythm should be preserved. In patients with cerebellar dysfunction, the rhythm is erratic. Myasthenia gravis results in fatigue with repetitive motion. Other syllables address other muscle groups. "Ta" tests the tip of the tongue, and "ga" tests the posterior tongue.[2] If dystonic jaw or tongue movements are present, determine which muscle groups are involved by having the patients actively open, close, protrude and laterally deviate the mandible. Similarly, if cervical tremor is noted, attempt to determine its direction (vertical vs. horizontal) and any improvement in voice with manual stabilization of the larynx. These maneuvers will assist with determining which management options may be appropriate (see management below).

Clinical uses for laryngeal electromyography and interpretation of findings

Diagnostic
- To assess laryngeal nerve integrity with vocal fold immobility
- If the electromyogram is normal, consider mechanical fixation process
- If vigorous interference pattern with immobility probable synkinesis
- To determine site of nerve injury
  - Assess differential activity in cricothyroid versus thyroarytenoid musculature
- To determine severity of paresis
- Complete nerve section → absent voluntary muscle activity
- Fibrillation potentials after 3 weeks → recovery unlikely
- Polyphasic action potentials → indicate reinnervation; however, potential for recovery uncertain

Therapeutic
- Botulinum toxin injections
- Spasmodic dysphonia (adductor and abductor)
- Essential tremor

11.1.6 Flexible Laryngoscopy

The nasal surface of the soft palate is assessed for tremor or spasmodic movements at rest, as may be present in essential tremor, palatal myoclonus, or dystonia. The patient is asked to swallow and say "kitty cat" to check symmetry and competence of velopharyngeal closure, which may be compromised in neurologic conditions like dystonia, bulbar palsy, stroke, or peripheral nerve injury.[7,8] The scope is advanced to visualize the tongue base and pharynx, with alternating phonation of /ee/ and /ah/ used to observe anterior and posterior tongue movements. The pharynx is observed for tremor, symmetry of contraction on swallowing and hypopharyngeal secretion pooling, which may be attributed to either motor or sensory abnormalities.

The vocal cords are assessed initially with the patient breathing quietly at rest. The patient is asked to phonate /ee/ to assess vocal fold adduction. The eee-sniff maneuver is used to assess symmetry of abduction/adduction and can detect fatigue in myasthenia gravis or evidence of paradoxical cord movement when performed rapidly. Subtle findings of vocal fold paresis include a widened ipsilateral ventricle and anterior tipping of the ipsilateral arytenoid cartilage, with resultant height mismatch of the vocal cords due to the vocalis process and posterior cord lying at a more inferior level. Superior laryngeal nerve weakness may manifest with psilateral deviation of the epiglottic petiole during high-pitched voice production.[9] The cough is a useful way to differentiate psychogenic stridor from true bilateral laryngeal paralysis.[7] Aphonic malingering patients may not adduct their vocal folds completely when asked to phonate; however, they adduct normally with cough. Tremor of laryngopharyngeal structures may be seen at rest (e.g., essential tremor) or with specific vocalization tasks (e.g., dystonic tremor).

Bowing of the vocal cords can be seen in PD, MSA, and as part of normal aging. To assess the superior laryngeal nerve, the patient is asked to perform a glissando, phonating from low to high pitch and back down. The pitch should rise as the vocal folds become longer and thinner due to cricothyroid muscle contraction.[7,8]

Distinguishing between a neurologic disorder and functional or psychiatric voice problems can be difficult. Some common hyperfunctional distortions include anteroposterior compression of the glottis, aryepiglottic fold contraction, and false vocal-fold adduction. These patients also characteristically elevate the larynx and speak with a low lung volume.[1] In addition, they often pause briefly prior to phonation to allow for laryngeal posturing, in contrast to adductor spasmodic dysphonia patients, who do not display this prephonatory posturing. However, hyperfunctional behaviors may be learned as a means of compensating for a neurologic defect and thus both can coexist. Stroboscopy should be performed as part of the laryngoscopic examination to examine the vocal cord mucosal wave.

11.2 Diagnosis

11.2.1 Ancillary Tests

Nonacoustic Analysis

The effect of a patient's disorder on quality of life is important to ascertain, as it can affect subsequent management. Validated scales to measure the degree of disability attributable to a voice disorder include the Voice Handicap Index (VHI), VHI-10, and the Voice-Related Quality of Life.[10]

Electromyography

Electromyography (EMG) uses needle electrodes inserted into laryngeal muscles to record spontaneous and voluntary muscular activity. The laryngeal muscles are never completely at rest and thus there will always be some degree of spontaneous activity. Topical anesthetic is not used because it can affect the electrical signal.[11] The thyroarytenoid muscle is approached via the cricothyroid membrane. There are two ways to enter the muscle. In our preferred method, the needle is angled approximately 30 to 45 degrees and is then directed superiorly and slightly laterally, piercing the skin just off midline (▶ Fig. 11.1). The needle location within the muscle is verified by asking the patient to phonate. In the other approach, the subglottic air space is entered in the midline and the needle is then diverted superiorly into the right or left vocal fold. A disadvantage of the latter approach is that it frequently stimulates coughing, due to activation of sensory receptors in the vocal fold mucosa. The posterior cricoarytenoid muscle (PCA) can also be approached by two methods. In our preferred method, the thyroid cartilage is grasped and its posterior lamina rotated to the ipsilateral side (▶ Fig. 11.2a). The EMG needle is inserted halfway between the midpoint of the posterior border of the thyroid cartilage and the cricoid cartilage and is advanced until it contacts the posterior cricoid lamina. Needle placement within the PCA is confirmed by sniffing. Patients can find this method difficult to tolerate due to discomfort from the degree of laryngeal rotation required. An alternative approach to the PCA is via the cricothyroid membrane. The needle is advanced intraluminally through the subglottis and posterior cricoid lamina until the PCA muscle is entered (▶ Fig. 11.2b). This method can be limited by cricoid cartilage calcification in older patients. The cricothyroid muscle is tested by inserting the needle in the midline, onto the superior edge of the cricoid cartilage. The tip of the needle is then "walked" over the cartilage, superiorly and laterally to avoid the strap muscles. To verify needle placement in the cricothyroid muscle, the patient is asked to perform a glissando from a comfortable pitch up to a falsetto.[12] Strap muscle injections should be made along the superior border of the thyroid cartilage, targeting the thyrohyoid muscle. Supraglottic injections are performed via the thyrohyoid membrane under direct flexible endoscopic visualization (▶ Fig. 11.3). Injections made too high can diffuse into tongue base musculature and cause significant dysphagia. Clinical uses of laryngeal EMG are summarized in the box "Clinical uses for laryngeal electromyography and interpretation of findings (p. 98)."

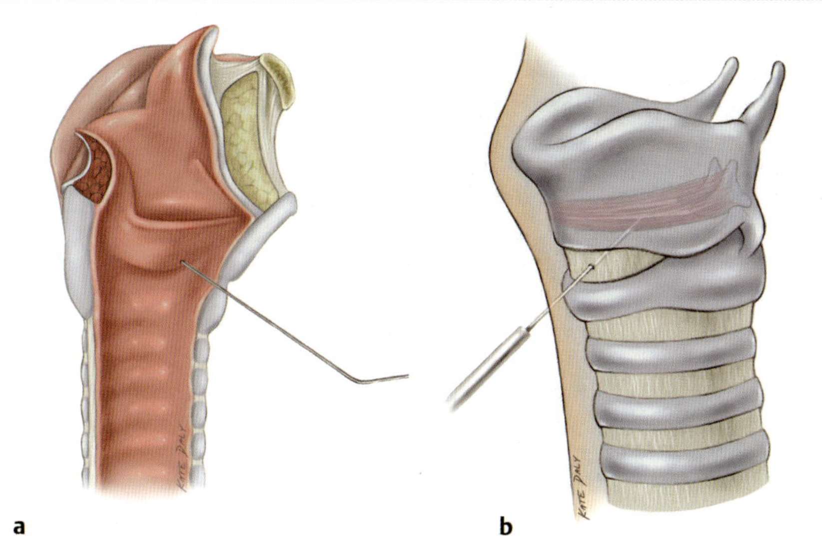

Fig. 11.1 (**a**) Transcricothyroid approach for thyroarytenoid muscle injections. (**b**) Transcricothyroid approach for thyroarytenoid muscle injections.

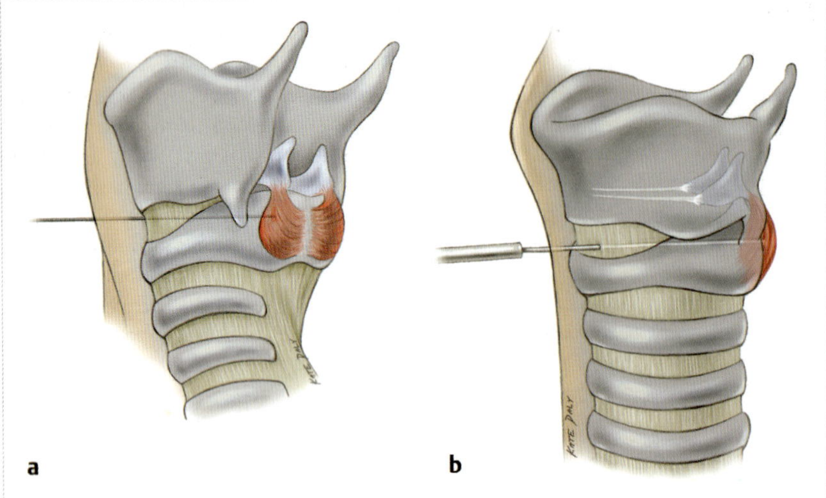

Fig. 11.2 (a) Posterior approach for posterior cricoarytenoid muscle injections. (b) Transcricoid approach to posterior cricoarytenoid muscle.

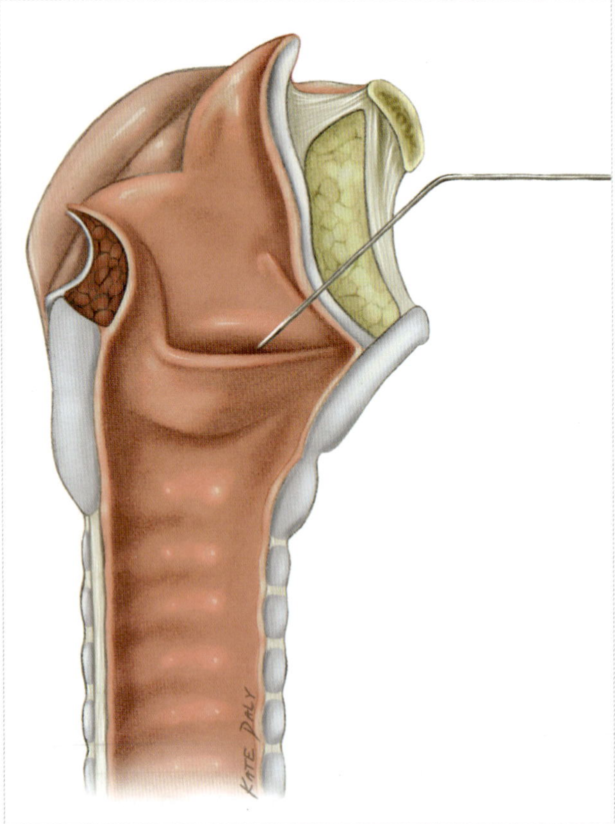

Fig. 11.3 Transhyoid approach, useful for supraglottic musculature injections.

Sensory Assessment

Laryngopharyngeal sensory testing can be useful for evaluating causes of aspiration. A pressure-controlled and duration-controlled air puff is delivered to various locations within the larynx via the port of a flexible fiberoptic laryngoscope. Duration of the air puff is held constant at 50 ms while air pressure is varied. Pressures necessary to elicit an adductor vocal cord reflex are compared to established normative values to help assess the severity of sensory loss.[13]

11.3 Treatment

In the following sections, management of some of the more common neurologic disorders that affect the larynx is discussed. The disorders can be classified into hyperfunctional, hypofunctional, and mixed movement disorders (see the box "Classification of laryngeal neurologic disorders (p. 100)"). Hyperfunctional disorders will often benefit from medications or treatments like botulinum toxin to reduce muscular activity, whereas hypofunctional disorders require augmentation strategies (local or systemic).

Classification of laryngeal neurologic disorders

Hyperfunctional
- Dystonia
- Tremor
- Tic disorders, Tourette syndrome
- Myoclonus
- Choreas
- Muscle tension dysphonia, posturing
- Psychogenic

Hypofunctional
- Vocal fold paresis/paralysis
- Neuromuscular junction disorders
- Myopathic diseases
- Parkinson disease
- Amyotrophic lateral sclerosis, multiple sclerosis, primary lateral sclerosis
- Stroke
- Psychogenic

Mixed
- Some cases of Parkinson disease
- Some cases of multiple sclerosis
- Sensory
- Vocal fold paresis/paralysis
- Stroke
- Parkinson disease
- Psychogenic
- Multiple sclerosis

11.3.1 Hyperfunctional Disorders

Dystonia

Dystonia is sustained or intermittent muscle contractions that cause twisting and repetitive movements or abnormal postures. It is broadly classified according to age of onset, etiology and clinical distribution (see the box "Classification of dystonia (p. 101)"). Laryngeal dystonia or spasmodic dysphonia (SD), is divided into adductor and abductor types. Females are affected twice as commonly as males, a positive family history of dystonia is present in approximately 12%, and the dystonia focally affects the larynx in 80%.[14,15] Adductor SD classically presents with strain-strangle phonation punctuated by voicing arrests (breaks or pauses) due to involuntary cocontraction of agonist and antagonist laryngeal musculature with hyperadduction of the vocal folds.[14,15] Abductor SD classically presents with a whispering, weak, breathy voice that is particularly notable at voicing onset due to contraction of the posterior cricoarytenoid muscles, resulting in inappropriate vocal fold abduction. Some diagnostic pitfalls include "compensatory abductor dysphonia" whereby patients with severe adductor SD produce a breathy voice by whispering or not contracting their vocal folds to prevent spasms and broken speech patterns; the much rarer "compensatory adductor dysphonia," in which abductor SD patients try to prevent breathiness by initiating speech with their vocal folds tightly contracted; and the rare adductor respiratory dystonia where patients get paradoxical adduction of the vocal folds in inspiration, causing stridor.[16,17,18]

Classification of dystonia

Etiology

Primary
- Hereditary
  - Autosomal dominant (*DYT1* gene)
  - X-linked recessive

Secondary
- Sporadic
- Associated with other hereditary neurologic diseases (e.g., Wilson disease, Huntington disease)
- Environmental (e.g., posttraumatic, toxic, tardive, vascular)
- Dystonia associated with Parkinson disease

Distribution
- Focal (e.g., blepharospasm, oromandibular dystonia, spasmodic dysphonia, cervical dystonia, writer's cramp)
- Segmental (e.g., Meige syndrome)
- Multifocal
- Generalized

Systemic pharmacotherapy is rarely beneficial for focal laryngeal dystonia. Other management strategies, such as recurrent laryngeal nerve section,[19,20] selective laryngeal denervation/reinnervation procedures[21] and myectomy/ myoplasty of various laryngeal muscles,[22,23] have shown limited long-term success. Botulinum toxin type A is the preferred management option for patients with all forms of SD, with many published series proving efficacy with low morbidity.[14,24] Needle placement for toxin injection uses the methods outlined earlier (▶ Fig. 11.1, ▶ Fig. 11.2). A 27-gauge monopolar hollow Teflon-coated recording/injecting needle is used to deliver the toxin. Response to treatment can be assessed by using a patient-rated SD-specific symptom questionnaire (see the box "Symptom questionnaire to assess response to botulinum toxin therapy (p. 102)"). For adductor SD, both cords can be injected at the same time, generally starting at 1 unit of toxin per cord and then adjusting subsequent doses based on the patient's response. A history of breathy voice for longer than 2 weeks after the initial injection suggests the need for subsequent dose reduction; conversely, lack of appropriate response with inadequate improvement of strain or breaks as measured on a patient rating scale suggests the need for dose increase. For abductor SD, one cord is injected at a time to minimize risk of airway compromise. Depending on the patient's response to that injection, the other cord can then be injected after 2 weeks (if < 50% improvement on patient symptom rating scale) or when symptoms recur (if good symptom control with single cord injection). The disease tends to fluctuate in symptom severity over time and thus botulinum toxin doses will need occasional readjustments, even when a patient has been on a seemingly stable dose regime for a number of years.

Tremor

Tremor is defined as "a series of involuntary, relatively rhythmic, purposeless, oscillatory movements" observed in axial, distal, or proximal musculature, or any combination thereof.[25,26] All people have normal physiologic tremor that occurs with a frequency of 6 to 12 hertz (Hz), whereas frequency of pathologic tremors indicating neurologic disease can range from 3 to 7 Hz.[26,27] Laryngeal tremor may accompany tremor observed elsewhere in the body, particularly the pharyngeal, respiratory and articulatory systems, or occur as an isolated phenomenon. It may be horizontal or vertical in direction. Essential tremor (ET) is the most common presentation of tremor affecting the larynx; approximately 10 to 20% of patients with limb ET will have a vocal component.[28,29] The tremor of ET is a regular, rhythmic oscillatory movement of 4- to 12-Hz frequency. It occurs due to reciprocal activation of antagonistic muscles, especially during sustained phonation, caused by oscillations in central pathways, particularly the olivocerebellorubral loop system.[30,31,32,33,34,35] Compared with limb ET, which is generally absent at rest, 74% of patients with laryngeal ET in a recent series had some degree of laryngeal tremor during quiet respiration.[29] Dystonic tremor shares many features with laryngeal ET, including voice instability and improvement with alcohol, and up to 25% of patients with SD may have a tremor component.[14] However, dystonic tremor is typically irregular and task-specific with a directional preponderance that occurs due to agonist–antagonist muscle contractions.[36] In adductor dystonic tremor, symptoms are provoked by phrases containing many voiced onsets (e.g., counting from 80 to 90), whereas ET affects the voice across all vocal tasks without regard to phonetic composition. Electromyographic patterns can help differentiate dystonic from essential tremor (▶ Fig. 11.4).[37,38,39] Vocal ET rarely responds to systemic medications like beta-blockers and anticonvulsants; however, botulinum toxin may benefit up to two-thirds of patients.[29,40] For predominantly horizontal laryngeal tremor, toxin is initially injected into the bilateral thyroarytenoid muscles. For vertical tremor, strap muscles are initially injected.

Symptom questionnaire to assess response to botulinum toxin therapy

BOTOX INJECTION PATIENT REPORT SHEET

FOR VOICE

Please fill this out if you have had a previous botox injection into the voice box.

NAME:____________________________

TODAY'S DATE:____________________

DATE OF LAST INJECTION:____________________

1. For how many weeks did you have an improved voice? In other words, how many weeks after your last injection did you start to get worse? ______________weeks
2. When your voice was at its very best, what percentage of function did you have? "100%" represents a completely normal voice and "0%" is a fully disabled voice with no functional ability.

No function

0% 5% 10% 15% 20% 25% 30%

Moderate function

40% 45% 50% 55% 60% 65%

Normal function

70% 75% 80% 85% 90% 95% 100%

3. How would you rate your voice today?

No function

0% 5% 10% 15% 20% 25% 30%

Moderate function

35% 40% 45% 50% 55% 60% 65%

Normal function

70% 75% 80% 85% 90% 95% 100%

4. Please list any bad effects you experienced after the last injection and how long they lasted:

Breathy/whispery voice for ____________ weeks/days

Trouble swallowing for ____________ weeks/days

Difficult breathing for ____________ weeks/days

Other for ____________ weeks/days

5. Please list what medications you take for mood or anxiety, neurologic, or psychiatric difficulties. If you are not sure, just list all of your medications:

______________________ ______________________

______________________ ______________________

______________________ ______________________

Tic Disorder

A tic is a sudden, rapid, nonrhythmic, recurrent stereotyped motor movement or vocalization that typically waxes and wanes in frequency and is often preceded by a premonitory urge or sensation.[41,42,43] Onset is usually in childhood; however, adult onset can occur. One characteristic of a tic disorder is that the movements or vocalizations can be voluntarily suppressed by the patient for minutes or hours, often followed by a flurry of movements afterward.[26] Gilles de la Tourette syndrome is the most severe form of tic disorder with involuntary vocalizations being the hallmark of the disease. However, for the majority of people with a tic disorder, vocalizations are more subtle and may manifest merely as a sniff or throat clearing. Vocal tics (including phonic tics, laryngeal tics, or coughing) can occur intermixed with speech or at rest, and the vocalizations may be articulate words or inarticulate sounds. All patients with a suspected tic disorder should be assessed by a neurologist, and the type of pharmacologic intervention is based on the patient's predominant symptoms, with clonidine or clonazepam being useful to treat the movement disorder and selective serotonin-reuptake inhibitors assisting in the treatment of comorbid conditions, such as obsessive–compulsive disorder.[41,43] Botulinum toxin injections have been utilized to manage rapid facial, vocal, and dystonic tics; however, the benefits are variable, likely due to the frequently complex nature of the involuntary movements.[44,45,46] Following injection, some patients with severe, persistent tics involving one group of muscles may report a decrease in the urge to make that particular movement, which suggests an effect of injection on the sensory component of the disorder.

Myoclonus

Myoclonus is a movement disorder in which involuntary, brief movements secondary to muscular contractions (positive myoclonus) or inhibitions (negative myoclonus, "asterixis") occur.[47,48,49] Laryngeal involvement can manifest with myoclonic movement of the laryngeal muscles or of the muscles of respiration. Singulus (hiccup) is the most common form of laryngeal myoclonus and occurs due to involuntary diaphragmatic contractions that result in sudden inspiration against a closed glottis. It is often stimulated by diaphragmatic irritation and the etiologies may be cortical, spinal, metabolic or peripheral (e.g., gastric irritation).[50] On electrophysiologic studies, hiccup frequency decreased with a rise in arterial pCO_2 and increased with its decline. Treatment may include physical maneuvers, such as breath holding, rapidly drinking liquid, breathing into a bag, and pharmacotherapy (e.g., baclofen, atropine, narcotics, gabapentin).

Stuttering

Stuttering is a CNS disorder characterized by involuntary and inappropriate use of speaking musculature, resulting in dysfluency in connected speech with associated cognitive effects of frustration, apprehension, and avoidance.[26,51,52] Stuttering often manifests in childhood and like dystonia, is action induced. Fluency can be increased by competing sensory stimulation or emotional arousal, motor actions, and using rhythmical patterns (e.g., metronome). Delayed auditory feedback that causes "deautomatization" of sensory processing can modify basal ganglia processing strategies and thereby improve fluency.[53,54] The primary management strategy is speech therapy.[55] For those who continue to experience dysfluency,

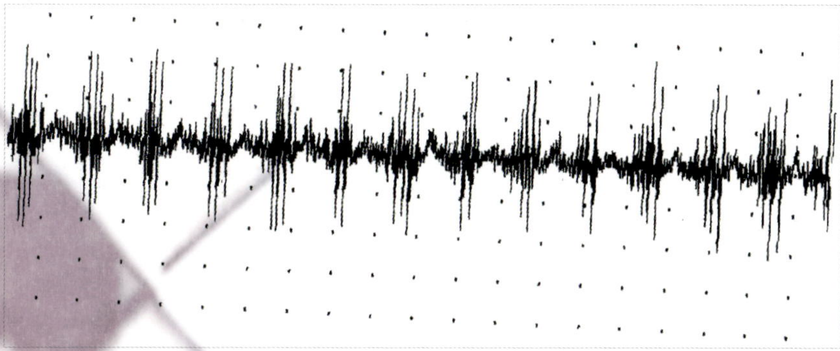

Fig. 11.4 Electromyographic tracing from a patient with essential tremor.

clomipramine can improve fluency and obsessive-compulsive behavioral comorbidities.[56,57] Botulinum toxin may lessen glottic stops occurring as part of the stuttering process; however, it will not restore fluency and few patients continue past 1 to 2 injections.[58]

Muscle Tension Dysphonia

Muscle tension dysphonia (MTD) often develops as a compensatory strategy for an underlying laryngeal pathology; however, it can exist as an isolated phenomenon. Laryngeal, perilaryngeal, suprahyoid, neck, and jaw muscles may be involved.[59,60,61] Pitch alterations and easy fatigue occur with chronic intermittent dysphonia. The voice may become breathy and harsh and mimic adductor SD. Management strategies include relaxation techniques, neck and shoulder positioning exercises, and speech therapy to improve vocal efficiency. Underlying laryngeal pathologies should be addressed where possible and nonsteroidal anti-inflammatory drugs (NSAIDs), massage, and physical therapy may provide some benefit.

Hypofunctional Disorders

(Vocal fold paralysis is not addressed here; see Chapter 9.)

Parkinson Disease

Parkinsonism is a neurologic syndrome manifested by any combination of tremor at rest, rigidity, bradykinesia, and loss of postural reflexes, with at least two of these four features being required for diagnosis.[26,62] Speech and laryngeal disability is common and can include hypophonia, monopitch, prosodic insufficiency, hypokinetic dysarthria, and discoordinated or paradoxical vocal fold motion.[63,64] Lee-Silverman Voice Treatment is effective in improving hypophonia associated with poor respiratory support.[65,66] In addition, vocal fold augmentation procedures may improve hypophonia in patients who have vocal fold atrophy/bowing and relatively normal pulmonary function test results. Patients with a Parkinson-plus syndrome, characterized by parkinsonism with autonomic and sensory disturbances (e.g., multiple system atrophy [MSA]), should not be offered vocal fold augmentation procedures. These patients have a high incidence of life-threatening obstructive airway issues and should instead be referred for sleep studies and consideration of continuous positive airway pressure (CPAP) or tracheostomy.[67]

Myasthenia Gravis

Myasthenia gravis (MG) is an autoimmune disorder of the neuromuscular junction that is characterized by fluctuating ocular or oropharyngeal weakness, often with limb weakness, that improves after administration of cholinergic medications. Oropharyngeal and laryngeal weakness causing ineffective cough predisposes patients to aspiration. Weakness of the posterior cricoarytenoid muscle can cause respiratory failure with airway obstruction. Diagnosis can be confirmed by injection of edrophonium, repetitive nerve stimulation, and acetylcholine receptor antibody titers. Management is with systemic cholinergic medications.

11.4 Treatment Failures

Most neurologic disorders involving the larynx also affect other body parts and should be managed by a multidisciplinary team consisting of a neurologist, otolaryngologist, and speech therapist. Excluding focal neurologic conditions localized to the larynx (e.g., SD), primary management is generally with systemic medications. The patient's neurologist manages medication choice, dose, and changes to medications for inadequate symptom control or disease progression, although close collaboration between specialties is important. For hyperkinetic disorders where symptomatic control can be achieved with botulinum toxin injection, effects are transient and subside once the toxin is destroyed after 3 to 4 months. Possible reasons for a suboptimal response to an injection may include

1. Inadequate Dose: Most of the laryngeal neurologic disorders wax and wane over time and thus the toxin dose required can also vary.
2. Too High a Dose: If suspected based on patient symptoms, subsequent doses can be reduced once effects subside after 3 to 4 months. Alternatively, strategies like treating one side of the larynx at a time can be implemented (see the above subsection, Dystonia)
3. Inaccurate Toxin Placement: Performing injections under EMG guidance minimizes the risk of needle misplacement.
4. Antibody Production: Although rare, if a patient remains consistently nonresponsive to botulinum toxin type A, it is possible he has developed antibodies to this strain of toxin. This is generally seen during the first year of treatment and can be managed by changing to botulinum toxin type B.

11.4.1 Key Points

- Movement disorders of the larynx can be divided into hypofunctional, hyperfunctional, mixed, and sensory categories.
- A team approach to these disorders including a neurologist is essential to ensure optimal diagnosis and management outcomes.
- Many neurologic disorders that affect the larynx also affect other body areas and may partially respond to systemic medications.
- Hyperfunctional disorders of the larynx may respond to injections of botulinum toxin.
- Hypofunctional disorders of the larynx can be managed with interventions that augment function.

References

[1] Woodson GE, Blitzer A, Alexander RE, Grant NN. Neurologic evaluation of the larynx and pharynx. In: Cummings Otolaryngology-Head and Neck Surgery. Philadelphia, PA: Elsevier; 2010: 832–836

[2] Aronson AE. Clinical Voice Disorders. New York, NY: Thieme Medical Publishers; 1985

[3] Baken RJ. Clinical Measurements of Speech and Voice. Boston, MA: College-Hill Press; 1987

[4] Nelson M, Cooper DM, Lawson W. Laryngeal sensory receptors. In: Blitzer A, Brin MF, Sasaki CT, Fahn S, Harris K, eds. Neurologic Disorders of the Larynx. New York, NY: Thieme Medical Publishers; 1992. 12–28

[5] Kirchner JA. Joseph H. Ogura Memorial Lecture. The vertebrate larynx: adaptations and aberrations. Laryngoscope 1993; 103: 1197–1201

[6] Sasaki CT. Electrophysiology of the larynx. In: Blitzer A, Brin MF, Sasaki CT, Fahn S, Harris K, eds. Neurologic Disorders of the Larynx. New York, NY: Thieme Medical Publishers; 1992: 45–56

[7] Woodson GE, Zwirner P, Murry T et al. Use of flexible fiberoptic laryngoscopy to assess patients with spasmodic dysphonia J Voice 1991; 5: 85–91

[8] Yanagisawa E. Physical examination of the larynx and videolaryngoscopy. In: Blitzer A, Brin MF, Sasaki CT, Fahn S, Harris K, eds. Neurologic Disorders of the Larynx. New York, NY: Thieme Medical Publishers; 1992

[9] Roy N, Smith ME, Houtz DR. Laryngeal features of external superior laryngeal nerve denervation: revisiting a century-old controversy. Ann Otol Rhinol Laryngol 2011; 120: 1–8

[10] Rosen CA, Lee AS, Osborne J, Zullo T, Murry T. Development and validation of the Voice Handicap Index-10. Laryngoscope 2004; 114: 1549–1556

[11] Chitkara A, Meyer T, Cultrara A, Blitzer A. Dose response of topical anesthetic on laryngeal neuromuscular electrical transmission. Ann Otol Rhinol Laryngol 2005; 114: 819–821

[12] Lovelace RE, Blitzer A, Ludlow CL. Clinical laryngeal electromyography. In: Blitzer A, Brin MF, Sasaki CT, Fahn S, Harris K, eds. Neurologic Disorders of the Larynx. New York, NY: Thieme Medical Publishers; 1992: 66–81

[13] Aviv JE, Martin JH, Jones ME et al. Age-related changes in pharyngeal and supraglottic sensation. Ann Otol Rhinol Laryngol 1994; 103: 749–752

[14] Blitzer A, Brin MF, Stewart CF. Botulinum toxin management of spasmodic dysphonia (laryngeal dystonia): a 12-year experience in more than 900 patients. Laryngoscope 1998; 108: 1435–1441

[15] Blitzer A. Spasmodic dysphonia and botulinum toxin: experience from the largest treatment series. Eur J Neurol 2010; 17 Suppl 1: 28–30

[16] Blitzer A, Brin MF. Laryngeal dystonia: a series with botulinum toxin therapy. Ann Otol Rhinol Laryngol 1991; 100: 85–89

[17] Brin MF, Fahn S, Blitzer A, Ramig LO, Stewart C. Movement disorders of the larynx. In: Blitzer A, Brin MF, Sasaki CT, Fahn S, Harris K, eds. Neurologic Disorders of the Larynx. New York, NY: Thieme Medical Publishers; 1992: 240–248

[18] Grillone GA, Blitzer A, Brin MF, Annino DJ, Saint-Hilaire MH. Treatment of adductor laryngeal breathing dystonia with botulinum toxin type A. Laryngoscope 1994; 104: 30–32

[19] Dedo HH, Izdebski K. Intermediate results of 306 recurrent laryngeal nerve sections for spastic dysphonia. Laryngoscope 1983; 93: 9–16

[20] Aronson AE, De Santo LW. Adductor spastic dysphonia: three years after recurrent laryngeal nerve resection. Laryngoscope 1983; 93: 1–8

[21] Berke GS, Blackwell KE, Gerratt BR, Verneil A, Jackson KS, Sercarz JA. Selective laryngeal adductor denervation-reinnervation: a new surgical treatment for adductor spasmodic dysphonia. Ann Otol Rhinol Laryngol 1999; 108: 227–231

[22] Shaw GY, Sechtem PR, Rideout B. Posterior cricoarytenoid myoplasty with medialization thyroplasty in the management of refractory abductor spasmodic dysphonia. Ann Otol Rhinol Laryngol 2003; 112: 303–306

[23] Koufman JA, Rees CJ, Halum SL, Blalock D. Treatment of adductor-type spasmodic dysphonia by surgical myectomy: a preliminary report. Ann Otol Rhinol Laryngol 2006; 115: 97–102

[24] Brin MF, Fahn S, Moskowitz C et al. Localized injections of botulinum toxin for the treatment of focal dystonia and hemifacial spasm. Mov Disord 1987; 2: 237–254

[25] DeJong RN. The Neurologic Examination. 3rd ed. New York. NY: Hueber; 1967

[26] Brin MF, Blitzer A, Velickovic M. Movement disorders of the larynx. In: Blitzer A, Brin MF, Ramig LO, eds. Neurologic Disorders of the Larynx. 2nd ed. New York, NY: Thieme Medical Publishers; 2009:160–195

[27] Marsden CD, Obeso JA, Rothwell JC. Benign essential tremor is not a single entity. In: Yahr MD, ed. Current Concepts in Parkinson's Disease. Amsterdam, The Netherlands: Excerpta Medica; 1983

[28] Lebrun Y, Devreux F, Rousseau JJ, Darimont P. Tremulous speech. A case report. Folia Phoniatr (Basel) 1982; 34: 134–142

[29] Sulica L, Louis ED. Clinical characteristics of essential voice tremor: a study of 34 cases. Laryngoscope 2010; 120: 516–528

[30] Davis CH, Kunkle EC. Benign essential (heredofamilial) tremor. Trans Am Neurol Assoc 1951; 56: 87–89

[31] Marshall J. Observations on essential tremor. J Neurol Neurosurg Psychiatry 1962; 25: 122–125

[32] Critchley E. Clinical manifestations of essential tremor. J Neurol Neurosurg Psychiatry 1972; 35: 365–372

[33] Marshall J. Pathology of tremor. In: Findley LJ, Capildeo R, eds. Movement Disorders: Tremor. New York. NY: Oxford University Press; 1984: 95–123

[34] Deuschl G, Elble RJ. The pathophysiology of essential tremor. Neurology 2000; 54 Suppl 4: S14–S20

[35] McIntyre CC, Savasta M, Walter BL, Vitek JL. How does deep brain stimulation work? Present understanding and future questions. J Clin Neurophysiol 2004; 21: 40–50

[36] Schaefer SD, Watson BC, Freeman FJ et al. Vocal tract electromyographic abnormalities in spasmodic dysphonia preliminary report. Trans Am Laryngol Assoc 1987; 108: 187–196

[37] Blitzer A, Lovelace RE, Brin MF, Fahn S, Fink ME. Electromyographic findings in focal laryngeal dystonia (spastic dysphonia). Ann Otol Rhinol Laryngol 1985; 94: 591–594

[38] Sataloff RT, Mandel S, Mann EA, Ludlow CL. Practice parameter: laryngeal electromyography (an evidence-based review). Otolaryngol Head Neck Surg 2004; 130: 770–779

[39] Maronian NC, Robinson L, Waugh P, Hillel AD. A new electromyographic definition of laryngeal synkinesis. Ann Otol Rhinol Laryngol 2004; 113: 877–886

[40] Hertegård S, Granqvist S, Lindestad PA. Botulinum toxin injections for essential voice tremor. Ann Otol Rhinol Laryngol 2000; 109: 204–209

[41] Jankovic J. Differential diagnosis and etiology of tics. Adv Neurol 2001; 85: 15–29

[42] Pringsheim T, Davenport WJ, Lang A. Tics. Curr Opin Neurol 2003; 16: 523–527

[43] Singer HS. Tourette's syndrome: from behaviour to biology. Lancet Neurol 2005; 4: 149–159

[44] Marras C, Andrews D, Sime E, Lang AE. Botulinum toxin for simple motor tics: a randomized, double-blind, controlled clinical trial. Neurology 2001; 56: 605–610

[45] Porta M, Maggioni G, Ottaviani F, Schindler A. Treatment of phonic tics in patients with Tourette's syndrome using botulinum toxin type A. Neurol Sci 2004; 24: 420–423

[46] Houeto JL, Karachi C, Mallet L et al. Tourette's syndrome and deep brain stimulation. J Neurol Neurosurg Psychiatry 2005; 76: 992–995

[47] Marsden CD, Hallett M, Fahs S. The nosology and pathophysiology of myoclonus. In: Marsden CD, Fahn S, eds. Movement Disorders. London, UK: Butterworth Scientific; 1982: 196–248

[48] Nirenberg MJ, Frucht SJ. Myoclonus. Curr Treat Options Neurol 2005; 7: 221–230
[49] Agarwal P, Frucht SJ. Myoclonus. Curr Opin Neurol 2003; 16: 515–521
[50] Shim C. Motor disturbances of the diaphragm. Clin Chest Med 1980; 1: 125–129
[51] Webster RL, Dorman MF. Changes in reliance on auditory feedback cues as a function of oral practice. J Speech Hear Res 1971; 14: 307–311
[52] Perkins WH, Kent RD, Curlee RF. A theory of neuropsycholinguistic function in stuttering. J Speech Hear Res 1991; 34: 734–752
[53] Van Riper C. The Nature of Stuttering. 1st ed. Englewood Cliffs, NJ: Prentice Hall; 1982
[54] Hargrave S, Kalinowski J, Stuart A, Armson J, Jones K. Effect of frequency-altered feedback on stuttering frequency at normal and fast speech rates. J Speech Hear Res 1994; 37: 1313–1319
[55] Bothe AK, Davidow JH, Bramlett RE, Ingham RJ. Stuttering treatment research 1970–2005: I. Systematic review incorporating trial quality assessment of behavioral, cognitive, and related approaches. Am J Speech Lang Pathol 2006; 15: 321–341
[56] Gordon CT, Cotelingam GM, Stager S, Ludlow CL, Hamburger SD, Rapoport JL. A double-blind comparison of clomipramine and desipramine in the treatment of developmental stuttering. J Clin Psychiatry 1995; 56: 238–242
[57] Stager SV, Ludlow CL, Gordon CT, Cotelingam M, Rapoport JL. Fluency changes in persons who stutter following a double blind trial of clomipramine and desipramine. J Speech Hear Res 1995; 38: 516–525
[58] Brin MF, Stewart C, Blitzer A, Diamond B. Laryngeal botulinum toxin injections for disabling stuttering in adults. Neurology 1994; 44: 2262–2266
[59] Morrison MD, Nichol H, Rammage LA. Diagnostic criteria in functional dysphonia. Laryngoscope 1986; 96: 1–8
[60] Koufman JA, Blalock PD. Functional voice disorders. Otolaryngol Clin North Am 1991; 24: 1059–1073
[61] Belafsky PC, Postma GN, Reulbach TR, Holland BW, Koufman JA. Muscle tension dysphonia as a sign of underlying glottal insufficiency. Otolaryngol Head Neck Surg 2002; 127: 448–451
[62] Fahn S. Parkinson's disease and other basal ganglion disorders. In: Asbury AK, McKhann GM, McDonald WI, eds. Diseases of the Nervous System: Clinical Neurobiology. Philadelphia, PA: Ardmore Medical Books; 1986: 1217–1228
[63] Aronson AE, Brown JR, Litin EM, Pearson JS. Spastic dysphonia. II. Comparison with essential (voice) tremor and other neurologic and psychogenic dysphonias. J Speech Hear Disord 1968; 33: 219–231
[64] Hanson DG, Gerratt BR, Ward PH. Cinegraphic observations of laryngeal function in Parkinson's disease. Laryngoscope 1984; 94: 348–353
[65] Logemann JA, Fisher HB, Boshes B, Blonsky ER. Frequency and cooccurrence of vocal tract dysfunctions in the speech of a large sample of Parkinson patients. J Speech Hear Disord 1978; 43: 47–57
[66] Ramig LO, Sapir S, Countryman S et al. Intensive voice treatment (LSVT) for patients with Parkinson's disease: a 2 year follow up. J Neurol Neurosurg Psychiatry 2001; 71: 493–498
[67] Munschauer FE, Loh L, Bannister R, Newsom-Davis J. Abnormal respiration and sudden death during sleep in multiple system atrophy with autonomic failure. Neurology 1990; 40: 677–679

12 Systemic and Endocrine Disorders of the Larynx

Edward J. Damrose and Mai Thy Truong

The impact of hormones on laryngeal development has long been recognized. As early as 400 BC, Aristotle described the effect of castration on the songbird.[1] Starting in the 16th century, males were castrated between the ages of 7 and 9 to preserve the unbroken voice; castrati had a strong presence in Italian opera and the choir of the Sistine Chapel for the next three centuries.[2] Hormones impact laryngeal development and function in many ways, and considering the larynx as being comprised of discrete target components can provide a framework for understanding how systemic and endocrine disorders can affect the larynx. These anatomic components include

- Extravascular spaces: Fluid shifts within these spaces, in response to hormonal fluctuations, can result in laryngeal edema or dehydration, which in turn can affect voice quality and function. These may be seen in states of hypothyroidism, acromegaly, and menopause.
- Epithelium and glandular cells: Dysfunction and changes in glandular secretion in response to hormonal states can lead to dehydration and dysphonia.[3]
- Muscles: Androgens cause hypertrophy of laryngeal striated muscle.[4] Muscle atrophy may be seen with other endocrine disorders.[5]
- Laryngeal framework: Androgens and growth hormone promote growth and calcification of cartilaginous structures of the larynx.
- Neurovascular structures: Laryngeal neuropathy may be secondary diabetic states.

Hormone receptors have been identified both in the nucleus and in the cytoplasm of vocal fold cells, with receptor differences depending on age and gender. Androgen receptors have been identified in glandular cell cytoplasm, estrogen receptors in epithelial cell cytoplasm, and progesterone receptors in glandular cell nuclei.[6] Thyroid hormone receptors have been found in the lamina propria, the cartilage, and the glandular elements of the larynx.[7] The interaction of these hormones with their receptors accounts for normal maturation, growth, and function of the larynx, and for derangement in vocal function in various pathological states.

A number of systemic disorders also affect laryngeal function. Many of these are autoimmune, such as rheumatoid arthritis (RA), systemic lupus erythematosus (SLE), and relapsing polychondritis (RP). Some are characterized by their histopathologic findings, such as the presence of granulomas in granulomatosis with polyangitis (GPA, formerly known as Wegener granulomatosis) or sarcoidosis, or the deposition of protein complexes, as is seen in amyloidosis. The impact of these systemic disorders can manifest in a variety of ways, with relatively mild symptoms, such as hoarseness and odynophonia, in some cases, to life-threatening airway obstruction in others. How these disease processes affect laryngeal function, their clinical presentation, and their management are discussed in this chapter.

12.1 Development and Puberty

Testosterone is produced in small amounts by the adrenal cortex. Later, the majority of testosterone is produced by the Leydig cells of the testes, controlled by the hypothalamic–pituitary–gonadal axis. The hypothalamus produces gonadotropin-releasing hormone (GnRH), which stimulates pituitary release of luteinizing hormone (LH), which in turn stimulates Leydig cells to produce testosterone. Testosterone binds directly to androgen receptors located in the cytoplasm of target cells. Testosterone may be converted by 5-alpha-reductase to dihydrotestosterone (DHT), which has even greater binding affinity for the androgen receptor. This complex translocates to the cell nucleus, wherein protein synthesis is initiated. Testosterone affects the maturation of secondary sex characteristics and genitalia, promotes muscle growth, and leads to the closure of growth plates. A small fraction (0.1%) of testosterone may be converted to estradiol by aromatase, which binds to estrogen receptors. Normal testosterone levels range from 300 to 1000 ng/dL in males, and 20 to 80 ng/dL in females.

12.1.1 Males

In males, pubertal changes take place between ages 9 and 17.[8,9] The factors that initiate puberty are not well understood. Anatomically, there is an increase in the anteroposterior length of the thyroid cartilage and the thyroid ala enlarges to produce a more prominent notch, resulting in an "Adam's apple." The vocal cords lengthen and become more rounded, the epithelium thickens and forms three distinct layers, laryngeal mucus becomes more viscous, the arytenoids grow, the thyroarytenoid ligaments become thicker, and the cricothyroid muscle broadens.[3,10] These changes are irreversible and result in an adult voice that is approximately one octave lower than that of a child.

Changes in the Male Larynx in Puberty[3,10]

- Growth of the cartilaginous framework and development of the thyroid prominence
- Descent of the larynx
- Lengthening and thickening of vocal folds
- Thickening of the epithelium of the vocal fold, forming three distinct layers
- Growth of the arytenoids
- Thickening of the thyroarytenoid ligaments
- Broadening of the cricothyroid muscle

With puberty, the larynx descends, lengthening the vocal tract —the distance from the lips to the glottis. Lengthening of the vocal tract produces changes in vocal timbre and resonance. The anteroposterior length of the vocal fold doubles and fundamental frequency slows, resulting in a deeper voice.[10] Baritones and bases tend to have longer vocal tracts.[11,12,13] Vocal fold elongation is greater in males, with an overall increase in length of 67% following puberty, compared to females, in whom the increase is only 24%.[14]

The drop in fundamental frequency of the male voice occurs later in puberty, between Tanner stages III and IV.[15] As the changes progress, the adolescent male voice cracks often. Several theories have been postulated to explain this: imbalance between the child-like glottis and the wind power of the adult thoracoabdominal structure, with fluctuations in power resulting in a yodeling voice[3]; the substitution of the chest voice (or heavy mechanism) for the head voice (or light mechanism) in an adolescent who is still speaking in a child-like voice[16]; and the natural learning curve of a maturing male adapting to the developing laryngeal muscles and their increase in strength and size.[8]

12.1.2 Females

Puberty in females occurs 1 to 3 years before it does in males. As in males, early development is dominated by androgen secretion by the adrenal cortex during adrenarche. Menarche marks the completion of the maturation of the reproductive system controlled by the hypothalamic–pituitary–gonadal axis. Cyclical secretion involves a positive feedback mechanism by which an increased estrogen level triggers the simultaneous release of LH and follicle-stimulating hormone (FSH), involved in ovulation and menses. The ovaries are the primary source of estradiol and also produce a small amount of testosterone. The average age of onset of menses is 12.6 years (range, 9.1 to 16.2 years old).[17]

A woman's voice is one-third of an octave lower than a child's voice. The female larynx is thought to develop gradually as a child ages, without the dramatic changes that are seen in a male larynx at puberty. Female vocal tract growth is steady throughout puberty and adulthood.[10] There is little development of the thyroid cartilage compared to what is seen in the male, and it reaches adult size by the onset of puberty. The vocal muscle remains small, although it may enlarge slightly.[3] In contrast to males, fundamental frequency in females drops progressively over ages 8 to 19, with steady expansion of the lower tonal range.[18]

12.2 Androgens

12.2.1 Physiology

Androgens play an important role in the maturation of the human male larynx.

Animal models have provided useful information detailing the impact of androgens (testosterone and dihydrotestosterone) on laryngeal growth and function. Androgen stimulation of the sheep larynx enlarges the thyroid cartilage framework, ultimately resulting in a lengthening of the vocal fold. The distance between the vocal process and the base of the arytenoid increases, as does the distance between the vocal and muscular processes.[19] Androgens stimulate the development of muscle and cartilage cells, with a concomitant increase in androgen receptor mRNA production,[5] while inhibition of androgen exposure prevents these developments.[5,20,21]

12.2.2 Androgen Deficiency

Numerous disorders of androgen physiology have been identified, but the laryngeal and phonatory impact has been detailed in relatively few. Androgen deficiency may have a negative impact on male laryngeal development and can be broadly characterized into three classes: failure of testosterone production, failure of testosterone secretion, and failure of testosterone action. In primary hypogonadism, the testes fail to develop normally (e.g., Klinefelter syndrome, bilateral anorchia, Leydig cell aplasia, Noonan syndrome), resulting in impaired levels of circulating androgens. Androgen insensitivity is characterized by a defect in the dihydrotestosterone receptor, impairing cellular response to androgens. Failure of normal hypothalamic–pituitary function accounts for the third major class of androgen hypofunction.

12.2.3 Idiopathic Hypogonadotropic Hypogonadism

Idiopathic hypogonadotropic hypogonadism (IHH) is a congenital disorder most commonly associated with deficient GnRH secretion. Hypogonadism, infertility, and absent or incomplete pubertal maturation are seen. A variation of this disorder is Kallman syndrome, an X-linked syndrome characterized by anosmia. Androgen therapy and supplementation have been investigated in various populations. Prior to treatment, IHH males have a mean fundamental frequency between normal male controls and normal female controls. After 3 months of androgen therapy, the fundamental frequency approaches that of normal males. These changes are likely secondary to permanent gains in laryngeal muscle mass.[22]

The differential diagnosis of hypothalamic–pituitary dysfunction includes neoplasia, ischemic changes (cerebrovascular accident), infiltrative processes (sarcoidosis, histiocytosis), and trauma. Patients should be evaluated for concomitant hypothyroidism and hypoadrenalism. If dysfunction occurs postpuberty, additional symptoms and signs may include impotence, decreased libido, and testicular atrophy.

12.2.4 Androgen Excess

Normal serum testosterone in women is 20 to 80 ng/dL. Androgen excess may be characterized by hirsutism, clitoral enlargement, facial acne, breast atrophy, and laryngeal virilization with deepening of the voice.[23] Evaluation involves discriminating between endogenous sources of excess androgens (ovarian neoplasia, polycystic ovary syndrome, Cushing disease, congenital adrenal hyperplasia) and exogenous sources (anabolic steroids, testosterone, metapyrone).[24]

In females, androgen exposure has broad effects, as shown in histological studies of the mouse model. When exposed to anabolic steroids, the thyroarytenoid muscle undergoes hypertrophy and hyperplasia. Histological changes of the epithelium also include basal cell hyperplasia, parakeratosis, and squamous metaplasia of the laryngeal mucosa. Hyperplasia of seromucinous glands and increased vascularity, vascular congestion, and edema can be seen in the connective tissue stroma. Ballooning and a characteristic signet ring appearance of the cartilage cells can be seen in laryngeal cartilage.[4] In females, laryngeal virilization is manifested by a deepening of the voice and enlargement of the thyroid cartilage (or Adam's apple), changes that are thought to be irreversible.[25] In female to male transsexuals, androgen exposure produces a reduction in mean fundamental frequency at about the third month of treatment.[26] A reduction of 100 Hz may be seen with injections of testosterone enthanate 200 mg bimonthly.

12.2.5 Congenital Adrenal Hyperplasia

Congenital adrenal hyperplasia (CAH) is an autosomal recessive disorder characterized by defects in hydroxylation of cortisol precursors, resulting in low levels of cortisol, increased levels of corticotropin (ACTH), and adrenal hyperplasia. In the most common form of the disease, absence of the 21-hydroxylase enzyme results in excess net production of androgens, with a subsequent virilizing effect. Normal mean fundamental frequency in female speech is between 165 to 255 Hz. In the virilized larynx, fundamental frequencies can be seen in the range of normal males (85 to 180 Hz).[26,27] Urinalysis will demonstrate elevated levels of dihydroepiandrosterone (DHEA), androsterone, and pregnanetriol. Treatment is with daily hydrocortisone or prednisolone. Early recognition and prompt treatment may prevent the voice problems seen in females with the disorder.

12.2.6 Puberphonia

Puberphonia (pubescent falsetto, mutational falsetto) is a functional voice disorder that must be distinguished from disorders of androgen insufficiency. Males exhibit an abnormally high speaking voice but demonstrate normal secondary sexual characteristics. The onset of the disorder is usually during the adolescent growth spurt. Pitch breaks, breathiness, and hoarseness may also be seen in addition to high pitch. The exact etiology is unclear, but underlying psychosocial factors are frequently identified during evaluation. Once organic causes like IHH are excluded, treatment is with voice therapy and is usually successful.[28,29] In refractory cases, treatment with botulinum toxin or with type 3 thyroplasty can also provide relief of symptoms.[30,31]

12.3 Estrogen and Progesterone

12.3.1 Physiology

Estrogens are reported to have a hypertrophic effect on the laryngeal mucosa and to increase secretion from laryngeal glandular cells. Estrogens cause a differentiation and maturation of fat cells. In periods of elevated estrogen, such as during pregnancy, the larynx has been described as hyperemic, with congested mucosa.[32] Estrogens act in cyclical fashion with progesterone. Progesterone has been reported to have an antiproliferative effect on mucosa, accelerating desquamation, decreasing glandular cell secretion while increasing viscosity and acidity, leading to dryness. Also, progesterone has been implicated in inhibiting capillary permeability, trapping extracellular fluid and causing edema. Some synthetic progesterones have been shown to have androgenic effects.[33] Estrogens can enhance development of the neuromuscular junction, while their absence impairs neuromuscular development.[34,35]

12.3.2 The Premenstrual Vocal Syndrome

Laryngopathia Premenstrualis

Vocal symptoms have been described during the premenstrual phase, mostly in trained vocal professionals, in a condition known as *laryngopathia premenstrualis*. The clinical entity is characterized by vocal fatigue, decreased range with loss of highest pitches, decreased power, and flat timbre.[35] It has been reported that 33% of nonprofessional voice users, and a higher percentage of professionals, experience these voice symptoms.[33,36] In the contracts of some vocalists, "grace days" are allotted for voice rest for this reason.[33] It has been reported that the elevations in estrogen and progesterone cause structural changes in laryngeal mucosa resulting in changes in vocal tone.

Premenstrual Vocal Syndrome Symptoms[33,36]

- Vocal fatigue
- Decreased range, with higher tones more susceptible for loss
- Loss of vocal power
- Decline in high harmonics

Prior to menstruation, estrogen elevation causes a thickening of mucus while rising progesterone levels increase the viscosity and acidity of glandular secretions. In the premenstrual period, the squamous mucosa of the vocal fold and the cervix appear cytologically similar and vocal fold changes closely resemble those seen in the cervix as menses progresses.[33] Videostroboscopy may demonstrate reduced tonicity of the laryngeal muscle, stiffer epithelium, reduced vibratory amplitude, vibratory asymmetry, edema of the vocal cords and venous dilation. Acoustic analysis may demonstrate increased jitter—a measurement of frequency variation during sustained phonation.[37] These premenstrual symptoms are more aggravated and more prevalent in vocal abusers.[38]

It is not clear whether laryngopathia premenstrualis represents a true pathological disorder or not. The syndrome may simply be a clinical entity that is more apparent to vocal professional with their greater vocal demand and who may therefore be more sensitive to vocal perturbations. Treatment generally involves support—education, emphasis on proper vocal hygiene, hydration, avoidance of abusive vocal behaviors, and rest.

12.3.3 Laryngopathia Gravidarum

Voice change associated with pregnancy is termed *laryngopathia gravidarum*. It is generally associated with vocal symptoms similar to those seen premenstrually as result of elevated levels of estrogen and progesterone. These voice changes have been reported in 15 to 20% of pregnant women and tend to occur in the last 5 months of pregnancy.[3] Vocal changes during pregnancy have also been attributed to abdominal distention, which interferes with abdominal muscle function and may exacerbate laryngopharyngeal reflux.[39]

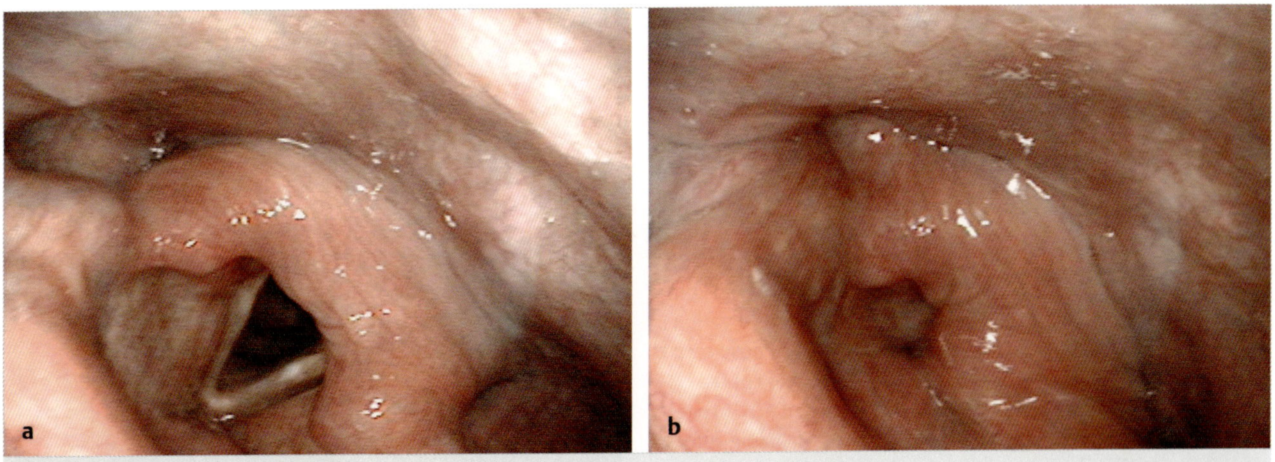

Fig. 12.1 Laryngeal findings in 30-year-old woman, 8 weeks gestation, with laryngopathia gravidarum. (a) Quiet inspiration demonstrating posterior laryngeal edema. (b) Forceful inspiration with prolapse of edematous tissue into laryngeal introitus.

Laryngopathia gravidarum has also been associated with pre-eclampsia. Generalized edema is seen commonly in women with severe pre-eclampsia. Edema of the larynx and upper airway may be mild or severe, with symptoms and signs ranging from hoarseness to dyspnea and stridor secondary to airway obstruction (▶ Fig. 12.1). Laryngeal edema may be the presenting symptom of severe pre-eclampsia.[40] Pre-eclamptic women who will be undergoing general anesthesia need careful airway assessment to avoid airway complications and difficult endotracheal intubation. Under direct visualization, awake or fiberoptic intubation may be considered.[41,42,43,44] Planned prolonged intubation and intensive care unit monitoring should also be considered until resolution of edema.[45] The disorder tends to resolve after delivery.[46]

12.3.4 Menopause and the Menopausal Vocal Syndrome

Menopause is defined as the cessation of menstruation, when ovarian follicles become atretic. In the United States, the average age of onset of menopause is 51. During menopause, there is a loss of ovarian sensitivity to gonadotropin stimulation, and estrogen production declines with the cessation of ovarian follicular activity. Serum gonadotropin concentrations increase in response, FSH rises more than LH. The ovary continues to secrete androgens because of the high serum LH concentrations. A major contribution to estrogen in the circulation then comes from the peripheral aromatization of androstenedione of both ovarian and adrenal origin. The decline in estrogen results in the classic symptoms of menopause, including "hot flashes," mood instability, and depression, as well as findings of vaginal, urethral, and cervical atrophy.[47]

The drop in estrogen and progesterone with the increase in androgens may result in menopausal vocal syndrome (MVS).[33] Vocal changes during menopause have long been reported, but few studies have been done to fully investigate these changes. Loss of glandular cells in laryngeal mucosa results in increased dryness, with concomitant dysphonia and vocal fatigue.[48] Clinical symptoms of MPS include decreased vocal intensity, vocal fatigue, decrease pitch range, and loss of timbre.[33]

Menopausal Vocal Syndrome Symptoms[33,49]

1. Lowering of vocal intensity
2. Vocal fatigue
3. Decreased range with loss in high notes
4. Change in timbre in spoken and singing voices
5. Loss of power
6. Loss of "brilliance"
7. Loss of stability
8. Huskiness

Boulet and Oddens evaluated voice changes in professional singers during the fifth decade of life in an effort to evaluate the impact of aging and of menopause on voicing. The authors found that 77% of women and 71% of men reported vocal changes. Compared to men, women reported more problems with huskiness, loss of range in high registers, and impaired steadiness of voice. Both sexes reported change in timbre.[49]

Abitbol et al evaluated 17 women with MVS.[33] Laryngeal and cervical smears with cytological analysis were performed. Cervical and laryngeal smears were nearly identical, revealing mucosal atrophy, basophil infiltration, and reduced glandular cells. Muscular atrophy, thinning of vocal fold mucosa, reduction of amplitude during phonation, asymmetry between right and left vocal folds, and a decreased vocal range were reported on laryngoscopy. Hormone replacement therapy (HRT) was successful in improving or alleviating symptoms in most patients, with restoration of muscular contour, vibratory amplitude, and vocal timbre.[33] Hormone replacement therapy also reverses the cytological changes seen on laryngeal and cervical smears in postmenopausal patients, with improvement in atrophy-dystrophy in those patients receiving HRT. Patients receiving HRT also report improvement in vocal symptoms, with decreased hoarseness, instability, and fatigue, and improved pitch and timbre.[50]

The phonatory effects of HRT in different combinations (estrogen-progestin versus estrogen-only) have also been evaluated. Both loudness and pitch are more effectively preserved in postmenopausal patients who receive HRT compared to those that do not, while those patients receiving estrogen-only therapy seem to report the fewest subjective symptoms.[51] The merits of HRT effects on the voice must be weighed against the possible side effects, which can include increased risk of heart disease, stroke, and breast cancer.

12.3.5 Oral Contraceptives

Oral contraceptives are hormonal preparations containing combinations of estrogen and progestin in varying concentrations. There is a traditional view that oral contraceptives pose a risk to vocal quality.[39] However, old formulations of oral contraceptives contained higher doses of hormones, particularly progestins, which may have had potentially greater virilizing effects on the larynx.[52] In contrast, modern oral contraceptives have significantly reduced levels of estrogens and progestins, and current research suggests that these low-dose formulations lack the virilizing effects noted with earlier generations of oral contraceptives. Recent literature suggests there is negligible impact on vocal function with the use of oral contraceptives, that long-term use is safe, and that oral contraceptives may actually confer advantages in pitch range and stability in patients taking oral contraceptives compared to those women who do not.[52,53,54,55,56]

12.4 Thyroid Function and the Larynx

12.4.1 Physiology

The thyroid gland has multiple effects on development, growth, and metabolism. The larynx has been shown to be a thyroid hormone target. Altman et al identified thyroid hormone receptors in the larynx of a human male and a human female cadaver.[7] Studies of *Xenopus laevis* have also revealed the key role thyroid hormone plays in androgen competency in the developing larynx. If thyroid hormone secretion is blocked, androgens cannot stimulate normal laryngeal growth. Developing *Xenopus laevis* laryngeal cartilage and muscle have been found to express thyroid receptor mRNA, and because these receptors are nuclear transcription factors, thyroid hormone has been implicated in playing a role in the development cascade in masculinization.[57]

12.4.2 Hypothyroidism

Hypothyroidism is a state of low production of thyroid hormone. Signs and symptoms of the disease vary in relation to the amount of hormone deficiency, and the acuteness with which the deficiency developed. If hypothyroidism is congenital and untreated, the state of cretinism has been associated with a small larynx. Hypothyroid states have been associated with hoarseness, vocal fatigue, muffling of the voice, loss of range, and a feeling of a lump in the throat (globus pharyngeus).[39] The dysphonia of hypothyroidism has been described as coarse or gravelly, and low pitched. Ataxic dysarthria and lingual articulatory imprecision due to tongue swelling and macroglossia are also described, and they aggravate laryngeal symptoms.[58] On clinical exam, muscle stiffness, dry epithelium with reduced vibratory amplitude, mucinous edema, cricoarytenoid joint stiffness, and pale vocal folds with edema of the Reinke space have been noted.[3]

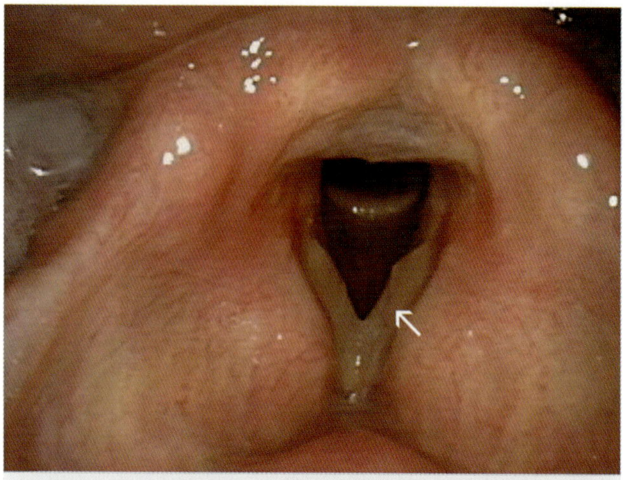

Fig. 12.2 Laryngeal findings of diffuse bilateral vocal fold edema in a 42-year-old hypothyroid man (*arrow* indicates vocal fold).

Hypothyroidism has been reported to cause myxedema of the laryngeal muscle and vocal folds, grossly similar to Reinke edema, with a resultant lowering of pitch (▶ Fig. 12.2). Biopsy shows mild exudation of fibrin and basophilic material with some proliferation of fibroblasts in the Reinke space.[59] An increased level of acid mucopolysaccarides has also been described submucosally in the vocal folds, resulting in an osmotic increase in fluid content, leading to edema and decreased vibration.[60] Severe hypothyroidism and myxedema have been reported to be associated with decreased vocal muscle strength and even vocal fold paralysis.[39] Hormone replacement generally resolves symptoms.

12.4.3 Hyperthyroidism

Hyperthyroidism is due to thyroid hormone overproduction. Mild hyperthyroidism is not likely associated with laryngeal pathology; however, severe thyrotoxicosis may cause submucosal vocal fold changes and muscle weakness, as well as symptoms similar to those seen in hypothyroid states.[39] Dysphonia has not been carefully described, but breathy voice quality and reduced loudness have been reported, presumably due to weakness of the laryngeal musculature.[58] Tremulousness of the voice and hoarseness have been associated with anxiety, while gastroesophageal reflux in the hyperthyroid state may worsen laryngeal symptoms. Clinically, examination of the larynx may demonstrate weakened vocal fold muscles and the presence of a glottic chink during phonation, resulting in a breathy, hoarse voice.[3] Treatment with propylthiouracil or ablation of the gland with restoration of euthyroidism generally resolve symptoms.

12.5 Diabetes and the Larynx

Laryngeal manifestations of diabetes have not been extensively characterized. Researchers have suggested a general neuropathy that, in a professional voice user, may result in impaired tactile and sensory information needed for vocal control. Unilateral and bilateral vocal cord paralysis has been attributed to diabetic neuropathy in various case reports, some reports documenting return of function with hyperglycemic control.[61,62,63,64] In general, diabetes is associated with an increased risk of infection. Infectious laryngitis, both bacterial and fungal, has been described in diabetics, and the infections may be severe. Symptoms may include hoarseness, pain, and stridor. In severe cases, airway obstruction requiring tracheostomy and radical airway debridement has been reported.[65] Chronic granulomatous infections from fungal sources like *histoplasmosis* or *cryptococcosis* can mimic carcinoma on presentation, leading to improper treatment and surgical excision.[66,67]

Diabetes may have a greater *indirect* impact on laryngeal disease beyond that described above. Patients with diabetes have a significant risk for cardiovascular disease and critical illness; a recent study has suggested that diabetics may be at increased risk of airway stenosis, perhaps related to a higher likelihood of critical illness with prolonged intubation.[68] This may be compounded by the association between diabetes and reflux.[69,70] Lower esophageal sphincter function, a key physiologic barrier against the refluxate of gastric contents, is impaired in diabetes.[71] Along with neural impairment of motility, as in gastric atony, these changes make laryngeal and pharyngeal damage from reflux more likely in diabetics.

12.6 Hypophyseal Disorders

12.6.1 Acromegaly

Acromegaly is the clinical syndrome that results from excessive secretion of growth hormone (GH). Its annual incidence is three to four cases per million persons. The mean age at diagnosis is 40 to 45 years; the characteristic findings are macrognathia and enlarged, swollen hands and feet, which result in increasing shoe and glove size and the need to enlarge rings. The facial features become coarse, with enlargement of the nose and frontal bones as well as the jaw, and the teeth become spread apart. The most common cause of acromegaly is a growth hormone-secreting adenoma of the anterior pituitary.[72]

Vocal changes have been described as a deepening of the voice with narrow register and intensity. Tissue from the oral cavity to the pharynx thickens, while the sinus cavities increase in volume, both leading to a change in vocal resonance. Clinically, the epiglottis and thyroid cartilage enlarge, the cricoarytenoid joint may demonstrate decreased mobility, and the vocal folds develop thickened epithelium.[3] True and false vocal cords thicken as well, and a widening of the larynx is associated with pitch changes.[73] The mean fundamental frequency in acromegalic patients is significantly lower than in normal controls. Interestingly, a rapid increase in fundamental frequency has been noted in patients following hypophysectomy, suggesting that the vocal changes are reversible.[74]

12.6.2 Amyloidosis

Amyloidosis is an abnormal deposition of insoluble protein fragments in tissues and organs. Any tissue may be affected, with signs and symptoms secondary to enlargement or dysfunction of the target tissue. Amyloidosis may be localized or systemic, primary or secondary. Although many amyloid proteins have been identified, AL, AA, and AB are the most common.[75] In AL (light chain), the protein is derived from the kappa or lambda immunoglobulin light chains of plasma cells. It may be localized or seen in association with myeloma. In AA (amyloid-associated), the protein is a nonimmunoglobulin of hepatic origin, is systemic, and is usually associated with chronic inflammatory or infectious diseases. AB is found in patients with Alzheimer disease, in which amyloid deposits or plaques develop within neurons. Symptoms vary depending on the tissue or organ affected. In the larynx, the most common presenting symptom is hoarseness, although dyspnea, hemoptysis, dysphagia, and airway obstruction have been reported.[76,77]

Most cases of laryngeal amyloidosis are localized and of the AL subtype. Sites of deposition include the ventricle, false cords, true cords, aryepiglottic folds, and subglottis (▶ Fig. 12.3). Diagnosis requires biopsy of affected tissues, with identification of the characteristic green birefringence of amyloid when tissues are stained with Congo red dye. Treatment generally involves conservative surgical excision of symptomatic lesions. Steroids have no benefit. Evaluation for systemic disease, including multiple myeloma, is recommended but is usually negative.

12.6.3 Sarcoidosis

Sarcoidosis is an idiopathic inflammatory disorder characterized by the development of noncaseating granulomas.[78] Lung involvement, with the development of mediastinal lymphadenopathy and pulmonary infiltrates, is seen in 90% of patients, but any organ system can be affected. The disease shows a predilection for adults 20 to 40 years of age, and otolaryngologic findings are present in about 10% of patients. Laryngeal involvement is rare (0.5–1.5% of cases).[79] Isolated laryngeal involvement is rarer still. Symptoms of laryngeal involvement include hoarseness, dyspnea, stridor, dysphagia, and cough. Some patients with laryngeal involvement are asymptomatic.

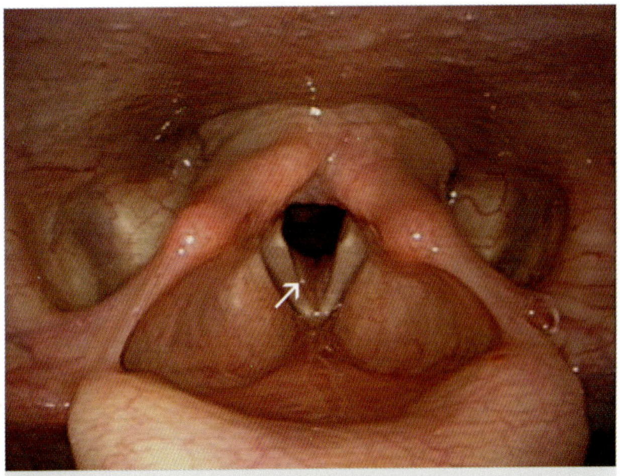

Fig. 12.3 Laryngeal findings in a 40-year-old woman with localized laryngeal amyloidosis (*arrow* indicates anterior subglottic amyloid deposits).

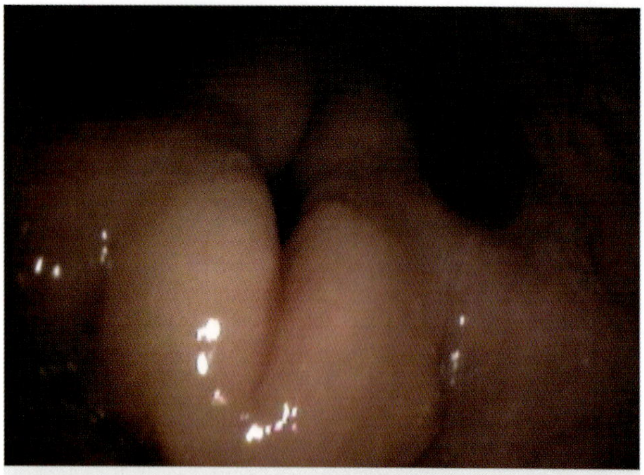

Fig. 12.4 Sarcoidosis affecting the supraglottis. (Courtesy of Michael Pitman, MD.)

When the larynx is involved, the supraglottis is the most commonly affected site (80–85%) (▶ Fig. 12.4). In 15 to 20% of cases, subglottic involvement occurs. Involvement of the glottis is rare (about 1%). Within the supraglottis, the most commonly involved subsites are the epiglottis, arytenoids, aryepiglottic folds, and ventricular folds. The involved tissue typically appears smooth, pale, and edematous.[79]

Workup includes biopsy, with histopathologic confirmation of noncaseating granulomas. Serum evaluation may demonstrate elevation in liver enzymes, creatinine, angiotensin-converting enzyme (ACE), and calcium levels. Angiotensin-converting enzyme is elevated only in 60% of patients with sarcoidosis; a negative finding therefore does not rule out the disease.

Treatment depends on symptoms. For asymptomatic patients, no treatment is needed. In the symptomatic patient, treatment is controversial. Prednisone, methotrexate, intralesional steroid injection, and inhaled budesonide have been used with mixed results. Endoscopic resection of involved tissue using the carbon dioxide (CO_2) laser may improve breathing in patients with dyspnea, although in severe cases tracheostomy may be required. Spontaneous remission of disease may occur over 12 to 36 months, and with this in mind, therapy should be supportive, rather than radically ablative.[78,79]

12.6.4 Granulomatosis with Polyangitis (GPA)

GPA is an idiopathic, multisystem disease characterized by necrotizing vasculitis and noncaseating granuloma formation.[80,81] The disorder can affect the upper airway, particularly the nose and larynx, the lung, and the kidneys. Arthritis manifests in 60% of patients, and rapidly progressive glomerulonephritis in 70%. Pulmonary nodules (coin lesions) are classically seen on chest x-ray. Crusting, bleeding, septal ulceration with perforation, and saddle nose deformity characterize the nasal findings.

In the larynx, patients may develop subglottic stenosis. Subglottic stenosis may develop in 10 to 15% of patients with WG.[80] Laryngeal involvement is usually characterized by hoarseness, cough, and stridor, with progressive dyspnea. Laryngoscopy will usually reveal subglottic and at times upper cervical tracheal stenosis (▶ Fig. 12.5). Tissue may appear friable. In some patients, the inflammatory process and cicatrix formation can involve the inferior aspect of the vocal folds and the anterior commissure.

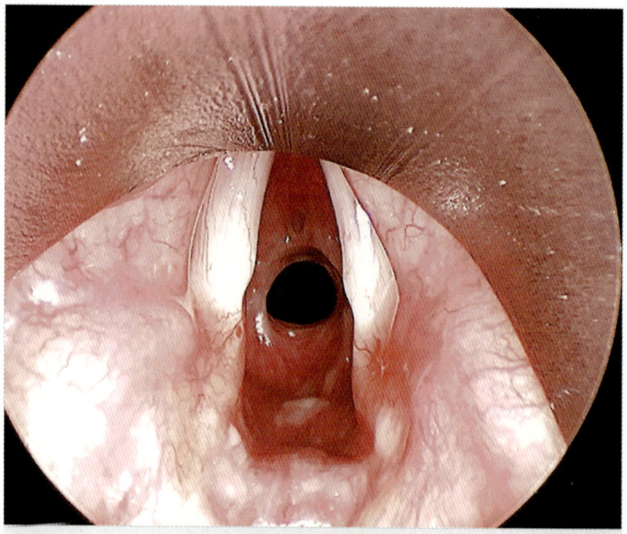

Fig. 12.5 Subglottic stenosis.

Diagnosis depends on a constellation of clinical and laboratory findings. The American College of Rheumatology has identified clinical criteria for GPA.[82] Laboratory analysis may reveal an elevated erythrocyte sedimentation rate (ESR) and C-reactive protein (CRP). Anti-neutrophil cytoplasmic autoantibodies (ANCAs) may be elevated. Cytoplasmic staining ANCAs (cANCA) are also elevated, although negative studies do not conclusively rule out disease.

American College of Rheumatology Criteria for Granulomatosis with Polyangitis[1]

- Nasal or oral inflammation (e.g., oral or nasal ulceration)
- Pulmonary abnormalities (e.g., nodules, infiltrates, cavities)
- Renal dysfunction (e.g., microhematuria, red cell casts)
- Tissue biopsy demonstrating noncaseating granulomas

(Source: Adapted from Leavitt RY, Fauci AS, Bloch DA, et al. The American College of Rheumatology 1990 criteria for the classification of Granulomatosis with Polyangitis (formerly, Wegner granulomatosis). Arthritis Rheum 1990; 33: 1101–1107.)

Systemic therapy, while not curative, is successful in controlling the disease. Corticosteroids, cyclophosphamide, methotrexate, azathioprine, and cotrimoxazole are helpful in managing systemic symptoms. Dilation of subglottic stenosis with local steroid application is helpful in alleviating dyspnea, although this may need to be repeated periodically to control symptoms. In severe cases, tracheostomy may be indicated.[80,81,82]

12.6.5 Rheumatoid Arthritis

Rheumatoid arthritis is a common autoimmune disorder and can involve the larynx in 26 to 53% of patients.[83] The cricoarytenoid joint is a diarthroidial synovial joint, and

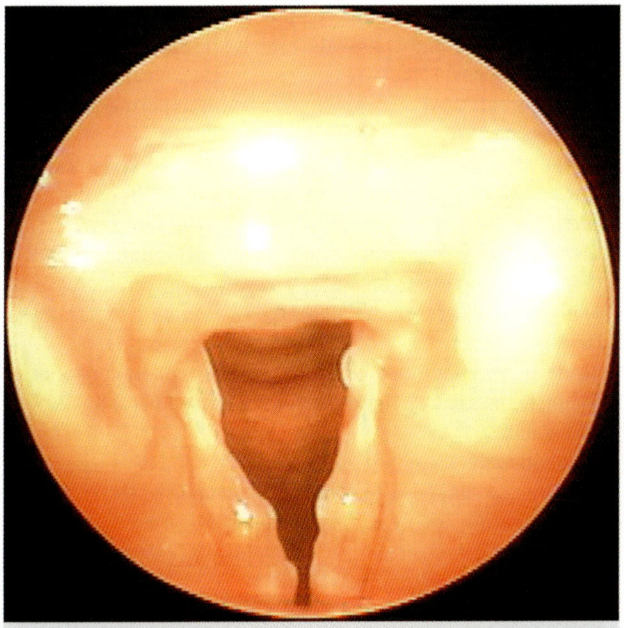

Fig. 12.6 Rheumatoid "bamboo" nodules in a patient with rheumatoid arthritis.

inflammation results in hoarseness, odynophagia, odynophonia, and referred otalgia. Joint inflammation can progress to ankylosis, with subsequent vocal fold paralysis. When bilateral, patients may develop dyspnea and stridor. Laryngoscopy may reveal edema and erythema in the region of the affected arytenoid. Hypomobility or immobility of one or both vocal folds may be observed.[84] Rheumatoid arthritis may cause an arteritis of the vasa nervorum of the vagus and laryngeal nerves, so some of the motion abnormalities observed may be secondary to neuropathy as well as arthritis.[85]

Rheumatoid nodules, also called "bamboo nodules," may present on the vocal folds and contribute to hoarseness (▶ Fig. 12.6). The nodules may be clinically difficult to distinguish from simple nodules, but histopathologically are characterized by a central zone of necrosis surround by histiocytes, monocytes, and fibroblasts.[86]

Serum evaluation may demonstrated elevated CRP, ESR, rheumatoid factor (RF), antinuclear antibody (ANA), and anti-cyclic citrullinated peptide (CCP). It is important to recognize the potential for airway compromise in patients with rheumatoid arthritis, particularly during acute exacerbations of the disease. Tracheostomy may be indicated for airway obstruction. With improvement in inflammation, improved mobility of the vocal folds may follow, allowing decannulation.

Approximately 25 to 40% of patients with rheumatoid arthritis will have subluxation at C1 and C2, with 2 to 5% of these patients demonstrating spinal cord compression.[83] Hyperextension of the neck during operative laryngoscopy or intubation may destabilize the cervical spine and result in acute cord compression with potentially devastating neurological sequelae. Lateral neck x-ray may be helpful to identify patients with subluxation and can help with surgical and anesthetic planning. In patients with subluxation, the minimization of neck extension and the use of fiberoptic intubation techniques may be indicated to minimize the risk of cord compression.

12.6.6 Relapsing Polychondritis

Relapsing polychondritis (RP) is a systemic autoimmune disorder characterized by recurrent progressive inflammatory destruction of cartilage.[87,88] The etiology is unknown, but development of autoantibodies to type II collagen has been implicated. The peak incidence is between the 4th and 6th decades of life, and there is a female to male ratio of 3:1. While the clinical manifestations may vary, 50% of patients have involvement of the respiratory tract. In the head and neck, the pinnae, nose, trachea, and larynx are affected. Hyaline cartilage of joints is affected, resulting in arthritis, but proteoglycan-rich structures like the eye, heart, vascular tree, and kidneys are also at risk.[88] Twenty-five to 35% of patients with RP have a second, concomitant autoimmune disorder.

Clinically, laryngeal involvement manifests as hoarseness, cough, dyspnea, and pain over the thyroid and tracheal cartilages. Mucosal edema involving the true vocal folds and subglottis may be observed on laryngoscopy. Computed tomography may reveal circumferential edema of the soft tissues of the larynx, as well as hypointensity of the cartilage.[87] Biopsy of cartilage may show erosion, and an acute on chronic inflammatory cell infiltrate. Laboratory analysis may reveal an elevation in inflammatory markers such as ESR and CRP. The McAdam Criteria are generally employed to confirm the diagnosis.[89]

McAdam Criteria for the Diagnosis of Relapsing Polychondritis[89]

- Bilateral auricular chondritis
- Nasal chondritis
- Respiratory tract chondritis
- Polyarthritis
- Occular inflammation (e.g., scleritis, episcleritis, conjunctivitis)
- Cochleovestibular inflammation (e.g., vertigo, neural hearing loss)
- A minimum of three findings is required for clinical diagnosis.

(Source: Adapted from McAdam LP, O'Hanlan MA, Bluestone R, Pearson CM. Relapsing polychondritis: Prospective study of 23 patients and a review of the literature. Medicine 1976; 55:193–215.)

There is no standardized medical treatment for RP. Mild acute inflammatory symptoms may be treated with nonsteroidal anti-inflammatory drugs, dapsone, or colchicine. More severe symptoms may necessitate systemic corticosteroids or immunosuppressive medications, such as methotrexate or azathioprine. Acute airway obstruction should be managed with endotracheal intubation or tracheostomy. For chronic airway fibrotic stenosis, formal laryngotracheal reconstruction has been undertaken with good results.[90]

12.6.7 Systemic Lupus Erythematosus

Systemic lupus erythematosus is a common autoimmune disorder characterized by systemic deposition of autoantibodies in tissues, resulting in a type III hypersensitivity reaction and inflammation. Essentially any organ system may be affected. The full spectrum of the disease is beyond the scope of this chapter, but its common manifestations include arthritis, fever, malaise,

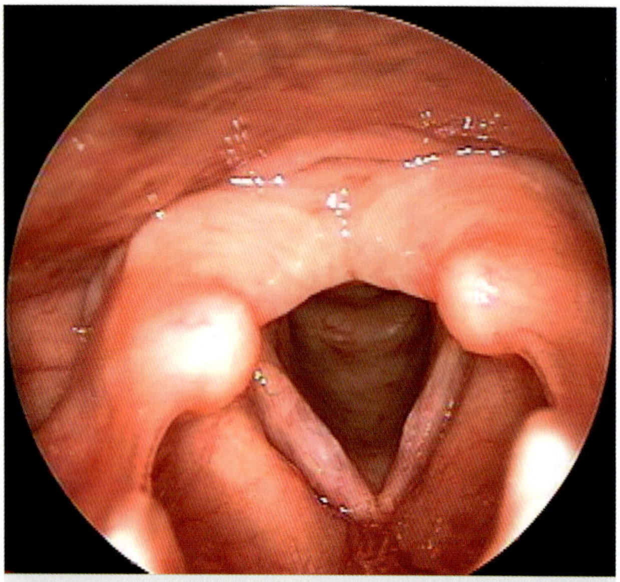

Fig. 12.7 Laryngeal exam findings in a patient with systemic lupus erythematosus.

and a malar or "butterfly" facial rash.[81,91] Laryngeal involvement may occur in 1 to 13% of patients (▶ Fig. 12.7). Symptoms may include hoarseness, odynophagia, and dyspnea. Subglottic stenosis, vocal cord paralysis, epiglottitis, laryngeal edema, and nodule formation have all been reported.[92,93]

As in other inflammatory disorders, markers like ESR and CRP may be elevated. Antinuclear antibody (ANA), antithyroglobulin antibody, and antithyroid microsomal antibody may all be elevated. Treatment depends on the severity of disease. Nonsteroidal anti-inflammatory medications and corticosteroids are helpful to reduce inflammatory symptoms. With more severe symptoms, immunosuppressive agents, such as methotrexate and cyclophosphamide, may be indicated.

12.7 Key Points

- Changes in the male larynx during puberty are the result of androgen stimulation, leading to lengthening and thickening of the vocal folds, causing lowering of the voice by an octave; puberty in the female is characterized by less dramatic changes in the larynx, with gradual, age-dependent changes resulting in a voice lowered by one-third of an octave.
- Androgen stimulation of the larynx causes irreversible changes, including hypertrophy and hyperplasia of muscle, thickening of the epithelium, growth of the cartilaginous framework, lengthening of the vocal folds, and lowering of the fundamental frequency. Estrogens have a hypertrophic effect on laryngeal mucosa and cause an increase in secretion of glandular cells. Progesterone has an antiproliferative effect, decreasing glandular secretion while increasing acidity and viscosity, leading to desquamation and dryness.
- Exogenous administration of androgens results in virilization of the female larynx and permanent changes in voice.
- Hormonal changes during pregnancy may result in laryngeal edema—laryngopathia gravidarum—with symptoms ranging from hoarseness to airway obstruction. Laryngeal evaluation is always indicated and may be important in perinatal planning.
- A premenstrual vocal syndrome has been described in professional singers, with vocal symptoms that result from the surge in estrogen and progesterone prior to menses.
- Menopause has been implicated in vocal symptoms due to the decrease in estrogen and progesterone and an increase in androgens, which may be alleviated by hormone replacement therapy.
- Modern formulations of oral contraceptives likely contribute to hormone stability that results in improved vocal quality and stability.
- Amyloidosis is known to affect the larynx and is usually localized. Biopsy is needed to confirm the diagnosis, and treatment generally involves conservative surgical excision of symptomatic deposits.

References

[1] Aristotle. Historia Animalium. Book 9. Vol. 4. In: Rambaud J. Theses de l'Ecole de Medicine de Paris. Paris, France: l'Ecole de Medicine de Paris; 1853

[2] Jenkins JS. The lost voice: a history of the castrato. J Pediatr Endocrinol Metab 2000; 13 Suppl 6: 1503–1508

[3] Abitbol J, Abitbol P. Endocrine disorders of the larynx. In: Ferlito A, ed. Diseases of the Larynx. New York, NY: Arnold; 2000: 311–334

[4] Talaat M, Talaat AM, Kelada I, Angelo A, Elwany S, Thabet H. Histologic and histochemical study of effects of anabolic steroids on the female larynx. Ann Otol Rhinol Laryngol 1987; 96: 468–471

[5] Tobias ML, Marin ML, Kelley DB. The roles of sex, innervation, and androgen in laryngeal muscle of Xenopus laevis. J Neurosci 1993; 13: 324–333

[6] Newman SR, Butler J, Hammond EH, Gray SD. Preliminary report on hormone receptors in the human vocal fold. J Voice 2000; 14: 72–81

[7] Altman KW, Haines GK, Vakkalanka SK, Keni SP, Kopp PA, Radosevich JA. Identification of thyroid hormone receptors in the human larynx. Laryngoscope 2003; 113: 1931–1934

[8] King A, Ashby J, Nelson C. Effects of testosterone replacement on a male professional singer. J Voice 2001; 15: 553–557

[9] Larsen PRKH, Melmed S, Polonsky KS. Williams Textbook of Endocrinology. New York, NY: Elsevier; 2003

[10] Fitch WT, Giedd J. Morphology and development of the human vocal tract: a study using magnetic resonance imaging. J Acoust Soc Am 1999; 106: 1511–1522

[11] Dmitriev L, Kiselev A. Relationship between the formant structure of different types of singing voices and the dimensions of supraglottic cavities. Folia Phoniatr (Basel) 1979; 31: 238–241

[12] Cleveland TF. Acoustic properties of voice timbre types and their influence on voice classification. J Acoust Soc Am 1977; 61: 1622–1629

[13] Hollien H, Green R, Massey K. Longitudinal research on adolescent voice change in males. J Acoust Soc Am 1994; 96: 2646–2654

[14] Kahane JC. Growth of the human prepubertal and pubertal larynx. J Speech Hear Res 1982; 25: 446–455

[15] Harries M, Hawkins S, Hacking J, Hughes I. Changes in the male voice at puberty: vocal fold length and its relationship to the fundamental frequency of the voice. J Laryngol Otol 1998; 112: 451–454

[16] Amy de la Bretèque B. La reeducation des troubles de la mue. Rev Laryngol Otol Rhinol (Bord) 1995; 116: 271–272

[17] WalshPC, Retick AB, Vaughan ED, et al. Campbell-Walsh Urology. 8th ed. Philadelphia, PA: WB Saunders; 2002

[18] Pedersen MF, Møller S, Krabbe S, Bennett P, Svenstrup B. Fundamental voice frequency in female puberty measured with electroglottography during continuous speech as a secondary sex characteristic. A comparison between

voice, pubertal stages, oestrogens and androgens. Int J Pediatr Otorhinolaryngol 1990; 20: 17–24
[19] Beckford NS, Rood SR, Schaid D, Schanbacher B. Androgen stimulation and laryngeal development. Ann Otol Rhinol Laryngol 1985; 94: 634–640
[20] Sassoon D, Kelley DB. The sexually dimorphic larynx of Xenopus laevis: development and androgen regulation. Am J Anat 1986; 177: 457–472
[21] Fischer LM, Catz D, Kelley DB. Androgen-directed development of the Xenopus laevis larynx: control of androgen receptor expression and tissue differentiation. Dev Biol 1995; 170: 115–126
[22] Akcam T, Bolu E, Merati AL, Durmus C, Gerek M, Ozkaptan Y. Voice changes after androgen therapy for hypogonadotrophic hypogonadism. Laryngoscope 2004; 114: 1587–1591
[23] Strauss RH, Liggett MT, Lanese RR. Anabolic steroid use and perceived effects in ten weight-trained women athletes. JAMA 1985; 253: 2871–2873
[24] Derman RJ. Effects of sex steroids on women's health: implications for practitioners. Am J Med 1995; 98 1A: 137S–143S
[25] Fürst-Recktenwald S, Dörr HG, Rosanowski F. Androglottia in a young female adolescent with congenital adrenal hyperplasia and 21-hydroxylase deficiency. J Pediatr Endocrinol Metab 2000; 13: 959–962
[26] Damrose EJ. Quantifying the impact of androgen therapy on the female larynx. Auris Nasus Larynx 2009; 36: 110–112
[27] Nygren U, Södersten M, Falhammar H, Thorén M, Hagenfeldt K, Nordenskjöld A. Voice characteristics in women with congenital adrenal hyperplasia due to 21-hydroxylase deficiency. Clin Endocrinol (Oxf) 2009; 70: 18–25
[28] Colton RH, Casper JK, Leonard R. Understanding Voice Problems: A Physiological Perspective for Diagnosis and Treatment. Philadelphia, PA: Lippincott Williams and Wilkins; 2006
[29] Dagli M, Sati I, Acar A, Stone RE, Dursun G, Eryilmaz A. Mutational falsetto: intervention outcomes in 45 patients. J Laryngol Otol 2008; 122: 277–281
[30] Woodson GE, Murry T. Botulinum toxin in the treatment of recalcitrant mutational dysphonia. J Voice 1994; 8: 347–351
[31] Remacle M, Matar N, Verduyckt I, Lawson G. Relaxation thyroplasty for mutational falsetto treatment. Ann Otol Rhinol Laryngol 2010; 119: 105–109
[32] Maceri DR. Head and neck manifestations of endocrine disease. Otolaryngol Clin North Am 1986; 19: 171–180
[33] Abitbol J, Abitbol P, Abitbol B. Sex hormones and the female voice. J Voice 1999; 13: 424–446
[34] Wu KH, Tobias ML, Kelley DB. Estrogen receptor expression in laryngeal muscle in relation to estrogen-dependent increases in synapse strength. Neuroendocrinology 2003; 78: 72–80
[35] Wu KH, Tobias ML, Kelley DB. Estrogen and laryngeal synaptic strength in Xenopus laevis: opposite effects of acute and chronic exposure. Neuroendocrinology 2001; 74: 22–32
[36] Davis CB, Davis ML. The effects of premenstrual syndrome (PMS) on the female singer. J Voice 1993; 7: 337–353
[37] Chae SW, Choi G, Kang HJ, Choi JO, Jin SM. Clinical analysis of voice change as a parameter of premenstrual syndrome. J Voice 2001; 15: 278–283
[38] Chernobelsky SI. A study of menses-related changes to the larynx in singers with voice abuse. Folia Phoniatr Logop 2002; 54: 2–7
[39] Sataloff RT. Professional Voice: The Science and Art of Clinical Care. San Diego, CA: Singular; 1997
[40] Perlow JH, Kirz DS. Severe preeclampsia presenting as dysphonia secondary to uvular edema. A case report. J Reprod Med 1990; 35: 1059–1062
[41] Heller PJ, Scheider EP, Marx GF. Pharyngolaryngeal edema as a presenting symptom in preeclampsia. Obstet Gynecol 1983; 62: 523–525
[42] Seager SJ, Macdonald R. Laryngeal oedema and pre-eclampsia. Anaesthesia 1980; 35: 360–362
[43] Brock-Utne JG, Downing JW, Seedat FF. Laryngeal oedema associated with pre-eclamptic toxaemia. Anaesthesia 1977; 32: 556–558
[44] Brimacombe J. Acute pharyngolaryngeal oedema and pre-eclamptic toxaemia. Anaesth Intensive Care 1992; 20: 97–98
[45] Rocke DA, Scoones GP. Rapidly progressive laryngeal oedema associated with pregnancy-aggravated hypertension. Anaesthesia 1992; 47: 141–143
[46] Höing R, Seitzer D. Zur Klinik der Laryngopathia gravidarum. Laryngol Rhinol Otol (Stuttg) 1988; 67: 564–566
[47] Mattingly RF, Huang WY. Steroidogenesis of the menopausal and postmenopausal ovary. Am J Obstet Gynecol 1969; 103: 679–693
[48] Buchsbaum HJ. The Menopause. New York, NY: Springer Verlag; 1983
[49] Boulet MJ, Oddens BJ. Female voice changes around and after the menopause —an initial investigation. Maturitas 1996; 23: 15–21
[50] Caruso S, Roccasalva L, Sapienza G, Zappalá M, Nuciforo G, Biondi S. Laryngeal cytological aspects in women with surgically induced menopause who were treated with transdermal estrogen replacement therapy. Fertil Steril 2000; 74: 1073–1079
[51] Lindholm P, Vilkman E, Raudaskoski T, Suvanto-Luukkonen E, Kauppila A. The effect of postmenopause and postmenopausal HRT on measured voice values and vocal symptoms. Maturitas 1997; 28: 47–53
[52] Wendler J, Siegert C, Schelhorn P et al. The influence of Microgynon and Diane-35, two sub-fifty ovulation inhibitors, on voice function in women. Contraception 1995; 52: 343–348
[53] Amir O, Kishon-Rabin L. Association between birth control pills and voice quality. Laryngoscope 2004; 114: 1021–1026
[54] Amir O, Biron-Shental T, Tzenker O, Barer T. Different oral contraceptives and voice quality—an observational study. Contraception 2005; 71: 348–352
[55] Gorham-Rowan M, Langford A, Corrigan K, Snyder B. Vocal pitch levels during connected speech associated with oral contraceptive use. J Obstet Gynaecol 2004; 24: 284–286
[56] Gorham-Rowan MM. Acoustic measures of vocal stability during different speech tasks in young women using oral contraceptives: a retrospective study. Eur J Contracept Reprod Health Care 2004; 9: 166–172
[57] Cohen MA, Kelley DB. Androgen-induced proliferation in the developing larynx of Xenopus laevis is regulated by thyroid hormone. Dev Biol 1996; 178: 113–123
[58] Aronson A. Clinical Voice Disorders. New York, NY: Decker, 1980
[59] Michaels L. Pathology of the Larynx. New York, NY: Springer-Verlag; 1984
[60] Ritter F. Otolaryngology. Philidelphia, PA: WB Saunders; 1973
[61] Sommer DD, Freeman JL. Bilateral vocal cord paralysis associated with diabetes mellitus: case reports. J Otolaryngol 1994; 23: 169–171
[62] Semiz S, Fişenk F, Akçurin S, Bircan I. Temporary multiple cranial nerve palsies in a patient with type 1 diabetes mellitus. Diabetes Metab 2002; 28: 413–416
[63] Kabadi UM. Unilateral vocal cord palsy in a diabetic patient. Postgrad Med 1988; 84: 53–, 55–56
[64] Shuman CRWB, Weissman B. Recurrent laryngeal nerve involvement as a manifestation of diabetic neuropathy. Diabetes 1968; 17: 302–02
[65] Klein AM, Tiu C, Lafreniere D. Malignant mimickers: chronic bacterial and fungal infections of the larynx. J Voice 2005; 19: 151–157
[66] Sulica L. Laryngeal thrush. Ann Otol Rhinol Laryngol 2005; 114: 369–375
[67] Schwartz JR, Nagle MG, Elkins RC, Mohr JA. Mucormycosis of the trachea: an unusual cause of acute upper airway obstruction. Chest 1982; 81: 653–654
[68] Ettema SL, Loerhl TA, Toohill RJ, Merati AL. The prevalence of diabetes in a series of patients with subglottic stenosis. Ear Nose Throat J 2007; 86: 687–690
[69] Nishida T, Tsuji S, Tsujii M et al. Gastroesophageal reflux disease related to diabetes: Analysis of 241 cases with type 2 diabetes mellitus. J Gastroenterol Hepatol 2004; 19: 258–265
[70] Lluch I, Ascaso JF, Mora F et al. Gastroesophageal reflux in diabetes mellitus. Am J Gastroenterol 1999; 94: 919–924
[71] Zhang Q, Horowitz M, Rigda R, Rayner C, Worynski A, Holloway RH. Effect of hyperglycemia on triggering of transient lower esophageal sphincter relaxations. Am J Physiol Gastrointest Liver Physiol 2004; 286: G797–G803
[72] Bengtsson BAES, Edén S, Ernest I, Odén A, Sjögren B. Epidemiology and long-term survival in acromegaly. A study of 166 cases diagnosed between 1955 and 1984. Acta Med Scand 1988; 223: 327–335
[73] Morewood DJBP, Belchetz PE, Evans CC, Whitehouse GH. The extrathoracic airway in acromegaly. Clin Radiol 1986; 37: 243–246
[74] Williams RG, Richards SH, Mills RG, Eccles R. Voice changes in acromegaly. Laryngoscope 1994; 104: 484–487
[75] Alaani A, Warfield AT, Pracy JP. Management of laryngeal amyloidosis. J Laryngol Otol 2004; 118: 279–283
[76] Barnes EL, Zafar T. Laryngeal amyloidosis: clinicopathologic study of seven cases. Ann Otol Rhinol Laryngol 1977; 86: 856–863
[77] Mitrani M, Biller HF. Laryngeal amyloidosis. Laryngoscope 1985; 95: 1346–1347
[78] Plaschke CC, Owen HH, Rasmussen N. Clinically isolated laryngeal sarcoidosis. Eur Arch Otorhinolaryngol 2011; 268: 575–580
[79] Mrówka-Kata K, Kata D, Lange D, Namysłowski G, Czecior E, Banert K. Sarcoidosis and its otolaryngological implications. Eur Arch Otorhinolaryngol 2010; 267: 1507–1514
[80] Solans-Laqué R, Bosch-Gil JA, Canela M, Lorente J, Pallisa E, Vilardell-Tarrés M. Clinical features and therapeutic management of subglottic stenosis in patients with Wegener's granulomatosis. Lupus 2008; 17: 832–836
[81] Loehrl TA, Smith TL. Inflammatory and granulomatous lesions of the larynx and pharynx. Am J Med 2001; 111 Suppl 8A: 113S–117S

[82] Leavitt RY, Fauci AS, Bloch DA et al. The American College of Rheumatology 1990 criteria for the classification of Wegener's granulomatosis. Arthritis Rheum 1990; 33: 1101–1107

[83] Brooker DS. Rheumatoid arthritis: otorhinolaryngological manifestations. Clin Otolaryngol Allied Sci 1988; 13: 239–246

[84] Woldorf NM, Pastore PN, Terz J. Rheumatoid arthritis of the cricoarytenoid joint. Arch Otolaryngol 1971; 93: 623–627

[85] Wolman L, Darke CS, Young A. The larynx in rheumatoid arthritis. J Laryngol Otol 1965; 79: 403–434

[86] Friedman BA. Rheumatoid nodules of the larynx. Arch Otolaryngol 1975; 101: 361–363

[87] Kim CM, Kim BS, Cho KJ, Hong SJ. Laryngotracheal involvement of relapsing polychondritis in a Korean girl. Pediatr Pulmonol 2003; 35: 314–317

[88] Letko E, Zafirakis P, Baltatzis S, Voudouri A, Livir-Rallatos C, Foster CS. Relapsing polychondritis: a clinical review. Semin Arthritis Rheum 2002; 31: 384–395

[89] McAdam LP, O'Hanlan MA, Bluestone R, Pearson CM. Relapsing polychondritis: prospective study of 23 patients and a review of the literature. Medicine (Baltimore) 1976; 55: 193–215

[90] Karaman E, Duman C, Cansz H, Ylmaz M, Ibrahimov MJ. Laryngotracheal reconstruction at relapsing polychondritis. J Craniofac Surg 2010; 21: 211–212

[91] Woo P, Mendelsohn J, Humphrey D. Rheumatoid nodules of the larynx. Otolaryngol Head Neck Surg 1995; 113: 147–150

[92] Teitel AD, MacKenzie CR, Stern R, Paget SA. Laryngeal involvement in systemic lupus erythematosus. Semin Arthritis Rheum 1992; 22: 203–214

[93] Toomey JM, Snyder GG, Maenza RM, Rothfield NF. Acute epiglottitis due to systemic lupus erythematosus. Laryngoscope 1974; 84: 522–527

13 Laryngeal Trauma

Philip A. Weissbrod

Laryngeal trauma can be divided broadly into two classes: blunt trauma and penetrating trauma. Appropriate management of these injuries can be life-saving interventions and timely treatment can have major consequences on future quality of life.

Blunt trauma includes motor vehicle accidents (MVAs), clothesline injuries, assaults, strangulations, sporting injuries, and other assorted accidents. Over the past 30 to 40 years in the United States, there have been significant decreases in the incidence of laryngeal trauma. This decline, in particular in the 1990s, can be attributed to the advent of more strict seatbelt laws, improved automobile safety devices, and decreasing violent crime in the United States.[1]

Laryngeal penetrating trauma most frequently results from gunshot or stab wounds, but also can occur from vocational injuries, animal bites, and other penetrating injury. The severity of injury relates to the size, velocity, and makeup of the projectile. High-velocity injuries often cause more severe injuries because of tissue loss and include injuries inflicted by military- and civilian-grade rifles.[2]

Laryngeal trauma is a rare event and many of the paradigms for management were established in the 1980s and 1990s. For the purpose of this chapter, the management protocols are reviewed and updated in consideration of advances in imaging, laryngoscopic evaluation, and endoscopic surgical techniques.

13.1 History and Physical Examination

13.1.1 History

In most scenarios, an otolaryngologist will be called to evaluate a laryngeal trauma patient after injury has been recognized. Typically, by the time of consultation, primary and secondary trauma surveys have been completed and C-spine and other injuries have been recognized. For the purposed of this chapter, it is assumed that this workup has been completed.

Irrespective of the type of laryngeal trauma, there are common pertinent points in assessing patient history. For both blunt and penetrating laryngeal trauma, understanding the mechanism of injury is of utmost importance, as it suggests the possible nature and severity of injury.

Patients can have a constellation of symptoms that includes voice change, cough, dysphagia, odynophagia, dyspnea, pain, and hemoptysis. Absence of the aforementioned symptoms does not exclude the possibility of laryngeal trauma, as some patients present with relatively few complaints. There also appears to be no correlation between symptom and severity of injury, with the exception of difficulty breathing, which correlates to more severe injuries.[1]

Delayed edema can also be of concern, especially where this is a significant amount of energy delivered to the neck, as seen in motor vehicle, clothesline, and strangulation injuries. Also, many patients with severe trauma arrive in the emergency department having been intubated in the field with emergent surgical airways, or are unable to communicate their symptoms. If this is the case, early diagnostic evaluation is encouraged to expedite corrective therapies.

13.1.2 Physical Examination

As with a primary trauma survey, the first step in evaluating laryngeal trauma is assessing the airway. Initial evaluation should address the oral and nasal cavities down to the subglottis and hypopharynx. Evaluation of the trachea and mainstem bronchi is of value, but likely should be deferred to avoid precipitation of laryngospam in an unstable airway in an uncontrolled setting.

Stridor, defined as noisy respiration, is an early sign of airway obstruction. Inspiratory stridor localizes obstruction to the glottis and above, expiratory stridor to the subglottis and below, and biphasic stridor to the glottis or subglottis. Other clues to impending respiratory compromise include recruitment of accessory respiratory muscles, rapid shallow breathing, supraclavicular contractions, intercostal retractions, and change in mental status.

Examination of the external neck should focus on signs of trauma, including ecchymosis, tenderness, subcutaneous air, palpable cartilage abnormalities such as blunting of the thyroid ala, bleeding, expanding hematoma, or evidence of penetrating injury. For motor-vehicle-related trauma, seatbelt marks on the neck and chest can indicate underlying injury. If there is noted airflow through a penetrating or open wound, no effort should be made to cover or close this, as it could potentiate airway obstruction.

Making note of the caudal cranial positioning of penetrating trauma as well as the vector in which the projectile traveled once it entered tissue is important because it dictates diagnostic and therapeutic pathways. Penetrating trauma is divided into three anatomical zones: zone I is from sternum to cricoid, zone II from cricoid to angle of mandible, and zone III from angle to skull base (▶ Table 13.1, ▶ Fig. 13.1). The pertinence of zone to workup and therapy is discussed further.

The presence of crepitus or subcutaneous air on palpation of the neck or chest indicates possible perforation of the pharynx, hypopharynx, trachea, or esophagous. With the presence of subcutaneous air, both pneumothorax and pneumomediastinum should be considered and evaluated carefully with chest auscultation and chest x-ray or computed tomography (CT).

Examination of the oral cavity should assess for any additional upper airway trauma or source of bleeding. If bloody secretions are noted, traumatic injury laceration or breach of mucosa from trauma should be suspected.

Careful neurologic evaluation with special attention to the cranial nerves can help define the location, extent, and severity of the injury. The neurologic examination should also include gross assessment of the spinal cord and brachial plexus. Palpation of the distal pulses should be performed, especially in the setting of penetrating trauma, to evaluate for vascular injury.

Flexible laryngoscopy is an essential component of a specialist's examination for all forms of trauma. With the advent of improved optics, high-resolution flexible laryngoscopic images

Table 13.1 Zones of penetrating injury

Injury zone	Structures at risk	Diagnostic modality
Zone I	Vascular: Common carotid artery; innominate artery, internal jugular vein; subclavian artery and vein; vertebral artery Nervous: Brachial plexus, phrenic, vagus, recurrent laryngeal nerve; spinal cord Other: Lung apex, thyroid, trachea, thoracic duct	CTA or angiogram; esophagram or esophagoscopy
Zone II	Vascular: Internal jugular vein, common carotid internal/external carotid, vertebral artery Nervous: Accessory, hypoglossal, marginal mandibular, phrenic, vagus, spinal cord Other: Hypopharynx, larynx, pharynx, submandibular gland, trachea	Surgical exploration if deep to the platysma, CTA or observation if stable; esophagram or esophagoscopy
Zone III	Vascular: Branches of external carotid, internal carotid, internal jugular vein, vertebral artery Nervous: Facial, glossopharyngeal, vagus, accessory, hypoglossal, spinal cord, sympathetic chain Other: Parotid gland Pharynx	CT angiography or angiogram

Abbreviations: CTA, computed tomography angiography.

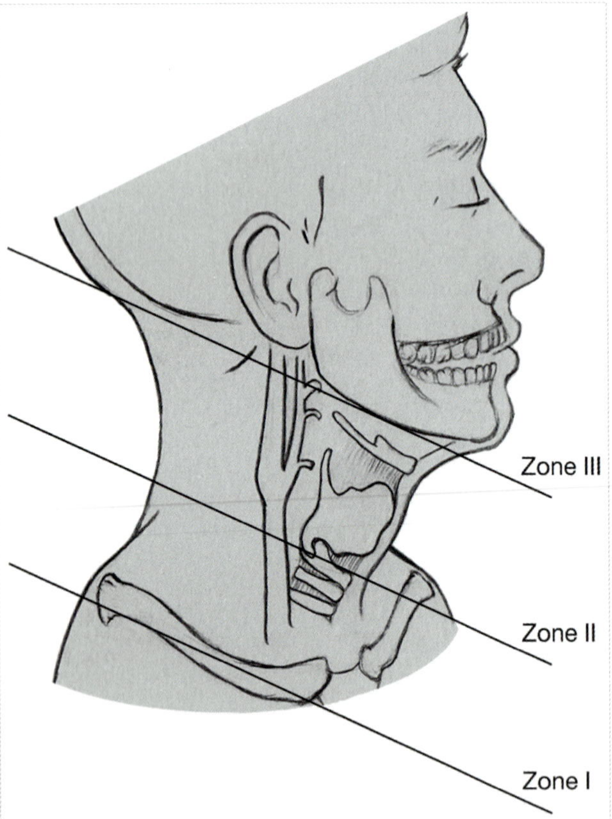

Fig. 13.1 Zones of penetrating injury.

can provide a detailed account of the traumatized larynx. Careful examination of the upper airway should include dynamic laryngeal evaluation for vocal fold mobility during respiration and phonation and documentation of mucosal disruption or laceration, cartilaginous exposure, laryngeal edema, airway narrowing, and the presence of blood or secretions.

Identification of the above findings is important because some models of treatment for laryngeal trauma dictate treatment protocols.[1] Other important findings include shortening of the aryepiglottic (AE) folds, arytenoid dislocation and subsequent displacement of the arytenoid vocal process, epiglottic fracture, height mismatch of the vocal processes, or other obvious anatomic alteration of the upper aerodigestive lumen.

Transglottic evaluation of the subglottis and trachea should likely be deferred, as this can cause laryngospasm and acute decompensation unless the patient is properly anesthetized, a process that can be challenging in this clinical scenario.

13.2 Diagnosis

In laryngeal trauma, if airway compromise is imminent, further diagnostic evaluation should be delayed until an airway is secured. The mainstay of diagnosis in blunt trauma, aside from physical examination, is CT. Historically, plain-film x-ray was used frequently as an initial study and it can still be of benefit if CT is unavailable. Free air in the soft tissue indicates aerodigestive tract injury and displaced framework fractures can be visualized on plain films.

Most emergency departments have access to high-resolution CT that can greatly aid in decision making in the stable blunt

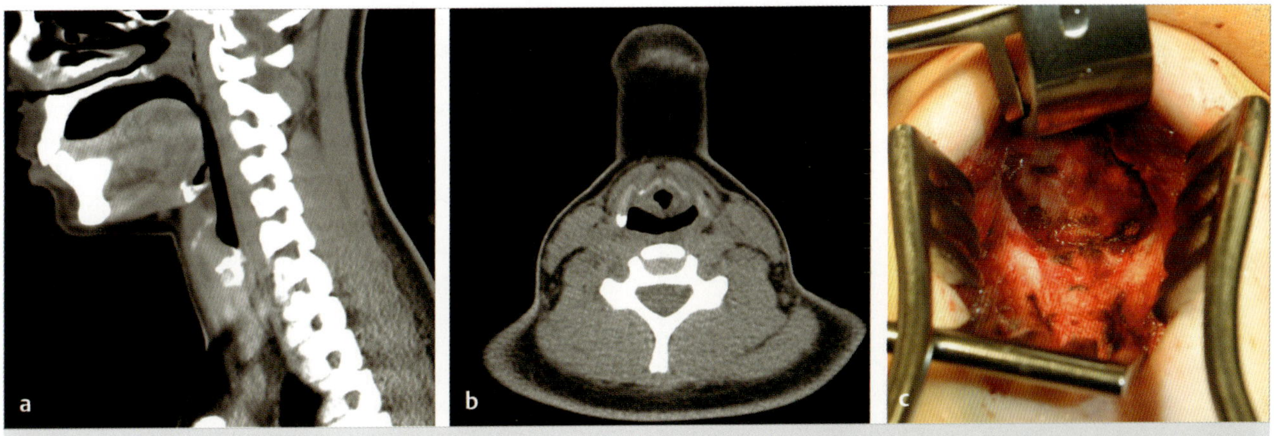

Fig. 13.2 (a) Sagittal and (b) axial computed tomography image of anterior blunt neck trauma that occurred during a fall onto a brick surface 6 weeks earlier. Note the posteriorly displaced thyroid cartilage fracture. (c) Intraoperative photo of the same depressed comminuted fracture.

airway trauma patient. Careful note should be made of the larygotracheal framework, which includes the trachea, cricoid, thyroid, arytenoid, and epiglottic cartilage as well as the hyoid bone (▶ Fig. 13.2). If there is a fracture present, notation of displacement or comminution is important as this can dictate treatment course. Other findings that should be noted that alter treatment course include hematoma, subcutaneous air, and compression or narrowing of the airway. For strangulation injury, the presence of subcutaneous bleeding, platysmal swelling, and hemorrhagic lymph nodes (on magnetic resonance imaging), can differentiate life- and non-life threatening injury.[3]

In penetrating trauma that extends beyond the platysma, the major vascular structures of the neck are the central component of evaluation. Failure to identify injury to one of the great vessels, major branches of the carotid, or vertebral artery, can have significant consequences including sentinel hemorrhage or stroke.

Up to 30% of major vascular injuries in zone I and up to 25% in zone III are asymptomatic.[4,5,6] Therefore, all zone I and zone III injuries, even if asymptomatic, require vascular investigation. Surgical exploration in these zones is infrequently done until postangiography because of increased difficulty in accessing structures due to sternal and mandibular and skull base structures for zones I and III, respectively.

Angiography is the gold standard in diagnosis of zone I and III injury. Although it is an excellent diagnostic tool and can also allow for therapeutic intervention, it is time consuming, expensive, and has a relatively high complication rate of up to 2%.[7] In some institutions, angiography has been replaced by CT angiography (CTA) due to the relative ease, cost-effectiveness, accuracy, and rapidity of administration.[8] Computed tomography angiography has been shown to reduce the need for exploratory surgery without compromising diagnostic sensitivity.[9,10] In a prospective study of 106 penetrating injuries by Inaba et al, CTA was 100% sensitive and 93.5% specific in diagnosing vascular injury.[11] An additional diagnostic alternative is color-flow Doppler imaging, which is highly sensitive but technician dependent.[12]

Classic diagnostic evaluation of zone II injury suggests surgical exploration is the preferred diagnostic modality for subplatysmal injury. It has been suggested that clinical examination alone can be an effective screening method, as opposed to more costly angiography, which does not alter the treatment course for this particular injury location.[13] Again, increased use of CTA is starting to alter diagnostic paradigms for zone II injury as well. Woo et al reviewed a 10-year history of penetrating zone II neck trauma that included 130 cases.[14] When CTA was used, there was a significant decrease in the total number of exploratory surgeries as well as negative exploratory surgeries. Given this somewhat conflicting data, diagnostic decision making currently is largely surgeon or institution dependent and the question of cost effectiveness likely warrants further exploration.

An esophagram also plays a significant role in evaluating blunt and penetrating trauma of the neck. Gastrograffin is typically used as it is less reactive in the mediastinum than barium should there be a leak. Esophageal imaging is particularly important for zone I penetrating injury, considering that the superior aspect of the zone is the cricoid, which marks the location of the cricopharyngeus and upper esophageal sphincter. Esophageal evaluation should be included in the evaluation of any trauma where pharyngeal, hypopharyngeal, tracheal, or esophageal luminal perforation is suspected.

Some practitioners use esophageal endoscopy rather than esophageal imaging. In the hands of a skilled endoscopist, this can be a good option; however, both rigid and flexible esophagoscopy have potential morbidity. In rigid endoscopy, mechanical injury can worsen a small tear or even create a perforation if there is pre-existing injury to the esophageal wall or mucosa. Conversely, flexible endoscopy requires pneumatic insufflation, which can cause barotrauma and create or worsen subcutaneous air accumulation if there is transluminal perforation. Sensitivity of both flexible/rigid esophagoscopy and esophogram is 80 to 90%,[15] and when they are used together, nears 100%.[16]

Diagnostic bronchoscopy is also a useful study, especially in cases where there is subcutaneous air present but negative esophageal studies. Flexible bronchoscope technology has largely made diagnostic rigid bronchoscopy obsolete in this particular setting, especially considering that there is no need for insufflation, as in the case of flexible esophagoscopy.

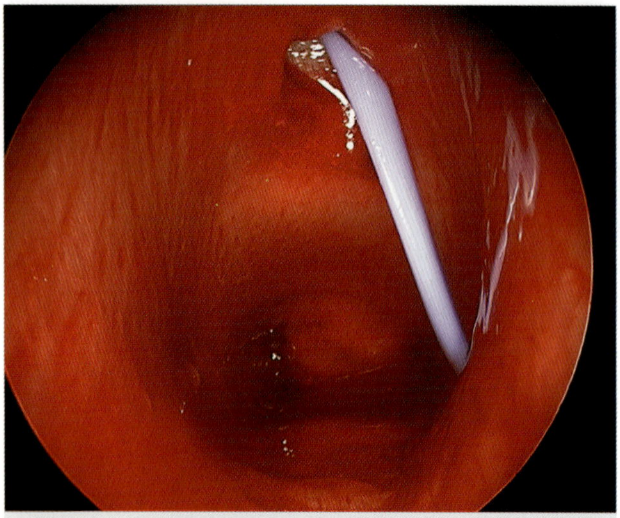

Fig. 13.3 A zero-degree endoscopic subglottic image of a zone II penetrating small-caliber bullet wound. The course of the bullet is marked by a vascular loop to better illustrate the trajectory of the projectile from the cricotracheal membrane to lateral tracheal wall. The bullet lodged in a cervical vertebrae, narrowly missing the carotid artery. Note the tracheotomy tube in the trachea distally.

Finally, direct laryngoscopy is another important and critical skill for diagnosing intralaryngeal injury. If an emergent airway has been secured, there is little morbidity to direct visualization of the larynx, although in select cases there can be further disruption of traumatized tissue or displaced cartilage. Using zero- and 70-degree telescopes is helpful in visualizing the endolarynx and subglottis (▶ Fig. 13.3). Alternative laryngoscopic methods should be considered as well, including use of vallecular scopes. such as a Lindholm laryngoscope, or using a Macintosh blade with the aid of rigid telescopes for visualization in cases where there is significant cartilage disruption or intralarngeal mucosal trauma.

13.3 Treatment

13.3.1 Blunt Trauma

Management of blunt trauma starts with a decision about the stability of the airway. If the airway is unstable, tracheotomy is the most reliable means for securing an airway. Intubation is possible, but should be performed only by a seasoned endoscopist. In general, endotracheal intubation is an acceptable option if the endolaryngeal mucous membrane is intact or if the laryngeal framework is only mildly displaced.[17]

If a surgical airway is indicated, tracheotomy below the second ring is preferable, but cricothyroidotomy is an acceptable alternative in emergent situations. Tracheotomy should be performed in an awake patient under local anesthesia to prevent any additional air extravasation into soft tissue from positive pressure if there is a transluminal breach, and to avoid potential airway obstruction in the sedated patient. If there is complete laryngotracheal separation, intubation is extremely perilous, because false passages are easily created, and bilateral vocal fold paralysis is not uncommon.

If the airway is stable and there is no impending obstruction, information accumulated during physical examination and diagnostic imaging can be used to guide treatment decisions. Complex mucosal lacerations, displaced cartilaginous framework fractures, or significant laryngeal edema are indicators for tracheotomy.[1,18]

Minor laryngeal edema, small hematoma, and nondisplaced fractures can be observed in a monitored setting, avoiding intubation and tracheotomy, as these injuries are at low risk for airway obstruction. Such patients should have minimal physical activity and keep to limited voice use to prevent worsening of hemorrhage and edema in the acute phase. Strangulation injuries should be monitored closely, even if initially asymptomatic, because airway obstruction can occur up to 24 hours after insult due to laryngeal edema.[19]

Medical management should focus on humidification and reduction or avoidance of further irritation. Humidification via facemask or face tent reduces crusting and presumably improves mucosal wound healing. Use of prophylactic antireflux medication, such as a proton pump inhibitor or H_2 blocker, and elevation of the head of the bed are suggested to minimize additional inflammation or irritation from laryngopharyngeal reflux. A corticosteroid, such as dexamethasone, is a valuable aid to reduce acute effects of swelling and should be used early. If there are mucosal abrasions, lacerations, or subcutaneous air, antibiotic coverage for upper aerodigestive tract flora should be implemented.

When cartilaginous fracture is present, diagnostic imaging helps dictate treatment planning. Nondisplaced fractures typically can be observed. Displaced and comminuted fractures, especially of the thyroid and cricoid cartilages, should be repaired via open reduction and internal fixation (ORIF). Early intervention and repair are preferable, as they are thought to improve clinical outcome.[1,20,21]Some authors advocate repair within 48 hours citing improved clinical outcomes, although the data are somewhat limited.[22,23]

Repair and fixation of cartilage fractures requires an open surgical approach via a horizontal cervical incision (▶ Fig. 13.4). In approaching laryngeal fractures, a number of core concepts should be considered during reconstruction. Ideally, the best outcome is restoring normal anatomy and function. In cases where there is tissue loss or restoring the original framework structure is not possible, consider the following two priorities for guidance: (1) The inferior rim of the thyroid cartilage provides most of the anteroposterior structural support of the larynx. Reconstructing it will allow for proper tension and symmetry of the vocal folds. (2) If the anterior commissure is disrupted or if a laryngofissure is required, failure to properly resuspend the anterior commissure will be detrimental to voice outcome.[24]

A simple displaced fracture should be reduced and fixed with a titanium miniplate. Newer plating systems have absorbable plates that are an alternative to titanium plates.[25] When plating, careful note should be made to ensure the screw does not penetrate the laryngeal mucosa. After reduction of fractures, multiple screws should be placed on each side of the fracture to

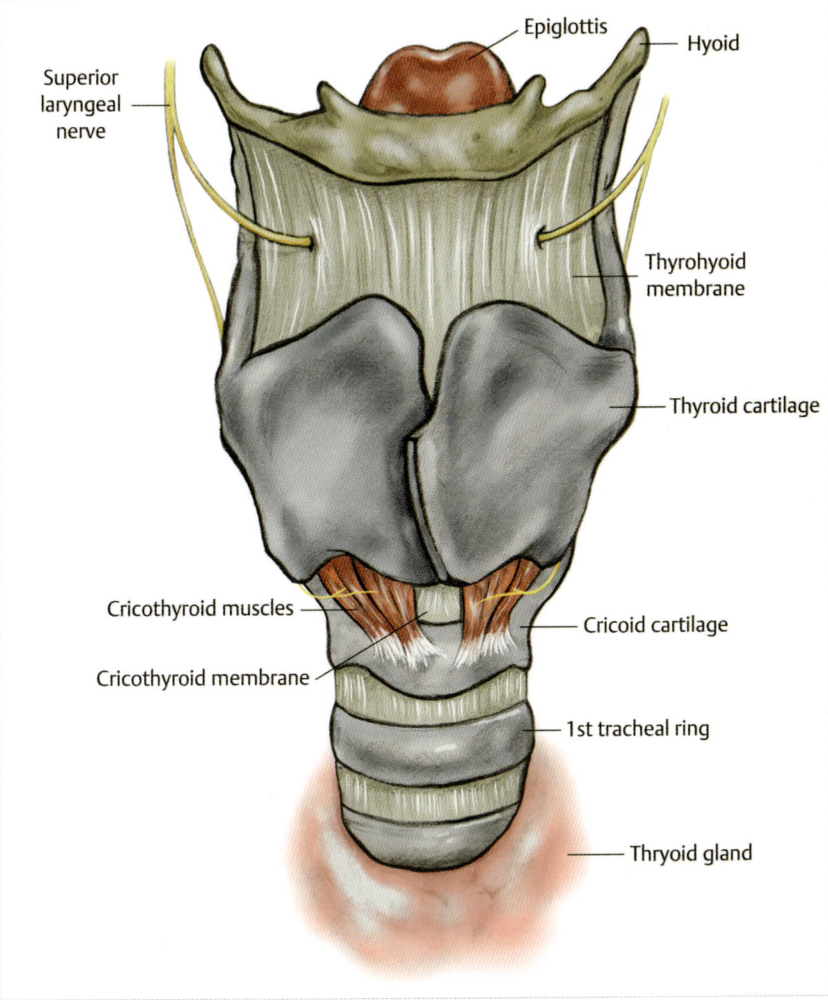

Fig. 13.4 Artist's rendering of displaced thyroid cartilage fracture requiring open reduction and internal fixation.

reduce the chances of subluxation during the healing process (▶ Fig. 13.5 and ▶ Fig. 13.6). For comminuted fractures, multiple plates or mesh can be utilized. In situations where there is severe comminution, tissue loss, or the cartilage is not calcified, nonabsorbable suture or wires are alternatives to plating systems. Attempts should be made to cover exposed cartilage with native tissue or skin graft to prevent granuloma formation.

Significant mucosal injuries should also be repaired if present. Failure to do so will create a higher likelihood of persistent voice alterations due to scar and vibratory irregularities. With improved endoscopic instrumentation, mucosal laceration and repair can be attempted via endoscopic techniques.[26] Use of an absorbable suture and endoscopic needle pusher can allow the skilled endoscopic surgeon to repair isolated mucosal lacerations from trauma or iatrogenic injury.

For repair of significant mucosal lacerations or significant stenosis, a thyrotomy is indicated. A thyrotomy is accomplished by incising the anterior cricotracheal apparatus from cricothyroid to thyrohyoid membrane in a vertical fashion. If there is no anterior vertical fracture, an oscillating saw should be used to make a vertical thyrotomy through the anterior thyroid cartilage from cricothyroid membrane to the thyroid notch. Alternatively, if there is a vertical thyroid cartilage fracture, it can be used for access instead of a midline thyroid cartilage cut. The mucosa should be incised with a blade or fine scissor (▶ Fig. 13.7). It is essential that the anterior commissure be transected at its midline. Failure to do so potentiates poor voice outcome after reconstruction.

Once the larynx is opened, the repair of mucosal laceration can be performed with absorbable suture. If there is significant tissue loss, a skin or mucosal graft can be used to reconstruct defects. If there has been significant loss of tissue at the anterior commissure, the use of a laryngeal keel can prevent anterior glottic webbing (▶ Fig. 13.8 and ▶ Fig. 13.9). The keel is left in place for 7 to 14 days depending on the severity of injury.

If the cartilaginous structural framework has been significantly disrupted, leading to airway column collapse, or if there is significant mucosal injury or tissue loss, laryngeal stents can be used to provide infrastructure during healing. Laryngeal stents come in a number of preformed shapes and sizes, such as the Montgomery laryngeal stent, which is available in childsize, or adult small, medium, and large. Alternatively, a stent can be fashioned by molding endotracheal tubes,[27] T-tubes, or Silastic blocks (▶ Fig. 13.10).

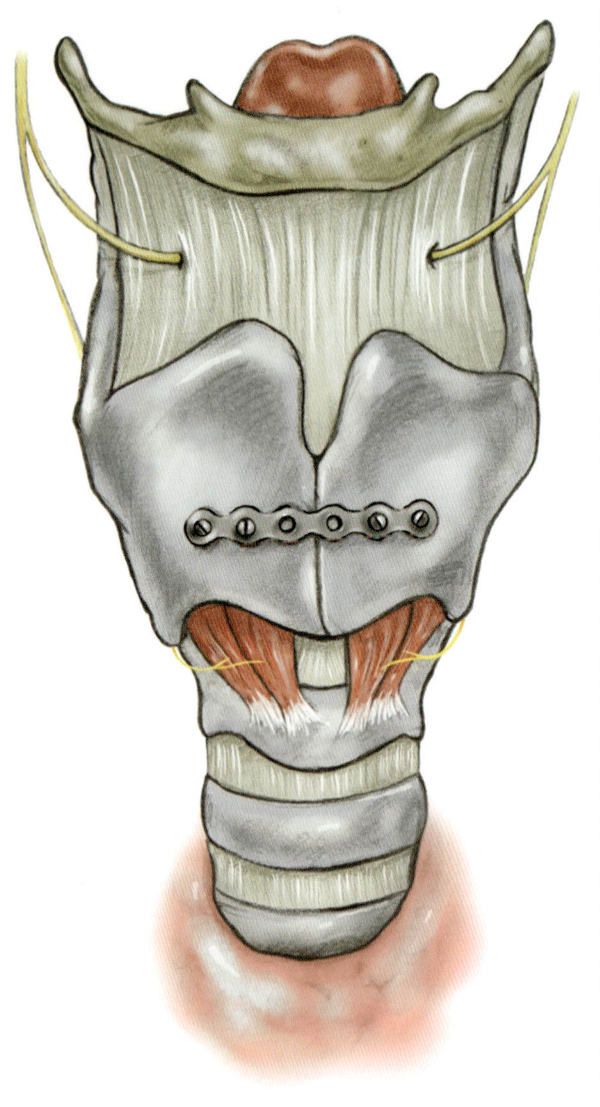

Fig. 13.5 Thyroid cartilage fracture post open reduction and internal fixation. Note multiple screws on each side of the fracture line.

Typically, stents should extend from the false vocal fold to the first tracheal ring. They may be extended higher or lower depending on the area of collapse, although this may precipitate more patient discomfort. Stents are secured in place by a nonabsorbable suture, which is passed through the skin, strap muscles, thyroid cartilage, stent, and back to the skin. Sutures are passed both above and below the vocal folds and secured to buttons overlying the skin (▶ Fig. 13.11). Similarly, if there is framework disruption of the cricoid infrastructure, stenting at this level can be employed as an alternative to cricotracheal resection.

Stented patients require a return to the operating room for endoscopic removal. Duration of stenting is controversial. Most authors cite a minimum of 2 weeks and a maximum of 6 weeks for optimal outcome. Comparison of studies and stent durations is difficult because most decisions to place stents are based on a more significant extent of injury and on personal experience, as opposed to an objective controlled study.

Closure of a laryngofissure should be done meticulously. The anterior vocal folds should be sutured to the outer thyroid cartilage perichondrium. The right and left should be sutured at the same level to avoid height mismatch, which leads to a poor voice outcome.

13.3.2 Penetrating Trauma

As mentioned above, diagnostic and therapeutic decision making for penetrating trauma is dictated by the location of the injury and the presumed course of the projectile. Zones I and III are similar in that there are numerous vital structures that are not easily accessible via surgical exploration. Despite difficult accessibility, if there is systemic instability, shock, airway obstruction, or rapidly expanding hematoma as a result of a penetrating neck injury, emergent surgical or interventional radiologic vascular intervention is necessary regardless of zone.

The most common injuries in zone I and frequently in zone III are vascular. Injury to a major vascular structure requires immediate repair in the unstable patient, and repair after diagnostic angiography or CTA in the stable patient. Hemorrhage should be initially controlled with direct pressure. Use of a Foley catheter can also be helpful for tamponade, by placing it in the wound. Probing of the wound or removal of clot or projectile should be delayed until in a controlled setting and the necessary instruments for repair of major vascular structures are available. Appropriate intravenous access is required in the event that there needs to be rapid resuscitation.

Repair of vascular injury can be done via open surgical repair, interventional radiologic stenting, or occlusion when appropriate.[28] For open surgical repair of major vessels, both proximal and distal vessel control is essential to prevent uncontrolled bleeding during attempted repair. If proximal control requires thoracic access or distal control requires intracranial exposure, a thoracic or neurosurgical consult should be obtained.

As a generalization, all venous structures can be ligated, although bilateral ligation of internal jugular veins should be avoided due to the possibility of significant vascular congestion and edema. Ligation of major arteries can be associated with acute and long-term complications, but should be done as a life-saving procedure. Ligation of the common or internal carotid is possible but is associated with cerebrovascular insufficiency, especially in the elderly.[29] Surgical ligation of the subclavian can cause acute upper extremity ischemia or claudication. Complications from ligation can be avoided by vascular repair or shunting; however, this may be beyond the skill set of most otolaryngologists and may require vascular surgery consultation.

Zone II injury that penetrates the platysma classically is explored, although there is now variability in clinical practice, as already discussed in this chapter. There is increasing evidence that the asymptomatic patient can be observed if there are no identifiable aerodigestive tract injuries noted on CTA or angiogram and esophageal evaluation.

Surgical exploration in zone II should focus on the anterior venous drainage system as well as exploration of the great

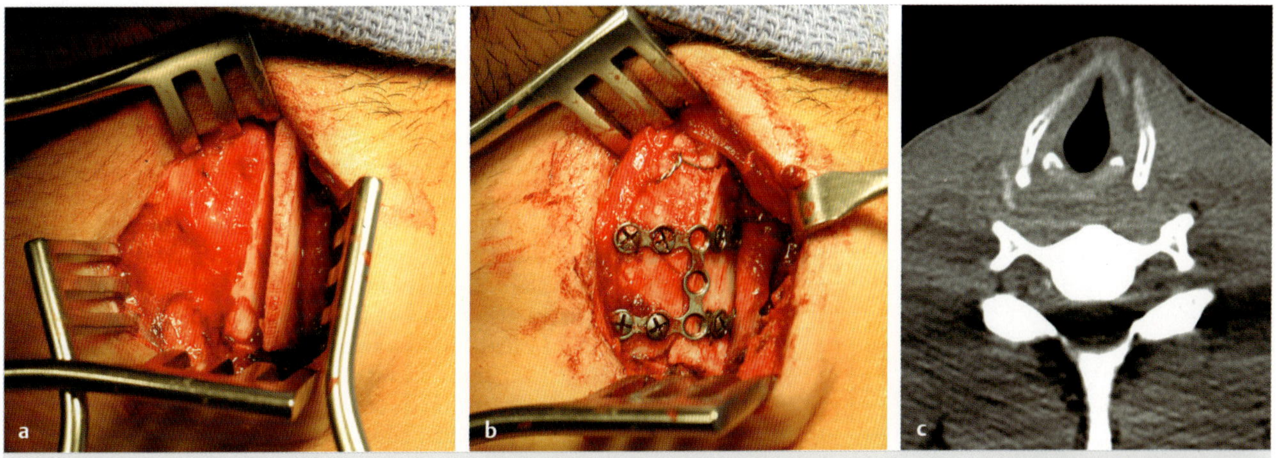

Fig. 13.6 Intraoperative images of (**a**) pre- and (**b**) post-open reduction and internal fixation and (**c**) corresponding axial computed tomography image of a thyroid cartilage fracture that occurred when a 20-year-old man hit a moving biker while riding a skateboard. The repair was done less than 36 hours after the fracture occurred. There was only a small vocal fold hematoma on fiberoptic laryngoscopic exam and no airway symptoms other than deepening of the voice. For repair, note the presence of both an H-plate with 4-mm rescue screws and a 25-gauge wire at the superior border of the thyroid cartilage.

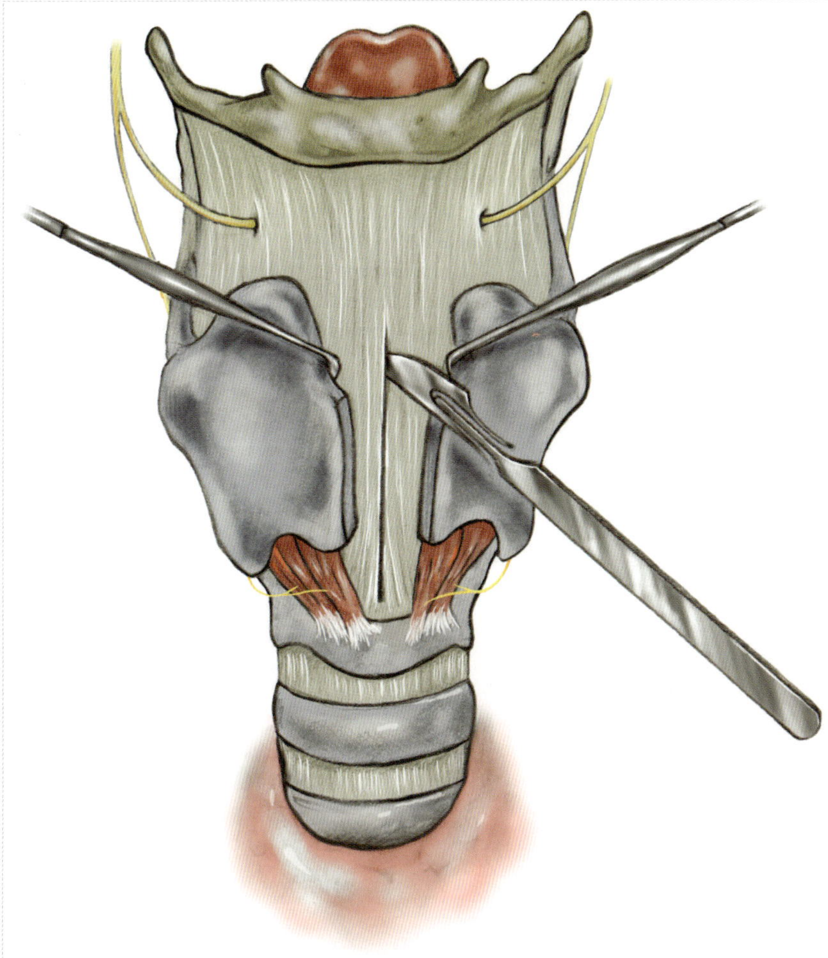

Fig. 13.7 Sharp transection of the anterior commissure.

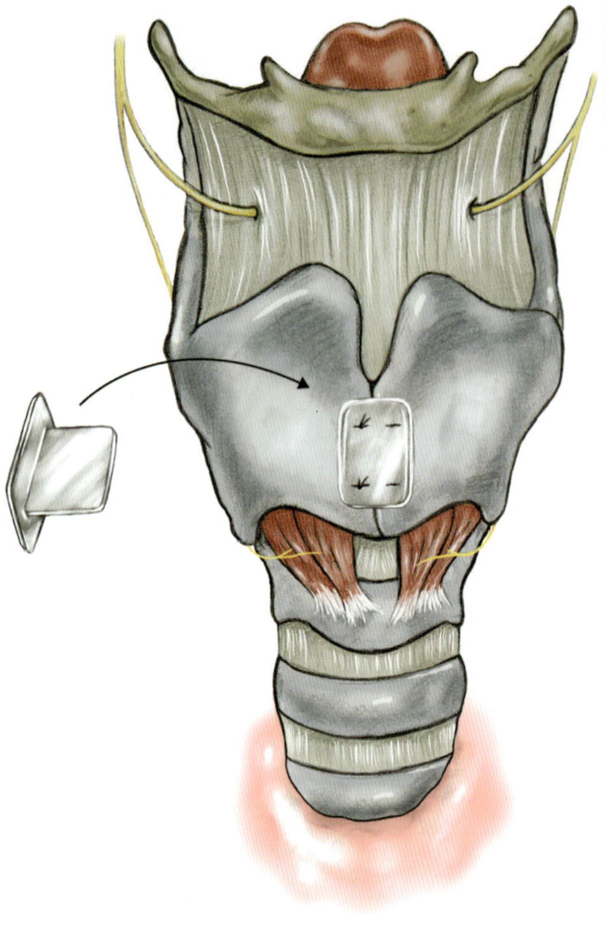

Fig. 13.8 The keel is placed into the anterior commissure region to prevent webbing during the healing process.

vessels and their major branches. If there is hemorrhage within the vascular sheath, it should be opened so that further visualization of the carotid, jugular, and vagus can be appreciated. Small lacerations of the vessels can be repaired primarily. Care should be taken not to narrow the diameter of the carotid during repair as it will reduce flow. Unilateral internal jugular ligation can be performed with little consequence. Similarly, the external carotid can be repaired or ligated if needed. If there is loss of tissue of the common or internal carotid, resection of the involved segment and reanastamosis of healthy vascular tissue is preferred to ligation because of associated morbidity.

In the event of transluminal perforation of the upper aerodigestive tract, conservative management, including maintenance of NPO (nothing taken orally) status and broad spectrum and anaerobic antibiotic coverage, should be the initial steps. If there is abscess formation or a large perforation is noted with extraluminal accumulation of secretions, external drainage should be employed, given the significance of developing mediastinitis or sepsis.

Vocal fold paralysis can occur with injury to the recurrent laryngeal nerve (RLN), or vagus. An RLN that is transected sharply can be repaired after the ends are freshened with microsurgical techniques. Although there may not be meaningful functional movement, repair of the nerve can allow for synkinetic reinnervation and tone. Alternatively, ansa cervicalis anastomosis to the RLN is another option, especially if there is a segmental loss of the RLN due to trauma.

Vertebral artery injury should evaluated for during workup, especially when there is an associated cervical spine injury or neurologic symptom. Neurologic sequelae are rare, but can be devastating due to posterior cerebral circulation ischemia and stroke. If vertebral artery injury is present, neurosurgical consultation is recommended, as management can range from observation or anticoagulation (if not contraindicated) to open or endovascular repair for high-grade or symptomatic injury.[30,31]

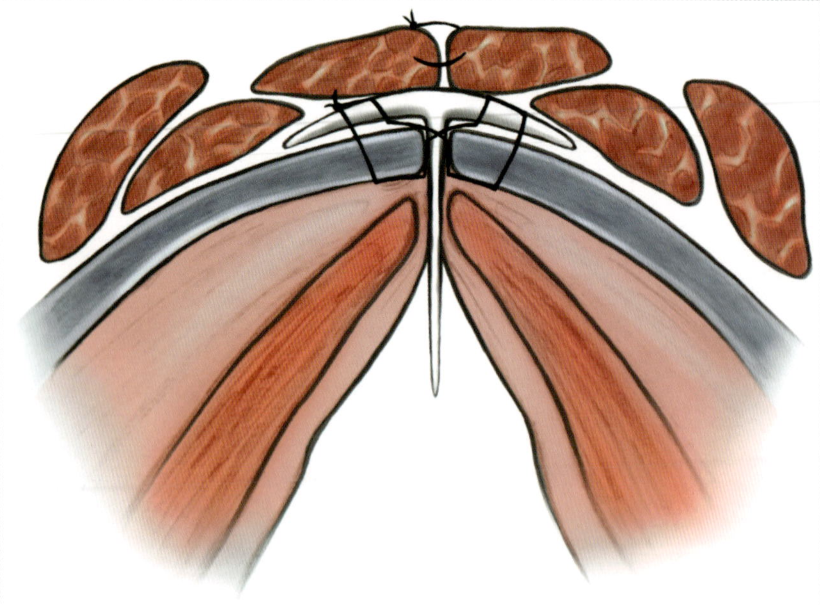

Fig. 13.9 The keel is secured into place with two figure-of-eight sutures. (Based on Montgomery WW. Surgery of the Larynx, Trachea, Esophagus, and Neck. 1st ed. Philadelphia: Saunders; 2002: Figures 15–17B.)

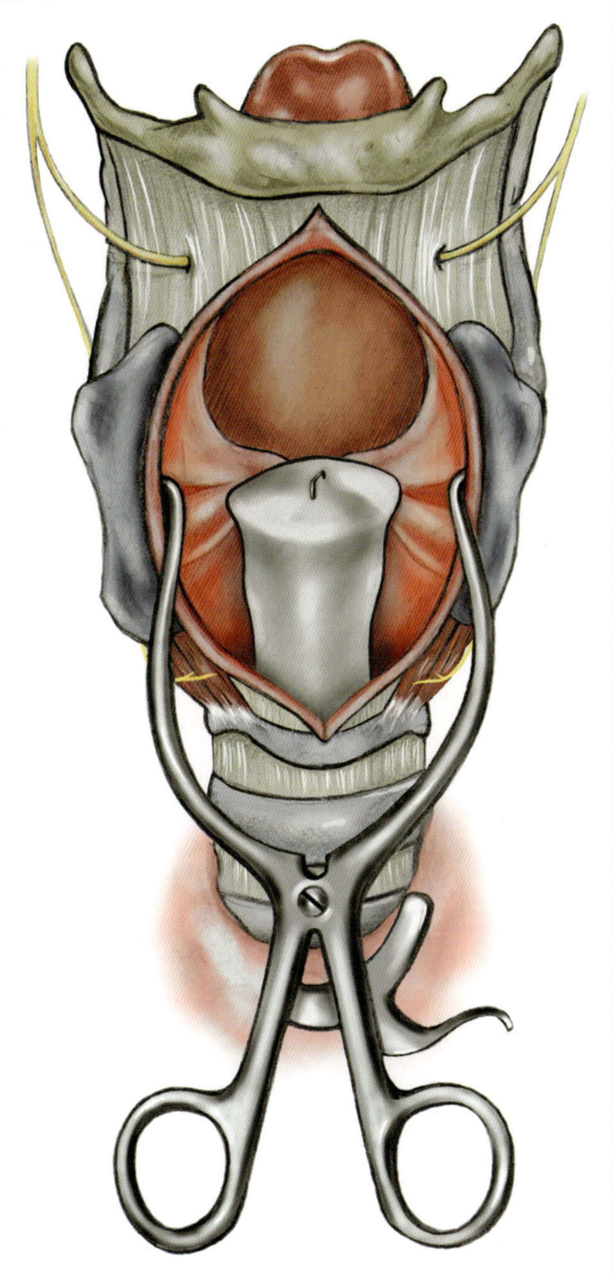

Fig. 13.10 A Montgomery laryngeal stent being placed through a laryngofissure.

13.4 What to Do When Treatment Fails

Treatment failure in laryngeal trauma can come in a variety of forms. Dividing failure into acute and long-term failure can be helpful for purposes of discussion. Acute failure can include airway obstruction, persistent bleeding, stroke, or other neurologic deficit, or manifestations of upper aerodigestive tract perforation. Long-term treatment failures include vocal fold paralysis, scarring, stenosis, dysphagia/aspiration, tracheotomy tube dependence, and complications from initial management strategies.

Management of acute failure involves revisiting many of the above treatment strategies or algorithms. The inclusion of specialists that focus on the area of failure is advisable.

Correction of long-term treatment failures can be a complicated and challenging prospect for many of the above issues. Treatment of dysphagia/aspiration, vocal fold immobility and laryngeal stenosis are discussed in Chapters 4, 9, and 10, respectively, but there are a few salient points that are worth mentioning here with respect to laryngeal trauma.

Typically, use of stents is reserved for the most extreme cases. Use of a stent can cause scarring of the vocal fold and is associated with granuloma formation. Granulomas can be resected with cold instrumentation, microdebridement, or laser. Triamcinolone injection, inhaled steroid[32] and systemic steroid administration, as well as reflux control, are also valuable in encouraging resolution.

For severe laryngeal trauma where there is significant framework disruption, there can be cartilaginous collapse post stent removal. Conservative treatment includes rigid or balloon dilation and treatment of scar with resection, mitomycin, and triamcinolone. In extreme cases, where the larynx is not functional or salvageable, supraglottic or total laryngectomy is an option.[33]

13.5 Key Points

13.5.1 Blunt Trauma

- If there is evidence of impending obstruction or significant laryngeal mucosal trauma, a tracheotomy is preferable to endotracheal intubation.
- If there are displaced thyroid or cricoid cartilage fractures, or significant mucosal defects, early repair improves outcomes.
- Nondisplaced fractures can be observed.
- Stenting is controversial, but it is indicated when there is significant loss of framework support.

13.5.2 Penetrating Trauma

- Esophageal injuries are often missed and should be evaluated by esophagram or esophageal endoscopy.
- Traditional dogma for zone II injury is exploration; however, with the increase in CTA, observation has become a more common practice and surgical exploration is not necessarily mandatory.
- If surgical exploration is indicated for vascular injury, the first step in surgical management should be proximal and distal control of the injured vessel.
- The external carotid and internal jugular vein can be ligated with little consequence.
- Vascular stenting should be considered for significant injury to the internal carotid and subclavian arteries if repair is not feasible.

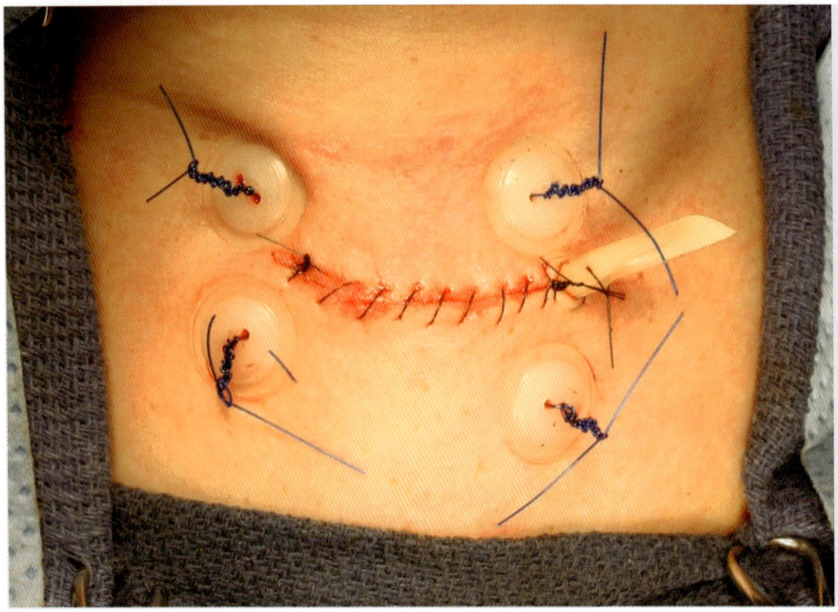

Fig. 13.11 Postoperative photo of a laryngeal stent secured by cervical buttons.

References

[1] Schaefer SD. The acute management of external laryngeal trauma. A 27-year experience. Arch Otolaryngol Head Neck Surg 1992; 118: 598–604

[2] Demetriades D, Theodorou D, Cornwell E et al. Transcervical gunshot injuries: mandatory operation is not necessary. J Trauma 1996; 40: 758–760

[3] Christe A, Thoeny H, Ross S et al. Life-threatening versus non-life-threatening manual strangulation: are there appropriate criteria for MR imaging of the neck? Eur Radiol 2009; 19: 1882–1889

[4] Rao PM, Ivatury RR, Sharma P, Vinzons AT, Nassoura Z, Stahl WM. Cervical vascular injuries: a trauma center experience. Surgery 1993; 114: 527–531

[5] Mansour MA, Moore EE, Moore FA, Whitehill TA. Validating the selective management of penetrating neck wounds. Am J Surg 1991; 162: 517–520, discussion 520–521

[6] Sclafani SJA, Cavaliere G, Atweh N, Duncan AO, Scalea T. The role of angiography in penetrating neck trauma. J Trauma 1991; 31: 557–562, discussion 562–563

[7] Múnera F, Soto JA, Palacio DM et al. Penetrating neck injuries: helical CT angiography for initial evaluation. Radiology 2002; 224: 366–372

[8] Burgess CA, Dale OT, Almeyda R, Corbridge RJ. An evidence based review of the assessment and management of penetrating neck trauma. Clin Otolaryngol 2012; 37: 44–52

[9] Bell RB, Osborn T, Dierks EJ, Potter BE, Long WB. Management of penetrating neck injuries: a new paradigm for civilian trauma. J Oral Maxillofac Surg 2007; 65: 691–705

[10] Osborn TM, Bell RB, Qaisi W, Long WB. Computed tomographic angiography as an aid to clinical decision making in the selective management of penetrating injuries to the neck: a reduction in the need for operative exploration. J Trauma 2008; 64: 1466–1471

[11] Inaba K, Munera F, McKenney M et al. Prospective evaluation of screening multislice helical computed tomographic angiography in the initial evaluation of penetrating neck injuries. J Trauma 2006; 61: 144–149

[12] Demetriades D, Theodorou D, Cornwell E et al. Penetrating injuries of the neck in patients in stable condition. Physical examination, angiography, or color flow Doppler imaging. Arch Surg 1995; 130: 971–975

[13] Jarvik JG, Philips GR, Schwab CW, Schwartz JS, Grossman RI. Penetrating neck trauma: sensitivity of clinical examination and cost-effectiveness of angiography. AJNR Am J Neuroradiol 1995; 16: 647–654

[14] Woo K, Magner DP, Wilson MT, Margulies DR. CT angiography in penetrating neck trauma reduces the need for operative neck exploration. Am Surg 2005; 71: 754–758

[15] Noyes LD, McSwain NE, Markowitz IP. Panendoscopy with arteriography versus mandatory exploration of penetrating wounds of the neck. Ann Surg 1986; 204: 21–31

[16] Armstrong WB, Detar TR, Stanley RB. Diagnosis and management of external penetrating cervical esophageal injuries. Ann Otol Rhinol Laryngol 1994; 103: 863–871

[17] Schafer SD. Laryngeal trauma. In: Stewart MG, ed. Head, Face, and Neck Trauma. 1st ed. New York, NY: Thieme; 2005: 207–222

[18] Schaefer SD, Close LG. Acute management of laryngeal trauma. Update. Ann Otol Rhinol Laryngol 1989; 98: 98–104

[19] Stanley RB, Hanson DG. Manual strangulation injuries of the larynx. Arch Otolaryngol 1983; 109: 344–347

[20] Kleinsasser NH, Priemer FG, Schulze W, Kleinsasser OF. External trauma to the larynx: classification, diagnosis, therapy. Eur Arch Otorhinolaryngol 2000; 257: 439–444

[21] Bent JP, Silver JR, Porubsky ES. Acute laryngeal trauma: a review of 77 patients. Otolaryngol Head Neck Surg 1993; 109: 441–449

[22] Butler AP, Wood BP, O'Rourke AK, Porubsky ES. Acute external laryngeal trauma: experience with 112 patients. Ann Otol Rhinol Laryngol 2005; 114: 361–368

[23] Cherian TA, Rupa V, Raman R. External laryngeal trauma: analysis of thirty cases. J Laryngol Otol 1993; 107: 920–923

[24] Castellanos PF. Acute laryngeal trauma. In: Eisle DW, McQuone SJ, eds. Emergencies of the Head and Neck. 1st ed. St. Louis, MO: Mosby; 2000: 168–182

[25] Sasaki CT, Marotta JC, Lowlicht RA, Ross DA, Johnson M. Efficacy of resorbable plates for reduction and stabilization of laryngeal fractures. Ann Otol Rhinol Laryngol 2003; 112: 745–750

[26] Bloom DC, Carvalho DS, Kearns DB. Endoscopic repair of pediatric traumatic laryngeal injury. Int J Pediatr Otorhinolaryngol 2001; 60: 243–247

[27] Schaefer SD, Carder HM. How I do it—head and neck. A targeted problem and its solution. Fabrication of a simple laryngeal stent. Laryngoscope 1980; 90: 1561–1563

[28] Cherian TA, Rupa V, Raman R. External laryngeal trauma: analysis of thirty cases. J Laryngol Otol 1993; 107: 920–923

[29] Scott BG. Approach to penetrating inuries of the neck. In: Stewart MG, ed. Head, Face, and Neck Trauma. 1st ed. New York, NY: Thieme; 2005:202–207

[30] Desouza RM, Crocker MJ, Haliasos N, Rennie A, Saxena A. Blunt traumatic vertebral artery injury: a clinical review. Eur Spine J 2011; 20: 1405–1416

[31] Demetriades D, Theodorou D, Asensio J et al. Management options in vertebral artery injuries. Br J Surg 1996; 83: 83–86

[32] Abo M, Fujimura M, Kibe Y, Kida H, Matsuda T. Beclomethasone dipropionate inhalation as a treatment for post-intubation tracheal stenosis. Int J Clin Pract 1999; 53: 217–218

[33] Consalici R, Dall'Olio D. Severe laryngeal fracture treated by supracricoid laryngectomy. J Laryngol Otol 2010; 124: 1239–1241

14 Laryngeal Malignancy

Andrew B. Tassler and Richard V. Smith

Cancer of the larynx represents between 1 and 5% of all human malignancy and is the second most common site of neoplastic disease within the upper aerodigestive tract, second only to cancers of the oral cavity.[1] Although laryngeal cancer accounts for approximately 25% of all head and neck cancers, its incidence in the United States is decreasing (▶ Fig. 14.1). This is likely secondary to decreased rates of smoking and tobacco usage in general. Despite the decreasing incidence, the relative 5-year survival of laryngeal cancer patients has remained essentially unchanged since the 1970s (▶ Fig. 14.2). Given the static nature of overall survival in laryngeal cancer patients, newer treatment strategies have focused on preservation of laryngeal function and quality of life, while maintaining equivalency in survival.

The demographics of laryngeal cancer are changing. In the United States, men are diagnosed with laryngeal cancer at a rate of approximately four times more often than women according to the National Cancer Institute's 2005–2009 Surveillance Epidemiology and End Results (SEER) data, a decrease from a 6:1 ratio in the early 1970s. The vast majority of laryngeal cancer cases (~85%) can be attributed to tobacco and alcohol exposure. Tobacco exposure plays a more significant role in the development of glottic cancers, while alcohol exposure is often a more significant finding in patients with supraglottic tumors. Exposure to both alcohol and tobacco has a synergistic effect. Radiation exposure, human papilloma virus- (HPV-) associated papillomatosis, and exposure to chemical, environmental, and industrial substances have also been linked to the development of laryngeal malignancies.

14.1 History and Physical Examination

A thorough history for laryngeal cancer patients, as for all patients, is fundamental in the initial encounter and evaluation. Specific and careful questioning regarding pain, dysphagia, dysphonia, and aspiration is vital and often provides strong indications and clues as to the specific primary location of a malignancy within the larynx or pharynx. As with any evaluation, the clinician must consider the possibility of malignancy before the diagnosis can be made. Based upon patient history, physical examination, and clinician experience, an index of suspicion for malignancy must be maintained and pursued.

The duration of symptoms plays a key role in the patient evaluation. Voice change, dysphagia, odynophagia, pharyngeal pain, otalgia, or the presence of a neck mass for more than 2 to 4 weeks in a patient, particularly those with risk factors for head and neck cancer, should prompt evaluation for malignancy. Questions regarding signs and symptoms of postnasal drainage, and laryngopharyngeal reflux, as well as any periodicity to the dysphonia or other symptoms, are important as well. The quality of the patient's voice, their ability to manage their own secretions, and any signs of upper airway obstruction

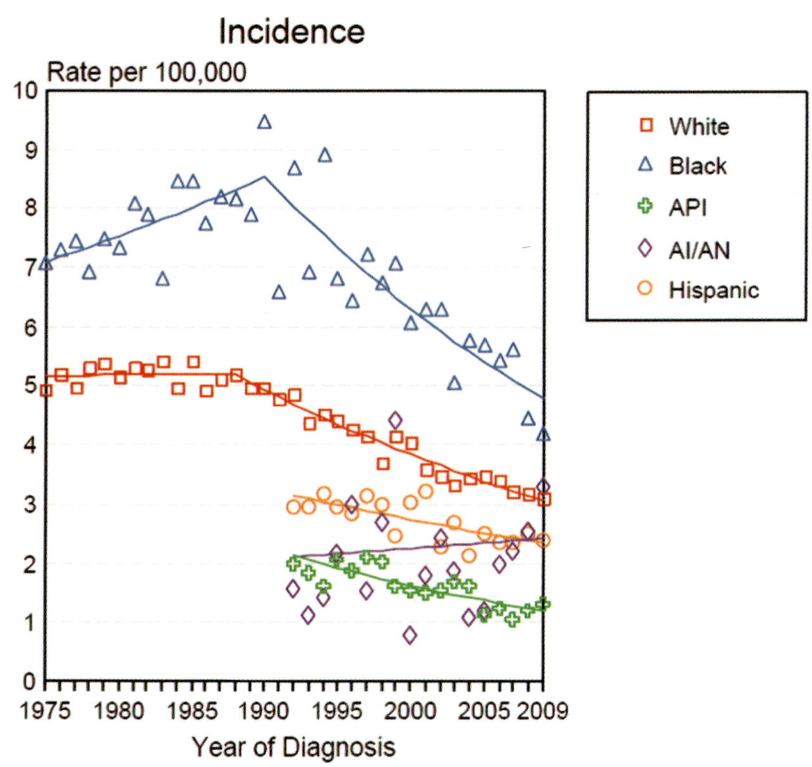

Fig. 14.1 The incidence of laryngeal cancer is declining across all races and ethnic groups. (Courtesy of www.seer.cancer.gov)

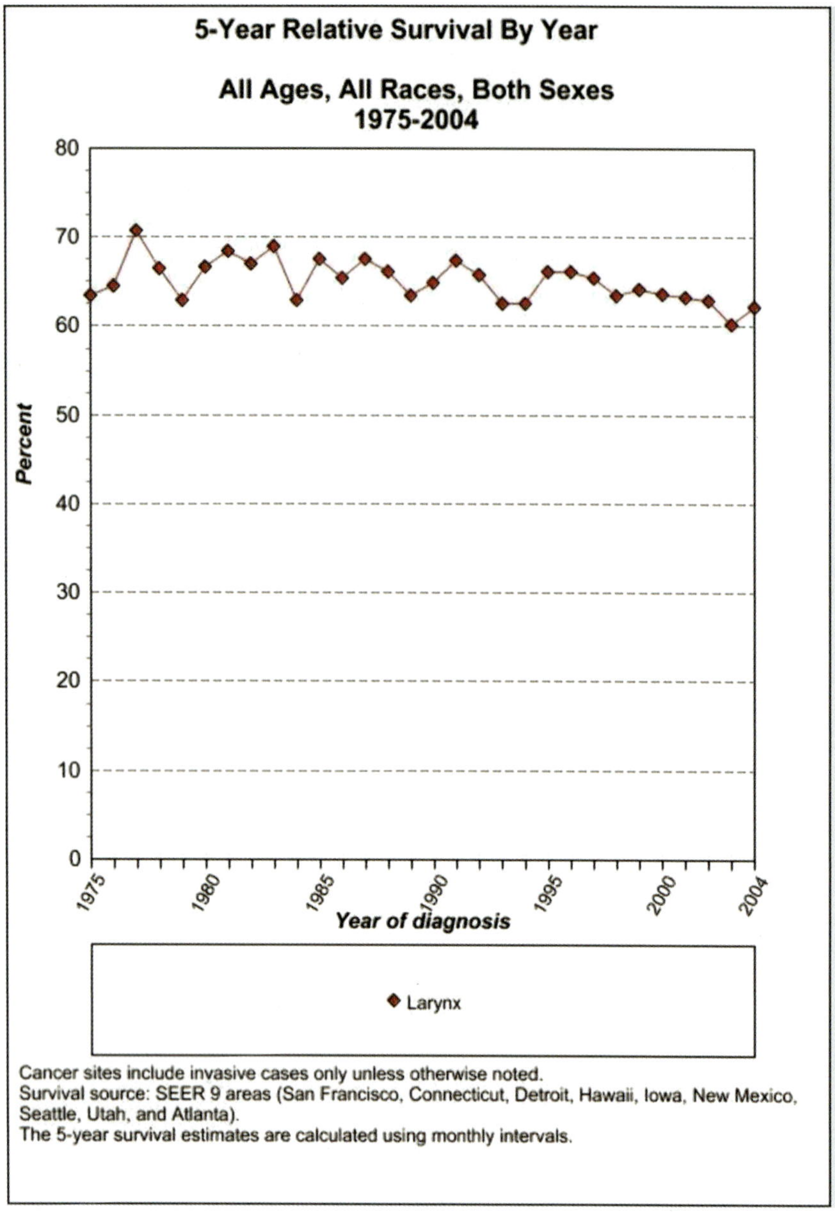

Fig. 14.2 Despite the decreasing incidence of laryngeal cancer, the relative 5-year survival remains essentially unchanged since the 1970s. The 5-year survival estimates are calculated using monthly intervals. Survival source: National Cancer Institute's Surveillance Epidemiology and End Results-9 (SEER 9) areas (San Francisco, Connecticut, Detroit, Hawaii, Iowa, New Mexico, Seattle, Utah, and Atlanta). (Courtesy of www.seer.cancer.gov.)

or stridor should be noted. Careful questioning regarding a patient's dysphagia and any possible aspiration should be pursued. The patient should be asked about weight loss and constitutional symptoms. Fortunately, the most common type of laryngeal cancer, glottic cancer, is often detected at an early stage given the common symptom of persistent voice change and hoarseness. Signs and symptoms of supraglottic and the rarer subglottic cancers can be more subtle and nonspecific, which can lead to a delay in diagnosis compared to glottic cancer.

A full head and neck examination is performed with careful evaluation of the larynx and hypopharynx either by mirror exam or flexible fiberoptic endoscopy. If a flexible technique is used, it is often helpful to capture static images of any lesions or ideally to record a dynamic video of the endoscopy. Videostroboscopy is a useful adjunct as well, particularly for lesions of the glottic larynx. Evaluation of the larynx should pay particular attention to both the location of any abnormal lesions and tissue as well the dynamic function and mobility of the larynx. The location and extent of the tumor are important not only for staging, but also in determining what the patient's presenting laryngeal function is and what partial laryngeal surgery may be possible. The next step in evaluation of a possible laryngeal malignancy is typically endoscopy with biopsy to establish a tissue diagnosis as well as to assess the extent of the tumor and the potential for endoscopic exposure.

The management of a patient with a suspected laryngeal malignancy prior to the initial endoscopy and biopsy represents a critical decision point for the initial treating physician. What may be viewed as a straightforward procedure to establish tissue diagnosis should be discouraged if the otolaryngologist is uncomfortable with, unfamiliar with, or simply does not often treat head and neck cancer. If a patient will likely be referred to another physician for either surgery and/or long-term follow-up, it is critically important that this treating physician be able to see the lesion(s) in question prior to instrumentation and biopsy. This is particularly important in patients who may be treated with nonoperative modalities as first-line therapy. Knowledge of the location and extent of the original tumor is fundamental to the ability to perform a partial laryngeal resection if the tumor persists or recurs following nonsurgical treatment with radiation, chemotherapy, or both.

14.2 Differential Diagnosis

The differential diagnosis of a laryngeal lesion suspicious for malignancy is not particularly vast, especially in the setting of patients with known environmental and social risk factors. Broadly speaking, lesions of the larynx can be divided into inflammatory, infectious, and neoplastic categories. The most common malignancy, squamous cell carcinoma, arises from the epithelium of the larynx and presents as a lesion emanating from the mucosa, often with signs of hyperkeratosis and ulceration.

Squamous cell carcinoma represents roughly 95% of all laryngeal malignancy, but does have variations and subtypes. The basaloid variant or basosquamous carcinoma of the larynx represents a more aggressive type of squamous cell cancer, which is typically poorly differentiated.[2] In contrast to HPV/P16 positive tumors of the oropharynx, which often have basaloid features and improved treatment response and outcomes, basosquamous tumors of the larynx are not often associated with HPV infection and are aggressive tumors that can be resistant to multimodality treatment. Verrucous carcinoma of the larynx is another variant of squamous cell carcinoma, which is estimated to account for 1 to 2% of laryngeal squamous cancers. Verrucous cancers are typically exophytic and hyperkeratotic in appearance, distinctly different from the more common leukoplakia or erythroplakia (▶ Fig. 14.3).

The diagnosis of a verrucous cancer requires a high index of suspicion based on the typical gross appearance of the lesion and close communication between the head and neck surgeon and pathologist. Verrucous cancers of the larynx are well differentiated, but locally aggressive tumors that have little metastatic potential. Surgery with clear margins is considered definitive treatment. An important defining feature of verrucous tumors is their relative radioresistance with high rates of local recurrence when treated with primary radiotherapy.[3]

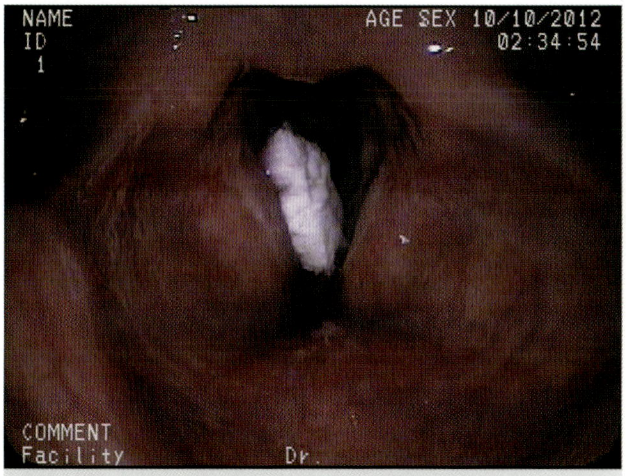

Fig. 14.3 Verrucous carcinoma of the right true vocal fold visualized with a flexible laryngoscope. Note the characteristic hyperkeratotic and exophytic appearance of the lesion.

Other less common malignancies of the larynx, such as tumors of minor salivary origin, granular cell tumors, and sarcomas have a more variable appearance. These more rare tumors may have a significant component that is submucosal in location. In this chapter, we will focus on the management of laryngeal squamous cell carcinoma.

Infectious lesions of the larynx are common, but often resolve quickly and are less suspicious for malignancy. The appearance of laryngeal infection on physical exam often reveals more diffuse changes of the larynx, with erythema and edema predominating. Laryngeal motion and function is typically intact. In contrast to neoplastic lesions, the onset of infection is typically more rapid and may accompany other systemic symptoms such as fever, chills, rhinorrhea, and cough, among others. Though typically acute, laryngeal infection can be chronic, particularly with the growing population of patients who are immunosuppressed for prolonged periods of time (human immunodeficiency virus [HIV], solid organ transplantation, and diabetes). Although uncommon, chronic viral, bacterial, and fungal infections of the larynx can be seen in this population and are often difficult to discern from malignant lesions without tissue diagnosis.[4]

Although inflammatory processes of the larynx, such as a vocal process granuloma, can be seen secondary to common clinical scenarios such as laryngopharyngeal reflux and intubation, other inflammatory lesions are often a manifestation of systemic inflammatory conditions. Systemic conditions such as sarcoidosis, amyloidosis, and granulomatosis with polyangitis (formerly known as Wegener granulomatosis) classically affect the larynx in supraglottic, glottic, and subglottic locations, respectively. In a similar fashion to infectious processes of the larynx, inflammatory lesions often demonstrate diffuse mucosal changes without frank ulceration or masses. The mucosa is often intact despite the abnormalities seen. Diagnosis of inflammatory laryngeal lesions often requires a high index of suspicion as well as close attention to other comorbid conditions and previously diagnosed systemic inflammatory conditions. Formal endoscopy and biopsy may be required to make a definitive diagnosis and rule out a neoplastic process.

14.3 Diagnosis

Diagnosis of any laryngeal malignancy requires histopathologic tissue evaluation and confirmation. Although some select lesions (and patients) may be able to undergo tissue biopsy under topical anesthesia in an office setting, the gold standard for evaluation and biopsy is formal endoscopy in the operating room.

14.3.1 Endoscopy

Close communication with the anesthesiologist is critically important when performing an initial endoscopy and biopsy of a patient with suspected laryngeal malignancy. As the patient's airway is truly being "shared" in such cases, a discussion and plan, however straightforward the case may seem, should be set prior to the induction of a general anesthetic. This is, of course, critically important in patients with obstructing lesions and potentially tenuous airways, but should be pursued prior to all cases. Whenever possible, our preference is general anesthesia with mask ventilation and rigid telescopic endoscopy performed prior to the placement of an endotracheal tube. Dynamic movement of the larynx can also be assessed prior to the administration of a paralytic agent. Once the airway has been secured, further endoscopy with 0-, 30-, 70-, and possibly 120-degree rigid endoscopes is then carried out, which allows a complete and panoramic evaluation of the larynx and the concerning lesions. Suspension laryngoscopy, either with an operating microscope or high-definition (HD) telescope, should be used liberally. The suspension technique allows complete evaluation of the larynx as soft tissues can be gently retracted, external pressure precisely applied, and careful telescope examination used to evaluate the extent of disease. Further, the use of a suspension technique provides useful information regarding a patients' laryngeal exposure and the extent of the lesion should an endoscopic resection be considered.

Representative biopsies of any suspicious lesions should be obtained using standard techniques and biopsy forceps. Frozen-section analysis can be useful if there is significant question as to the diagnosis and/or whether a biopsy contains representative tissue. A frozen section that yields a negative result and leads to further biopsy that confirms malignancy is obviously of significant value. A frozen section may also allow confirmation of malignancy if an oncologic resection of a lesion is pursued at the initial endoscopy.

If a resection will be performed at a later date, pathologic mapping of a tumor can also be performed at the initial endoscopy. This technique involves taking biopsies of both abnormal tissue (tumor) as well as adjacent normal-appearing tissue. The pathologic confirmation of an essentially "negative" margin prior to a definitive resection makes the extent of resection, and associated morbidity, more predictable. In addition, the biopsy of visually normal tissues may reveal significant dysplasia or even additional malignancy, which may change the patient's treatment plan. A patient with diffuse dysplasia or malignancy can sometimes be seen with significant tobacco and/or other environmental exposures. Such patients with diffuse epithelial changes or "field cancerization" present a therapeutic challenge, but recognition of the pathologic situation is of primary importance.

14.3.2 Imaging

Although physical examination and rigid endoscopy provide excellent evaluation of the extent of mucosal disease in patients with laryngeal cancer, the depth and extent of disease involvement can be underestimated.[5]

The management of early-stage glottic cancer, with normal vocal fold motion and no anterior commissure involvement is unlikely to be changed based on comuted tomography (CT) or magnetic resonance imaging (MRI). As will be discussed in the treatment section regarding neck staging and management, there is little potential for lymph node involvement in this scenario and thus the need for imaging in all patients with early glottic cancer is debatable. This exception aside, any supraglottic or subglottic carcinoma should be evaluated by CT or MRI prior to initial treatment. The threshold to perform a CT on a patient with a glottic tumor with impaired vocal fold motion or anterior commissure extension should be minimal; extension to the paraglottic or pre-epiglottic spaces as well as early cartilage invasion will upstage what were initially thought to be early (T1 or T2) stage tumors.

Anatomical cross-sectional imaging of the larynx and neck with either CT or MRI is the standard at this time. Although MRI may provide slightly better detail of cartilaginous involvement, the availability and speed of CT scanning often make it the most common imaging modality used. Computed tomography now commonly allows multiplanar reconstruction, which was previously considered to be a significant advantage of MRI. Contrast should be added to imaging studies whenever feasible as this will aid in the identification of enhancing tumor; intravenous (IV) contrast also allows for clear delineation of the cervical vasculature as well as suspicious or obviously metastatic lymphadenopathy. Cross-sectional imaging allows close inspection of the laryngeal cartilage(s) both from the standpoint of calcification and osseous changes as well as tumor involvement.

Though its use is not yet standardized, positron emission tomography (PET) scanning is increasingly used in the initial treatment planning and extensively in the posttreatment surveillance of head and neck cancer patients. Although the anatomical detail of PET alone is rarely sufficient to alter the assessment (T stage) of a primary tumor, PET is now frequently combined with diagnostic CT to improve the anatomical detail of the scan.[6] However, where PET and PET-CT may be most useful is in the detection of nodal and distant metastases. We will routinely use this modality in patients with pathological lymphadenopathy, with a primary tumor location (supraglottic or subglottic) with high potential for occult cervical metastases, or with T3 and T4 laryngeal cancers.

14.4 Treatment

As is undoubtedly clear from other chapters in this text, the larynx is a unique organ that has a central and profound use and meaning in human lives. Besides its fundamental purpose of separating and protecting the airway from the digestive tract, the larynx is a critical element of our ability to interact with others and communicate our feelings. These unique facts about the human larynx are a critical and significant consideration in the treatment of laryngeal cancer both for patients and clinicians. The desire to eradicate cancer while maintaining function has been a driving force in the evolution of laryngeal cancer treatment.

As with other squamous cell carcinomas of the upper aerodigestive tract, the treatment options for laryngeal cancer include surgery, radiation, and chemotherapy. For early stage (I and II) disease, single-modality therapy (surgery or radiation) is often adequate. For more advanced-stage disease (III and IV), multimodality treatment is often indicated.

Combinations of chemotherapy and radiotherapy are now routinely employed in the care of patients with locoregionally advanced (stage III and IV) laryngeal cancer. The landmark Veterans' Affairs (VA) Laryngeal Cancer Study was the first randomized trial to demonstrate the efficacy of nonsurgical therapy in preventing total laryngectomy; although this trial demonstrated equivalent survival for patients with advanced laryngeal cancer treated with either primary total laryngectomy or induction chemotherapy followed by definitive radiation for those patients responding to the initial chemotherapy, approximately two-thirds of patients treated with initial nonsurgical therapy were able to avoid laryngectomy without compromising survival.[7] The subsequent landmark RTOG 91–11 trial demonstrated optimal laryngeal preservation with concomitant chemotherapy and radiotherapy in comparison to induction chemotherapy followed by radiation.[8] As a result of this stepwise evolution in research, concurrent chemoradiotherapy has become the most common nonoperative treatment modality for locoregionally advanced laryngeal cancer.

Although there is emerging data regarding the use of chemotherapy as a single modality for very highly selected patients with early to intermediate-stage laryngeal cancer,[9,10] this should not be considered a standard approach. However, chemotherapy as a single modality is often reserved for palliation of symptoms associated with incurable recurrence or for distant metastases or to improve survival in this setting. The most common curative-intent treatment algorithms for laryngeal cancer combine chemotherapy with radiation either as an initial treatment strategy as described above or for high-risk patients in a postoperative setting.[11,12]

14.4.1 Staging

Laryngeal cancer staging follows the standard American Joint Committee on Cancer (AJCC) T (tumor) N (node) M (metastases) system; nodal and metastatic disease is staged similarly to other head and neck cancer subsites. T staging of laryngeal cancer, however, represents one of the more unique and often confusing classification systems among human malignancies (see the box "AJCC tumor staging for laryngeal cancer based on subsite of origin (p. 131)"). Laryngeal cancer is first classified by its site of origin: supraglottis, glottis, and subglottis. Glottic cancer represents the most common subsite within the larynx and accounts for 50 to 75% of all laryngeal cancer. Supraglottic tumors account for the majority of the other laryngeal malignancies (30 to 40%). The subglottis is a rare site for primary laryngeal cancer and represents less than 5% of all laryngeal cancer.

AJCC tumor staging for laryngeal cancer based on subsite of origin

- **TX** Primary tumor cannot be assessed.
- **T0** No evidence of primary tumor
- **T** Carcinoma in situ

Supraglottis
- **T1** Tumor limited to one subsite of supraglottis with normal vocal cord mobility.
- **T2** Tumor invades mucosa of more than one adjacent subsite of supraglottis or glottis or region outside the supraglottis (e.g., mucosa of base of tongue, vallecula, medial wall of pyriform sinus) without fixation of the larynx.
- **T3** Tumor limited to larynx with vocal cord fixation and/or invades any of the following: postcricoid area, pre-epiglottic space, paraglottic space, and/or inner cortex of thyroid cartilage.
- **T4a** Moderately advanced local disease
- Tumor invades through the thyroid cartilage and/or invades tissues beyond the larynx (e.g., trachea, soft tissues of neck including deep extrinsic muscle of the tongue, strap muscles, thyroid, or esophagus).
- **T4b** Very advanced local disease
- Tumor invades prevertebral space, encases carotid artery, or invades mediastinal structures.

Glottis
- **T1** Tumor limited to the vocal cord(s) (may involve anterior or posterior commissure) with normal mobility
- **T1a** Tumor limited to one vocal cord
- **T1b** Tumor involves both vocal cords.
- **T2** Tumor extends to supraglottis and/or subglottis and/or with impaired vocal cord mobility.
- **T3** Tumor limited to the larynx with vocal cord fixation and/ or invasion of paraglottic space and/or inner cortex of the thyroid cartilage
- **T4a** Moderately advanced local disease
- Tumor invades through the outer cortex of the thyroid cartilage and/or invades tissues beyond the larynx (e.g., trachea, soft tissues of neck including deep extrinsic muscle of the tongue, strap muscles, thyroid, or esophagus).
- **T4b** Very advanced local disease
- Tumor invades prevertebral space, encases carotid artery, or invades mediastinal structures.

Subglottis
- **T1** Tumor limited to the subglottis
- **T2** Tumor extends to vocal cord(s) with normal or impaired mobility.
- **T3** Tumor limited to larynx with vocal cord fixation
- **T4a** Moderately advanced local disease
- Tumor invades cricoid or thyroid cartilage and/or invades tissues beyond the larynx (e.g., trachea, soft tissues of neck including deep extrinsic muscles of the tongue, strap muscles, thyroid, or esophagus).
- **T4b** Very advanced local disease.
- Tumor invades prevertebral space, encases carotid artery, or invades mediastinal structures.

Source: Adapted from Edge SB, Byrd DR, Compton CC et al, eds. Larynx. In: AJCC Cancer Staging Manual. 7th ed. New York, NY: Springer; 2010: 57–62.

Further characterization of a primary laryngeal tumor is related to the subsites within the larynx involved by the tumor, the functional changes created by the tumor, and extension outside of the larynx itself. Although tumors of increasing T stage are undoubtedly more advanced, have more infiltrative growth, and are associated with decreased survival, what makes the staging system of laryngeal cancer challenging is the occasional incongruity between T staging and available surgical options. As an example, a tumor that is "transglottic," meaning it involves the supraglottic, glottic, and subglottic larynx, may require a total laryngectomy, but could be staged as a T2 lesion assuming normal vocal fold mobility. On the other hand, a T4 lesion confined to the supraglottic larynx may be resectable with a partial laryngectomy such as a supraglottic or supracricoid laryngectomy. This example of a lesser T-stage tumor requiring a more radical surgery underscores the unique anatomy and function of the larynx, the knowledge of which is essential to understanding the treatment options and decision making for laryngeal malignancy. Although stage does not always correlate with surgical options, it does correlate with survival and the types of nonsurgical therapy offered.

Overall, staging takes into account all components of the TNM to place a given tumor and patient from stages 1 through 4. Overall and disease-free survival is reduced with increasing stage. Charts that closely detail the different TNM configurations and stages are readily available at www.cancer.gov, but some basic facts regarding overall staging are helpful to remember. First, the overall stage cannot be less than the T stage—a T4N0 carcinoma is a stage 4 cancer. Second, any tumor with nodal disease is a stage 3 (N1 disease) or stage 4 (N2 or N3 disease) cancer. Finally, any tumor with distant metastatic disease is a stage 4 cancer regardless of the other criteria. Using these rules, one can readily stage tumors and begin to delineate treatment options based on whether a patient has early (stage 1 or 2) or more advanced (stage 3 or 4) disease. As mentioned previously, early-stage tumors can often be treated with single modality therapy, whereas more advanced lesions typically require multimodality treatment plans.

14.4.2 Neck Staging and Management

Staging of neck metastases for laryngeal cancer follows the AJCC nodal staging system, which is used for all head and neck cancers with the exception of nasopharyngeal primary tumors (see the box "AJCC nodal staging system for laryngeal cancer (p. 132)"). The first echelon of nodal drainage for the larynx is typically to levels 2, 3, and 4 and may be bilateral, even in an apparently well-lateralized tumor. Level 6 (paratracheal) nodes may also be a primary drainage basin and must be considered as well, particularly in tumors with subglottic involvement.

AJCC nodal staging system for laryngeal cancer

- **N0** No regional lymph node metastasis
- **N1** Metastasis in a single ipsilateral lymph node: ≤ 3 cm in maximum dimension
- **N2** Metastasis in a single ipsilateral lymph node: > 3 cm but 6 cm in greatest dimension
- Metastases in multiple ipsilateral lymph nodes: none > 6 cm in greatest dimension.
- Metastases in bilateral or contralateral lymph nodes: none > 6 cm in greatest dimension
- **N2a** Metastasis in a single ipsilateral lymph node: > 3 cm but ≤ 6 cm in greatest dimension
- **N2b** Metastases in multiple ipsilateral lymph nodes: none > 6 cm in greatest dimension
- **N2c** Metastases in bilateral or contralateral lymph nodes: none > 6 cm in greatest dimension
- **N3** Metastasis in a lymph node: none > 6 cm in greatest dimension

Source: Adapted from Edge SB, Byrd DR, Compton CC et al, eds. Larynx. In: AJCC Cancer Staging Manual. 7th ed. New York, NY: Springer; 2010: 57–62.

For thorough descriptions of the distribution of lymphatics within the larynx one is referred to the writings of otolaryngologists such as John Kirchner and his seminal work on laryngeal specimens.[13] In practical terms, the supraglottic and subglottic portions of the human larynx contain rich lymphatics as compared to the glottic larynx, which is essentially devoid of lymphatic drainage. The implications of these differences are that tumors located within subsites that are rich in lymphatics spread to involve the cervical lymph nodes much more readily than do glottic tumors. In demonstration of this fact, one retrospective analysis of T1 and T2 glottic cancers revealed a nodal metastasis rate of 0%.[14]

On the other hand, even in the absence of nodal metastasis either by physical examination or imaging (N0 neck), the propensity of tumors located in the supraglottic and subglottic larynx to metastasize to cervical nodes is so significant (30–70%) that these areas of nodal drainage must be addressed in nearly any treatment plan, whether surgical (neck dissection) or nonsurgical (radiation ± chemotherapy).[15]

14.4.3 Partial Laryngeal Surgery

The evolution of surgical management of laryngeal cancer began first with the thyrotomy in the 1850s, which progressed to the vertical partial laryngectomy in the latter part of the 19th century. The mid-20th century saw the development of the open supraglottic laryngectomy and later the supracricoid partial laryngectomy. Though these techniques are less commonly performed in current clinical practice, their anatomical basis and technical features represent important knowledge for anyone providing comprehensive surgical treatment for laryngeal cancer.

In properly selected patients and in centers familiar with the postoperative rehabilition, the outcomes of open partial laryngeal surgery can be excellent. The majority of lesions amenable to open resection can, however, also be removed through a transoral technique with comparable oncologic outcomes and improved morbidity. Endoscopic resection can be performed without the need for a tracheotomy in the vast majority of cases, as compared to the open partial resections in which a tracheotomy is commonly performed. In addition, the dysphagia following endoscopic resection appears to be less than in open procedures. Other known complications of open resections, such as fistula, are extremely rare in transoral surgery.

The primary challenge and limitation that accompanies partial laryngeal surgery is proper patient selection. This exists first in terms of specific tumor anatomy, which may be amenable to partial laryngectomy. Determination of what type of partial laryngeal resection a given tumor may be amenable to underscores the critical need for the oncologic surgeon to perform the initial endoscopy of the patient. Furthermore, patient understanding of what such a procedure will entail and motivation to participate in what is often intensive postoperative speech and swallowing rehabilitation is of critical importance. Finally, patients with poor pulmonary function and the inability to tolerate any amount of aspiration are poor candidates for partial procedures.

The specific indications and details of open procedures such as vertical partial, supraglottic, and supracricoid partial laryngectomies are beyond the scope of this chapter. Given the narrow indications and often intensive rehabilitation required postoperatively, the application of open partial laryngeal resections should be limited to surgeons who perform the procedures most commonly and centers that have speech-language pathologists familiar with the postoperative rehabilitation of such patients.

14.4.4 Transoral Surgery

Transoral resection has now become the most common modality for performing partial laryngeal resections. This is most commonly performed as transoral laser microsurgery (TLM), but can also take the form of transoral robotic resection (TORS). Glottic resections are usually performed using the TLM techniques, and the procedure is performed under general anesthesia with placement of a small, laser-safe-type endotracheal tube. As mentioned, tracheotomy is rarely needed. The glottis is then exposed and suspended to rigidly fixate the operative field with subsequent laser resection. The carbon dioxide (CO_2) laser is most commonly used due to its favorable depth of penetration and cutting characteristics. The surgeon views the operative field through a binocular microscope and the laser is often mounted on the microscope itself. The limitation of this technique is the need for direct line of sight for the microscope and laser to the operative site. Recent developments in the field of laser surgery now offer a fiber-based laser system that can be fed through a curved or even malleable introducer. When combined with an endoscopic visualization, resection can now be performed without the need for direct line of sight.

As implied with the term *microsurgery*, dissection is performed either under microscopic or high-definition visualization, which allows careful examination of the tissues. This gives the surgeon the ability to resect tumor with close but negative margins. Dependent upon the size and location of a given tumor, the laryngeal exposure may need to be adjusted throughout the procedure to allow visualization of different subsites of the larynx. Unlike the classic en bloc resection technique, TLM can be performed in a piecemeal fashion if needed; the tumor can be divided using the CO_2 laser and different portions of the malignancy removed separately, to carefully assess the margins, without any negative effect on the oncologic outcome.[16]

No formal reconstruction is performed at the time of TLM resection and the surgical site heals by secondary intention. Once the larynx has healed and felt to be cancer free, reconstruction can be performed in a delayed fashion if necessary for vocal function. The details of postoperative reconstructive techniques go beyond the scope of this chapter, but most surgeons will wait 6 months or more from the time of resection before considering formal reconstruction.[17] Reconstruction can be in the form of injection laryngoplasty, lysis of synechial bands, or more formal laryngeal framework surgery such as thyroplasty, if needed. However, the majority of patients, despite significant resection defects, will have serviceable vocal function after complete healing.

14.4.5 Chemotherapy

Although current National Comprehensive Cancer Network (NCCN) guidelines offer several chemotherapy regimens, the most commonly employed agent (preferred by the NCCN) is cisplatin, which has potent antitumor and radiosensitizing effects.[18] The regimen approved by the NCCN (and used in the Radiation Therapy Oncology Group RTOG 91–11 study) is 100 mg/m^2 administered intravenously on days 1, 22, and 43 of radiotherapy. In addition to being myelosuppressive and highly emetogenic, cisplatin is frequently associated with nephrotoxicity, ototoxicity, and neurotoxicity. Carboplatin is a less nephrotoxic agent that can be utilized in the setting of cisplatin-induced renal dysfunction. Patients who have impaired renal function may also be considered for radiosensitization by cetuximab, a chimeric monoclonal antibody targeting the epidermal growth factor receptor (EGFR). The recommended regimen is a 400 mg/m^2 IV loading dose starting 1 week prior to initiation of radiotherapy, followed by 250 mg/m^2 weekly doses during radiotherapy.[17] Cetuximab does not cause myelosuppression and is infrequently associated with nausea or vomiting. However, it is commonly associated with generally tolerable papulopustular skin rash of the face, chest and back, diarrhea, and rarely, severe hypersensitivity reactions.

During chemotherapy and chemoradiotherapy, patients must receive adequate enteral and IV hydration, antiemetic prophylaxis, and close clinical follow-up to evaluate for and manage toxicity.

14.4.6 Radiation Therapy

Radiation therapy, either alone or combined with chemotherapy, can offer both high local control and laryngeal preservation rates, even among select advanced (T3–T4) patients.

In the definitive setting, radiation therapy to the larynx, regardless of the subsite of disease, is given to a total dose of 70 Gy to the primary lesion. It is typically given in 1.8 to 2.0 Gy treatments (called "fractions"). A dose of 60 Gy is typically utilized for high-risk lymph node regions of suspected microscopic involvement of the necks, while a dose of 54 Gy is used to address lower-risk lymph node regions.

Early-stage cancers (T1–T2) of the glottic larynx can be treated with local radiation therapy to the larynx without treating the lymph node regions. However, typically T3 and T4 glottic tumors are treated not only to the primary lesion, but also to the bilateral necks. As previously mentioned, the supraglottic larynx is rich in lymphatics and malignant tumors arising from the supraglottis are more likely to spread to regional lymph nodes. Therefore, the cervical node regions at risk are included in the radiation fields even in the absence of obvious nodal disease.[19]

Most institutions now use intensity modulated radiation therapy (IMRT), as opposed to more traditional two- or three-dimensional planning, to treat cancers of the head and neck, including those of the larynx. Intensity modulated radiation therapy has the ability to produce highly conformal dose distributions with steeper gradients, allowing for maximum coverage of target tissues while sparing nearby normal structures, such as the parotids and constrictor muscles.[20]

Radiotherapy is associated with frequent acute toxicities and occasionally debilitating chronic morbidities. Acute toxicities of head and neck radiotherapy include mucositis, taste changes and in-field dermatitis; long-term toxicities include xerostomia, dysphagia, hypothyroidism, and potential for radionecrosis.

14.5 Specific Laryngeal Lesions

14.5.1 Glottic Carcinoma in Situ

Carcinoma in situ (CIS) implies high-grade dysplasia, indistinguishable from carcinoma, but without invasion below the level of the epithelial lining or involvement of the superficial lamina propria. Glottic CIS can be treated operatively with narrow margin excision, regardless of technique, or with external beam radiation. Both modalities offer excellent local control and disease-free survival rates (▶ Table 14.1).

The authors tend to favor surgical management of CIS as this reserves laryngeal radiation for later usage if necessary. Further, salvage procedures for recurrence can often be less invasive if the larynx has not previously been irradiated. If a lesion is truly CIS, the voice outcome with both surgery and radiation is typically very good, leaving the patient with the ability to phonate and communicate effectively.

14.5.2 T1 Glottic Carcinoma

A T1 carcinoma of the glottic larynx is a tumor with multiple presentations. A T1 lesion of the glottis is limited to the true vocal folds themselves and the motion of the vocal folds is unimpaired; T1a lesions are limited to one vocal fold (▶ Fig. 14.4) and T1b lesions involve both vocal folds with the most common presentation being that of a "horseshoe" lesion extending across the anterior commissure (▶ Fig. 14.5).

The treatment options for T1 glottic cancer, as was the case for CIS, are generally surgical resection or external beam radiation. Resection is performed either with cold knife technique, or more commonly, using TLM techniques. External beam radiation

Table 14.1 Treatment results comparing transoral laser microsurgery and radiotherapy for glottic carcinoma in situ

Author	*N*	Treatment	DFS (%)	LC (%)	Recurrence (*N*)
Peretti et al 2010	71	TLM	100	93	16 (1 TL)
Roedel et al 2009	35	TLM	100	93	4
Damm et al 2000	29	TLM	100	87	4 – TLM or RT salvage
Smee et al 2010	24	RT	87.5	75	2 –TL salvage
Garcia-Serra et al 2002	30	RT	100	88	3 – all had TL salvage
Spayne et al 2001	67	RT	100	98	1 – TL salvage

Abbreviations: DFS, disease free survival; LC, local control; RT, radiotherapy; TL, total laryngectomy; TLM, transoral laser microsurgery.
Sources: Data from Peretti G, Piazza C, Cocco D, et al. Transoral CO_2 laser treatment for Tis-T3 glottic cancer: The University of Brescia experience on 595 patients. Head Neck 2010; 32:977–983. Roedel RM, Christiansen H, Mueller RM, Matthias C. Transoral laser microsurgery for carcinoma in situ of the glottic larynx. A retrospective follow-up study. ORL J Otorhinolaryngol Relat Spec 2009; 71(1):45–49. Damm M, Sittel C, Streppel M, Eckel HE. Transoral CO_2 laser for surgical management of glottic carcinoma in situ. Laryngoscope 2000; 110(7):1215–1221. Smee RI, Meagher NS, Williams JR, Broadley K, Bridger GP. Role of radiotherapy in early glottic carcinoma. Head Neck 2010; 32(7):850–859. Garcia-Serra A, Hinerman RW, Amdur RJ, Morris CG, Mendenhall WM. Radiotherapy for carcinoma in situ of the true vocal cords. Head Neck 2002; 24(4):390–394. Spayne JA, Warde P, O'Sullivan B, et al. Carcinoma-in-situ of the glottic larynx: results of treatment with radiation therapy. Int J Radiat Oncol Biol Phys 2001; 49(5):1235–1238.

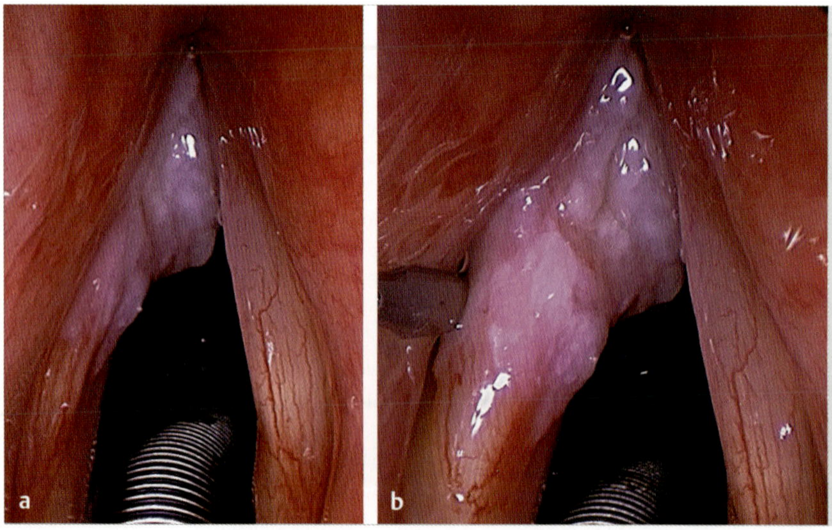

Fig. 14.4 **(a)** Intraoperative views of a T1a left vocal fold carcinoma extending to the anterior commissure. **(b)** Note the small laser-safe endotracheal tube passing into the proximal trachea.

for a glottic lesion can be performed in a focused, narrow field fashion given the extremely low probability of regional lymph node involvement. Open resection of a T1 glottic cancer is now rarely performed with the primary indication being anterior commissure disease that cannot be removed endoscopically.

Both endoscopic resection and radiation offer excellent and comparable local control and disease-free survival (▶ Table 14.2). Considerations for treatment choice often include tumor location, treatment tendencies of a given service, as well as patient preference. The primary consideration in terms of post-treatment quality of life (QOL) for such lesions is voice quality and vocal outcome. Sjogren et al investigated 34 patients, all with a similar T1a midcord squamous cell carcinoma and compared their vocal outcomes with either TLM or radiation. They found no significant differences when evaluating the two groups in acoustic, perceptual, aerodynamic, or stroboscopic analysis.[21] There were no differences between the two groups when evaluated with the Voice Handicap Index (VHI).

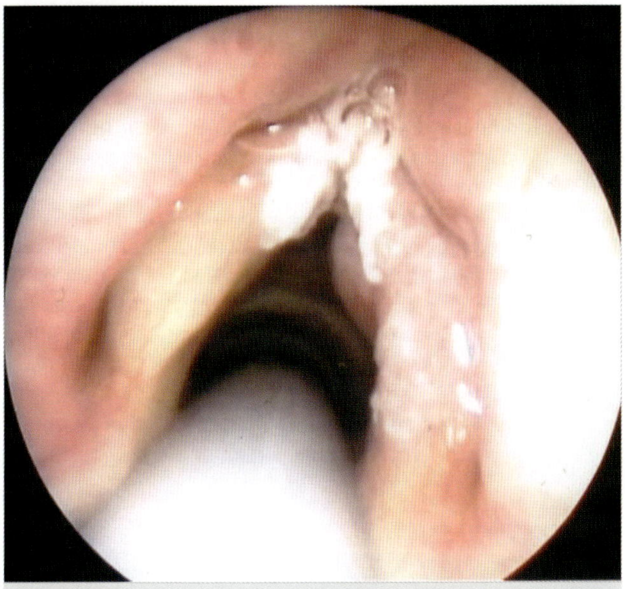

Fig. 14.5 Intraoperative view of a T1b carcinoma of the right true vocal fold crossing the anterior commissure to involve the left true vocal fold.

Lesions involving the anterior commissure can be either T1a tumors (not involving the contralateral vocal fold) or T1b (horseshoe lesions involving both folds) and should be evaluated with imaging prior to planned TLM resection. The anterior commissure tendon (Broyle ligament) represents an area where the anterior portions of the vocal tendons condense with the thyroepiglottic ligament. The important anatomical characteristic of this area is the lack of inner perichondrium, which offers less resistance to spread of anterior glottic tumors. An early-stage glottic cancer can extend to involve the inner aspect of the thyroid cartilage (T3) or completely penetrate through the cartilage (T4) with only a few millimeters of growth. Such tumors can be understaged if only evaluated endoscopically and thus preoperative imaging is recommended for this location.

Management of anterior commissure involvement remains a controversial aspect of the treatment of early laryngeal cancer. Both endoscopic exposure and adequate resection in this area requires technical skill and experience. Roedel et al reviewed their experience with TLM involving the anterior commissure over an 18-year period (1986–2004) and found consistently higher rates of local recurrence for both T1a and T1b tumors with anterior commissure involvement.[22] Radiation therapy for tumors with anterior commissure involvement is also associated with increased rates of recurrence suggesting that such tumors are either difficult to target with radiation, are understaged initially, or both. Open partial surgery such as a vertical partial laryngectomy offers excellent oncologic clearance of the anterior commissure, but generally has a longer recovery and worse functional outcome.

Table 14.2 Treatment results comparing transoral laser microsurgery and radiotherapy for T1 glottic carcinoma

Author	*N*	Treatment	OS (%)	DFS (%)	LC (%)	Recurrence (*N*)
Peretti et al						
2010	404	TLM		99	95	54 (8 TL)
Motta et al						
2005	432	TLM	85	97	96	58
Stoeckli et al 2003	91	TLM	85	96	86	
		RT	88	93	85	
Sjögren et al						
2008	189	TLM (70)	84	99	89	7
		RT (108)	80	92	75	34

Abbreviations: DFS, disease free survival; LC, local control; OS, overall survival; RT, radiotherapy; TL, total laryngectomy; TLM, transoral laser microsurgery.
Sources: Data from Peretti G, Piazza C, Cocco D, et al. Transoral CO_2 laser treatment for Tis-T3 glottic cancer: The University of Brescia experience on 595 patients. Head Neck 2010; 32:977–983. Motta G, Esposito E, Motta S, Tartaro G, Testa D. CO_2 laser surgery in the treatment of glottis cancer. Head Neck 2005; 27:566–574. Stoeckli SJ, Schnieper I, Huguenin P, Schmid S. Early glottis carcinoma: Treatment according pateint's preference? Head Neck 2003; 25(12):1051–1056. Sjogren EV, van Rossum, MA, Langeveld TP, et al. Voice outcome in T1a midcord glottic carcinoma: laser surgery vs. radiotherapy. Arch Otolaryngol Head Neck Surg 2008; 134(9):965–972.

14.5.3 T2 Glottic Carcinoma

T2 glottic cancer will have spread to involve the supraglottis and/or subglottis and/or have some impairment of vocal fold motion, a largely subjective characteristic. Given the wide range that exists within T2 tumors, the treatment of a given tumor is obviously related to its size and location when considering what type of a defect would be created by surgical resection and the local control outcomes with radiotherapy.

The local control and disease-free survival for both TLM and radiation of T2 glottic cancers are comparable (▶ Table 14.3) and thus the treatment decision is primarily related to patient and physician/institution preference as well as a thorough assessment of a given tumor and what deficits would be created by a surgical resection. If a T2 glottic tumor can be removed with a minimal laser resection this may offer the patient the benefit of single modality therapy, good function postoperatively (vocal quality and swallowing), and would reserve radiation therapy for recurrence and/or second tumors of the larynx. On the other hand, a larger T2 glottic tumor may be more suitable for radiotherapy if the predicted surgical defect would leave the patient with significant dysphonia and possible aspiration.

Though the presence or absence of impaired vocal fold mobility is a largely subjective matter, meta-analyses of T2 glottic tumors treated with initial radiotherapy shows significant differences in local control between tumors with and without vocal fold motion impairment. A subclassification of T2 glottic tumors to T2a (without vocal fold motion impairment) and T2b (with impairment) has been suggested given these findings.[23]

14.5.4 T3 Glottic Carcinoma

T3 glottic carcinoma demonstrates deeper penetration of the tumor either laterally into the paraglottic space or anterolaterally to minimally involve the thyroid cartilage. A glottic tumor with vocal fold fixation is, at a minimum, a T3 lesion and suggests deep infiltration of the larynx (paraglottic space) or cricoarytenoid joint involvement by the primary tumor. It is important to keep in mind that a T3 glottic tumor, even in the absence of nodal disease, represents a stage 3 or advanced laryngeal cancer. As detailed earlier, advanced stage (stage 3 or 4) laryngeal cancer is typically managed with multimodality therapy with concurrent chemoradiation being the standard of care for nonsurgical management.[8]

In terms of surgical management of T3 glottic cancer, the gold standard for resection is a total laryngectomy, which offers excellent local contro,l but is less commonly performed as primary treatment given the relative success of organ-preservation treatment strategies. For low-volume T3 glottic tumors, TLM can be performed with similar results to chemotherapy and radiotherapy. Given these issues, however, the case numbers for TLM of T3 glottic tumors are lower (▶ Table 14.4), but do show a trend toward improved local control as compared to primary radiotherapy as single-modality therapy. Success of radiation as a single modality treatment in T3 glottic cancers has been shown to be related to overall tumor volume. Mendenhall et al noted local control of 87% for tumors with total volume < $3.5\ cm^3$ compared with 29% local control for volumes > $3.5\ cm^3$.[24] The current standard of care for nonoperative treatment of T3 glottic cancer is concurrent chemoradiotherapy.

Table 14.3 Treatment results comparing transoral laser microsurgery and radiotherapy for T2 glottic carcinoma

Author	*N*	Treatment	OS (%)	DFS (%)	LC (%)	Recurrence (*N*)
Peretti et al 2010	109	TLM		98	87	24 (5 TL)
Motta et al 2005	236	TLM	77	86	87	84
Grant et al 2007	21	TLM	93	93	93	1
Stoeckli et al 2003	39	TLM	83	83	89	
		RT	78	88	67	
Smee et al 2010	142	RT		85	72	40 (24 TL)
Frata et al 2005	256	RT	59	86	73	62
Garden et al 2003	230	RT	73	92	72	67

Abbreviations: DFS, disease free survival; LC, local control; OS, overall survival; RT, radiotherapy; TL, total laryngectomy; TLM, transoral laser microsurgery.
Sources: Data from Peretti G, Piazza C, Cocco D, et al. Transoral CO_2 laser treatment for Tis-T3 glottic cancer: The University of Brescia experience on 595 patients. Head Neck 2010; 32:977–983. Motta G, Esposito E, Motta S, Tartaro G, Testa D. CO_2 laser surgery in the treatment of glottis cancer. Head Neck 2005; 27:566–574. Grant DG, Salassa JR, Hinni ML, Pearson BW, Hayden RE, Perry WC. Transoral laser microsurgery for untreated glottic carcinoma. Otolaryngol Head Neck Surg 2007; 137(3):482–486. Stoeckli SJ, Schnieper I, Huguenin P, Schmid S. Early glottis carcinoma: treatment according pateint's preference? Head Neck 2003; 25 (12):1051–1056. Smee RI, Meagher NS, Williams JR, Broadley K, Bridger GP. Role of radiotherapy in early glottic carcinoma. Head Neck 2010; 32(7):850–859. Frata P, Cellai E, Magrini SM, et al. Radical radiotherapy for early glottic cancer: results in a series of 1087 patients from two Italian radiation oncology centers. II. The case of T2N0 disease. Int J Radiat Oncol Biol Phys 2005; 63(5):1387–1394. Garden AS, Forster K, Wong PF, Morrison WH, Schechter NR, Ang KK. Results of radiotherapy for T2N0 glottic carcinoma: does the '2' stand for twice-daily treatment? Int J Radiat Oncol Biol Phys 2003; 55(2):322–328.

Table 14.4 Treatment results comparing transoral laser microsurgery and radiotherapy for T3 glottic carcinoma

Author	N	Treatment	OS (%)	DSS (%)	LC (%)	Recurrence
Vilaseca et al 2010	51	TLM	73	86	88	27 (25 TL)
Motta et al 2005	51	TLM	64	72	70	21
Grant et al 2007	10	TLM (T3/T4)	64	40	45	6
Mendenhall et al - 1997	75	RT	51	78	63	25
Johansen et al - 2002	128	RT	43	63	63	62

Abbreviations: DFS, disease free survival; LC, local control; OS, overall survival; RT, radiotherapy; TL, total laryngectomy; TLM, transoral laser microsurgery.
Sources: Data from Vilaseca I, Bernal-Sprekelsen M, Luis Blanch J. Transoral laser microsurgery for T3 laryngeal tumors: Prognostic factors. Head Neck. 2010; 32 (7):929–938. Motta G, Esposito E, Motta S, Tartaro G, Testa D. CO_2 laser surgery in the treatment of glottis cancer. Head Neck *2005; 27:566–574. Grant DG, Salassa JR, Hinni ML, Pearson BW, Hayden RE, Perry WC. Transoral laser microsurgery for untreated glottic carcinoma. Otolaryngol Head Neck Surg 2007; 137 (3):482–486.* Mendenhall WM, Parsons JT, Mancuso AA, Pameijer FJ, Stringer SP, Cassisi NJ. Definitive radiotherapy for T3 squamous cell carcinoma of the glottic larynx. J Clin Oncol *1997; 15(6):2394–2402. Johansen LV, Grau C, Overgaard J. Glottic carcinoma–patterns of failure and salvage treatment after curative radiotherapy in 861 consecutive patients. Radiother Oncol 2002; 63(3):257–267.*

14.5.5 T4 Glottic Carcinoma

T4 glottic cancer is further subdivided into T4a (locally advanced, but resectable) and T4b (very advanced and typically "unresectable"). T4a glottic cancer extends either through the thyroid cartilage or via other anatomic pathways to involve adjacent soft tissue and structures of the neck. Although some T4a tumors may be resectable with a partial laryngeal surgery, the indications and results for this procedure go beyond the scope of this chapter.

Resectable T4 glottic cancer is generally best treated with total laryngectomy followed by postoperative radiation or chemoradiation. Despite the low incidence of nodal metastases in purely glottic cancer, the threshold to perform bilateral neck dissections, including the central neck, should be quite low. There is minimal morbidity to the addition of bilateral lymphadenectomy in experienced hands and it provides definitive surgical treatment in addition to important staging information. As an aside, thorough paratracheal (central neck/ level VI) node dissection is an important aspect of nearly every total laryngectomy; recurrence/persistence of disease in such nodes is a likely cause of peristomal recurrence in the majority of cases in which this occurs. This is of particular important in recurrent tumors and/or tumors with subglottic involvement.

There is disagreement regarding the optimal primary treatment of T4 laryngeal cancer which will be touched upon further in the subsection, Advanced Laryngeal Cancer and Total Laryngectomy. Although some argue that all T4 laryngeal cancers are best treated with total laryngectomy,[25] others feel this depends more upon the bulk of disease and the extent of cartilage destruction. In this context, it is worth noting that the RTOG 91–11 study excluded patients with "large volume T4 disease" defined as tumor extending through cartilage or more than 1 cm into the base of tongue.

14.5.6 Supraglottic Carcinoma

Much like glottic carcinomas, T stage of supraglottic tumors is related to involved subsites and functional impairment (see the box "AJCC tumor staging for laryngeal cancer based on subsite of origin (p. 131)). The basic subsites of the supraglottic larynx are the epiglottis (which has an infrahyoid and suprahyoid subsite), the arytenoid cartilages, the false vocal folds, and the aryepiglottic (AE) folds. Unlike the glottic larynx, the supraglottic larynx is rich in lymphatics as mentioned in the section regarding general management of the neck. This difference is thought to have an embryologic origin as the st"ructures of the supraglottis arise from the primitive buccopharyngeal region, which then meets the glottis and subglottis derived from the tracheobronchial tree. The implications of this have already been mentioned, but treatment of the neck is mandatory for nearly all supraglottic tumors, even in the absence of clinically or radiographically positive lymphadenopathy.

14.5.7 T1 Supraglottic Carcinoma

A T1 supraglottic tumor involves only one subsite of the supraglottic larynx and has no impairment of vocal fold motion. The local control and disease-free survival for an early-stage supraglottic tumor are excellent with either endoscopic resection or primary radiotherapy. There are no randomized trials comparing endoscopic resection with primary radiation, but a review of larger series does show a trend toward improved local control with TLM resection techniques (▶ Table 14.5).

In the absence of clear nodal disease, the treatment options for an early stage supraglottic cancer at our institution are TLM or robotic resection with bilateral neck dissection of levels 2a, 3, and 4, or definitive external-beam radiation to the primary tumor and nodal drainage basins. If the patient is treated with initial surgery, further adjuvant therapy is given based on the

Table 14.5 Treatment results comparing transoral laser microsurgery and radiotherapy for T1 supraglottic carcinoma

Author	*N*	Treatment	OS (%)	DFS (%)	LC (%)	Recurrence (*N*)
Grant et al 2007	8	TLM	100	80	100	1
Motta et al 2004	45	TLM	91	97	98	12
Iro et al 1998	39	TLM		86		8
Johansen et al 2002	154	RT	55	71	67	56
Daugaard & Sand 1998	220	RT			50	
Nakfoor et al 1998	24	RT		78	96	

Abbreviations: DFS, disease free survival; LC, local control; OS, overall survival; RT, radiotherapy; TL, total laryngectomy; TLM, transoral laser microsurgery.
Sources: Data from Grant DG, Salassa JR, Hinni ML, Pearson BW, Hayden RE, Perry WC. Transoral laser microsurgery for carcinoma of the supraglottic larynx. Otolaryngol Head Neck Surg 2007; 136(6):900–906. Motta G, Esposito E, Testa D, Iovine R, Motta S. CO_2 laser treatment of supraglottic cancer. Head Neck *2004; 26(5):442–446. Iro H, Waldfahrer F, Altendorf-Hofmann A, Weidenbecher M, Sauer R, Steiner W. Transoral laser surgery of supraglottic cancer: follow-up of 141 patients. Arch Otolaryngol Head Neck Surg 1998; 124(11):1245–1250. Johansen LV, Grau C, Overgaard J. Supraglottic carcinoma: patterns of failure and salvage treatment after curatively intended radiotherapy in 410 consecutive patients. Int J Radiat Oncol Biol Phys 2002; 53(4):948–958. Daugaard BJ, Sand* HH. Primary radiotherapy of carcinoma of the supraglottic larynx–a multivariate analysis of prognostic factors. Int J Radiat Oncol Biol Phys *1998; 41(2):355–360. Nakfoor BM, Spiro IJ, Wang CC, Martins P, Montgomery W, Fabian R. Results of accelerated radiotherapy for supraglottic carcinoma: a Massachusetts General Hospital and Massachusetts Eye and Ear Infirmary experience. Head Neck 1998; 20(5):379–384.*

characteristics (perineural and lymphovascular invasion) and margins of the primary tumor as well as the pathologic evaluation of the cervical node dissection. Given the rich lymphatics of the supraglottis, what are thought to be early-stage tumors can often have nodal metastases and require postoperative radiation or chemoradiation.

14.5.8 T2 Supraglottic Carcinoma

The treatment options for a T2 supraglottic tumor are similar to a T1 lesion, but the resection is likely to be more extensive and the postoperative morbidity, primarily in the form of dysphagia, may be significant. In similar fashion to patients undergoing open partial laryngeal surgery, those being considered for endoscopic resection either with a TLM technique or robotic resection should be able to tolerate some degree of aspiration and be motivated to engage in speech and swallow rehabilitation postoperatively. Although the dysphagia results from endoscopic resections appear to be improved compared with open partial resections, patient selection remains an important consideration.

T2 supraglottic tumors frequently have nodal metastases, making them advanced stage (III or IV) tumors, which may require multimodality therapy. This fact is an important treatment consideration for supraglottic tumors in general: If a patient is likely to require postoperative radiation or chemoradiation based on their neck disease, this must be taken into consideration when considering surgical resection as primary therapy. It may not make sense to expose such a patient to the possible morbidity of surgery without conferring survival benefit if they may require radiation or chemoradiation in the postoperative period based on the extent of their pretreatment locoregional disease.

14.5.9 T3 Supraglottic Carcinoma

There are several surgical options for T3 supraglottic tumors. They can often be successfully managed with a supraglottic laryngectomy and bilateral neck dissection, particularly if the T3 designation is based upon pre-epiglottic space invasion. In that circumstance, either a TLM or TORS approach is appropriate, as described above for T2 lesions. Total laryngectomy with bilateral neck dissection and postoperative therapy may also be indicated. However, similar to T3 glottic cancer, this is less commonly performed as primary treatment given the relative success of nonoperative therapies and the ability to successfully salvage recurrences with a total laryngectomy.[26,27]

14.5.10 T4 Supraglottic Carcinoma

T4 supraglottic tumors are divided into T4a and T4b tumors in similar fashion to glottic T staging. For advanced tumors of the larynx, regardless of subsite, the mainstay of surgical treatment is total laryngectomy. Depending on the depth and degree of primary tumor extension, some supraglottic tumors treated with primary laryngectomy may require either a regional or free microvascular flap closure, particularly if there is significant extension to the base of tongue and/or lateral pharyngeal wall.

Some select T4 supraglottic tumors may be managed with partial laryngeal resections of either an open (supraglottic or supracricoid) or endoscopic variety, but these instances represent the exception as opposed to the rule. Nonsurgical management of a T4 supraglottic cancer should be with combined modality therapy (chemoradiation), but such lesions may achieve the best oncologic outcomes with primary surgery.[25]

14.5.11 Subglottic Carcinoma

Primary subglottic carcinoma represents an uncommon site of laryngeal cancer and likely accounts for less than 5% of all laryngeal tumors. Subglottic carcinomas will most commonly present with symptoms of hoarseness and/or airway obstruction and are often of an advanced T stage at diagnosis. T staging of subglottic carcinoma is similar to that of glottic carcinoma, with extension superiorly to the vocal folds or vocal fold motion impairment rendering a tumor a T2 lesion and fixation of a vocal fold again representing T3 disease. Highly selected early-stage subglottic carcinoma may be amenable to endoscopic resection, but the majority of subglottic cancers are managed with either initial nonoperative treatment (radiation or chemoradiation) or total laryngectomy.

14.5.12 Advanced Laryngeal Cancer and Total Laryngectomy

Even though many patients who undergo total laryngectomy develop functional alaryngeal speech and swallow without difficulty, the removal of a patient's larynx and creation of a permanent stoma is a life-changing event with long-term consequences. Not surprisingly, laryngeal preservation is preferred by most, particularly when the survival offered with initial nonsurgical treatment is comparable.

Retrospective analysis of laryngeal cancer treatment trends from 1985 to 2001 revealed an increase in initial nonsurgical management of laryngeal cancer—in particular for patients with locally advanced disease that would require total laryngectomy. Further analysis of particular tumor stages revealed a statistically significant decrease in survival for patients with T3N0 cancer of both the larynx (all subsites) and the glottis when they were treated nonoperatively.[26] In this review, however, nonoperative management included both patients treated with chemoradiation as well as radiation alone as a single modality. When the patients treated with initial chemoradiotherapy, the current standard of care for nonoperative treatment of advanced laryngeal cancer, were compared to surgery with or without postoperative radiation, the statistical significance of the survival difference was resolved. These findings further validate the use of concurrent therapy as the standard of care from an organ preservation standpoint.

There is a lack of consensus regarding which patients are best served by initial total laryngectomy. Although some argue that all T4 tumors should be treated with initial laryngectomy, others believe only certain T4 tumors are best suited by initial resection. It is undoubtedly true, however, that there are patients who present with advanced laryngeal cancers that are best managed with total laryngectomy prior to further treatment. Factors that should be considered in such cases are tumor volume, degree of cartilage destruction/penetration, and depth of invasion into surrounding structures. Perhaps most important, however, is the key factor of presenting functional status. If a patient requires a tracheotomy, gastrostomy tube, or both prior to initial treatment, the functional status of their larynx is significantly reduced and should lead one to consider primary surgical treatment. Despite the obvious issues associated with the creation of a permanent stoma, total laryngectomy can often provide improved function both in terms of swallowing and rehabilitated speech in such patients.

14.5.13 Voice Rehabilitation Following Total Laryngectomy

The loss of natural voice can be a devastating prospect for patients undergoing total laryngectomy. A decreased ability to communicate in an effective and fluid manner can lead to a significantly decreased QOL. The ability to rehabilitate and create alaryngeal speech is thus a critical component in the overall treatment of patients requiring total laryngectomy.

Total laryngectomy entails disconnection of the normally combined aerodigestive tract. The neopharynx is created either through primary closure or with the use of regional or free-flap reconstruction. The junction of the neopharynx and the proximal cervical esophagus functions as the neolarynx with vibration of the mucosal tissues functioning as the source of sound in alaryngeal speech.

Three means of speech rehabilitation exist for patients after total laryngectomy: the artificial larynx, esophageal speech, and tracheoesophageal puncture (TEP). The artificial larynx, or electrolarynx, is a handheld device that is typically placed against the neck and transmits a vibratory sound into the tissues and the pharynx; the remaining portions of the pharynx and oral cavity (palate, tongue, and lips) then articulate the sound into words. The electrolarynx has the advantage of easy acquisition and can also be used early in a patient's postoperative course. Although patients often use the artificial larynx for their long-term speech rehabilitation, negatives of its use include a mechanical voice, lack of hands-free speech, and the continuous need for battery power.

Esophageal speech is the opposite of the electrolarynx in that it allows for hands-free speech, requires no device or prosthesis, and is difficult to acquire and master. The details and methods of esophageal speech go beyond the scope of this chapter, but the mechanics of such speed production involve autoinsufflation of the esophagus and subsequent cephalad airflow through the pharyngoesophageal junction. Mucosal vibration within this area produces sound that is further augmented within the oropharynx and oral cavity. Once learned, esophageal speech produces speech with fluency and excellent voice quality. Esophageal speech, however, often has a long acquisition period and is difficult to master. Success in acquiring esophageal speech often requires extensive work with speech-language pathologists. These characteristics make esophageal speech the least commonly used form of alaryngeal speech following total laryngectomy.

The trachea–esophagus procedure (TEP), first described by Blom and Singer in 1980, makes use of the vibratory potential of the pharyngoesophageal junction in a similar fashion to esophageal speech.[27] The TEP was initially described as a secondary procedure performed endoscopically following a successful laryngectomy, but is now commonly performed at the time of laryngectomy (primary) as well as in a delayed fashion (secondary). The procedure creates a communication between the tracheostoma and the cervical esophagus inferior to the upper esophageal sphincter. A prosthesis that functions as a one-way valve is then introduced into the controlled fistula. The valve allows air to flow from the lungs into the esophagus below the pharyngoesophageal junction and then creates mucosal vibration, which is further augmented as in other forms of alaryngeal speech. A functioning valve does not allow aspiration of pharyngeal secretions into the tracheostoma.

The TEP is now the most commonly used method of alaryngeal speech rehabilitation. The procedure has a high rate of success when performed both as a primary or secondary procedure with larger series showing acquisition rates over 90% for primary TEP and 75 to 85% success for secondary TEP.[28,29] TEP speech is associated with improved speech outcomes both in terms of objective measures as well as patient satisfaction when compared to other methods of speech rehabilitation and communication.[30]

Primary TEP is now commonly performed in patients requiring salvage laryngectomy after radiation or chemoradiation failures. The procedure may also be performed in patient's requiring flap closure for partial or total pharyngeal defects with good results.[31]

A full discussion regarding the management of prosthesis and failures of TEP speech goes beyond the scope of this chapter. However, if one thinks of the requirements for TEP speech to be a driving force of airflow (the patient's lungs and general abilities) as well as pliable tissues, which can serve as a vibratory surface within the neopharynx the causes of TEP speech failures derive directly from these requirements. Patients with severe chronic obstructive pulmonary disorder, malnutrition, and the inability to perform the complex steps to produce alaryngeal speech are unable to produce the driving force for TEP speech. On the other hand, patients with strictured, previously radiated, and/or bulky, nonpliable flaps may experience difficulty from less than ideal vibratory tissues.

14.6 Recurrence and Salvage

Inherent to the increased use of nonoperative treatment for laryngeal cancer— in particular, advanced laryngeal cancer—is the need for surgical salvage should the initial treatment strategy fail and the patient present with persistent or recurrent tumor. Though some patients with persistent or recurrent disease may be managed with partial laryngeal resection, the majority is treated with total laryngectomy. Determination of which patients may be managed with a partial surgery goes beyond the scope of this chapter, but of critical importance to such situations is that the surgeon who will perform the salvage surgery has seen and evaluated the patient, ideally with formal endoscopy, prior to the administration of radiation or chemoradiation. In the absence of this detailed knowledge of the initial tumor, the surgeon is often left with operative descriptions and imaging studies in an effort to reconstruct the extent of the presenting tumor.

Survival data for recurrent laryngeal cancer treated with salvage surgery reveal superior outcomes[32] compared with other head and neck subsites.[33] The success of salvage surgery for laryngeal cancer is, not surprisingly, related to the recurrent tumor stage. In a small series ($N = 43$) of initial T1 and T2 cancers of the glottis treated by radiotherapy and requiring salvage surgery (both partial laryngectomy and total laryngectomy), Ganly et al from Memorial Sloan Kettering (New York, NY) demonstrated significantly improved disease-specific and overall survival for patients with recurrent disease of T stages 1 or 2 as compared to stages 3 and 4.[34]

The data for retrospective analyses, however, is typically pooled data and includes nonuniform patient populations. In terms of laryngeal cancer, this may include many patients treated only with radiation as opposed to chemoradiation as is now more commonplace. Although there is less data regarding the ability to salvage patients who have failed chemoradiation, it is reasonable to expect slightly worsened results with tumors that have endured multimodality therapy; consequently, they may display more aggressive and resistant behavior.

The effects of nonoperative therapy also complicate the success of salvage laryngeal surgery. Secondary to microvascular changes of radiation and the potentiating effect of concurrent chemotherapy, the tissue characteristics and wound-healing potential of patients treated with radiation and chemoradiation are severely compromised.[35] Not surprisingly, this results in significantly increased rates of wound complications and pharyngocutaneous fistulas; in addition, patients undergoing salvage surgery often develop postoperative strictures, which can lead to dysphagia and speech-rehabilitation difficulties. These increased complication rates, in particular pharyngocutaneous fistulas, have led to increased use of either regional or free-tissue transfer in salvage laryngectomy.

The most commonly used regional flap, the pectoralis major myocutaneous flap, can be used with either a skin paddle integrated into the anterior aspect of the pharyngeal closure or as a muscle-only flap used to reinforce a primarily closed pharynx. Although there is some debate as to whether such a strategy results in lower fistula rates or improved healing of fistulas that occur at the expected rate, the use of such flaps in salvage procedures is increasing.[36]

Free tissue transfer has also been increasingly used in salvage laryngectomies with decreased fistula rates as well. Free flaps can be used in a similar fashion to pectoralis major flaps as either a reinforcing flap or as one integrated into the pharyngeal closure. The introduction of vascular, pliable, nonradiated tissue may not only improve the immediate postoperative wound healing in salvage procedures, but may also lead to improved functional outcomes in terms of swallowing and speech rehabilitation.[37]

14.7 Key Points

- The unique characteristics of the human larynx and preservation of those functions and features are the driving force behind treatment of laryngeal malignancy.
- The incidence of laryngeal cancer is decreasing, but the overall 5-year survival rate has remained essentially unchanged since the 1970s.
- Careful history taking with attention to symptoms of pain, dysphagia, and dysphonia provides important information regarding which aspect of the larynx is affected by a malignancy.
- Patients with suspected laryngeal malignancy should be promptly referred to the likely treating institution or physician(s) for initial imaging and endoscopy.
- Close communication with anesthesia colleagues and careful examination with angled endoscopes provide the safest and most thorough examination of the larynx.

- Tumor staging of laryngeal cancer is unique and requires detailed knowledge of anatomy and function for proper staging and treatment,
- Early-stage (1 and 2) disease can often be treated by single-modality therapy; advanced-stage disease (3 and 4) typically requires multimodality therapy.
- Local control and voice outcomes for early glottic cancer treated with TLM and radiation are comparable.
- Compromised laryngeal function and the need for either tracheotomy or gastrostomy tube placement at presentation are important considerations when formulating a treatment plan and attempting nonoperative therapy for a locally advanced laryngeal cancer.
- Salvage surgery after chemotherapy and radiotherapy has a much higher incidence of wound complications, and tissue transfer should be routinely considered.

References

[1] Curado MP, Hashibe M. Recent changes in the epidemiology of head and neck cancer. Curr Opin Oncol 2009; 21: 194–200

[2] Bahar G, Feinmesser R, Popovtzer A et al. Basaloid squamous carcinoma of the larynx. Am J Otolaryngol 2003; 24: 204–208

[3] Huang SH, Lockwood G, Irish J et al. Truths and myths about radiotherapy for verrucous carcinoma of larynx. Int J Radiat Oncol Biol Phys 2009; 73: 1110–1115

[4] Tami TA, Ferlito A, Rinaldo A, Lee KC, Singh B. Laryngeal pathology in the acquired immunodeficiency syndrome: diagnostic and therapeutic dilemmas. Ann Otol Rhinol Laryngol 1999; 108: 214–220

[5] Thabet HM, Sessions DG, Gado MH, Gnepp DA, Harvey JE, Talaat M. Comparison of clinical evaluation and computed tomographic diagnostic accuracy for tumors of the larynx and hypopharynx. Laryngoscope 1996; 106: 589–594

[6] Branstetter BF, Blodgett TM, Zimmer LA et al. Head and neck malignancy: is PET/CT more accurate than PET or CT alone? Radiology 2005; 235: 580–586

[7] Wolf G, Hong K, Fisher S et al. The Department of Veterans Affairs Laryngeal Cancer Study Group. Induction chemotherapy plus radiation compared with surgery plus radiation in patients with advanced laryngeal cancer. N Engl J Med 1991; 324: 1685–1690

[8] Forastiere AA, Goepfert H, Maor M et al. Concurrent chemotherapy and radiotherapy for organ preservation in advanced laryngeal cancer. N Engl J Med 2003; 349: 2091–2098

[9] Holsinger FC, Kies MS, Diaz EM et al. Durable long-term remission with chemotherapy alone for stage II to IV laryngeal cancer. J Clin Oncol 2009; 27: 1976–1982

[10] Holsinger FC, Lin HY, Bassot V, Laccourreye O. Platin-based exclusive chemotherapy for selected patients with squamous cell carcinoma of the larynx and pharynx. Cancer 2009; 115: 3909–3918

[11] Cooper JS, Pajak TF, Forastiere AA et al. Radiation Therapy Oncology Group 9501/Intergroup. Postoperative concurrent radiotherapy and chemotherapy for high-risk squamous-cell carcinoma of the head and neck. N Engl J Med 2004; 350: 1937–1944

[12] Bernier J, Domenge C, Ozsahin M et al. European Organization for Research and Treatment of Cancer Trial 22931. Postoperative irradiation with or without concomitant chemotherapy for locally advanced head and neck cancer. N Engl J Med 2004; 350: 1945–1952

[13] Kirchner JA, Carter D. Intralaryngeal barriers to the spread of cancer. Acta Otolaryngol 1987; 103: 503–513

[14] Yang CY, Andersen PE, Everts EC, Cohen JI. Nodal disease in purely glottic carcinoma: is elective neck treatment worthwhile? Laryngoscope 1998; 108: 1006–1008

[15] Lindberg R. Distribution of cervical lymph node metastases from squamous cell carcinoma of the upper respiratory and digestive tracts. Cancer 1972; 29: 1446–1449

[16] Ambrosch P. The role of laser microsurgery in the treatment of laryngeal cancer. Curr Opin Otolaryngol Head Neck Surg 2007; 15: 82–88

[17] Cavanagh JP, Hart RD, Brown T, Trites JRB, Brake M, Taylor SM. Laryngeal reconstruction following CO2 laser surgery for glottic cancer. Head Neck 2009; 31: 1369–1376

[18] National Comprehensive Cancer Network (NCCN) Guidelines 2012

[19] Garden AS, Morrison WH, Ang KK. Larynx and hypopharynx cancer. In: Gunderson LL, Tepper JE, eds. Clinical Radiation Oncology. 3rd ed. Philadelphia, PA: Elsevier Saunders: 2012; 639–664

[20] Feng FY, Kim HM, Lyden TH et al. Intensity-modulated chemoradiotherapy aiming to reduce dysphagia in patients with oropharyngeal cancer: clinical and functional results. J Clin Oncol 2010; 28: 2732–2738

[21] Sjögren EV, van Rossum MA, Langeveld TP et al. Voice outcome in T1a midcord glottic carcinoma: laser surgery vs radiotherapy. Arch Otolaryngol Head Neck Surg 2008; 134: 965–972

[22] Rödel RM, Steiner W, Müller RM, Kron M, Matthias C. Endoscopic laser surgery of early glottic cancer: involvement of the anterior commissure. Head Neck 2009; 31: 583–592

[23] McCoul ED, Har-El G. Meta-analysis of impaired vocal cord mobility as a prognostic factor in T2 glottic carcinoma. Arch Otolaryngol Head Neck Surg 2009; 135: 479–486

[24] Mendenhall WM, Parsons JT, Mancuso AA, Pameijer FJ, Stringer SP, Cassisi NJ. Definitive radiotherapy for T3 squamous cell carcinoma of the glottic larynx. J Clin Oncol 1997; 15: 2394–2402

[25] Gourin CG, Conger BT, Sheils WC, Bilodeau PA, Coleman TA, Porubsky ES. The effect of treatment on survival in patients with advanced laryngeal carcinoma. Laryngoscope 2009; 119: 1312–1317

[26] Hoffman HT, Porter K, Karnell LH et al. Laryngeal cancer in the United States: changes in demographics, patterns of care, and survival. Laryngoscope 2006; 116 Suppl 111: 1–13

[27] Singer MI, Blom ED. An endoscopic technique for restoration of voice after laryngectomy. Ann Otol Rhinol Laryngol 1980; 89: 529–533

[28] Kao WW, Mohr RM, Kimmel CA, Getch C, Silverman C. The outcome and techniques of primary and secondary tracheoesophageal puncture. Arch Otolaryngol Head Neck Surg 1994; 120: 301–307

[29] Chone CT, Gripp FM, Spina AL, Crespo AN. Primary versus secondary tracheoesophageal puncture for speech rehabilitation in total laryngectomy: long-term results with indwelling voice prosthesis. Otolaryngol Head Neck Surg 2005; 133: 89–93

[30] Clements KS, Rassekh CH, Seikaly H, Hokanson JA, Calhoun KH. Communication after laryngectomy. An assessment of patient satisfaction. Arch Otolaryngol Head Neck Surg 1997; 123: 493–496

[31] Yu P, Lewin JS, Reece GP, Robb GL. Comparison of clinical and functional outcomes and hospital costs following pharyngoesophageal reconstruction with the anterolateral thigh free flap versus the jejunal flap. Plast Reconstr Surg 2006; 117: 968–974

[32] Weber RS, Berkey BA, Forastiere AA et al. Outcome of salvage total laryngectomy following organ preservation therapy: the Radiation Therapy Oncology Group trial 91-11. Arch Otolaryngol Head Neck Surg 2003; 129: 44–49

[33] Agra IM, Carvalho AL, Ulbrich FS et al. Prognostic factors in salvage surgery for recurrent oral and oropharyngeal cancer. Head Neck 2006; 28: 107–113

[34] Ganly I, Patel SG, Matsuo J et al. Results of surgical salvage after failure of definitive radiation therapy for early-stage squamous cell carcinoma of the glottic larynx. Arch Otolaryngol Head Neck Surg 2006; 132: 59–66

[35] Paydarfar JA, Birkmeyer NJ. Complications in head and neck surgery: a meta-analysis of postlaryngectomy pharyngocutaneous fistula. Arch Otolaryngol Head Neck Surg 2006; 132: 67–72

[36] Gil Z, Gupta A, Kummer B et al. The role of pectoralis major muscle flap in salvage total laryngectomy. Arch Otolaryngol Head Neck Surg 2009; 135: 1019–1023

[37] Withrow KP, Rosenthal EL, Gourin CG et al. Free tissue transfer to manage salvage laryngectomy defects after organ preservation failure. Laryngoscope 2007; 117: 781–784

15 Chronic Aspiration

Ahmad I. Al Omari and C. Kwang Sung

In addition to managing respiration and vocalization, the major function of the larynx is protection of the airway during swallowing through several mechanisms. The vocal folds adduct to seal the glottis, and the arytenoids tilt forward to contact the epiglottis base before the opening of the upper esophageal sphincter.[1,2] The hyoid bone and the larynx are pulled upward and forward by contraction of the suprahyoid muscles and the thyrohyoid muscle. The epiglottis tilts backward to seal the laryngeal vestibule. At times these mechanisms fail, leading to aspiration.

Aspiration is defined as passage of secretions, ingested solids and liquids, or refluxed or regurgitated gastric contents below the level of the true vocal folds.[3] In contrast, laryngeal penetration occurs when material enters the larynx above the true vocal folds, but does not go beyond.[4] Laryngeal penetration is sometimes observed in normal individuals. Aspiration of microscopic quantities also occurs in normal individuals; however, aspiration that is visible on fluoroscopy or endoscopy is pathologic and associated with an increased risk of aspiration pneumonia or airway obstruction and requires careful assessment and management to prevent life-threatening complications.[5]

15.1 Causes of Aspiration

Aspiration is due to impairment of the laryngeal airway protective mechanism that results from loss of motor activity and/or sensation of the larynx. Aspiration may be an isolated event due to temporary impairment of the airway protective mechanism, as found in alcohol-, drug-, seizure-, or anesthesia-related decreased level of consciousness. Chronic or intractable pulmonary aspiration refers to the repeated or long-term inhalation of foreign material into the tracheobronchial tree,[6] which is most commonly seen in neurologic disorders, with stroke being the most frequent, especially those involving the brainstem with bilateral cranial nerve palsies. The box "Common causes of chronic aspiration (p. 142)" lists the common causes of chronic aspiration.[7]

15.2 History

Patients with chronic aspiration may present with cough and frequent throat clearing, recurrent chest infections and fever, voice changes, and weight loss. Airway obstruction, laryngospasm, pulmonary abscess, sepsis, and death all are possible. Many factors determine the consequences of aspiration, including the volume of aspirate, the pH of the aspirate (more acidic is more damaging to the lungs, producing chemical pneumonitis), the depth of the aspiration material in the airway and the status of the pulmonary clearance mechanism.[8] A detailed history of associated symptoms such as dysphagia, regurgitation, weakness, tremor, and loss of coordination will help to identify the underlying cause of aspiration. It is mandatory to inquire about previous history of neurologic and neuromuscular disorders, trauma, head and neck cancer, surgery, and radiotherapy. A full list of medications should be obtained.

Common causes of chronic aspiration

Cerebrovascular accidents
- Ischemic
- Hemorrhagic

Degenerative neurologic disorders
- Parkinson disease
- Amyotrophic lateral sclerosis
- Progressive supranuclear palsy
- Multiple sclerosis
- Huntington disease

Dementia
- Alzheimer disease
- Lewy body dementia
- Vascular dementia

Neuromuscular and muscular disorders
- Myasthenia gravis
- Poliomyelitis
- Muscular dystrophies

Peripheral nerve disorders
- Guillain-Barre syndrome
- Postviral neuropathy

Trauma
- Traumatic brain injury
- Hematoma
- Neck trauma

Tumors
- Brain tumors
- Peripheral nerve tumors

Iatrogenic
- Head and neck cancer surgery
- Anterior cervical spine surgery
- Thyroid/parathyroid surgery
- Cardiothoracic surgery

Pharyngeal disorders
- Neoplasms
- Postradiation changes
- Cricopharyngeal dysfunction
- Zenker diverticulum
- Stricture
- Cervical osteophytosis

Esophageal disorders
- Neoplasms
- Stricture
- Achalasia
- Esophageal dysmotility
- Gastroesophageal reflux

15.3 Physical Examination

A thorough examination of the of the head and neck should focus on the anatomical integrity of the upper aerodigestive tract with careful assessment of cranial nerve function, including tongue movement, wasting and fasciculation, as well as absence of the gag and cough reflexes, and loss of the pharyngeal and laryngeal sensation. Indirect mirror laryngoscopy or flexible nasolaryngoscopy are used to examine the pharynx and larynx. Pooling of secretion in the vallecula, pyriform sinuses, and postcricoid region should be noted. Careful assessment of vocal fold mobility and glottic competence is extremely important as aspiration occurs in 44% of patients with unilateral vocal fold immobility and 57% of those with bilateral vocal fold immobility.[9] The examiner should then move on to the general physical examination to assess for any pulmonary complications of aspiration as well as find any evidence of neurologic disease or possible underlying causes for aspiration. The general condition of the patient should be noted to determine the severity of aspiration and the need for urgent management.

15.4 Diagnostic Testing

An understanding of the possible underlying cause of aspiration may emerge after a complete history and physical examination; however, for precise diagnosis and management of aspiration, diagnostic studies are required to complete the workup. The order in which tests may be carried out will depend on the clinical findings. The highest clinical yield tests for evaluating patients with an incompetent larynx are videofluoroscopic swallowing study and fibroptic endoscopic evaluation of swallowing.

15.4.1 Chest Radiography

A number of patterns of pulmonary infiltrates may be seen in a patient with chronic aspiration complicated by aspiration pneumonia. Consolidation in a dependent lung segment is usually seen. The basal segments of the lower lobes are typically involved if the patient was in the upright position during aspiration, while the posterior segments of the upper lobes or apical segments of lower lobes are involved if the patient was in the supine position.[8]

15.4.2 Videofluoroscopic Swallowing Study

Also known as modified barium swallow (MBS), videofluoroscopic swallowing study (VFSS) allows the visualization of bolus trajectory in relation to structures throughout the upper aerodigestive tract in real time. The details of VFSS are described in other chapters of this book. In brief, various volumes and textures of liquid and food mixed with barium contrast are administered and a clinical impression of swallowing is obtained from the fluoroscopic images (▶ Fig. 15.1).[10,11] The VFSS can be used to develop a treatment plan for patients with impaired swallow function. When the pharyngeal swallow is initiated, five mechanical events that protect the airway and clear the pharynx can be observed by VFSS: elevation and retraction of the soft palate, elevation and anterior displacement of the larynx and hyoid bone, laryngeal closure, pharyngeal contraction, and opening of the pharyngoesophageal region.[12] The Penetration-Aspiration Scale is often used to assess the presence and the severity of aspiration.[13]

15.4.3 Fiberoptic Endoscopic Evaluation of Swallowing

Fiberoptic endoscopic evaluation of swallowing (FEES) allows assessment of the competency of airway protection as well as the effectiveness of compensatory maneuvers, postures, bolus modifications, and sensory encouragements in improving the safety of swallowing.[14,15] The examination includes anatomical and physiological evaluation to identify any potential bolus obstruction or abnormal movement (e.g., tremor, myoclonus). Pre-swallow aspiration is usually a result of posterior oral spillage and/or delay in swallowing initiation. Aspiration during the swallow typically occurs because of the failure of one or more of the laryngeal closure mechanisms. Aspiration after the

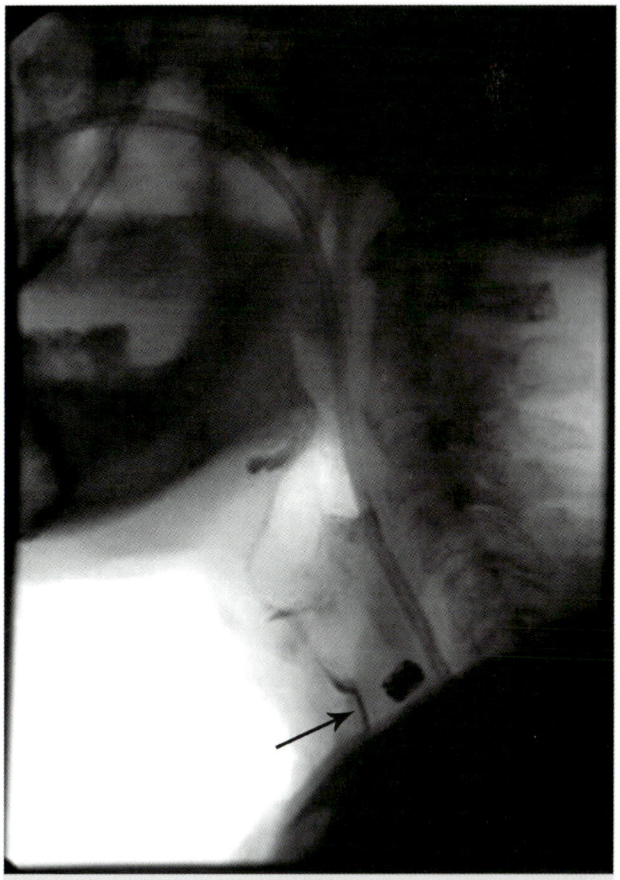

Fig. 15.1 Aspiration of thin liquid. Note barium along anterior tracheal wall (*arrow*).

swallow occurs when residue in the vallecula or pyriform sinuses falls into the airway after the swallow is finished.[16]

15.4.4 Fiberoptic Endoscopic Evaluation of Swallowing with Sensory Testing

Fiberoptic endoscopic evaluation of swallowing with sensory testing (FEESST) combines the established endoscopic evaluation of swallowing with sensory testing using modified equipment that determines laryngopharyngeal sensory discrimination thresholds by delivering air pulse stimuli to the mucosa innervated by the superior laryngeal nerve.[17]

15.4.5 Bolus Scintigraphy

Bolus scintigraphy is a technique that permits both a functional and a semiquantitative study to estimate the amount of inhaled bolus.[18,19] It is limited by poor definition in visualizing anatomical structures and low specificity.

15.5 Conservative Management of Aspiration

The primary intent of the clinical evaluation of patients with swallowing disorders and chronic aspiration is to define the presence and cause of aspiration, and to determine a plan to improve swallowing efficacy and safety to prevent its life-threatening complications. The treatment plan can utilize compensatory strategies or surgical procedures depending on the individual patient, the characteristic of swallowing impairment, and the severity of aspiration. Conservative management of aspiration typically begins with trial of compensatory strategies.

15.5.1 Swallow Posture Adjustments

Changes in head or body posture are compensatory techniques that may be recommended to reduce aspiration or pharyngeal residue. They have been shown to eliminate aspiration of at least one bolus of liquid in up to 77% of patients.[20] However, the efficacy of posture techniques can differ with the type of swallowing disorder.[21] These positions may be used individually or in combination to improve swallowing and prevent aspiration.

Chin Tuck

This is also referred to as "chin down." The patient is asked to touch the chin to the chest while swallowing, which causes narrowing of the laryngeal entrance. This improves airway protection and is useful for patients with decreased laryngeal elevation, reduced tongue base movement, and decreased laryngeal vestibule closure.[22] It has been reported to eliminate aspiration in 72% of patients with various medical diagnoses.[21]

Head Rotation

The patient is instructed to rotate the head toward the weak side. This closes the side of the pharynx toward which the head is rotated and bolus flow is directed primarily toward the normal side. It is useful in cases of unilateral pharyngeal wall paresis or paralysis or unilateral laryngeal paralysis to decrease residue after swallow.[21,23] Either performed alone or with other postural changes, it is effective in reducing aspiration in postsurgical head and neck cancer patients up to 71% of the time.[24]

Head Tilt

This position is used if the patient has trouble with the oral transit and pharyngeal impairment on the same side. The patient tilts the head toward the stronger side to direct the bolus down with the gravity away from the weak side.[20]

15.5.2 Swallowing Maneuvers

Various maneuvers can be used by patients to control the pharyngeal phase of swallowing and decrease the risk of aspiration. The efficacy of the maneuvers in preventing aspiration is often assessed as part of the VFSS or FEES.

Supraglottic Swallow Maneuver

The patient is instructed to breathe in and hold the breath immediately prior to swallowing. The breath hold continues during the swallow and the patient is asked to cough immediately after the swallow to expel any residue from the larynx, then repeat the swallow.[12] This maneuver results in earlier cricopharyngeal opening, prolonged pharyngeal swallow, change in extent of vertical laryngeal position before the swallow, and prolonged airway closure.[23]

Supersupraglottic Swallow Maneuver

The supersupraglottic swallow includes the same steps as the supraglottic swallow, but during the voluntary breath hold the patient is asked to bear down, increasing the effort of closure resulting in earlier cricopharyngeal opening, prolonging pharyngeal swallow, increasing laryngeal valving and changing the vertical laryngeal position before swallow. These changes are more effective and maintained longer than in the supraglottic swallow.[15] It is useful for patients who have undergone supraglottic laryngectomy[25] as well as patients who have received radiotherapy to the head and neck.[26]

Effortful Swallow Maneuver

During this maneuver, the patient is asked to maximally squeeze all of the muscles of swallowing. This increases the force of tongue propulsion and contact against the posterior pharyngeal wall,[27] improving bolus clearance from the vallecula.[12] The effortful swallow results in further anterior excursion of the hyoid in the superior direction, longer duration of laryngeal vestibule closure, and upper esophageal sphincter opening, and decreased oral residue.[28] It may be used with patients who have reduced tongue strength, reduced pharyngeal contraction, reduced laryngeal elevation, reduced laryngeal vestibular closure, or cricopharyngeal dysfunction.[29]

Mendelsohn Maneuver

The Mendelsohn maneuver is a voluntary prolongation of laryngeal excursion at the midpoint of the swallow.[30] This increases the extent and duration of laryngeal elevation, thus increasing the duration and width of cricopharyngeal opening and improving the overall coordination of the swallow.[12] The patient is instructed to swallow normally. At the middle of swallow, when the larynx is felt to elevate, the patient is instructed to keep the larynx elevated for 2 seconds and then relax.[31] The Mendelsohn maneuver is useful for patients with reduced laryngeal movement, delayed or reduced cricopharyngeal opening, or discoordinated swallow.[32]

15.5.3 Bolus Size and Diet Modification

The risk of aspiration in the dysphagic patient can be mitigated by changing diet consistency and bolus volume. Thickened liquid diets are popular to manage aspiration and often used in conjunction with a chin-tuck posture.[32,33] Large bolus volumes may provide better sensory awareness of the bolus in the oral cavity,[34] while smaller bolus sizes are more useful in patients who require multiple swallows to clear a single bolus.[35]

If initial compensatory maneuvers and bolus modifications fail to eliminate aspiration, management should include more aggressive treatment to prevent life-threatening pulmonary complications. This may include antibiotics, chest physiotherapy, and frequent suctioning of secretions from the mouth and pharynx. In addition, prevention of further aspiration can be assisted with interventions that maintain the nutritional status of the patient by alternative routes.

Nasogastric (NG) feeding tubes are a time proven technique to provide nutritional support; although its prolonged use can lead to complications such as injury to the nose or nasal cavity, sinusitis, gastroesophageal reflux and aspiration pneumonia.[36] Its efficacy in reducing aspiration is equivocal, and some studies suggest that NG tubes may actually increase the risk aspiration.[37]

Percutaneous endoscopic gastrostomy (PEG) is a safe and effective means of direct feeding to the stomach. It is generally used when there is need for prolonged enteral nutrition,[38] and results in longer survival time and less risk of aspiration compared with NG tubes. PEG tubes are generally larger caliber than NG feeding tubes, which leads to less interruption of nutrition.[39]

Tracheostomy tubes have not proven to be an effective treatment for eliminating aspiration, although they can minimize aspiration.[40] Tracheostomy tubes are useful for improving pulmonary toilet,[41] but may disturb hyoid movement and laryngeal elevation during swallowing.[42]

15.6 Surgical Management for Chronic Aspiration

When a patient continues to aspirate despite conservative management techniques, surgical treatment may be indicated. The timing and surgical procedure chosen are based on the underlying cause of aspiration, patient condition, and prognosis. Ideally, the procedure should have minimal possible complications and be reversible if the underlying cause of aspiration is eliminated.

15.6.1 Vocal Fold Medialization

Vocal fold medialization techniques are indicated when chronic aspiration results from glottic insufficiency secondary to unilateral vocal fold immobility or paralysis. Aspiration is most

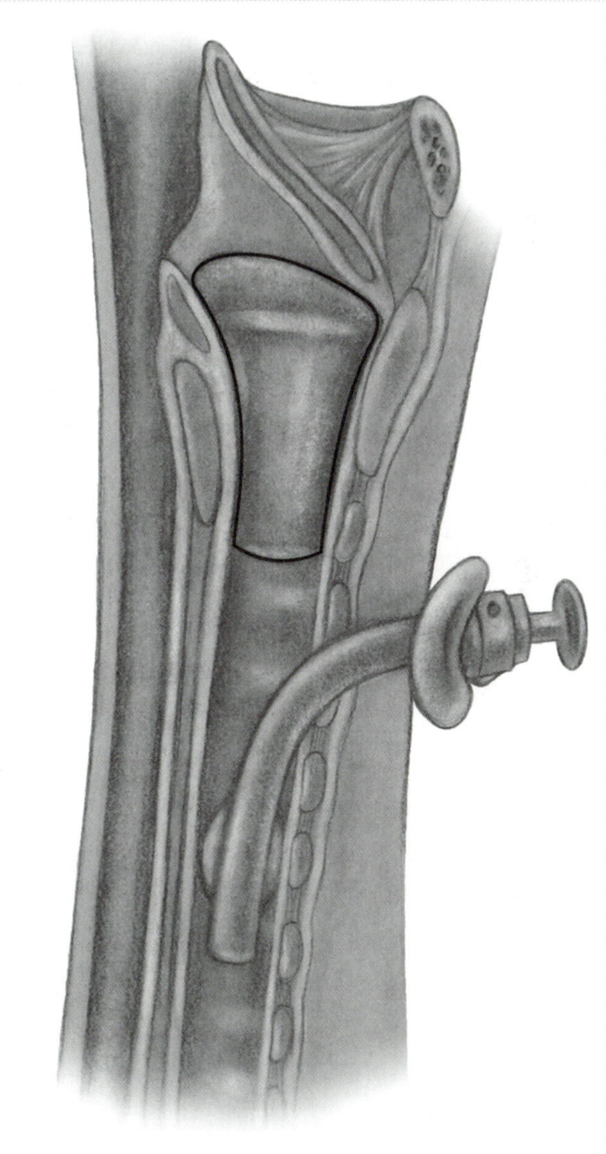

Fig. 15.2 Endolaryngeal stent with tracheostomy tube.

likely when a vocal fold paralysis is combined with laryngeal sensory deficit. This may result from a high vagal lesion or with simultaneous superior and recurrent laryngeal nerve injury. A variety of surgical procedures are available to medialize the immobile vocal fold to achieve adequate glottal closure. Techniques include injection laryngoplasty, medialization laryngoplasty (type I thyroplasty), and laryngeal reinnervation. These techniques are addressed in detail in Chapter 9 of this book.

15.6.2 Endolaryngeal Stent

Placement of an endolaryngeal stent is a reversible procedure where aspiration can be eliminated initially and temporarily by obturating the glottis using a solid silicon stent inserted endoscopically and secured using transcervical sutures (▶ Fig. 15.2).[43] Alternatively, a vented stent that has a hollow lumen and slit at the apex allows some phonation.[44] Both types of stents require a tracheostomy. Continued aspiration, granulation tissue formation, patient discomfort, and lack of appropriate sizes have limited the application of stents.[45]

15.6.3 Narrow Field Laryngectomy

In patients for whom there is no anticipation of reversal of the underlying cause of life-threatening aspiration, a narrow-field laryngectomy is an option to prevent aspiration-associated pulmonary infection. This involves removal of the laryngeal skeleton with sparing of the hyoid bone and strap muscles, a high tracheal transection and preservation of a maximum amount of pharyngeal mucosa (▶ Fig. 15.3a). A vertical midline incision is made from the hyoid bone to the upper extent of the tracheotomy site. The strap muscles are elevated away from laryngeal framework to expose the thyroid and cricoid cartilages and a permanent tracheostomy is performed at the first or second tracheal ring. The cricoid is then lifted upward and separated from the postcricoid mucosa as much as possible. The pharynx is entered at the level of the arytenoid cartilages and a limited infrahyoid pharyngotomy is performed to expose the epiglottis with maximum preservation of the mucosa in postcricoid area. The aryepiglottic folds and the vallecula are preserved as well to help minimize the size of the pharyngeal opening. The pharyngeal closure is supported with the strap muscle as a second layer and a permanent tracheostomy is formed (▶ Fig. 15.3b). The wound is closed in layers and drained with a small penrose drain. The patient is fed via NG tube for 5 to 10 days until he or she is ready for oral feeding.[46]

15.6.4 Subperichondrial Cricoidectomy

This irreversible procedure was developed by Cummings in 1987 and reported by Eisele et al in 1995 as an alternative to total and narrow field laryngectomy for patients with intractable aspiration and no anticipated recovery.[47] A vertical midline incision is performed to expose the cricoid cartilage and the upper trachea. After a tracheotomy is made, the outer cricoid cartilage perichondrium is opened vertically and elevated to the posterior cricoid lamina. The inner cricoid perichondrium is elevated circumferentially and the cricoid cartilage is then removed piecemeal bilaterally using a biting forceps with preservation of the posterior cricoid lamina. The inner cricoid perichondrium and the subglottic mucosa are transected

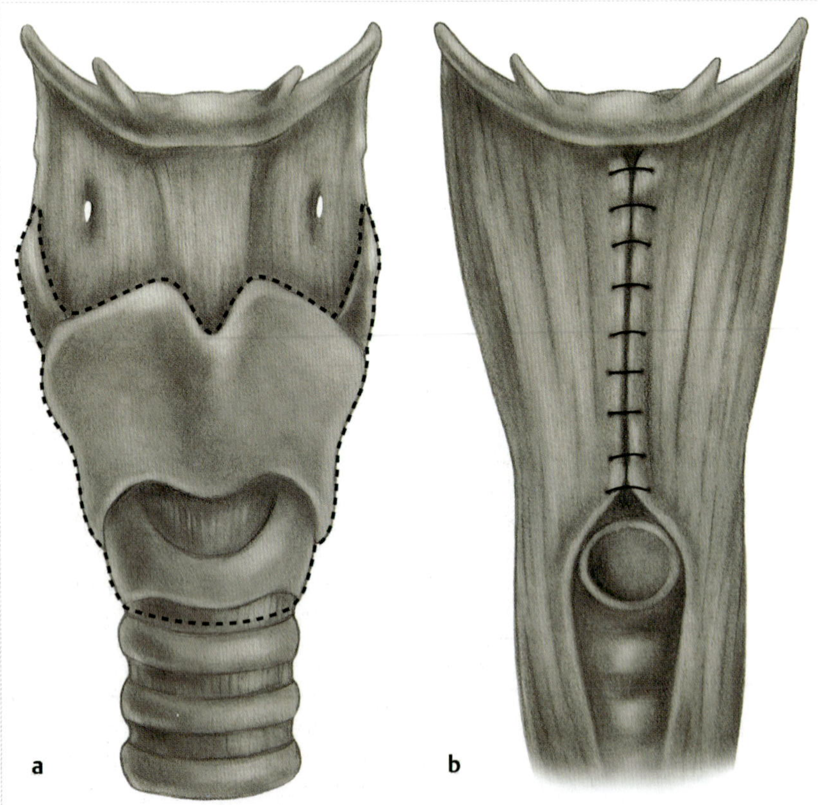

Fig. 15.3 Narrow field laryngectomy. (**a**) Laryngeal structures to be removed. (**b**) Pharyngeal closure bolstered with sternohyoid muscles.

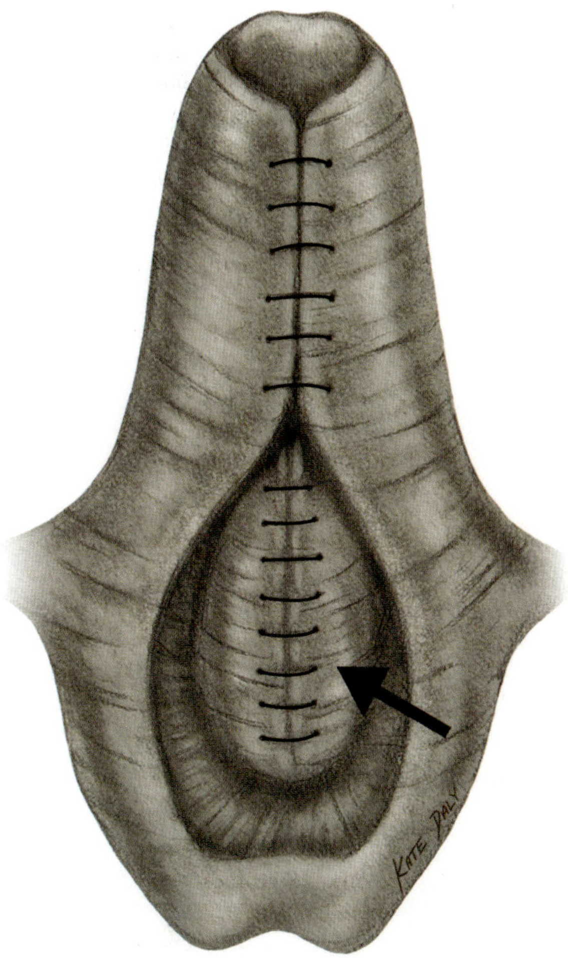

Fig. 15.4 Vertical laryngoplasty with intralaryngeal mucosal closure and extralaryngeal mucosal closure. The *arrow* indicates closure of intralaryngeal mucosa layer. The extralaryngeal mucosa is partially closed in this figure.

horizontally and the ends are closed horizontally using interrupted inverting absorbable sutures. The strap muscles are approximated and the wound is closed in layers with a drain and tracheostomy in place. The main disadvantages of this procedure are the need for tracheostomy and the inability to phonate.

15.6.5 Vertical Laryngoplasty

This procedure, also referred to as tubed laryngoplasty, was described by Biller et al in 1983 as a means to eliminate aspiration in the patients after glossectomy.[48] It was then adapted to patients with other causes of aspiration.[49] A tracheotomy is fashioned, then a continuous mucosal incision is made around the edge of epiglottis, onto the aryepiglottic folds, arytenoids, and interarytenoid mucosa, and a mucosa flap is elevated. The supraglottic laryngeal mucosa and epiglottic mucosa are then closed and plicated into a vertical tube with an intralaryngeal layer and an extralaryngeal layer, respectively (▶ Fig. 15.4). Phonation may be possible in this procedure, but a tracheostomy is still needed. A modification of the Biller technique designed to decrease dehiscence called the *steamboat technique* was described in which the epiglottic cartilage is trimmed and a tibial periosteal graft is inserted to reinforce closure of the mucosa, creating an arrangement resembling a Chinese steamboat.[50]

15.6.6 Epiglottopexy

This is a reversible procedure using an epiglottis flap to close the laryngeal inlet. The laryngeal inlet is closed via an infrahyoid approach with denuding of the epiglottis, aryepiglottic folds, and arytenoids, then suturing the denuded epiglottis posteriorly to the aryepiglottic folds and arytenoids.[51] In addition to achieving protection of the laryngeal inlet, it can allow preservation of speech through a small laryngeal inlet that can be fashioned posteriorly.[52] Because of the elasticity of the epiglottic cartilage the risk of flap dehiscence is quite high. Scoring of the epiglottic cartilage at the base can decrease this risk.[53]

15.6.7 Glottic Closure

A glottic closure procedure was suggested by Montgomery for patients with loss of laryngeal sphincter function. The operation sacrifices phonatory function and requires tracheostomy. Through a transthyrotomy approach to the glottis, the mucosa of the true and false vocal folds is stripped and the true folds and false vocal folds are closed in two layers.[54] A third layer of closure may be added by rotation of a sternohyoid muscle into the supraglottis.[55] A new modification of the procedure featured reduction of the entire structure of the larynx. To reduce the laryngeal space, both edges of the cut thyroid cartilage are excised and sutures are made collectively in the false vocal folds and true vocal folds, with no need for insertion of a hinged muscle flap. This laryngeal closure technique has been shown to completely eliminate aspiration.[56]

15.6.8 Tracheoesophageal Diversion and Laryngotracheal Separation

The tracheoesophageal diversion procedure was suggested by Lindeman for the patients with intractable aspiration in whom recovery is expected only after a prolonged period. This is an effective and reversible procedure in which a separation of the upper respiratory tract from the digestive tract is performed with a tracheoesophageal anastomosis and accompanying tracheostomy, diverting aspirated saliva or food into the esophagus (▶ Fig. 15.5).[57]

The procedure begins with a horizontal division of the trachea at the fourth and fifth tracheal rings. The proximal tracheal segment is anastomsed to an opening in the anterior esophagus in an end-to-side fashion. The distal tracheal segment is then sutured to the skin to create a tracheostoma. For those patients with a pre-existing tracheostomy, which is usually located in a more proximal position, Lindeman developed the laryngeotracheal separation procedure. Here the short proximal tracheal stump is oversewn as a blind pouch and the closure is supported with a sternothyroid muscle flap (▶ Fig. 15.6).[58,40]

Surgical reversal of laryngotracheal separation has been reported in selected patients with the return of phonation and

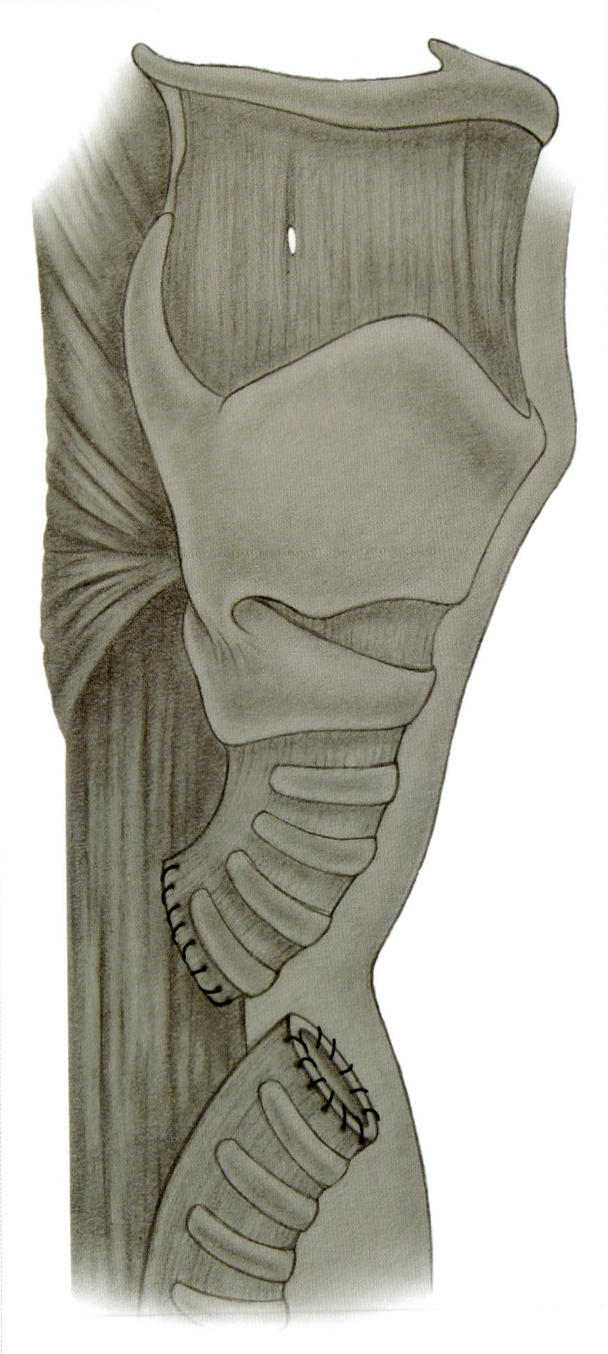

Fig. 15.5 Tracheoesophageal diversion.

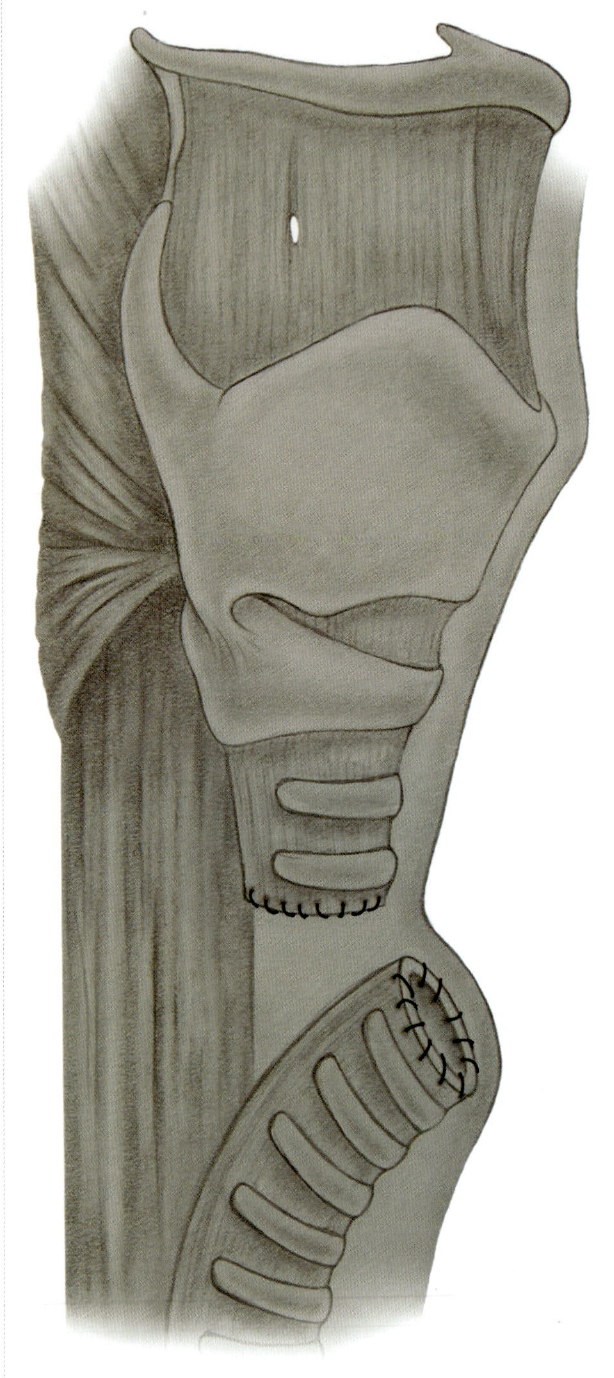

Fig. 15.6 Laryngotracheal separation.

swallowing,[59,60] but with a significant risk of complications and inefficacy.[61] Because of potential risk of complications caused by chronic pooling of saliva and food in the proximal tracheal blind pouch, a modified laryngeotracheal separation with tracheoesophageal diversion despite a high tracheotomy level was described by Krespi.[62] In this modification the proximal anterior tracheal cartilage with the inferior half of the cricoid is removed. This leaves a mucosal flap that is anastomosed with the anterior esophagus.[40,62]

15.6.9 Total Laryngectomy

Total laryngectomy separates the respiratory and digestive tracts, and has been considered as the procedure of choice for the definitive treatment of the patient with life-threatening aspiration. Although total laryngectomy remains the most reliable and definitive way to achieve complete cessation of aspiration, it has no potential for reversal and has a significant negative psychological effect for the patient and family.[3]

15.7 Key Points

- Chronic aspiration is a complicated problem with a variety of etiologies and a wide range of diagnostic treatment options.
  - It is most commonly seen in neurologic disorders, with stroke being the most frequent, especially involving the brainstem with bilateral cranial nerve palsies.
- Complications from intractable pulmonary aspiration can result in life-threatening pulmonary infections.
  - Diagnostic efforts should aim to determine the mechanism of aspiration and to find reversible causes.
  - Initial conservative management includes postural adjustments, swallowing maneuvers, and enteral feeding tubes.
- Patients with continued life-threatening aspiration despite conservative measures are deemed candidates for surgical management.
  - Thorough patient counseling is vital, as most procedures will require tracheostomy and loss of voice function.
  - Surgical approaches involve separation of the upper respiratory tract and digestive tract.
    - Several procedures, including tracheoesophageal diversion and laryngotracheal separation, are considered simple, effective and reversible.

References

[1] Shaker R, Dodds WJ, Dantas RO, Hogan WJ, Arndorfer RC. Coordination of deglutitive glottic closure with oropharyngeal swallowing. Gastroenterology 1990; 98: 1478–1484

[2] Ohmae Y, Logemann JA, Kaiser P, Hanson DG, Kahrilas PJ. Timing of glottic closure during normal swallow. Head Neck 1995; 17: 394–402

[3] Pletcher SD, Eisele DW. Chronic aspiration. In: Flint PW, ed. Cummings Otolaryngology—Head and Neck Surgery. 5th ed. Philadelphia, PA: Mosby; 2010: 925–932

[4] Matsuo K, Palmer JB. Anatomy and physiology of feeding and swallowing: normal and abnormal. Phys Med Rehabil Clin N Am 2008; 19: 691–707

[5] Marik PE. Aspiration pneumonitis and aspiration pneumonia. N Engl J Med 2001; 344: 665–671

[6] Logeman J. Aspiration: review of etiologies. In: Evaluation and Treatment of Swallowing Disorders. San Diego, CA: College-Hill Press; 1983: 64–69

[7] Chevretton EB. Management and treatment of intractable aspiration. In: Pengilley Z, ed. Scott-Brown's Otorhinolaryngology Head and Neck Surgery. 7th ed. London, England: Hodder Arnold; 2008: 2094–2104

[8] Palmer JB, Drennan JC, Baba M. Evaluation and treatment of swallowing impairments. Am Fam Physician 2000; 61: 2453–2462

[9] Leder SB, Ross DA. Incidence of vocal fold immobility in patients with dysphagia. Dysphagia 2005; 20: 163–167, discussion 168–169

[10] Logemann JA. A Manual for the Videofuoroscopic Evaluation of Swallowing. Boston,MA: College-Hill Press; 1986

[11] Dodds WJ, Logemann JA, Stewart ET. Radiologic assessment of abnormal oral and pharyngeal phases of swallowing. AJR Am J Roentgenol 1990; 154: 965–974

[12] Logemann JA. Evaluation and Treatment of Swallowing Disorders. Austin, TX: ProEd; 1998

[13] Rosenbek JC, Robbins JA, Roecker EB, Coyle JL, Wood JL. A penetration-aspiration scale. Dysphagia 1996; 11: 93–98

[14] Donzelli J, Brady S. The effects of breath-holding on vocal fold adduction: implications for safe swallowing. Arch Otolaryngol Head Neck Surg 2004; 130: 208–210

[15] Ohmae Y, Logemann JA, Kaiser P, Hanson DG, Kahrilas PJ. Effects of two breath-holding maneuvers on oropharyngeal swallow. Ann Otol Rhinol Laryngol 1996; 105: 123–131

[16] Hiss SG, Postma GN. Fiberoptic endoscopic evaluation of swallowing. Laryngoscope 2003; 113: 1386–1393

[17] Aviv JE, Kim T, Sacco RL et al. FEESST: a new bedside endoscopic test of the motor and sensory components of swallowing. Ann Otol Rhinol Laryngol 1998; 107: 378–387

[18] Fattori B, Grosso M, Ursino F et al. Clinical applications of oro-pharyngo-oesophageal scintigraphy in the study of dysphagia. Acta Otorhinolaryngol Ital 2007; 27: 192–199

[19] Silver KH, Van Nostrand DL. The use of scintigraphy in the management of patients with pulmonary aspiration. Dysphagia 1994; 9: 107–115

[20] Rasley A, Logemann JA, Kahrilas PJ, Rademaker AW, Pauloski BR, Dodds WJ. Prevention of barium aspiration during videofluoroscopic swallowing studies: value of change in posture. AJR Am J Roentgenol 1993; 160: 1005–1009

[21] Ohmae Y, Karaho T, Hanyu Y, Murase Y, Kitahara S, Inouye T. [Effect of posture strategies on preventing aspiration] Nippon Jibiinkoka Gakkai Kaiho 1997; 100: 220–226

[22] Welch MV, Logemann JA, Rademaker AW, Kahrilas PJ. Changes in pharyngeal dimensions effected by chin tuck. Arch Phys Med Rehabil 1993; 74: 178–181

[23] Lazarus C, Logemann JA, Gibbons P. Effects of maneuvers on swallowing function in a dysphagic oral cancer patient. Head Neck 1993; 15: 419–424

[24] Logemann JA, Kahrilas PJ, Kobara M, Vakil NB. The benefit of head rotation on pharyngoesophageal dysphagia. Arch Phys Med Rehabil 1989; 70: 767–771

[25] Logemann JA, Gibbons PJ, Rademaker AW et al. Mechanisms of recovery of swallow after supraglottic laryngectomy. J Speech Hear Res 1994; 37: 965–974

[26] Logemann JA, Pauloski BR, Rademaker AW, Colangelo LA. Super-supraglottic swallow in irradiated head and neck cancer patients. Head Neck 1997; 19: 535–540

[27] Langmore SE. Endoscopic Evaluation and Treatment of Swallowing Disorders. New York, NY: Thieme; 2001

[28] Hind JA, Nicosia MA, Roecker EB, Carnes ML, Robbins J. Comparison of effortful and noneffortful swallows in healthy middle-aged and older adults. Arch Phys Med Rehabil 2001; 82: 1661–1665

[29] Pauloski BR. Rehabilitation of dysphagia following head and neck cancer. Phys Med Rehabil Clin N Am 2008; 19: 889–928

[30] Kahrilas PJ, Logemann JA, Krugler C, Flanagan E. Volitional augmentation of upper esophageal sphincter opening during swallowing. Am J Physiol 1991; 260: G450–G456

[31] Lazarus CL. Management of dysphagia. In: Bailey BJ, Johnson JT, Newlands SE, eds. Head and Neck Surgery—Otolaryngology. Philadelphia, PA: Lippincott Williams &Wilkins; 2006; 713–720

[32] Logemann JA. Treatment of oral and pharyngeal dysphagia. Phys Med Rehabil Clin N Am 2008; 19: 803–816, ix

[33] Castellanos VH, Butler E, Gluch L, Burke B. Use of thickened liquids in skilled nursing facilities. J Am Diet Assoc 2004; 104: 1222–1226

[34] Lazarus CL, Logemann JA, Rademaker AW et al. Effects of bolus volume, viscosity, and repeated swallows in nonstroke subjects and stroke patients. Arch Phys Med Rehabil 1993; 74: 1066–1070

[35] Logemann JA. Behavioral management for oropharyngeal dysphagia. Folia Phoniatr Logop 1999; 51: 199–212

[36] Bastow MD. Complications of enteral nutrition. Gut 1986; 27 Suppl 1: 51–55

[37] Alessi DM, Berci G. Aspiration and nasogastric intubation. Otolaryngol Head Neck Surg 1986; 94: 486–489

[38] Löser C, Aschl G, Hébuterne X et al. ESPEN guidelines on artificial enteral nutrition—percutaneous endoscopic gastrostomy (PEG). Clin Nutr 2005; 24: 848–861

[39] Dwolatzky T, Berezovski S, Friedmann R et al. A prospective comparison of the use of nasogastric and percutaneous endoscopic gastrostomy tubes for long-term enteral feeding in older people. Clin Nutr 2001; 20: 535–540

[40] Petring OU, Adelhøj B, Jensen BN, Pedersen NO, Lomholt N. Prevention of silent aspiration due to leaks around cuffs of endotracheal tubes. Anesth Analg 1986; 65: 777–780

[41] Eisele DW. Surgical approaches to aspiration. Dysphagia 1991; 6: 71–78

[42] Jung SJ, Kim DY, Kim YW, Koh YW, Joo SY, Kim ES. Effect of decannulation on pharyngeal and laryngeal movement in post-stroke tracheostomized patients. Ann Rehabil Med 2012; 36: 356–364

[43] Weisberger EC, Huebsch SA. Endoscopic treatment of aspiration using a laryngeal stent. Otolaryngol Head Neck Surg 1982; 90: 215–222
[44] Eliachar I, Nguyen D. Laryngotracheal stent for internal support and control of aspiration without loss of phonation. Otolaryngol Head Neck Surg 1990; 103 5pt 1: 837–840
[45] Wisdom G, Krespi YP, Blitzer A. Surgical Therapy for Chronic Aspiration. Op Tech Otolaryngol 1997; 8: 199–208
[46] Krespi YP, Blitzer A. Laryngectomy for aspiration: Narrow field technique. Oper Tech Otolaryngol–Head Neck Surg 1997; 8: 227–230
[47] Eisele DW, Seely DR, Flint PW, Cummings CW. Subperichondrial cricoidectomy: an alternative to laryngectomy for intractable aspiration. Laryngoscope 1995; 105: 322–325
[48] Biller HF, Lawson W, Baek SM. Total glossectomy. A technique of reconstruction eliminating laryngectomy. Arch Otolaryngol 1983; 109: 69–73
[49] Blitzer A. Evaluation and management of chronic aspiration. N Y State J Med 1987; 87: 154–160
[50] Ku PK, Abdullah VJ, Vlantis AC, Lee KY, van Hasselt AC, Tong MC. 'Steam-boat' supraglottic laryngoplasty for treatment of chronic refractory aspiration: a modification of Biller's technique. J Laryngol Otol 2009; 123: 1360–1363
[51] Habal MB, Murray JE. Surgical treatment of life-endangering chronic aspiration pneumonia. Use of an epiglottic flap to the arytenoids. Plast Reconstr Surg 1972; 49: 305–311
[52] Brookes GB, McKelvie P. Epiglottopexy: a new surgical technique to prevent intractable aspiration. Ann R Coll Surg Engl 1983; 65: 293–296
[53] Strome M, Fried MP. Rehabilitative surgery for aspiration. A clinical analysis. Arch Otolaryngol 1983; 109: 809–811
[54] Montgomery WW. Surgery to prevent aspiration. Arch Otolaryngol 1975; 101: 679–682
[55] Sasaki CT, Milmoe G, Yanagisawa E, Berry K, Kirchner JA. Surgical closure of the larynx for intractable aspiration. Arch Otolaryngol 1980; 106: 422–423
[56] Takano S, Goto T, Kabeya M, Tayama N. Surgical closure of the larynx for the treatment of intractable aspiration: surgical technique and clinical results. Laryngoscope 2012; 122: 1273–1278
[57] Lindeman RC. Diverting the paralyzed larynx: a reversible procedure for intractable aspiration. Laryngoscope 1975; 85: 157–180
[58] Yarington CT, Sutton D. Clinical experience with the tracheoesophageal anastomosis for intractable aspiration. Ann Otol Rhinol Laryngol 1976; 85: 609–612
[59] Snyderman CH, Johnson JT. Laryngotracheal separation for intractable aspiration. Ann Otol Rhinol Laryngol 1988; 97: 466–470
[60] Pletcher SD, Mandpe AH, Block MI, Cheung SW. Reversal of laryngotracheal separation: a detailed case report with long-term followup. Dysphagia 2005; 20: 19–22
[61] Zocratto OB, Savassi-Rocha PR, Paixão RM, Salles JM. Laryngotracheal separation surgery: outcome in 60 patients. Otolaryngol Head Neck Surg 2006; 135: 571–575
[62] Krespi YP, Quatela VC, Sisson GA, Som ML. Modified tracheoesophageal diversion for chronic aspiration. Laryngoscope 1984; 94: 1298–1301

16 Care of the Professional Voice*

Robert T. Sataloff, Johnathan B. Sataloff, and Mary J. Hawkshaw

Although singers and actors inspired many of the advances that have altered the standard of care for all patients with voice disorders, many other patients also are professional voice users. Clergy, attorneys, politicians, physicians, teachers, telephone receptionists, sports coaches, factory supervisors and many others depend upon vocal quality, volume, and endurance for their livelihoods. Because voice quality is essential for transmitting information and establishing credibility in our society, the majority of our patients are voice professionals; and all patients should be treated as such. In many ways, singers are the most demanding voice patients because they require outcomes that are not just normal, but that approach "perfect", especially classical operatic singers. However, they do not necessarily have the greatest demands for endurance among our many groups of voice professionals. An operatic singer typically performs once or twice a week. Rock singers may perform six nights a week on tour; Broadway singers perform eight shows a week; and elementary and middle school teachers have voice demands that may be even greater in some cases. Therefore, it is important for us to understand not only the skills required to recognize subtle problems with singers, but also the vocal demands of professionals in any voice-intensive endeavor. This subject is extensive and has filled entire books.[1,2,3,4] This chapter will be concise and limited to selected topics relevant to professional voice users that are not covered elsewhere in this book; it will focus primarily on singers because when otolaryngologists are skilled at caring for these especially challenging patients they usually are able to care for nearly all voice professionals.

16.1 Patient History

Obtaining extensive historical background information is necessary for a thorough evaluation of the voice patient, and the otolaryngologist who sees professional voice patients (especially singers and actors). A history questionnaire can be extremely helpful in documenting all the necessary information, helping the patient sort out and articulate his or her problems, and saving the clinician time recording information (see the Appendix).[5,6] Additional useful quality of life information also can be obtained from validated instruments such as the Vocal Health Index (VHI),[7] the VHI-10[8], and the VHI-S.[8] No history questionnaire is a substitute for direct, penetrating questioning by the physician; however, the direction of most useful inquiry can be determined from a glance at a questionnaire. This obviates the need for extensive writing, which permits the physician greater eye contact with the patient and facilitates rapid establishment of the close rapport and confidence that is vital in treating voice patients. The physician is also able to supplement initial impressions and historical information from the questionnaire with seemingly leisurely conversation during the physical examination. The use of the history questionnaire adds substantially to the efficiency, consistent thoroughness, and ease of managing these delightful, but often complex, patients.

The following questions should be explored with the patient.

16.1.1 How Old Are You?

Serious vocal endeavor may start in childhood and continue throughout a lifetime. As the vocal mechanism undergoes normal maturation, the voice changes. Age-related vocal training is controversial, especially training of children and pubescent voices. Nevertheless, performers and other voice professionals include patients of all ages; otolaryngologists and their voice teams should acquire the special knowledge and skills required to treat voice professionals of any age. This complex topic is beyond the scope of this chapter.

The clinical effects of aging in older adults seem more pronounced in female singers, although vocal fold histologic changes may be more prominent in males.[9,10] Nevertheless, excellent male singers occasionally extend their careers into their 70 s or beyond. However, some degree of breathiness, decreased range, and other evidence of aging should be expected in elderly voices. Nevertheless, many of the changes we typically associate with elderly singers (wobble, flat pitch) are due to lack of conditioning, rather than inevitable changes of biological aging. These aesthetically undesirable concomitants of aging often can be reversed.

16.1.2 What Is Your Specific Voice Problem?

Careful questioning as to the onset of vocal problems is needed to separate acute from chronic dysfunction. Often an upper respiratory tract infection will send a patient to the physician's office; however, penetrating inquiry, especially in singers and actors, may reveal a chronic vocal problem that is the patient's real concern. Identifying acute and chronic problems before beginning therapy is important so that both the patient and physician may have realistic expectations and make optimal therapeutic selections.

The specific nature of the vocal complaint can provide a great deal of information. *Hoarseness* is a coarse or scratchy sound that is most often associated with abnormalities of the leading edge of the vocal folds such as laryngitis or mass lesions. *Breathiness* is a vocal quality characterized by excessive loss of air during vocalization. Any condition that prevents full approximation of the vocal folds can be responsible. Possible causes include vocal fold paralysis, a mass lesion separating the leading edges of the vocal folds, arthritis of the cricoarytenoid joint, arytenoid dislocation, scarring of the vibratory margin, senile vocal fold atrophy (presbyphonia), psychogenic dysphonia, malingering, and other conditions.

Fatigue of the voice is inability to continue to speak or sing for extended periods without change in vocal quality and/or

* Reprinted in part with permission from Sataloff RT, Professional Voice: The Science and Art of Clinical Care. 3rd ed. San Diego, CA: Plural Publishing Inc.; 2005.

control. The voice may show fatigue by becoming hoarse, losing range, changing timbre, breaking into different registers, or exhibiting other uncontrolled aberrations. A well-trained singer should be able to sing for several hours without vocal fatigue. Fatigue is often caused by misuse of abdominal and neck musculature, oversinging, singing too loudly, or too long. However, we must remember that vocal fatigue may be a sign not only of general tiredness or vocal abuse (sometimes secondary to structural lesions or glottal closure problems), but also of serious illnesses such as myasthenia gravis. So, the importance of this complaint should not be understated.

Volume disturbance may manifest as inability to sing loudly or inability to sing softly. Each voice has its own dynamic range. Within the course of training, singers learn to sing more loudly by singing more efficiently. They also learn to sing softly, a more difficult task, through years of laborious practice. Actors and other trained speakers go through similar training. Most volume problems are secondary to intrinsic limitations of the voice or technical errors in voice use, although hormonal changes, aging, and neurologic disease are other causes. Superior laryngeal nerve paralysis also impairs the ability to speak or sing loudly.

Most highly trained singers require only about 10 to 30 minutes to "warm up the voice." Prolonged warm-up time, especially in the morning, is most often caused by reflux laryngitis. Tickling or choking during singing is most often a symptom of an abnormality of the vocal fold's leading edge. The symptom of tickling or choking should contraindicate singing until the vocal folds have been examined. Pain while singing can indicate vocal fold lesions, laryngeal joint arthritis, laryngeal tendonitis, infection, or gastric acid reflux irritation of the arytenoid region. However, pain is much more commonly caused by voice abuse with excessive muscular activity in the neck rather than an acute abnormality on the leading edge of a vocal fold. Sudden onset of pain (usually sharp pain) while singing may be associated with a mucosal tear or a vocal fold hemorrhage and warrants voice conservation pending laryngeal examination.

16.1.3 Do You Have Any Pressing Voice Commitments?

If a singer or professional speaker (e.g., actor, politician) seeks treatment at the end of a busy performance season and has no pressing engagements, management of the voice problem should be relatively conservative and designed to insure long-term protection of the larynx, the most delicate part of the vocal mechanism. However, the physician and patient rarely have this luxury. Most often, the voice professional needs treatment within a week of an important engagement and sometimes within less than a day. Caring for voice complaints in these situations requires highly skilled judgment and bold management.

16.1.4 Tell Me about Your Vocal Career, Long-Term Goals, and the Importance of Your Voice Quality and Upcoming Commitments

To choose a treatment program, the physician must understand the importance of the patient's voice and his or her long-term career plans, the importance of the upcoming vocal commitment, and the consequences of canceling the engagement. Injudicious prescription of voice rest can be almost as damaging to a vocal career as injudicious performance. For example, canceling a concert at the last minute may seriously damage a performer's reputation. Although a singer's voice is usually his or her most important commodity, other factors distinguish the few successful artists from the multitude of less successful singers with equally good voices. These include musicianship, reliability, and "professionalism." Reliability is especially critical early in a singer's career. Moreover, an expert singer often can modify a performance to decrease the strain on his or her voice. No singer, actor, or speaker should be allowed to perform in a manner that will permit serious injury to the vocal folds; nevertheless, in the frequent borderline cases, the condition of the larynx must be weighed against other factors affecting the singer or actor as an artist. Similar considerations apply to all professional voice users such as teachers, politicians, attorneys, clergy, motivational speakers, and others.

16.1.5 How Much Voice Training Have You Had?

Establishing how long a singer or actor has been performing seriously is important, especially if his or her active performance career predates the beginning of vocal training. Active untrained singers and actors frequently develop undesirable techniques that are difficult to modify. Extensive voice use without training or premature training with inappropriate repertoire may underlie persistent vocal difficulties later in life. The number of years a performer has been training his or her voice and the number of teachers during that time may be fair indices of vocal proficiency, but other factors also must be considered.

16.1.6 Under What Kinds of Conditions Do You Use Your Voice?

The Lombard effect is the tendency to increase vocal intensity in response to increased background noise. A well-trained singer learns to compensate for this tendency and to avoid singing at unsafe volumes. Singers of classical music usually have such training and frequently perform with only a piano, a situation in which the balance can be controlled well. However, singers performing in large halls, with orchestras, or in operas early in their careers tend to over-sing and strain their voices. Similar problems occur during outdoor concerts because of the lack of auditory feedback. This phenomenon is seen even more among pop singers. Often, despite little vocal training, they enjoy great artistic and financial success and endure extremely stressful demands on their time and voices. They are required to sing in large halls or outdoor arenas not designed for musical performance, amid smoke and other environmental irritants, accompanied by extremely loud background music. One frequently neglected key to survival for these singers is the proper use of monitor speakers. These direct the sound of the singer's voice toward the singer on the stage and provide auditory feedback. Determining whether the pop singer uses monitor speakers and whether they are loud enough for the singer to hear is important.

Amateur singers are often no less serious about their music than are professionals, but generally they have less ability to compensate technically for illness or other physical impairment. Rarely does an amateur suffer a great loss from postponing a performance or permitting someone to sing in his or her place. In most cases, the amateur singer's best interest is served through conservative management directed at long-term maintenance of good vocal health.

A great many of the singers who seek physicians' advice are primarily choral singers. They often are enthusiastic amateurs, untrained but dedicated to their musical recreation. They should be handled as amateur solo singers, educated specifically about the Lombard effect, and cautioned to avoid the excessive volume so common in a choral environment.

Like singers, actors require superior vocal quality, flexibility, and endurance; they often have to work under very challenging circumstances. Understanding the performance and rehearsal environment for actors is as important to providing informed laryngological care as it is for singers. For both, it is also important for physicians to determine whether the professional voice user is also engaged in a "day job." Some such endeavors required to earn money are very vocally demanding. These may include positions as waiters, receptionists, tour guides, sales personnel, babysitters, part-time teachers, and others. In evaluating actors, the physician needs to know whether the person works on stage (proscenium or in-the-round), camera (television and/or film), in nightclubs, comedy clubs, or other venues. Each has its own special vocal demands and hazards. Inquiries also should include information about the length of the working day and associated vocal demands, travel, special voice requirements (character voices, voice-overs, aging during the course of a play, etc.), special voice gestures required (screaming, sobbing, laughing), costumes that affect the voice (heavy hats or helmets, corsets that limit breathing and others), makeup that causes allergies or limits facial motion, stage fog or smoke, and many other factors. More information on this topic is available elsewhere.[11]

16.1.7 How Much Do You Practice and Exercise Your Voice?

Vocal exercise is as essential to the vocalist as exercise and conditioning of other muscle systems is to the athlete. Proper vocal practice incorporates scales and other specific exercises designed to maintain and develop the vocal apparatus. Simply acting or singing songs and giving performances without routine studious concentration on vocal technique is not adequate for the vocal performer.

16.1.8 How, When, and Where Do You Use Your Voice?

The physician should be aware of common habits and environments that are often associated with abusive voice behavior and should ask about them routinely. Screaming at sports events and at children is among the most common. Extensive voice use in noisy environments also tends to be abusive. These include noisy rooms, cars, airplanes, sports facilities, and other locations where background noise or acoustic design impairs auditory feedback. Dry, dusty surroundings may alter vocal fold secretions through dehydration or contact irritation, altering voice function. Activities such as cheerleading, teaching, choral conducting, amateur singing, and frequent communication with hearing-impaired persons are likely to be associated with voice abuse, as is extensive professional voice use without formal training.

16.1.9 Are You Aware of Misusing or Abusing Your Voice During Speaking or Singing?

Voice abuse and/or misuse should be suspected particularly in patients who complain of voice fatigue associated with voice use, whose voices are worse at the end of a working day or week, and in any patient who is chronically hoarse. Technical errors in voice use may be the primary etiology of a voice complaint, or they may develop secondarily due to a patient's effort to compensate for voice disturbance from another cause. Often, they are correctable through expert therapy and training.[12]

16.1.10 What Kind of Physical Condition Are You In?

Phonation is an athletic activity that requires good conditioning and coordinated interaction of numerous physical functions. Maladies of any part of the body may be reflected in the voice. Failure to maintain good abdominal muscle tone and respiratory endurance through exercise, is particularly harmful because deficiencies in these areas undermine the power source of the voice. Patients generally attempt to compensate for such weaknesses by using inappropriate muscle groups, particularly in the neck, causing vocal dysfunction. Similar problems may occur in the well-conditioned vocalist in states of generalized fatigue. These are compounded by mucosal changes that accompany excessively long hours of hard work. Such problems may be seen even in the well-trained voice professionals shortly before important engagements.

16.1.11 Have You Noted Voice or Bodily Weakness, Tremor, Fatigue, or Loss of Control?

Even minor neurologic disorders may be extremely disruptive to vocal function. Specific questions should be asked to rule out neuromuscular and neurologic diseases such as myasthenia gravis, Parkinson disease, tremors, other movement disorders, spasmodic dysphonia, multiple sclerosis, central nervous system neoplasm, and other serious maladies that may be present with voice complaints.

16.1.12 Do You Have Allergy or Cold Symptoms?

Acute upper respiratory tract infection causes inflammation of the mucosa, alters mucosal secretions, and makes the mucosa more vulnerable to injury. Coughing and throat clearing are particularly traumatic vocal activities and may worsen or provoke hoarseness associated with a cold. Postnasal drip and allergy may produce the same response. Infectious sinusitis associated with discharge and diffuse mucosal inflammation, results in similar problems, and may actually alter the sound of a voice, especially the patient's own perception of his or her voice. Futile attempts to compensate for disease of the supraglottic vocal tract, in an effort to return the sound to normal, frequently result in laryngeal strain. The expert singer or speaker should compensate by monitoring technique by tactile rather than by auditory feedback, or singing "by feel" rather than "by ear."

16.1.13 Do You Have Breathing Problems, Especially after Exercise?

Respiratory problems are especially important in voice patients. Mild respiratory dysfunction may adversely affect the power source of the voice.[13] Likewise, more severe respiratory dysfunction such as occult asthma may be particularly troublesome.[14] A complete respiratory history should be obtained in most patients with voice complaints, and pulmonary function testing is often advisable.

16.1.14 Have You Been Exposed to Environmental Irritants?

Environmental pollution is responsible for the presence of toxic substances and conditions encountered daily. Inhalation of toxic pollutants may affect the voice adversely by direct laryngeal injury, by causing pulmonary dysfunction that results in voice maladies, or through impairments elsewhere in the vocal tract. Ingested substances, especially those that have neurolaryngologic effects may also adversely affect the voice. Nonchemical environmental pollutants such as noise can cause voice abnormalities, as well. Otolaryngologists should be familiar with the laryngologic effects of the numerous potentially irritating substances and conditions found in the environment, as well as special pollution problems encountered by performers. Numerous materials used by artists to create sculptures, drawings, and theatrical sets are toxic and have adverse voice effects. In addition, performers are exposed routinely to chemicals encountered through stage smoke and pyrotechnic effects, as discussed elsewhere.[15,16,17] Although it is clear that some of the "special effects" result in serious laryngologic consequences, much additional study is needed to clarify the nature and scope of these occupational problems.

Mucosal irritants can disrupt the delicate vocal mechanism in almost any setting; however, performers are often in high-risk environments even in the absence of stage fogs and pyrotechnics. Allergies to dust and mold are aggravated commonly during rehearsals and performances in concert halls, especially older theaters and concert halls, because of numerous curtains, backstage trappings, and dressing room facilities that are rarely cleaned thoroughly. A history of recent travel suggests other sources of mucosal irritation. The air in airplanes is extremely dry, and airplanes are noisy, and one must be careful to avoid talking loudly and to maintain good hydration and nasal breathing during air travel.

16.1.15 Do You Smoke, Live With a Smoker, and/or Work around Smoke?

The deleterious effects of primary and secondary exposure to smoke are well known and should be considered in evaluation of the professional voice user.

16.1.16 Do Any Foods Seem to Affect Your Voice?

Various foods may affect the voice. Traditionally, many singers avoid milk products before performances. In many people, these foods seem to increase the amount and viscosity of mucosal secretions. Allergy and casein have been implicated. In some cases, restriction of these foods from the diet before a voice performance may be helpful. Chocolate and other foods (mint, eucalyptus, alcohol, fatty foods, and others) may have the same effect in some individuals and should be viewed similarly. Eating foods that cause or aggravate reflux prior to a performance may cause symptoms that interfere with the voice, as discussed later in this chapter. Such behaviors may explain symptoms in some voice professionals, especially the many who are unaware that they have laryngopharyngeal reflux and have a need to control their diets.

16.1.17 Do You Have Morning Hoarseness, Bad Breath, Excessive Phlegm, a Lump in Your Throat, and/or Heartburn?

Laryngopharyngeal reflux (LPR) is especially common among singers and trained speakers because of lifestyle and the high intra-abdominal pressure associated with proper support. Singers frequently perform at night, and many vocalists refrain from eating before performances because a full stomach can compromise effective abdominal support. They typically compensate by eating heartily at postperformance gatherings late at night and then go to bed with a full stomach. Although laryngopharyngeal reflux typically occurs while the patient is upright, nocturnal reflux may be precipitated by large meals prior to bedtime. Chronic irritation of arytenoid and vocal fold mucosa by reflux of gastric secretions may be associated occasionally with dyspepsia or heartburn. However, the key features of this malady are bitter taste and halitosis on awakening in the morning, a dry or "coated" mouth, often a scratchy sore throat or a feeling of a "lump in the throat", hoarseness, and the need for prolonged vocal warm-up. LPR occurs typically while patients are upright. So, symptoms are noted during the day rather than predominantly at night. The physician must be alert to these symptoms and ask about them routinely; otherwise, the diagnosis will often be overlooked because people who have had this problem for many years or a lifetime do not even realize it is abnormal.

16.1.18 Do You Have Trouble With Your Bowels or Belly?

Any condition that alters abdominal function, such as muscle spasm, constipation, or diarrhea, interferes with support and may result in a voice complaint. These symptoms may accompany infection, anxiety, various gastroenterological diseases, and other maladies, and they are common in performers who travel to numerous countries.

16.1.19 Are You under Particular Stress or in Therapy?

The human voice is an exquisitely sensitive messenger of emotion. Highly trained voice professionals learn to control the effects of anxiety and other emotional stress on their voices under ordinary circumstances. However, in some instances, this training may break down or a performer may be inadequately prepared to control the voice under specific stressful conditions. Preperformance anxiety is the most common example, but insecurity, depression, and other emotional disturbances are also generally reflected in the voice. Other publications have highlighted the complexity and importance of psychological factors associated with voice disorders.[18]

16.1.20 Do You Have Problems Controlling Your Weight? Are You Excessively Tired? Are You Cold When Other People Are Warm?

Endocrine problems warrant special attention. The human voice is extremely sensitive to endocrinological changes. Many of these are reflected in alterations of fluid content of the lamina propria just beneath the laryngeal mucosa. This causes alterations in the bulk and shape of the vocal folds and results in voice change. Hypothyroidism is a well-recognized cause of such voice disorders. Hoarseness, vocal fatigue, muffling of the voice, loss of range, and a sensation of a lump in the throat may be present even with mild hypothyroidism.

16.1.21 Do You Have Menstrual Irregularity, Cyclical Voice Changes Associated with Menses, Recent Menopause, or Other Hormonal Changes or Problems?

Voice changes associated with sex hormones are encountered commonly in clinical practice and have been investigated more thoroughly than have other hormonal changes. Although a correlation appears to exist between sex hormone levels and depth of male voices (higher testosterone and lower estradiol levels in basses than in tenors),[19] the most important hormonal considerations in males occur during or are related to puberty. Voice problems related to sex hormones are more common in female singers.

16.1.22 Do You Have Jaw Joint or Other Dental Problems?

Dental disease, especially temporomandibular joint (TMJ) dysfunction, introduces muscle tension in the head and neck, which is transmitted to the larynx directly through the muscular attachments between the mandible and the hyoid bone and indirectly as generalized increased muscle tension. These problems often result in decreased range, vocal fatigue, and change in the quality or placement of a voice. Such tension often is accompanied by excess tongue muscle activity, especially pulling of the tongue posteriorly. This hyperfunctional behavior acts through hyoid attachments to disrupt the balance between the intrinsic and extrinsic laryngeal musculature.

16.1.23 Do You or Your Blood Relatives Have Hearing Loss?

Hearing loss is often overlooked as a source of vocal problems. Auditory feedback is fundamental to speaking and singing. Interference with this control mechanism may result in altered vocal production, particularly if the person is unaware of the hearing loss. Distortion, particularly pitch distortion (diplacusis) may also pose serious problems for the singer. This appears to be due not only to aesthetic difficulties in matching pitch, but also to vocal strain that accompanies pitch shifts.[20]

In addition to determining whether the patient has hearing loss, inquiry should also be made about hearing impairment occurring in family members, roommates, and other close associates. Speaking loudly to people who are hard-of-hearing can cause substantial, chronic vocal strain. This possibility should be investigated routinely when evaluating voice patients.

16.1.24 Have You Suffered Whiplash or Other Bodily Injury?

Various bodily injuries outside the confines of the vocal tract may have profound effects on the voice. Whiplash, for example, commonly causes changes in technique, with consequent voice fatigue, loss of range, difficulty singing softly, and other problems. These problems derive from the neck muscle spasm, abnormal neck posturing secondary to pain, and consequent hyperfunctional voice use. Lumbar, abdominal, head, chest, supraglottic, and extremity injuries may also affect vocal technique and be responsible for the dysphonia that prompted the voice patient to seek medical attention.

16.1.25 Did You Undergo Any Surgery Prior to the Onset of Your Voice Problems?

A history of laryngeal surgery in a voice patient is a matter of great concern. It is important to establish exactly why the surgery was done, by whom it was done, whether intubation was necessary, and whether voice therapy was instituted pre- or postoperatively if the lesion was associated with voice abuse (vocal nodules). If the vocal dysfunction that sent the patient to the physician's office dates from the immediate postoperative period, surgical trauma must be suspected. Other operations also may cause voice dysfunction even without laryngeal incision, including tonsillectomy, surgery of the neck such as thyroidectomy, thoracic and abdominal surgery, and other surgical procedures.

16.1.26 What Medications and Other Substances Do You Use?

A history of alcohol abuse suggests the probability of poor vocal technique. Intoxication results in incoordination and decreased awareness, which undermine vocal discipline designed to optimize and protect the voice. The effect of small amounts of alcohol is controversial.

Patients frequently acquire antihistamines to help control "postnasal drip" or other symptoms. The drying effect of antihistamines may result in decreased vocal fold lubrication, increased throat clearing, and irritability leading to frequent coughing. Antihistamines may be helpful to some voice patients, but they must be used with caution.

A history of using any medications is important in evaluating voice professionals including antibiotics, diuretics, hormones, cocaine, pain medications (including aspirin and ibuprofen), psychotropic medications, and others.[21]

16.2 Physical Examination

Physical examination of any voice patient must include a thorough ear, nose, and throat evaluation, and assessment of general physical condition. The physician must remember that maladies of almost any body system may result in voice dysfunction, and the doctor must remain alert for conditions outside the head and neck. If the patient uses his or her voice professionally for singing, acting, or other vocally demanding professions, physical examination also should include assessment of the patient during typical professional vocal tasks; for example, a singer should be asked to sing, or a member of the clergy should be asked to deliver part of a sermon.

16.2.1 General Ear, Nose, and Throat Examination

Examination of the ears must include assessment of hearing acuity. Hearing loss in a spouse or significant other may be problematic as well if the voice professional strains vocally to communicate. The conjunctivae and sclerae should be observed routinely for erythema that suggests allergy or irritation, for pallor that suggests anemia, and for other abnormalities such as jaundice. These observations may reveal the problem reflected in the vocal tract even before the larynx is visualized. The nose should be assessed for patency of the nasal airway, character of the nasal mucosa, and nature of secretions, if any. A patient who is unable to breathe through the nose because of anatomic obstruction is forced to breathe unfiltered, unhumidified air through the mouth. Examination of the oral cavity should be complete. Xerostomia is particularly important because dryness of the oral and laryngeal mucosa is very disturbing to voice professionals; often the etiology can be identified and the problem, resolved. The presence of scalloping of the lateral aspects of the tongue should be noted. This finding is caused commonly by tongue thrust and may be associated with inappropriate tongue tension and muscle tension dysphonia. Dental examination should focus not only on oral hygiene but also on the presence of wear facets suggestive of bruxism. This suggests bruxism is a clue to excessive tension and may be associated with dysfunction of the temporomandibular joints, which also should be assessed routinely. Thinning of the enamel of the central incisors in a normal or underweight patient may be due to bulimia. However, it also may result from excessive ingestion of lemons, which some singers eat to help thin their secretions.

The neck should be examined for masses, restriction of movement, excess muscle tension and/or spasm, and scars from prior neck surgery or trauma. Laryngeal vertical mobility is also important. For example, tilting of the larynx produced by partial fixation of cervical muscles cut during previous surgery may produce voice dysfunction, as may fixation of the trachea to overlying neck skin. Examination of posterior neck muscles and range of motion should not be neglected. The cranial nerve function also should be assessed.

16.2.2 Laryngeal Examination

Examination of the larynx begins when the singer or other voice patient enters the physician's office. The range, ease, volume, and quality of the speaking voice should be noted. If the examination is not being conducted in the patient's native language, the physician should be sure to listen to a sample of the patient's mother tongue as well. Voice use is often different under the strain or habits of foreign language use. Rating scales used to describe the speaking voice more consistently may be helpful.[22,23] The classification proposed by the Japanese Society of Logopedics and Phoniatrics is one of the most widely used. It is known commonly as the GRBAS Voice Rating Scale.[24]

Physicians are not usually experts in voice classification. However, the physicians should at least be able to discriminate substantial differences in range and timbre, such as between bass and tenor, or alto and soprano. Although the correlation between speaking and singing voices is not perfect, a speaker with a low, comfortable bass voice who reports that he is a tenor may be misclassified and singing inappropriate roles with consequent voice strain. This judgment should be deferred to an expert, but the observation should lead the physician to make the appropriate referral.

Any patient with a voice complaint should be examined by indirect laryngoscopy at a minimum. Stroboscopic examination adds substantially to diagnostic abilities allowing visualization of small mucosal disruptions and hemorrhages that may be significant, but overlooked otherwise. This technique also allows photography of the larynx. The author evaluates all new voice patients with both flexible and rigid (telescope) laryngoscopy for optimal assessment of laryngeal dynamics and vibratory margin structure and function. In some patients, videokymography or high-speed video is valuable, as well. Rigid endoscopy under general anesthesia may be reserved for the rare patient whose vocal folds cannot be assessed adequately by other means or for patients who need surgical procedures to remove or biopsy laryngeal lesions.

16.2.3 Objective Tests

Reliable, valid, objective analysis of the voice is extremely important and is an essential part of a comprehensive physical examination. It is as valuable to the laryngologist as audiometry is to the otologist. Familiarity with some of the measures and technological advances currently available is helpful. This information is covered elsewhere.[25]

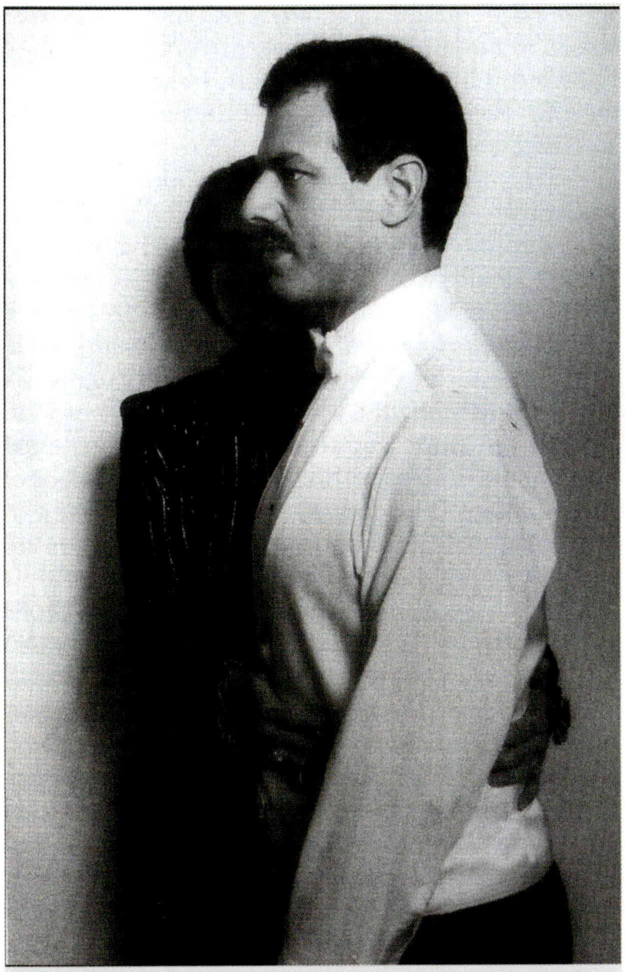

Fig. 16.1 Bimanual palpation of the support mechanism. The singer should expand posteriorly and anteriorly with inspiration. Muscles should tighten prior to onset of the sung tone. (Used with permission from Sataloff RT. Professional Voice: The Science and Art of Clinical Care. 3rd ed. San Diego, CA: Plural Publishing Inc.; 2005.)

16.2.4 Laryngeal Electromyography

Electromyography (EMG) requires an electrode system, an amplifier, an oscilloscope, a loudspeaker, and a recording system.[26] Electrodes are placed transcutaneously into laryngeal muscles. Electromyography can be extremely valuable in confirming cases of vocal fold paresis, in differentiating paralysis from arytenoid dislocation, distinguishing recurrent laryngeal nerve paralysis from combined recurrent and superior nerve paralysis, diagnosing other more subtle neurolaryngological pathology, and documenting functional voice disorders and malingering. It is also recommended for needle localization when using botulinum toxin for treatment of spasmodic dysphonia and other conditions.

16.2.5 Outcomes Assessment

Measuring the impact of a voice disorder has always been challenging. However, recent advances have begun to address this problem. Validated instruments such as the Voice Handicap Index (VHI)[7,8,27] are helpful in assessing the impact of the patient's voice disorder on the quality of life.

16.2.6 Voice Impairment and Disability

Quantifying voice impairment and assigning a disability rating (percentage of whole person) remain controversial. This subject is still not addressed comprehensively even in the most recent edition (6th edition, 2008) of the American Medical Association's *Guidelines for the Evaluation of Impairment and Disability*.[28] The *Guidelines* still do not take into account the person's profession when calculating disability. Alternative approaches have been proposed, and advances in this complex arena are anticipated over the next few years.[29]

16.2.7 Evaluation of the Singing Voice

The physician must be careful not to exceed the limits of his or her expertise especially in caring for singers. However, if voice abuse or technical error is suspected, or if a difficult judgment must be reached on whether to allow a sick singer to perform, a brief observation of the patient's singing may provide invaluable information. This is accomplished best by asking the singer to stand and sing scales either in the examining room or in the soundproof audiology booth. Similar maneuvers may be used for professional speakers, including actors (who can vocalize and recite lines), clergy and politicians (who can deliver sermons and speeches), and virtually all other voice patients. The singer's stance should be balanced, with the weight slightly forward. The knees should be bent slightly and the shoulders, torso, and neck should be relaxed. The singer should inhale through the nose whenever possible allowing filtration, warming, and humidification of inspired air. In general, the chest should be expanded, but most of the active breathing is abdominal. The chest should not rise substantially with each inspiration, and the supraclavicular musculature should not be involved obviously in inspiration. Shoulders and neck muscles should not be tensed even with deep inspiration. Abdominal musculature should be contracted shortly before the initiation of the tone. This may be evaluated visually or by palpation (). Muscles of the neck and face should be relaxed. Economy is a basic principle of all art forms. Wasted energy and motion and muscle tension are incorrect and usually deleterious.

The singer should be instructed to sing a scale (a five-note scale is usually sufficient) on the vowel /Y/, beginning on any comfortable note. Technical errors are usually most obvious as contraction of muscles in the neck and chin, retraction of the lower lip, retraction of the tongue, or tightening of the muscles of mastication. The singer's mouth should be open widely, but comfortably. When singing /Y/, the singer's tongue should rest in a neutral position with the tip of the tongue lying against the back of the singer's mandibular incisors. If the tongue pulls back or demonstrates obvious muscular activity as the singer performs the scales, improper voice use can be confirmed on the basis of positive evidence (▶ Fig. 16.2). The position of the larynx should not vary substantially with pitch changes. Rising of the larynx with ascending pitch is evidence of technical dysfunction. This examination also gives the physician an opportunity to observe any dramatic differences between the qualities and ranges of the patient's speaking voice and the singing voice.

Remembering the admonition not to exceed his or her expertise, the physician who examines many singers can often glean

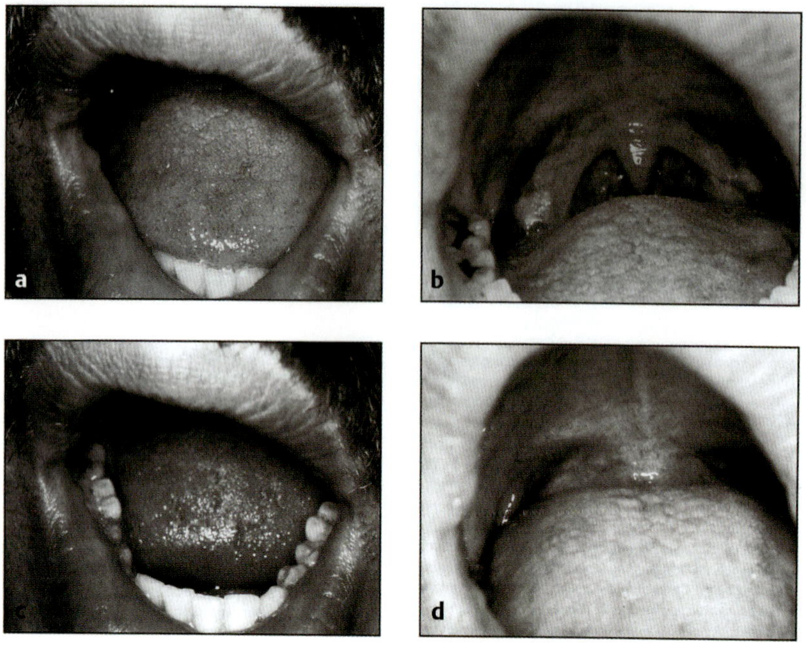

Fig. 16.2 Proper relaxed position of the (**a**) anterior and (**b**) posterior portions of the tongue. Common improper use of the tongue (**c**) pulled back from the teeth and (**d**) raised posteriorly. (Used with permission from Sataloff RT. Professional Voice: The Science and Art of Clinical Care. 3rd ed. San Diego, CA: Plural Publishing Inc.; 2005.)

valuable information from a brief attempt to modify an obvious technical error. For example, deciding whether to allow a singer with mild or moderate laryngitis to perform is often difficult. On the one hand, an expert singer has technical skills that allow him or her to compensate safely. On the other hand, if a singer does not sing with correct technique and does not have the discipline to modify volume, technique, and repertoire as necessary, the risk of vocal injury may be increased substantially even by mild inflammation of the vocal folds. In borderline circumstances, observation of the singer's technique may greatly help the physician in making a judgment. Details of appropriate observations and cautious therapeutic interventions may be found in other literature.[30]

16.3 Additional Examinations

A general physical examination should be performed whenever the patient's systemic health is questionable. Debilitating conditions such as mononucleosis may be noticed first by the singer as vocal fatigue. Neurologic and pulmonary assessments may be particularly revealing. Laryngologic manifestations of systemic disease, and common diagnoses and treatments in voice professionals, are beyond the scope of this brief chapter and are reviewed elsewhere in this book and in other literature.[1,2]

It is extremely valuable for the laryngologist to assemble an arts–medicine team that includes not only a speech-language pathologist, singing voice specialist, acting voice specialist, and voice scientist, but also medical colleagues in other disciplines. Collaboration with an expert neurologist, pulmonologist, endocrinologist, psychologist, psychiatrist, internist, physiatrist, and others with special knowledge of, and interest in, voice disorders is invaluable in caring for patients with voice disorders and provide expanded history and physical examination expertise that is outside the scope of otolaryngology, but essential to the comprehensive team assessment of professional voice users. Such interdisciplinary teams have not only elevated the standard of care in voice evaluation and treatment, but they are also largely responsible for the rapid and productive growth of voice as a subspecialty.

16.4 Appendix

Appendix: Sample questionnaire.

Used with permission from Sataloff RT. Professional Voice: The Science and Art of Clinical Care. 3rd ed. San Diego, CA: Plural Publishing Inc.; 2005.

PATIENT HISTORY: SINGERS

NAME ______________________________ AGE ______ SEX ______ RACE ______

HEIGHT ______ WEIGHT ______ DATE ______________

VOICE CATEGORY: ___ soprano ___ mezzo soprano ___ alto

___ tenor ___ baritone ___ bass

(If you are not currently having a voice problem, then please skip to Question # 3)

PLEASE CHECK OR CIRCLE CORRECT ANSWERS

1. How long have you had your present voice problem?

   Who noticed it? **myself, family, voice teacher, critics, everyone, other:** ______________

   Do you know what caused it? ___ **Yes** ___ **No**

   If yes, what?

   Did it come on slowly or suddenly? ___ **Slowly** ___ **Suddenly**

   Is it getting: ___ **Worse,** ___ **Better, or** ___ **Same?**

2. Which symptoms do you have? (Please check all that apply.)

   ___ Hoarseness (coarse or scratchy sound)

   ___ Fatigue (voice tires or changes quality after singing for a short period of time)

   ___ Volume disturbance (trouble singing ___ softly ___ loudly)

   ___ Loss of range (___ high ___ low)

   ___ Change in classification (example: voice lowered from soprano to mezzo)

   ___ Prolonged warm-up time (over half-hour needed to warm up voice)

   ___ Breathiness

   ___ Tickling or choking sensation while singing

   ___ Pain in throat while singing

   ___ Other; please specify: ______________________________

3. Do you have an important performance soon? ___ **Yes** ___ **No**

   Date(s): ______________________________

4. What is the current status of your singing career?

   ___ Professional ___ Amateur

5. What are your long-term career goals in singing?

___ Premiere operatic career

___ Premiere pop music career

___ Active avocation

___ Classical

___ Pop

___ Other; please specify: ________________________________

___ Amateur performance (choral or solo)

___ Amateur singing for own pleasure

6. Have you had voice training? ___ **Yes** ___ **No** If yes, at what age did you begin? _____
7. Have there been periods of months or years without lessons in that time?

   ___ **Yes** ___ **No**
8. How long have you studied with your present teacher?

   Teacher's name:

   Teacher's address:

   Teacher's telephone number:
9. Please list previous teachers and years during which you studied with them:
10. Have you ever had training for your speaking voice? ___ **Yes** ___ **No**

    Acting voice lessons? ___ **Yes** ___ **No**

    How many years? _______

    Speech therapy? ___ **Yes** ___ **No**

    How many months? _______
11. Do you have a job in addition to singing?

    ___ **Yes** ___ **No**

    If yes, does it involve extensive voice use?

    ___ **Yes** ___ **No**

    If yes, what is it? [actor, announcer (television/radio/sports arena), athletic instructor, attorney, clergy, politician, physician, sales person, stock broker, teacher, telephone operator or receptionist, waiter, waitress, secretary, other: ________________________]
12. In your performance work, in addition to singing, are you frequently required to speak?

    ___ **Yes** ___ **No**

...to dance? ___ **Yes** ___ **No**

13. How many years did you sing actively before beginning voice lessons initially?

14. What types of music do you sing? (Please check all that apply.)

___ Classical	___ Show
___ Nightclub	___ Pop/Rock

___ Other; please specify: ___________________________

15. Do you regularly sing in a sitting position (such as from behind a patio or drum set)?

___ **Yes** ___ **No**

16. Do you sing outdoors or in large halls, or with orchestras? (If yes, circle which one.)

___ **Yes** ___ **No**

17. If you perform with electrical instruments or outdoors, do you use monitor speakers?

___ **Yes** ___ **No**

If yes, can you hear them? ___ **Yes** ___ **No**

18. Do you play a musical instrument(s)? ___ **Yes** ___ **No**

If yes, please check all that apply:

___ Keyboard (Piano, Organ, Harpsichord, other: ___________________)

___ Violin, Viola

___ Cello

___ Bass

___ Plucked Strings (Guitar, Harp, other: ___________________)

___ Brass

___ Wind with single reed

___ Wind with double reed

___ Flute, Piccolo

___ Percussion

___ Bagpipes

___ Accordion

___ Other; please specify: ___________________________

19. How often do you practice?

Scales: **[daily, few times weekly, once a week, rarely, never]**

If you practice scales, do you do them all at once or do you divide them up over the course of the day?

[all at once, two or three sittings]

On days when you do scales, how long do you practice them?

[15, 30, 45, 60, 75, 90, 105, 120, over 120] minutes

Songs: **[daily, few times weekly, once a week, rarely, never]**

How many hours per day?

[0.5, 1, 1.5, 2, 2.5, 3, over 3]

Do you warm up your voice before you sing? ___ **Yes** ___ **No**

Do you warm up your voice after you have finished singing? ___ **Yes** ___ **No**

20. How much are you singing at present (average hours per day, total including practice time)?

Rehearsal:

Performance:

21. Please check all that apply to you:

___ Voice worse in the morning

___ Voice worse later in the day, after it has been used.

___ Sing performances or rehearsals in the morning

___ Speak extensively (teacher, clergy, attorney, telephone, work, other: ________________)

___ Cheerleader

___ Speak extensively backstage or at post-performance parties

___ Choral conductor

___ Frequently clear your throat

___ Frequent sore throat

___ Jaw joint problems

___ Bitter or acid taste, or bad breath first thing in the morning

___ Frequent "heartburn" or hiatal hernia

___ Frequent yelling or loud talking

___ Frequent whispering

___ Chronic fatigue

___ Work around extreme dryness

___ Frequent physical exercise (weight lifting, aerobics, etc.)

___ Frequently thirsty, dehydrated

___ Hoarseness first thing in the morning

___ Chest cough

___ Eat late at night

___ Ever used antacids

___ Under particular stress at present (personal or professional)

___ Frequent bad breath

___ Live, work or perform around smoke or fumes

___ Traveled recently: when: ________________________________

where: ________________________________

Eat/drink any of the following before singing?

___ Chocolate ___ Coffee ___ Spiced foods

___ Nuts ___ Alcohol ___ Milk or ice cream

___ Other; please specify: ___

Any specific vocal technical difficulties?

[trouble singing soft, trouble singing loud, poor pitch control, support problems, problems at register transitions, other: ___]

Any problems with your singing voice recently prior to the onset of the problem that brought you here?

[hoarseness, breathiness, fatigue, loss of range, voice breaks, pain singing, other: ___]

Any voice problems in the past that required a visit to a physician? **[e.g. laryngitis, nodules, polyps, hemorrhage, cancer, other]** If yes, please describe problem(s) and treatment(s):

22. Your family doctor's name, address and telephone number:

23. Your laryngologist's name, address and telephone number:

24. Recent cold? ___ **Yes** ___ **No**
25. Current cold? ___ **Yes** ___ **No**
26. Have you been exposed to any of the following chemicals frequently (or recently) at home or at work: (please check all that apply)

    ___ Carbon monoxide ___ Arsenic

    ___ Mercury ___ Aniline dyes

    ___ Insecticides ___ Industrial solvents

    ___ Lead ___ Industrial solvents (benzene, etc.)

    ___ Stage smoke
27. Have you been evaluated by an allergist? ___ **Yes** ___ **No**

    If yes, what allergies do you have: (medication allergies are covered in Question # 44)

    [none, dust, mold, trees, cat, dog, foods, other: ___]

    If yes, give name and address of allergist:

28. How many packs of cigarettes do you smoke per day? ________

    Smoking history:

    ___ Never

    ___ Quit. When? ________

    ___ Had smoked about ________ packs per day for ________ years.

    ___ Currently smoke; have smoked for ________ years.

29. Do you work in a smokey environment? ___ **Yes** ___ **No**

30. How much alcohol do you drink? **[none, rarely, a few times per week, daily]** If daily, or few times per week, on the average, how much do you consume? **[1, 2, 3, 4, 5, 6, 7, 8, 9, 10, more than 10]**

    Did you previously drink more heavily? ___ **Yes** ___ **No**

31. How many cups of coffee, tea, cola, or other caffeinated drinks do you drink per day? _____

32. List all recreational drugs you use **[marijuana, cocaine, amphetamines, barbiturates, heroin, other: ________________________________]**

33. Have you noticed any of the following? (Please check all that apply)

    ___ Hypersensitivity to heat or cold

    ___ Excessive sweating

    ___ Change in weight: gained/lost ______ lbs. in ______ weeks or ______ months

    ___ Change in skin or hair

    ___ Palpitation (fluttering) of the heart

    ___ Emotional liability (swings of mood)

    ___ Double vision

    ___ Numbness of the face or extremities

    ___ Tingling around the mouth or face

    ___ Blurred vision or blindness

    ___ Weakness or paralysis of the face

    ___ Clumsiness in arms or legs

    ___ Confusion or loss of consciousness

    ___ Difficulty with speech

    ___ Difficulty with swallowing

    ___ Seizure (epileptic fit)

    ___ Pain in the neck or shoulder

    ___ Shaking or tremors

    ___ Memory change

    ___ Personality change

    For females:

Are you pregnant? ___ **Yes** ___ **No**

Are your menstrual periods regular? ___ **Yes** ___ **No**

Have you undergone hysterectomy? ___ **Yes** ___ **No**

Were your ovaries removed? ___ **Yes** ___ **No**

At what age did you reach puberty? ____________

Have you gone through menopause? ___ **Yes** ___ **No**

If yes, when? ____________

34. Have you ever consulted a psychologist or psychiatrist? ___ **Yes** ___ **No**

    Are you currently under psychological or psychiatric treatment? ___ **Yes** ___ **No**

35. Have you injured your head or neck (whiplash, etc.)? ___ **Yes** ___ **No**
36. Describe any serious accidents related to this visit, if any:

37. Are you involved in legal action involving problems with your voice? ___ **Yes** ___ **No**
38. List name(s) of spouse and children, if any:

39. Brief summary of ENT problems, some of which may or may not be related to your present complaint: (Please check all that apply.)

___ Hearing loss
___ Ear noises
___ Dizziness
___ Facial paralysis
___ Nasal obstruction
___ Nasal deformity
___ Mouth sores
___ Jaw joint problem
___ Eye problem
___ Ear pain
___ Facial pain
___ Stiff neck
___ Lump in the neck
___ Lump in the face or head
___ Trouble swallowing
___ Excess eye skin
___ Excess facial skin
___ Other; please specify:

40. Do you have or have you ever had:

___ Diabetes
___ Hypoglycemia
___ Thyroid problems
___ Syphilis
___ Seizures
___ Psychiatric therapy
___ Frequent bad headaches
___ Ulcers

___ Gonorrhea
___ Herpes
___ Cold sores (fever blisters)
___ High blood pressure
___ Severe low blood pressure
___ Intravenous antibiotics or diuretics
___ Heart attack
___ Angina
___ Irregular heartbeat
___ Other heart problems
___ Rheumatic fever
___ Tuberculosis
___ Glaucoma
___ Multiple sclerosis
___ Kidney disease
___ Urinary problems
___ Arthritis or skeletal problems
___ Cleft palate
___ Asthma
___ Lung or breathing problems
___ Unexplained weight loss
___ Cancer (of ______________________)
___ Other tumor (______________________)
___ Blood transfusion
___ Hepatitis
___ AIDS
___ Meningitis
___ Other illness; please specify:

41. Do any blood relatives of yours have:

___ Diabetes
___ Hypoglycemia
___ Cancer (of ______________________)
___ Heart disease
___ Other major medical problems such as those above; please specify:

42. Describe serious accidents not directly related to your visit here:

___ none
___ Occurred with head injury, loss of consciousness or whiplash
___ Occurred without head injury, loss of consciousness or whiplash. Describe:

43. List all your current medications and doses (include birth control pills and vitamins).

44. Medication allergies

___ none
___ Penicillin
___ Sulfa
___ Tetracycline
___ Novocaine
___ Iodine
___ Codeine
___ Adhesive tape

___ Erythromycin ___ Aspirin

___ Keflex/Ceclor/Ceftin ___ X-ray dyes

___ Other; please specify:

45. List operations

___ Tonsillectomy (at age _____) ___ Adenoidectomy (at age _____)

___ Appendectomy (at age _____) ___ Heart surgery (at age _____)

___ Other; please specify:

46. List toxic drugs or chemicals to which you have been exposed:

___ Lead

___ Streptomycin, Neomycin, Kanamycin

___ Mercury

___ Other; please specify:

47. Have you had x-ray treatments to your head or neck (including treatments for acne or ear problems as a child, treatments for cancer, etc.)? ___ **Yes** ___ **No**

48. Describe any serious health problems of your spouse and/or children:

References

[1] Sataloff RT. Professional Voice: The Science and Art of Clinical Care. 3rd ed. San Diego, CA: Plural Publishing; 2005

[2] Rubin J, Sataloff RT, Korovin G. Diagnosis and Treatment of Voice Disorders. 3rd ed. San Diego, CA: Plural Publishing; 2006

[3] Benninger MS, Jacobson BH, Johnson AF, eds. Vocal Arts Medicine: The Care and Prevention of Professional Voice Disorders. New York, NY: Thieme Medical Publishers; 1994

[4] Fried MP, Ferlito A, eds. The Larynx. 3rd ed. Vol I. San Diego, CA: Plural Publishing; 2009

[5] Sataloff RT, Hawkshaw MJ, Anticaglia J. Patient history. In: Sataloff RT. Professional Voice: The Science and Art of Clinical Care. 3rd ed. San Diego, CA: Plural Publishing; 2005: 323–338

[6] Sataloff RT. Professional Voice: The Science and Art of Clinical Care. 3rd ed. San Diego, CA: Plural Publishing; 2005:1537–1732

[7] Jacobson BH, Johnson A, Grywalski C et al. The Voice Handicap Index (VHI): development and validation. Am J Speech Lang Pathol 1997; 6: 66–70

[8] Rosen CA, Murry T. Voice Handicap Index in singers. J Voice 2000; 14: 370–377

[9] Sataloff RT, Linville SE. The effects of age on the voice. In: Sataloff RT. Professional Voice: The Science and Art of Clinical Care. 3rd ed. San Diego, CA: Plural Publishing; 2005: 497–512

[10] Benninger MS, Abitbol J. The aging voice. In: Chalian AA, ed. Primary Care Otolaryngology for the Geriatric Patient. Washington, DC: American Academy of Otolaryngology Head and Neck Surgery; 2006: 66–85

[11] Raphael BN. Special considerations relating to members of the acting profession. In: Sataloff RT. Professional Voice: The Science and Art of Clinical Care. 3rd ed. San Diego, CA: Plural Publishing; 2005: 339–341

[12] Sataloff RT. Professional Voice: The Science and Art of Clinical Care. 3rd ed. San Diego, CA: Plural Publishing; 2005: 961–1060

[13] Spiegel JR, Cohn JR, Sataloff RT et al. Respiratory function in singers: medical assessment, diagnoses, and treatments. J Voice 1988; 2: 40–50

[14] Cohn JR, Sataloff RT, Spiegel JR et al. Airway reactivity-induced asthma in singers (ARIAS). J Voice 1991; 5: 332–337

[15] Sataloff RT. Pollution and its effect on the voice. In: Sataloff RT. Professional Voice: The Science and Art of Clinical Care. 3rd ed. San Diego, CA: Plural Publishing; 2005: 729–736

[16] Opperman D. Pyrotechnics in the entertainment industry: an overview. In: Sataloff RT. Professional Voice: The Science and Art of Clinical Care. 3rd ed. San Diego, CA: Plural Publishing; 2005: 737–750

[17] Rossol M. Pyrotechnics: health effects. In: Sataloff RT. Professional Voice: The Science and Art of Clinical Care. 3rd ed. San Diego, CA: Plural Publishing; 2005: 751–756

[18] Rosen DC, Sataloff RT. Psychology of Voice Disorders. San Diego, CA: Singular Publishing Group; 1997: 639–642

[19] Meuser W, Nieschlag E. [Sex hormones and depth of voice in the male (author's transl)] Dtsch Med Wochenschr 1977; 102: 261–264

[20] Sundberg J, Prame E, Iwarsson J. Replicability and accuracey of pitch patterns in professional singers. In: Davis PJ, Fletcher NH, eds. Vocal Fold Physiology: Controlling Chaos and Complexity. San Diego, CA: Singular Publishing Group; 1996: 291–306

[21] Sataloff RT, Hawkshaw MJ, Anticaglia J. Medications and the voice. In: Sataloff RT. Professional Voice: The Science and Art of Clinical Care. 3rd ed. San Diego, CA: Plural Publishing; 2005: 905–924

[22] Fuazawa T, Blaugrund SM, El-Assuooty A, Gould WJ. Acoustic analysis of hoarse voice: a preliminary report. J Voice 1988; 2: 127–131

[23] Gelfer MP. Perceptual attributes of voice: development and use of rating scales. J Voice 1988; 2: 320–326

[24] Hirano M. Clinical Examination of the Voice. New York, NY: Springer Verlag; 1982: 83–84

[25] Heuer RJ, Hawkshaw MJ, Sataloff RT. The clinical voice laboratory. In: Sataloff RT. Professional Voice: The Science and Art of Clinical Care. 3rd ed. San Diego, CA: Plural Publishing; 2005: 355–394

[26] Sataloff RT, Mandel S, Heman-Ackah YD, Manon-Espaillat R, Abaza M. Laryngeal Electromyography. 2nd ed. San Diego, CA: Plural Publishing; 2006

[27] Rosen CA, Lee AS, Osborne J, Zullo T, Murry T. Development and validation of the voice handicap index-10. Laryngoscope 2004; 114: 1549–1556

[28] Rondinelli R, ed. Guides to the Evaluation of Permanent Impairment. 6th ed. Chicago, IL: American Medical Association; 2008

[29] Sataloff RT. Voice impairment, disability, handicap, and medical-legal evaluation. In: Sataloff RT. Professional Voice: The Science and Art of Clinical Care. 3rd ed. San Diego, CA: Plural Publishing; 2005: 1427–1432

[30] Sataloff RT. Physical examination. In: Sataloff RT. Professional Voice: The Science and Art of Clinical Care. 3rd ed. San Diego, CA: Plural Publishing; 2005: 343–354

17 Principles of Phonosurgery

Nausheen Jamal and Gerald S. Berke

With publication of the landmark articles on the morphological structure of the vocal cord along with the elegant description of thyroplasty and its phonosurgical applications in 1974, Hirano and Isshiki lay the groundwork for the development of modern-day phonosurgery. To this day, our understanding of vocal fold vibration revolves around the "body-cover" hypothesis, which continues to guide microlaryngeal surgical technique.[1,2,3]

It is critical for the laryngeal surgeon to grasp a physiological understanding of vocal fold anatomy. Based on Hirano's histological analysis, we know that the vocal fold is a multilayer structure consisting of the stratified squamous epithelium and lamina propria ("cover"), the vocal ligament, and thyroarytenoid (TA), or vocalis, muscle ("body"). The lamina propria, which is immediately deep to the epithelium, is further divided into three layers: (1) the superficial lamina propria, also known as the Reinke space, which consists of loose fibrous tissue and hyaluronic acid; (2) the intermediate lamina propria, with longitudinally arranged elastin fibers and increasing quantities of hyaluronic acid; and (3) the deep layer of the lamina propria, with cross-linked collagen fibers as well as numerous fibroblasts. The conus elasticus lies in between the lamina propria and the TA muscle, and its free edge forms the vocal ligament in combination with the deep layers of the lamina propria. Deep to this lies the vocalis muscle, providing a gradually increasing gradient of vocal fold stiffness that makes up the basis of the mucosal wave.[4]

A good understanding of vocal fold anatomy is imperative for anyone performing phonosurgery. For a more thorough and detailed review of vocal fold anatomy and physiology, please refer to Chapters 1 and 2 of this book.

17.1 Patient Factors

As the economy of our society continues to evolve, more of our population is migrating away from labor-based employment and toward communication-based careers. As a result, dysphonia and aphonia have become ever more debilitating, affecting at least 28 million workers in the United States on a daily basis —many of whom perceive a negative impact on their jobs due to their vocal issues.[5] The definition of a voice professional has expanded from the singer and actor to include a more broad spectrum of people who need their voice to lead a productive life. The significance of voice communication for any given individual has grown in magnitude. Appropriate management of individuals with dysphonia begins with a thorough history and physical examination, including onset, duration, frequency, and variability of dysphonia; presence of symptoms of acid reflux; consumption of tobacco and alcohol; coexistent medical conditions along with their associated medication regimens, and a qualitative and quantitative assessment of voice use and misuse. Examination should go beyond a basic mirror or flexible laryngoscopic examination to include videostroboscopy. The authors prefer rigid stroboscopic examination, although examination using a transnasal distal chip flexible laryngoscope is equally valuable.

The combination of history and physical examination will typically reveal the cause of the patient's dysphonia, which can almost always be categorized as benign or malignant disease on the basis of examination alone. However, if there is any doubt, biopsy should be performed in an expedient manner. Any malignant disease process should be managed according to established protocols, preferably using a multidisciplinary approach.

17.2 Phonomicrosurgery: Indications

Benign epithelial disease can and should be approached in a conservative manner. The laryngeal surgeon must realize that the very presence of a discrete lesion does not constitute a reason to operate. Rather, the etiology of the lesion should be identified and addressed, and medical management of contributing comorbid conditions should be maximized. Further, the surgeon must ascertain whether the identified lesion is actually the etiology of the patient's vocal complaint and consider the effect on voice that removal of the lesion might have. Many singers, for example, have nodules that provide a unique characteristic to their voices, or that cause no problems with performance.[6] Treatment that leads to resolution of these nodules would adversely affect, rather than benefit, these patients.

In addition to addressing comorbidities, such as tobacco use and hypothyroidism, consideration should also be given to initiating an antireflux regimen and directed voice therapy. Often, these treatments alone will lead to sufficient improvement in the patient's voice. Furthermore, severe reflux will often obscure the presence or true severity of coexistent vocal fold pathology; therefore, re-evaluation after 6 to 8 weeks of an antireflux regimen is prudent. Detailed written instructions on a low-acid diet and appropriate use of proton pump inhibitors with or without H_2 blocking agents, as dictated by severity, are beneficial for patient education. Critical in this discussion is patient understanding with regard to the disease process, and the time needed to respond to appropriate therapy.

After maximal medical therapy is given, follow-up visits should assess for both subjective and objective improvement. If the mass lesion has resolved, surgery is clearly no longer indicated. In some cases, the lesion and the patient's voice quality may show significant improvement, but without resolution, such as in the case of cysts and polyps.[7] If conservative management has not been fully implemented (i.e., adherence to a low acid diet, antireflux medication regimen, and voice therapy

Table 17.1 Standard treatment regimen by lesion type

Intervention typically unnecessary	Likely to resolve with conservative management[a]	Likely to require surgery[b]
Vascular ectasias	Nodules (early)	Nodules (mature)
	Polyps (small)	Polyps
	Granulomas	Granulomas (very large)
		Cysts
		Papilloma

[a]Conservative management may include voice therapy, an antireflux regimen, and chemodenervation.
[b]Even lesions that are likely to require surgery often benefit from initial conservative management.

techniques, with adequate treatment of medical comorbidites), then the importance of these items should be stressed with the patient, with more time given for these methods to exert their beneficial effects. However, once maximization of medical therapy has been achieved with either incomplete or no improvement, and it is clear that the identified lesion is causing or contributing to the patient's dysphonia, it is appropriate to proceed with surgical intervention.

Of note, whereas some lesions, such as nodules and granulomas, may respond well to nonoperative interventions, others, such as polyps and cysts, are less likely to resolve completely without surgery. This should be taken into consideration in the decision-making process, when assessing for response to conservative measures (▶ Table 17.1).

17.3 Phonomicrosurgery: Preoperative Considerations

As with any surgery, preoperative planning is the key to intra- and postoperative phonosurgical success. This begins with an open discussion of the risks and benefits of the proposed procedure, which is meant to educate, but not frighten, the patient. Risks that should be discussed with the patient include the very small possibility (1–2%) that there may be no improvement and even a worsening of vocal quality, and that surgical outcomes are never 100% predictable. This should be accompanied by a general explanation of what the surgery entails, and the high probability of success. He or she should also be counseled on any necessary adjustment of medications perioperatively. Nonsteroidal anti-inflammatory drugs and blood thinners should be stopped prior to surgery, barring any medical contraindication, and duration of the medication hold is dictated by the pharmacologic effect of the specific medication.[8]

Next, in addition to an explanation of what to expect on the day of surgery, the patient should also be given clear postoperative instructions prior to surgery. These may include diet recommendations, prescribed medication regimens, and instructions on the degree and length of voice rest, if indicated.

Finally, the surgeon should review the most recent stroboscopic examination just prior to surgery. This will help correlate stroboscopic and surgical findings to allow for appropriate surgical decision-making.

Beginning with the next section, discussion of operative preparation and technique will be divided into two broad categories: endolaryngeal, or phonomicrosurgery; and extralaryngeal, or framework surgery, focusing on type I (medialization) thyroplasty and arytenoid adduction.

17.4 Phonomicrosurgery: Intraoperative Considerations

17.4.1 Equipment

As its name suggests, phonomicrosurgery entails great detail and delicacy in technique. As such, it is critical to ensure that the appropriate equipment is available prior to beginning the operation. Standard laryngoscopic equipment, as used for diagnostic endoscopies for head and neck cancers, is not sufficient.

It is helpful to have a variety of laryngoscopes at one's disposal, to enable adequate exposure with any variation of anatomy. A wide aperture facilitates a binocular view in addition to bimanual operation, although this is not possible with every patient. More narrow scopes may provide better visualization, but compromise bimanual operation or binocular view. A wide range of available laryngoscopes is imperative, with a range from wide to narrow ocular and laryngeal openings. A typical collection of laryngoscopes might include a Lindholm, Dedo, Jako, Benjamin-Slimline, and a Holinger anterior commissure laryngoscope, although this list should be tailored to the surgeon's preference (▶ Fig. 17.1). Similarly, an appropriate suspension apparatus should be available for each laryngoscope type.

Adequate visualization also requires use of an appropriate microscope and set of telescopes. The microscope used should be of sufficient complexity to allow for comfortable, ergonomic visualization at a focal length of 400 mm. One that can be used for delicate middle ear surgery is appropriate.[4] Ideally, the microscope should also be able to accommodate a carbon dioxide (CO_2) laser micromanipulator attachment, should the surgeon wish to employ a CO_2 laser in any procedure.

Telescopes are also quite useful in microlaryngeal surgery. A zero-degree Hopkins rod telescope measuring 4 to 5 mm diameter and 30 cm in length is needed at a minimum. Angled telescopes (30 and 70 degree) may also be useful in visualization of the subglottis and anterior commissure.

The surgeon should confirm the availability of adequate instrumentation prior to beginning any operation. This will help avoid unnecessary waiting and frustration intraoperatively. Critical equipment include various sized suctions (Frasier and velvet tips, small and large), cup forceps of various sizes and angles, an endoscopic needle (a modified butterfly needle may also be used) for intralaryngeal injection, blunt microelevators, alligator forceps, microscissors of various angles and directions, and a sharp sickle knife (▶ Fig. 17.2).

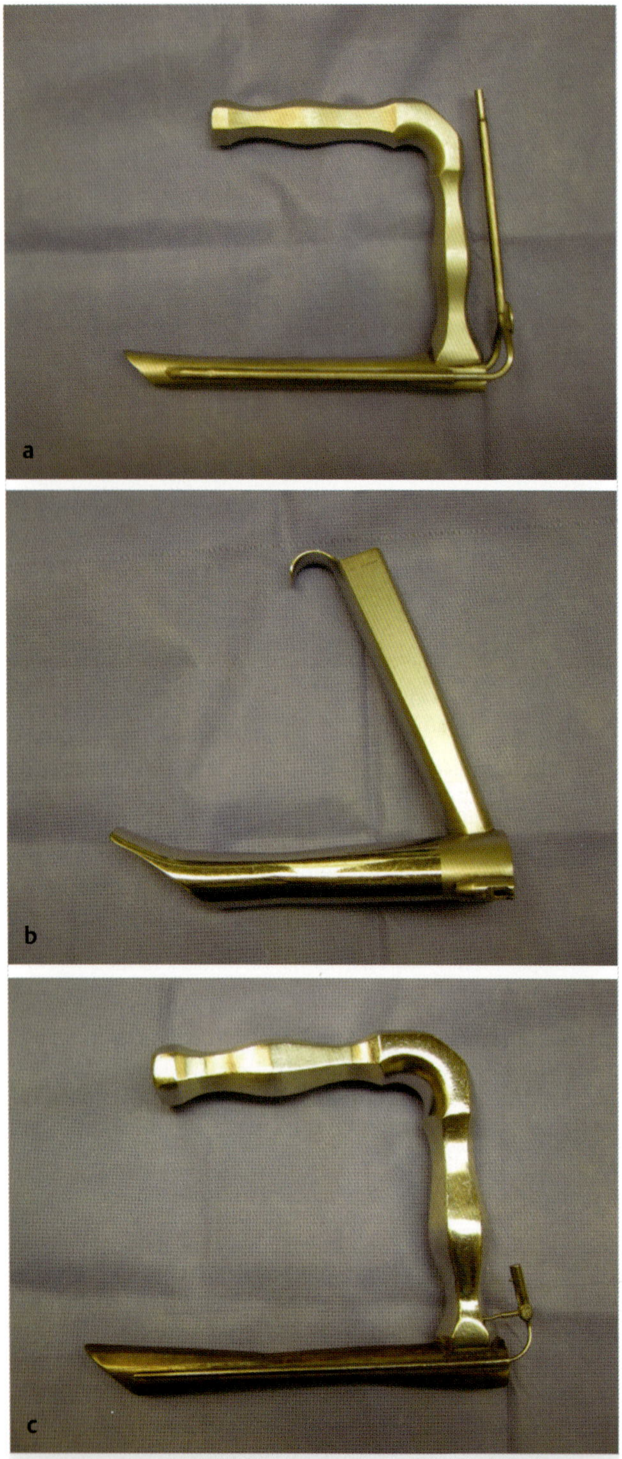

Fig. 17.1 (a) Dedo laryngoscope. (b) Lindholm laryngscope. (c) Holinger anterior commissure laryngoscope.

Finally, comfort and stability during these operations cannot be overemphasized. As such, the surgeon may wish to use an operating chair with arms that can be used to rest and stabilize the elbows or forearms during surgery.

17.4.2 Anesthesia

Excellent communication and teamwork with anesthesiology colleagues is paramount in laryngeal surgery. Prior to surgery, the case should be discussed with the anesthesia team. When possible, photographic documentation from a recent office visit greatly facilitates this conversation. If the patient is to be intubated, the size (typically 5.0 or 5.5) and type of endotracheal tube should be mutually agreed upon. For example, if use of the CO_2 laser is expected, an appropriate laser-safe tube should be selected. It may be preferable at times for the phonosurgeon to perform the intubation, as in the case of difficult anatomy, a large obstructive lesion, or a voice professional mandating an extremely experienced laryngoscopist for intubation. Occasionally, the surgeon may prefer operating while the patient is apneic, with or without use of jet ventilation. This should be discussed well in advance of surgery, so that an anesthesiologist who is well experienced and comfortable with these methods may be scheduled.

17.4.3 Technique

Positioning

After administration of antibiotics and steroids (10 mg of dexamethasone), the first key to successful phonomicrosurgery is adequate positioning. The ideal position is to put the patient into a "sniffing" position, with the head extended and neck flexed. A shoulder roll is not necessary when this position is used. On occasion, however, traditional neck extension with a shoulder roll allows for best exposure. Next, care should be taken to protect the maxillary alveolar ridge and dentition. This may be done with a dental guard, or with wet gauze in the edentulous patient.

Next, select the largest laryngoscope that is appropriate for the patient's anatomy, and insert it atraumatically. The distal tip of the laryngoscope should be positioned just superior to the lesion, with the false vocal folds pushed laterally by the sides of the scope. Avoid contacting the surface of the true vocal fold with the laryngoscope, as this will alter the appearance of both the pathology and of the vocal fold itself. The laryngoscope should then be fixed in place with a suspension apparatus of the surgeon's choice, taking care not to apply excess pressure on the maxillary ridge. Similarly, suspension should be used to stabilize the view, and not to improve it. Excessive upward rotation of the distal laryngoscope will lead to too much pressure on the teeth, thus risking a fracture of the dentition.

When an anterior view is difficult to achieve, cricoid pressure may be useful. This may be obtained using 3-inch silk tape, secured at either side of the operating table such that posterior and superior pressure is applied over the neck with the larynx under simultaneous visualization. A piece of gauze may be placed under the tape to protect the skin. The tape is then secured to the bed on either side of the patient's head. Another method to improve visualization includes altering neck position by applying more flexion. Next, the head of the bed should be elevated and the table should be lowered such that the larynx may be easily viewed through the microscope at a comfortable

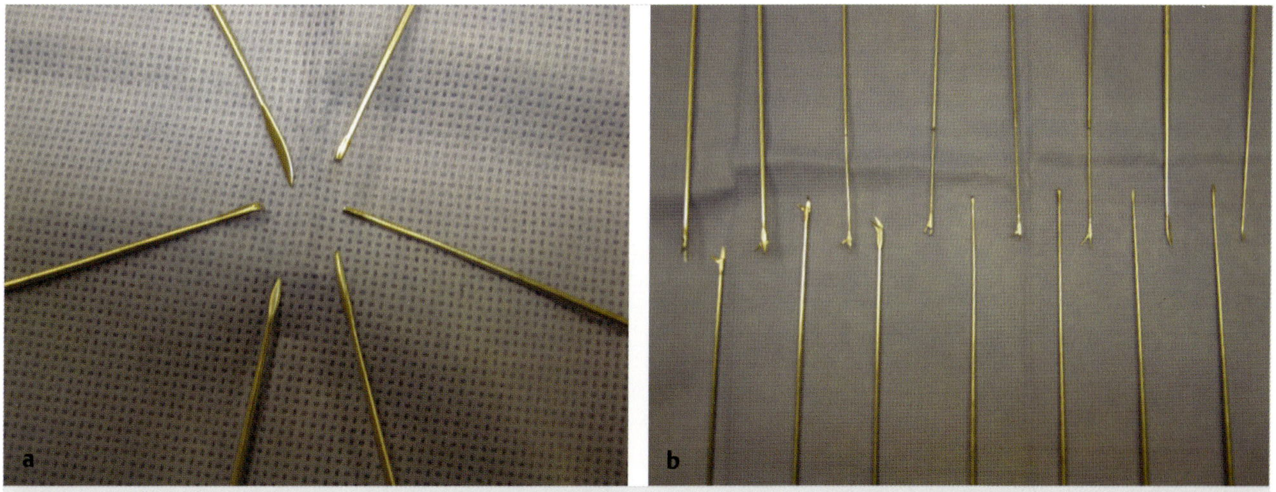

Fig. 17.2 (a) Laryngeal microdissection equipment. (b) Laryngeal micro-cup forceps and scissors. Note the various angles and directions of the instruments to facilitate dissection.

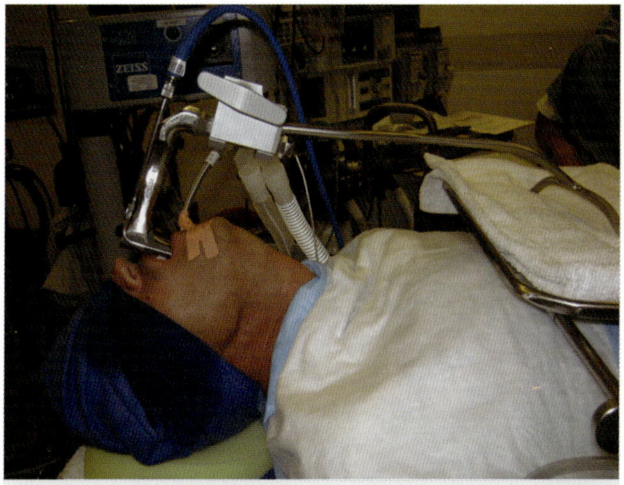

Fig. 17.3 Patient in position following laryngoscopy and suspension. Note the use of a metal endotracheal tube in this patient who is about to undergo laser laryngeal surgery.

angle. Alternatively, the patient can be placed in a reverse Trendelenberg position (▶ Fig. 17.3).

At this point, after administration of topical anesthesia, the zero-degree telescope can be used to assess the larynx and its pathology. Preoperative photographs are taken at this time. Next, the microscope should be brought in and set at a focal length of 400 mm; fine adjustments may be made to establish a clear and crisp binocular view.

Microflap: General Surgical Technique

The microflap technique may be applied to a number of different intracordal pathologies. A general description is provided here, followed by technique modifications according to specific pathologies.

First, a sickle knife is used to make an incision parallel to the vocal fold edge, just over or immediately lateral to the lesion (▶ Fig. 17.4). The knife should just enter epithelium, as indicated by a subtle "give" as pressure is applied. The knife can then be pulled back slightly to tent up epithelium and avoid damaging deeper structures as the incision is extended. Extension may also be performed using up-angled microscissors.

Next, a blunt instrument, such as a curved elevator, is used to gently dissect the lesion away from the surrounding tissue; the most important part of dissection is to identify and dissect the plane just lateral to the lesion, freeing it away from the vocal ligament (▶ Fig. 17.5). Microscissors may be used to cut any remnant-adherent fibrous bands. The mass can then be removed and passed off the field as specimen. The epithelial microflap is simply redraped. Hemostasis is easily achieved with topical vasoconstriction, such as with 4% cocaine or phenylephrine. Following lesion excision, the vocal fold edge should be straight and smooth in appearance. If not, the area of the microflap should be re-examined for remnant portions of the lesion.

Occasionally, dissection may be facilitated by hydrodissection. This is performed by a subepithelial injection of 1% lidocaine with 1:100,000 epinephrine. This can ease the identification and protection of the lamina propria and ligament. However, hydrodissection should be performed with caution, as injection may obscure the borders of the lesion, and this may result in inadequate resection.

The microsurgical technique described above is applicable for most intracordal lesions. However, it does not apply as a whole to all pathologies. Specific exceptions are briefly addressed on an individual basis below. For a detailed review of each of these lesions, please refer to Chapter 7.

17.5 Intracordal Cysts

Cysts are epithelial-lined structures that present in the mid-membranous vocal fold (▶ Fig. 17.6). Although the exact etiology is unclear, they are thought to arise as a result of vocal misuse, upper respiratory infection, or acid reflux.[9] Although they may decrease in size with voice rest or after voice therapy, they do not completely resolve spontaneously. As such, excision is often necessary. The microflap described above is an appropriate approach. However, the cyst is often attached to the superior epithelial surface (i.e., the microflap undersurface). As a result, it is best to excise the adherent epitheium to avoid incomplete excision or cyst rupture. This is done by making anterior and posterior cuts of the vocal fold epithelium, taking care to avoid disruption of the vocal ligament. The pathology can then be removed "en bloc" with the overlying epithelium using a small cup forceps (▶ Fig. 17.7). The vocal fold will re-epithelialize normally if the ligament is intact. This re-epithelialization is present as soon as 2 weeks postoperatively, at the patient's first follow-up. It is critical to remove the entire cyst to prevent scarring or sulcus formation.[6]

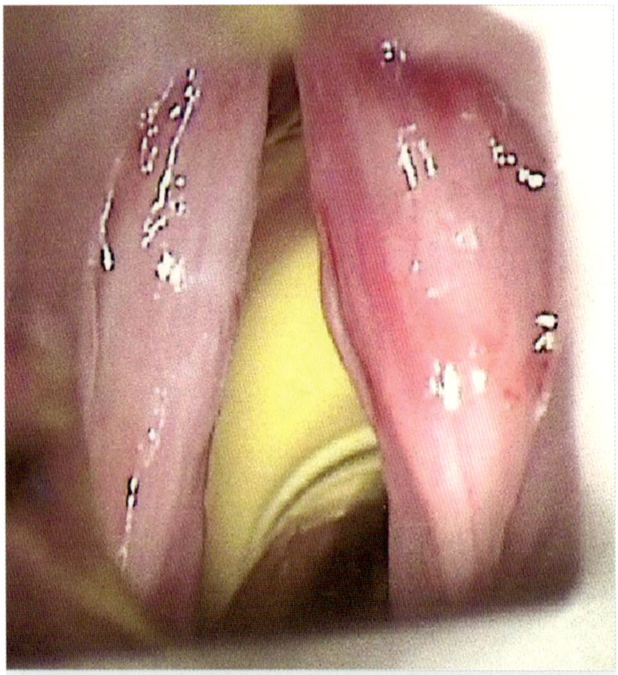

Fig. 17.4 Incision made lateral to vocal fold lesion.

17.6 Nodules

Vocal fold nodules are bilateral, symmetrical swellings of the anterior true vocal folds associated with impedance of complete glottal closure that are known to be the result of phonatory trauma associated with voice misuse (▶ Fig. 17.8).[6,10] Therefore, the cornerstone of treatment is voice therapy. Many patients demonstrate resolution of their nodules after maintaining healthy phonatory behaviors. In cases of chronic, mature subepithelial scar deposition, voice therapy alone may not be enough to reduce the size of these lesions. In these cases, phonomicrosurgery is a useful adjunct.

Unlike with cysts, a subepithelial approach is not necessary for nodules. The goal of nodule surgery is to attain a straight vocal fold edge. This is accomplished by conservative resection of the superficial exophytic aspect of the nodule by sharp excision. Thereafter, resumption of voice therapy will lead to resolution of any remnant lesion.

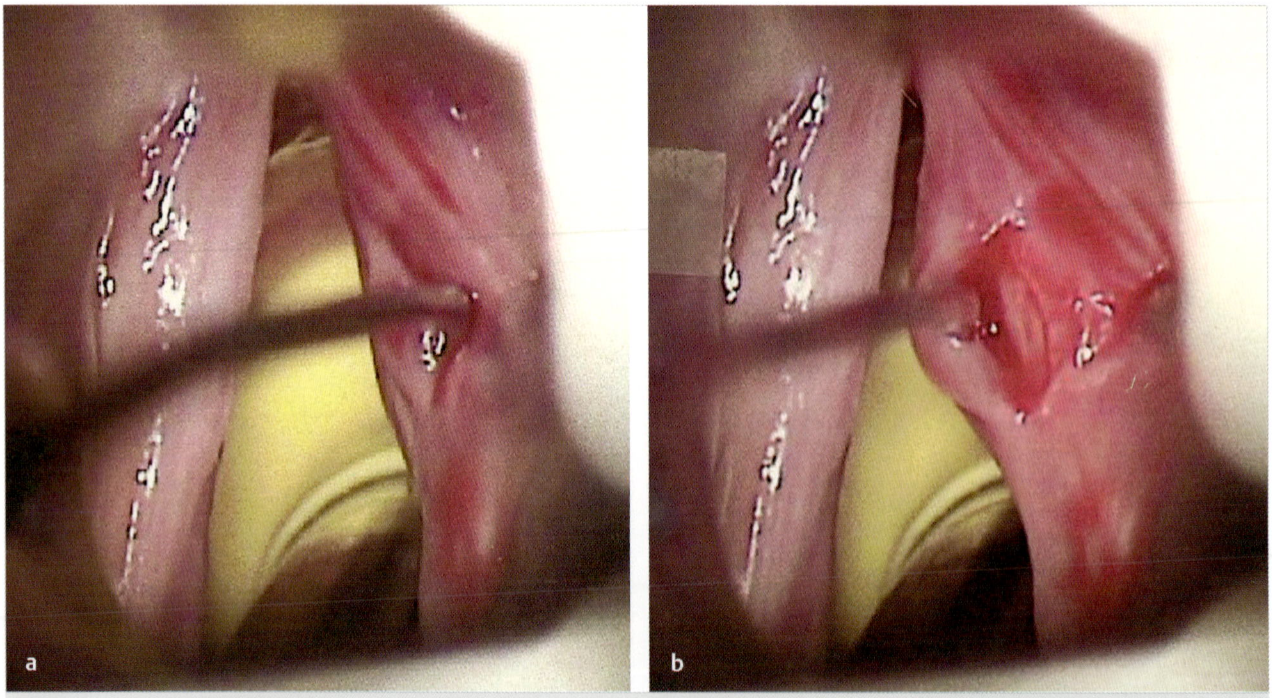

Fig. 17.5 (a, b) Dissection lateral to lesion, separating it from the vocal ligament.

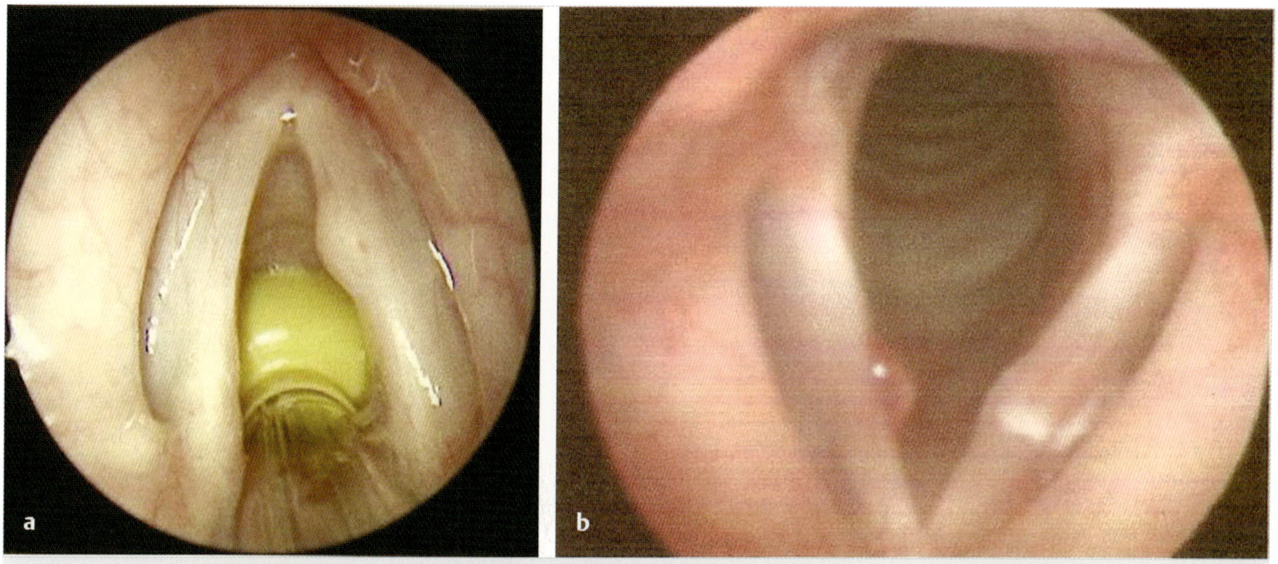

Fig. 17.6 (a) Typical appearance of a vocal fold cyst. (b) Hemorrhagic vocal fold cyst.

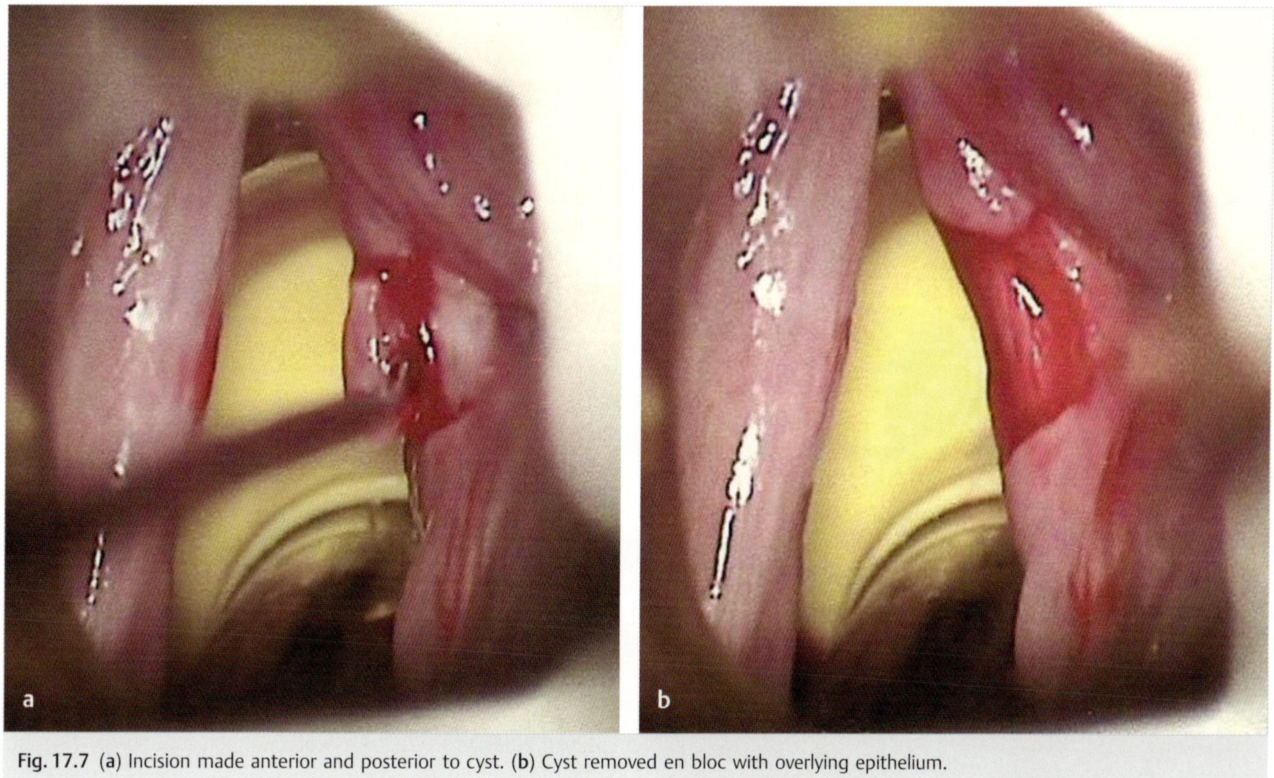

Fig. 17.7 (a) Incision made anterior and posterior to cyst. (b) Cyst removed en bloc with overlying epithelium.

17.7 Polyps

As approximately 90% of polyps fail conservative management, surgical removal is the norm.[11] In our practice, small polyps are typically removed in the office. Their exophytic nature lends them toward straightforward removal via transnasal endoscopy under local anesthesia. In the case of larger polyps, or when removal in the office is not otherwise possible, excision may be performed under general anesthesia via direct transoral laryngoscopy. Extent of dissection is dictated by the size and nature of the lesion. One may use a small cup forceps for pedunculated lesions or microscissors with aid of a Bouchayer forceps to retract the lesion laterally for wide-based polyps. Excess epithelium may need to be trimmed to ensure a straight vocal fold edge following excision. Care is taken not to violate the underlying vocal fold ligament.

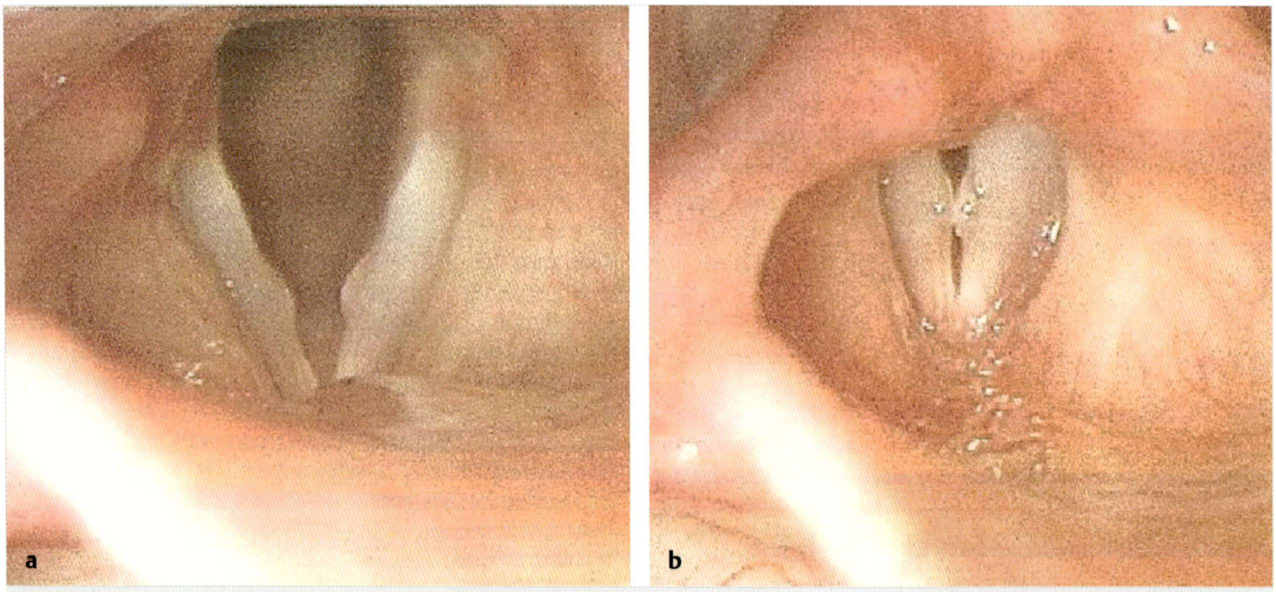

Fig. 17.8 (a, b) Vocal fold nodules.

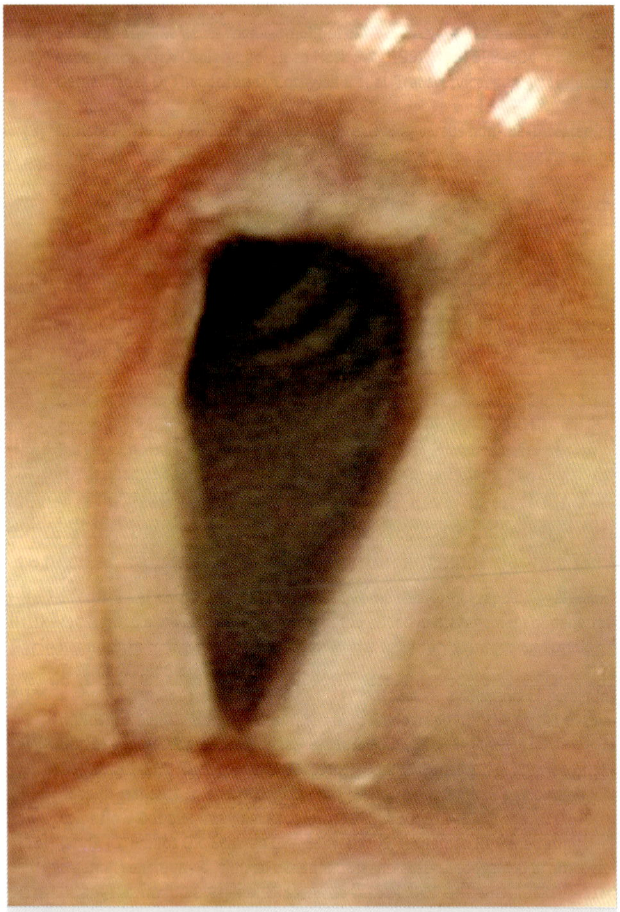

Fig. 17.9 Posterior commissure edema and mild left vocal process granulation tissue associated with severe laryngopharyngeal reflux. Videostroboscopy also demonstrated mucosal wave alteration due to mild Reinke edema, not appreciable with a halogen light source.

17.8 Vocal Process Granulomas

Granulomas form as a result of laryngeal trauma, usually in the form of intubation, laryngopharyngeal reflux, or compensation for glottal insufficiency due to paresis or presbylarynges (▶ Fig. 17.9).[6,12]

Excision is fraught with recurrence, and a decision for surgery should be undertaken very cautiously. Conservative treatment is the rule, with a low acid diet, maximized antireflux medication regimen, voice therapy, avoidance of the valsalva maneuver, as well as chemically induced paralysis using botulinum toxin.[13] An effort should be made to rule out an underlying glottal incompetency, which has been found in over half of patients with vocal process granulomas.[12] When even paralysis will not prevent contact of large bilateral contact ulcers, or when a malignant diagnosis cannot be excluded based on physical exam, surgical excision is warranted (▶ Fig. 17.10). Excision should be conservative, minimizing any further irritation of the perichondiurm.[14] Application of steroids has been described, but its application may not prevent recurrence.[4]

17.9 Vascular Ectasias

Vascular ectasias are the result of small developmental vascular anomalies within the vocal fold. Typically, they do not affect one's singing or speaking voice. As such, we have adopted a conservative approach toward these lesions, consisting of antireflux precautions, and voice therapy for abnormal laryngeal posturing. In the absence of a significant ectasia-associated dysphonia, phonomicrosurgery to address the lesion is more likely to harmfully affect the voice than the lesion itself.

The primary indication for surgical intervention for these lesions is in the event of bleeding. Once a bleeding event occurs, the patient is place on strict antireflux and voice rest precautions, in addition to a course of oral steroids. After

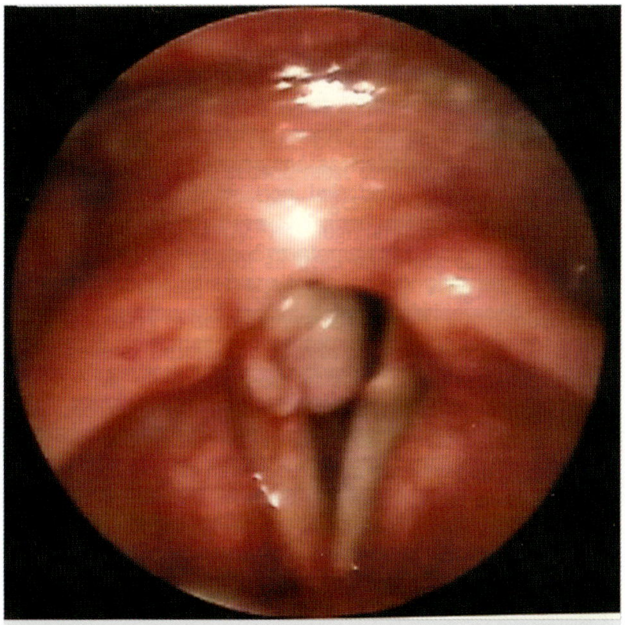

Fig. 17.10 Large vocal process granuloma that is unlikely to resolve with conservative medical management. This lesion was excised with long-term resolution of the granuloma.

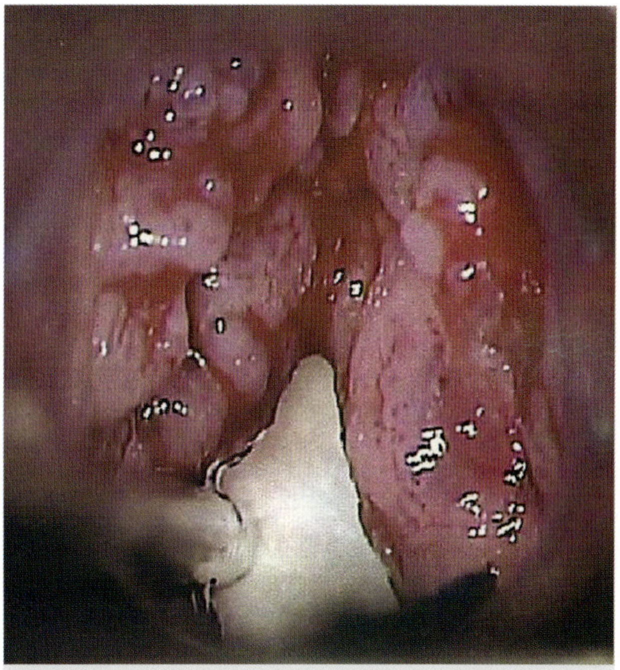

Fig. 17.11 Severe laryngeal papillomatosis requiring ablation under general anesthesia.

approximately one month, the patient is taken to the operating room and placed under general anesthesia. Following laryngoscopy and exposure, the carbon dioxide laser is used at a setting of 3 to 4 Watts with a defocused beam, and the affected areas are addressed. These lesions may also safely be treated in the office setting with a photoangiolytic laser, found more often in a facility that sees a high volume of voice patients.

Postoperatively, the patient is placed again on oral steroids, antireflux precautions, and voice rest. Serial videostroboscopic examinations are performed to assess for recovery.

17.10 Recurrent Respiratory Papillomatosis

Laryngeal papillomas are caused by infection with human papilloma virus (HPV), subtypes 6 and 11. It has an easily recognizable exophytic appearance with vascular stippling on stroboscopy, with definitive diagnosis obtained on pathologic section. Treatment of this condition is difficult, as much of the infected patient's larynx appears normal despite harboring subclinical infection. Long-term monitoring of recurrent respiratory papillomatosis (RRP) is critical, both for protection of the airway as well as assessment for development of malignancy, which occurs in approximately 2% of patients.[6]

Surgery is not curative for these patients, and therefore should not be overly aggressive. Mild-to-moderate disease can be treated under local anesthesia using the pulse-dye laser or potassium-titanyl-phosphate laser. If the patient cannot tolerate the procedure under local anesthesia, or if the disease is bulky and severe, it should be addressed under general anesthesia with an experienced anesthesiologist (▶ Fig. 17.11).

Available techniques include cold knife, microdebrider, and CO_2 laser. If using the CO_2 laser, our recommendations are as follows: the guiding beam should be diffused and set at 4 to 6 Watts, on a continuous setting. Unlike with the pulse-dye laser, extra care must be taken to avoid thermal injury to normal tissue. Additionally, one must avoid using the laser on directly apposing vocal fold edges and at the anterior commissure. Resection in these areas should be staged to avoid web formation and laryngeal stenoses.

Cidofovir can be considered for injection at the end of the procedure as an adjunctive measure in severe disease; however, this requires a preoperative discussion of the risks and benefits of this medication, in addition to its off-label use. A review of the literature has demonstrated a 2.7% malignant degeneration rate of laryngeal papilloma treated with cidofovir. Although this is similar to the rate of spontaneous malignant degeneration (2–3%) of laryngeal papilloma, the carcinogenic potential must be made known to the patient.[15] There is a dose-dependent risk of vocal fold scarring that is irreversible at high doses, as demonstrated in a canine model.[16] Patients who are of a child-bearing age should also be aware of possible side effects of infertility or teratogenicity.

17.11 Medialization Thyroplasty: Indications

After Payr's original description of laryngeal framework surgery for treatment of a paralyzed vocal fold in 1915, medialization thyroplasty resurfaced in the literature in the 1970s after publication of Isshiki's canine experiments and regained popularity in the late 1980s as an alternative to Teflon injection as a treatment for vocal fold paralysis.[2,17]

Indications for type I, or medialization, thyroplasty have expanded beyond simple paralysis. It can also be quite helpful in cases of vocal fold atrophy as well as paresis. A simple way to assess for potential improvement is by performing a manual compression test. This involves using the examiner's fingers to place pressure on one side of the larynx while having the patient phonate, and then compare the vocal quality to the voice produced by the larynx at baseline. The noncalcified larynx compresses quite easily. An improvement in quality or projection is indicative of the therapeutic potential of thyroplasty.

Another way to assess for potential benefit is by performing an injection laryngoplasty. It is less invasive than thyroplasty with temporary results, giving the surgeon an idea of whether open surgery is a feasible option for the patient. It is especially helpful in cases of immobility where vocal fold function is expected to recover, as in the case of recent surgery or upper respiratory infection where the recurrent laryngeal nerve's anatomical integrity is known to be intact. This procedure can be performed under local anesthesia in the office, and is described in further detail in Chapter 23.

Either medialization thyroplasty or arytenoid adduciton can be used to achieve equivalent phonatory quality in the patient with glottal incompetence.[18] However, in evaluation of the patient with marked bowing, or in a young patient in whom vocalis muscle atrophy is expected over time, a better consideration may be to perform an arytenoid adduction with laryngeal re-innervation.[19] Arytenoid adduction should particularly be considered in the patient with a large posterior gap that is contributing to the patient's dysphonia. Consultation with an experienced laryngologist is advised for either of these procedures.

17.12 Medialization Thyroplasty: Preoperative Considerations

Preoperative considerations for laryngeal framework surgery are essentially the same as those for phonomicrosurgery. Patient counseling should extend to include a discussion of postoperative care, particularly if the surgeon plans to place a drain or admit for overnight observation.

17.13 Medialization Thyroplasty: Intraoperative Considerations

Isshiki first described his type I thyroplasty as an actual incision and repositioning of the thyroid lamina on the affected side, such that the paralyzed vocal fold was brought closer to the midline without use of an implant.[2] Since the original description of thyroid cartilage framework surgery for vocal fold medialization, a number of modifications have been described, most notably with regard to use of foreign material as an implant to medialize the vocal fold. Several materials are available. A popular preformed implant choice is the Montgomery Thyroplasty Implant System (Boston Medical Products, Westborough, MA). Common customizable implant choices are porous expanded polytetrafluoroethylene ribbon and hand-carved silastic blocks. The most important consideration in selecting an implant is to choose an inert material with a straight edge that medializes at the appropriate level (i.e., at the level of the true vocal folds without medializing the false vocal folds).

To accurately judge the amount of medialization required, it is optimal to perform the surgery with the patient awake. This allows the intraoperative voice to guide implant sizing. As such, a preoperative discussion with the anesthesiologist regarding the steps of this surgery, with an understanding of when the patient will need to be able to follow commands, will help avoid frustration and confusion throughout the procedure.

Prior to beginning surgery, the patient should receive a dose of antibiotics. Furthermore, adequate local anesthesia should be administered, as it is critical for patient comfort. Ten cc's of 1% lidocaine with 1:100,000 epinephrine buffered with 8.4% sodium bicarbonate is our preferred anesthetic agent. This should be injected after a shoulder roll has been placed and landmarks have been marked, several minutes prior to making an incision.

Although not required for the operation, the surgeon may opt for concurrent endoscopic visualization. A transnasal fiberoptic laryngosope can be properly positioned by the surgeon and held in place by an assistant or by a scope-holding mechanism of the surgeon's choice (▶ Fig. 17.12).[20] This can then be connected to a camera and projected onto a monitor, as is done for endoscopic sinus surgery. If the surgeon has adequate assistance, the fiberoptic laryngoscope may also be introduced once the cartilage window has been created and estimation of implant size is performed.

Following sterile preparation and draping of the neck, a 4- to 5-cm incision is made over the thyroid cartilage, centered over the side of the vocal fold paralysis. Limited subplatysmal flaps are elevated. Then, the strap muscles are divided along the midline raphe, and only the muscles on the side of interest are elevated off of the thyroid cartilage perichondrium. Dissection should proceed superiorly and inferiorly to expose the limits of the thyroid cartilage and at least as far posteriorly as the oblique line. If an arytenoid adduction is to be performed, the posterior thyroid ala must be exposed, as described in the following section.

Next, the location of the window should be outlined. If a preformed implant is being used, an appropriate window sizer is employed to mark the cartilage. Otherwise, specific laryngeal landmarks are identified. The superior border of the window should be parallel to the inferior edge of the thyroid cartilage, and located halfway between the thyroid notch and the inferior edge. The inferior border should be approximately 2–3 mm above the inferior edge of the cartilage. The anterior border should be 5–7 mm behind the midline of the thyroid cartilage, and the posterior border should be just anterior to the oblique line (▶ Fig. 17.13).

Once the window has been marked, it is ready to be excised. This can be done with a knife, if the cartilage is soft. If it is calcified, a sagittal saw or otologic drill may be used instead. We

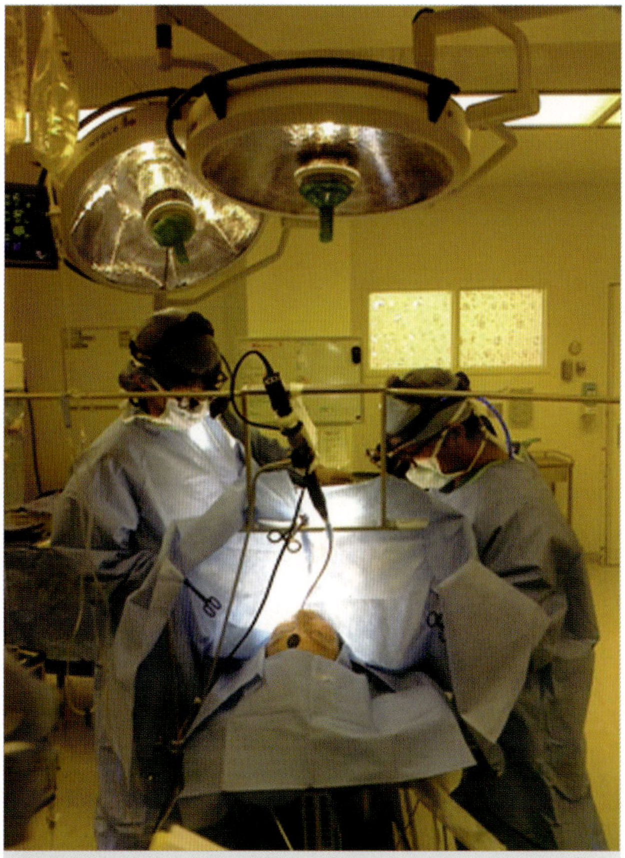

Fig. 17.12 Flexible laryngoscope secured to an orthopedic bar and connected to a digital camera. (Courtesy of Dinesh Chhetri, MD.)

usually excise the inner perichondrium with the cartilage window (▶ Fig. 17.14). With the patient awake and responsive, a blunt-tipped instrument such as a freer-elevator can be used to medialize the soft tissue as the patient phonates. A judgment is made on the degree of medialization needed to produce a strong voice, and an implant is fashioned accordingly.

We prefer to carve laryngeal implants from a Silastic block (▶ Fig. 17.15). Part of fashioning the implant involves designing external phalanges on the anterior and posterior aspects. These phalanges rest outside of the thyroid cartilage with a low profile. They are used to secure the implant in place using a permanent monofilament suture (▶ Fig. 17.16).

After irrigation of the surgical site, a Penrose drain is placed. The strap muscles and skin are closed over the drain in multiple layers. Following surgery, the patient may be admitted overnight for observation, or discharged home with follow-up the next day for drain removal. The risk of postoperative airway obstruction is extremely low, unless an arytenoid adduction is performed simultaneously.

17.14 Arytenoid Adduction

Although medialization thyroplasty usually provides sufficient vocal fold medialization, in certain instances, arytenoid adduction can provide either an alternate surgical option, or a means of augmenting an otherwise insufficient medialization achieved via thyroplasty. This method is particularly useful in cases of a large posterior gap, such as in men, whose larynges tend to be larger than those of women, and in cases of a vocal fold-level mismatch.[21]

The most common method of adduction, and the technique favored in our practice, is the use of an arytenoid adduction suture. This suture is used to mimic the action of the thyroarytenoid-lateral cricoarytenoid muscular complex.[22] In doing this, the vocal process of the arytenoid is rotated in a medial and caudal direction, leading to both dramatic medialization and increased tension of the vocal fold. When combined with laryngeal reinnervation, which leads to improved vocal fold tone, this procedure results in remarkable, long-term improvement in vocal quality.[19] In contrast, when performed in young patients, medialization thyroplasty alone may result in diminished vocal quality over the course of several years, as the vocalis muscle atrophies.

Although adduction is performed by some with the patient under local anesthesia, our preference is to use general anesthesia, as the procedure can be quite uncomfortable.[21] An incision is made midway between the thyroid notch and inferior margin of the thyroid cartilage in the anterior neck and should extend beyond the posterior margin of the cartilage on the paralyzed side. After raising subplatysmal flaps, the thyroid cartilage is exposed. The inferior constrictor and thyrohyoid muscles are released from the oblique line and divided to expose the posterior lamina (▶ Fig. 17.17a). The next step of arytenoid adduction involves identification of the arytenoid cartilage, specifically the muscular process. To accomplish this, the pyriform sinus mucosa is gently elevated with utmost caution, in order not to perforate the airway. The muscular process is then palpated as a small prominence at the level of the vocal fold. If not yet palpable, the posterior lamina of the thyroid cartilage may need to be partially resected. Once identified, two small monofilament nonabsorbable polypropylene sutures are then passed through the muscular process (the surrounding soft tissue or the cricoarytenoid tendon may be used if needed) (▶ Fig. 17.17b). These sutures are then passed anteromedially through the thyroid cartilage, to exit just anterior to the inferior tubercle. A drill may be needed here in very calcified cartilages. The sutures are then secured over a small bolster or microplate (▶ Fig. 17.17c). Very little tension is needed to achieve adequate adduction. Excessive tension will lead to a limited airway and strained vocal quality. In fact, although others have described separation of the cricoarytenoid joint prior to suture placement, this increases the risk of symptomatic postoperative airway restriction.[21] Following irrigation of the surgical bed, a Penrose drain is typically

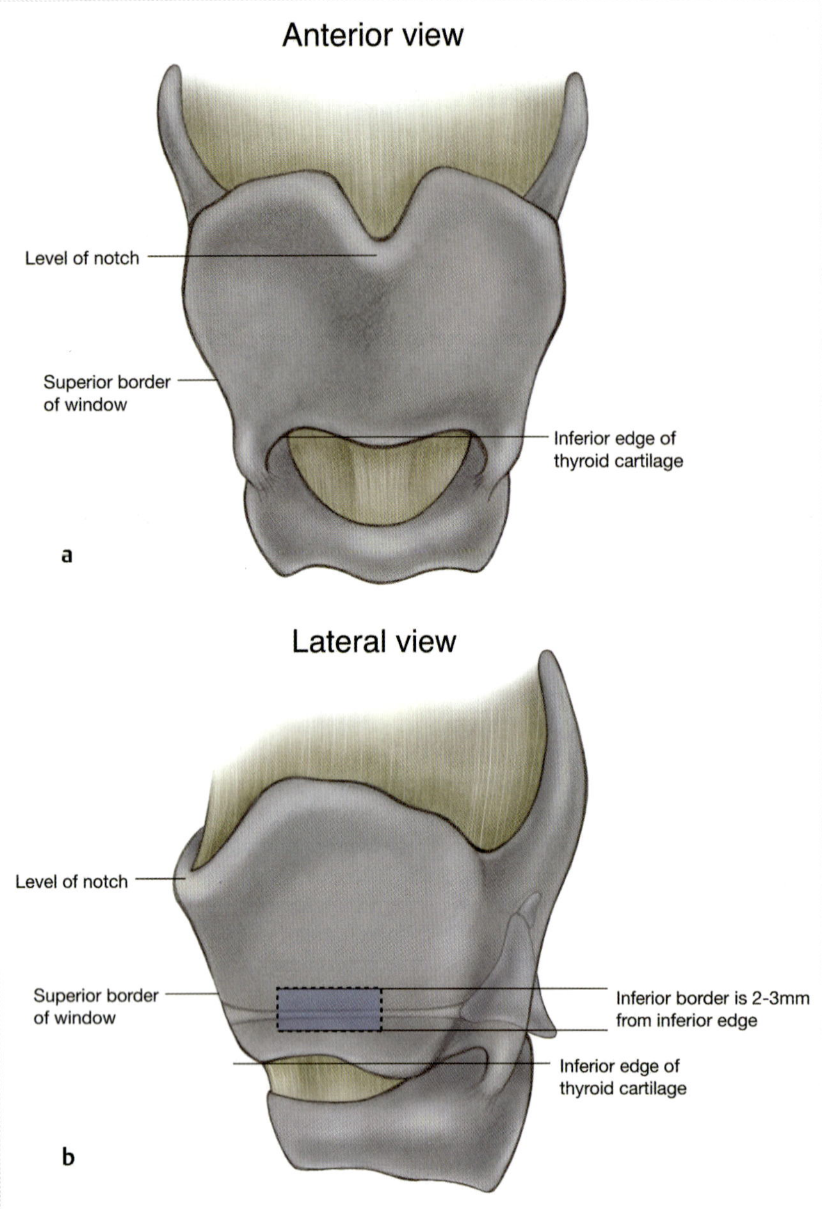

Fig. 17.13 (**a**) Thyroid cartilage landmarks, anterior view. (**b**) Thyroplasty landmarks, lateral view. (Courtesy of Jennifer Bergeron, MD.)

placed, and the operative site is closed in multiple layers. The patient is then observed overnight for airway monitoring.

17.15 Postoperative Considerations

Prior to discharge, the patient should be reminded of all postoperative instructions, including the medication regimen. Generally, the patient is given four prescriptions: antibiotics, steroids, an analgesic, and a proton pump inhibitor.

The postoperative discussion should also include a review of low-acid diet and voice rest instructions. Depending on the type and extent of surgery, voice rest may be strict or modified (i.e., limited to soft speaking only). Voice rest may range from a period of 2 to 14 days. Typically, the patient is seen in the office 2 weeks postoperatively and evaluated via videostroboscopy. Strict voice rest is then transitioned to limited, soft voice use. This is then gradually expanded to free speaking at about 6 weeks after surgery. Singers should be counseled to avoid singing for 1 to 2 months, and then resume under the guidance of a vocal coach. Following the healing process, voice therapy may be initiated at the surgeon's discretion.

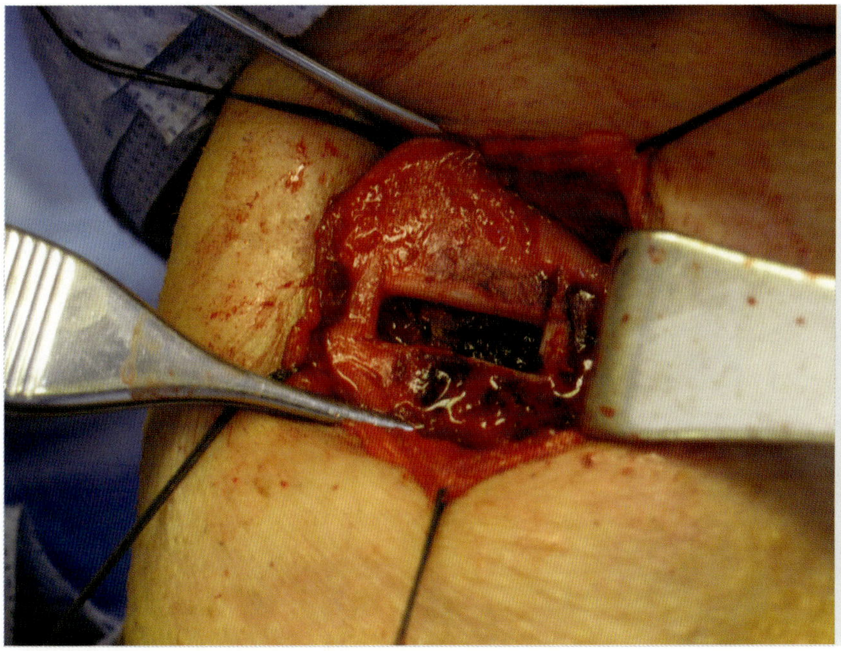

Fig. 17.14 Thyroplasty window excised from left thyroid lamina.

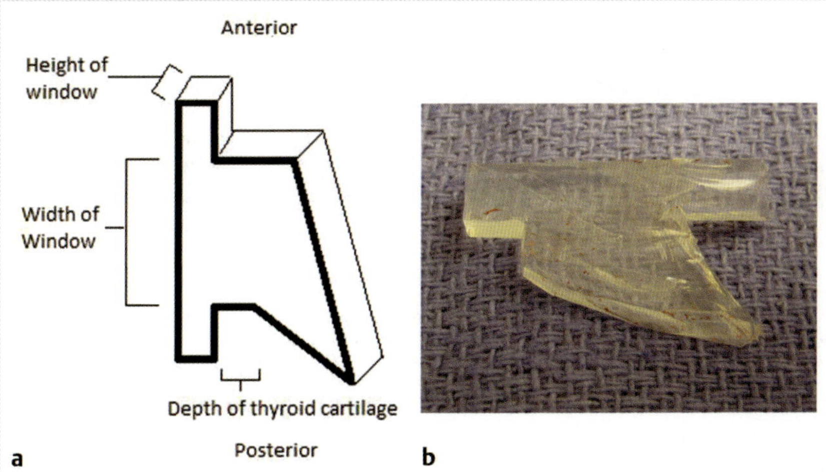

Fig. 17.15 (**a**) Schematic of Silastic implant. Courtesy of Jennifer Bergeron, MD. (**b**) Hand-carved Silastic implant.

17.16 Complications

Although complications are uncommon, even a perfectly executed surgery may yield imperfect results. Immediate intraoperative complications are variable and include injury to the dentition from laryngoscopy; pressure-induced injury to the lingual nerve, resulting in tongue numbness and parasthesia; injury or dislocation at the temporomandibular joint; laryngeal ecchymoses and edema; and postoperative pharyngitis. All of these possibilities should be discussed with the patient preoperatively, as mentioned previously. They primarily require supportive care and patient reassurance.

Long-term follow-up of phonomicrosurgery will occasionally demonstrate scar formation. Early postoperative voice rest control of acid reflux will usually help prevent scar, but this is not always predictable or avoidable. Some advocate steroid injection at the conclusion of vocal fold surgery, but there is no evidence to confirm the utility of this practice. The finding of vocal fold scarring is predicted by persistent or worsening dysphonia on surgical follow-up. Early diagnosis may help limit further degradation by enabling early revision or steroid injection in the office.[23] A well-developed scar or sulcus vocalis is very challenging to treat. A minithyrotomy approach has been described to address lesions consisting of lamina propria deficiency, although we advocate maximal reflux therapy with addition of type I thyroplasty as needed.[24] Overly aggressive use of the CO_2 laser may also result in formation of glottic webs. Treatment can be very challenging, as lysis often leads to recurrence of synechiae (▶ Fig. 17.18).

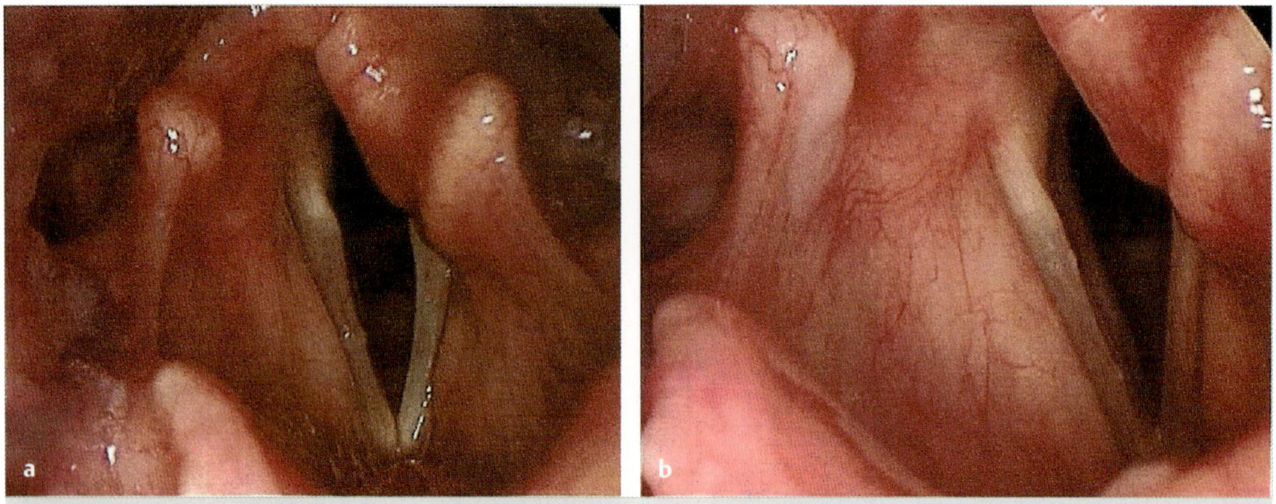

Fig. 17.16 (**a**) Left vocal fold paralysis and bowing approximately one year after thyroid surgery. (**b**) Straightened contour of left vocal fold following medialization thyroplasty, allowing glottic closure and improved phonation and deglutition.

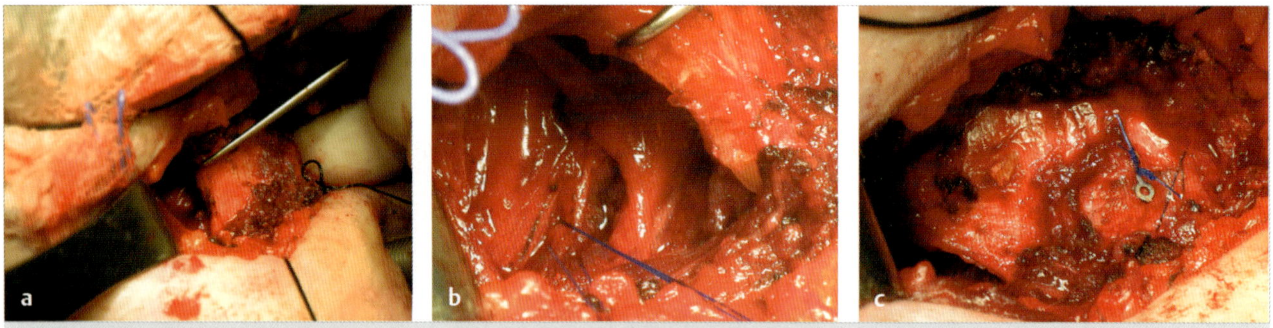

Fig. 17.17 (**a**) The posterior lamina of the thyroid cartilage has been exposed, and the pyriform sinus mucosa has been partially dissected away. (**b**) One polypropylene suture has been placed in the muscular process. It is being pulled away from the thyroid cartilage for demonstration purposes. (**c**) Both sutures have been passed through the anterior surface of the cartilage and secured over a two-hole microplate.

Prolonged, strict voice rest is not necessary following thyroplasty. Usually, just 1 to 2 days of voice rest, followed by restricted voice use, has been sufficient in our experience. A "final" voice result is usually attained approximately 1 to 2 months after surgery. A voice that is perceived as "strained" at this point is often due to an implant that is either too large or too superiorly placed, the latter causing false vocal fold medialization. If the voice has not improved after allowing for an adequate healing period, the implant should be removed or revised. Due to capsule formation around the implant, removal may afford sufficient medialization without need for further intervention (▶ Fig. 17.19).

A voice that remains breathy following medialization surgery may be undercorrected for two reasons. First, the implant placed may be too small. Intraoperative edema may lead the surgeon to falsely believe that a small implant has adequately medialized the vocal fold. Second, breathiness may be due to a persistent posterior glottic gap. A thyroplasty implant cannot medialize the vocal fold posterior to the vocal process (the location of which is approximated by the oblique line on

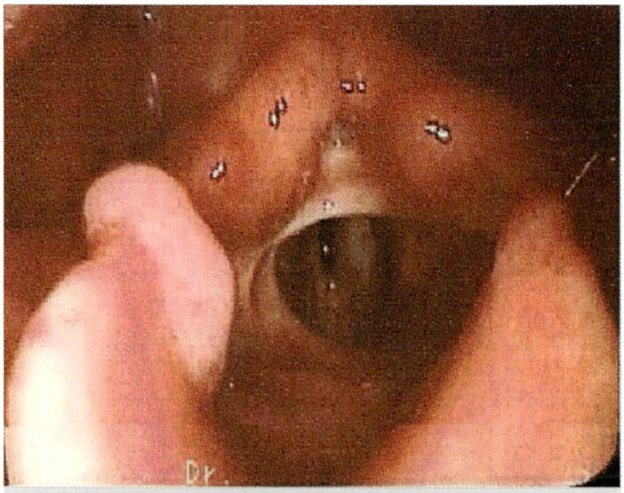

Fig. 17.18 Example of posterior glottic scarring and arytenoid tethering due to long-term, aggressive use of the CO_2 laser at an outside facility in a patient with recurrent respiratory papillomatosis.

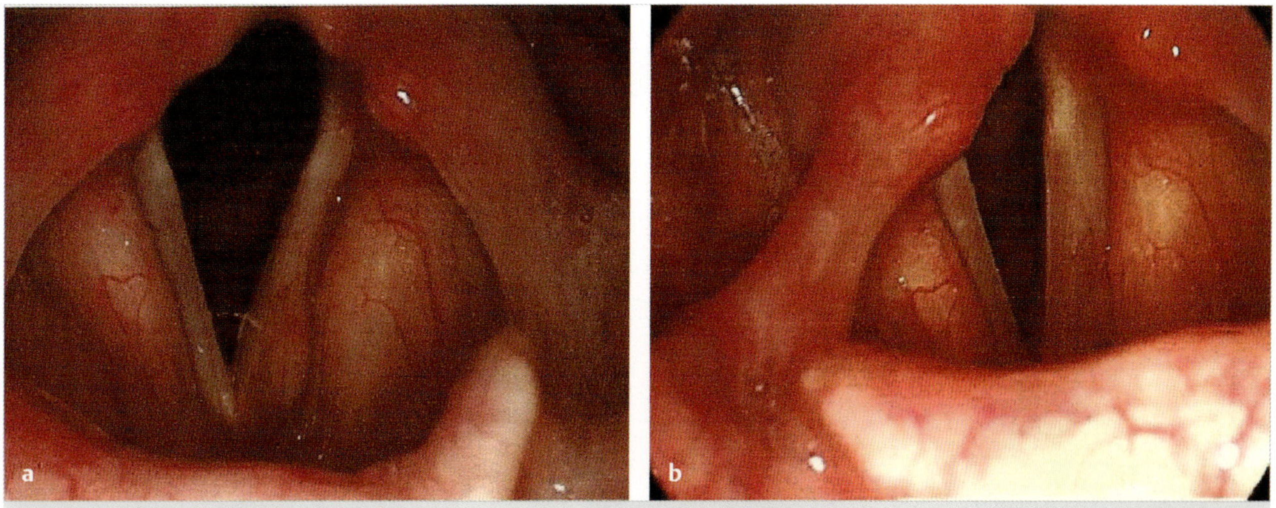

Fig. 17.19 (**a**) Overcorrection in the anterior left vocal fold, 3 months after medialization thyroplasty. (**b**) Following removal of the implant, the vocal fold healed nicely and all erythema and edema resolved. The capsule that had developed around the implant resulted in adequate medialization without implant replacement, with an excellent voice result.

the external thyroid lamina). In these cases, the patient may benefit from addition of an arytenoid adduction.

17.17 Conclusion

Phonosurgery has the ability to dramatically improve an individual's quality of life, particularly in those individuals who rely upon their voices for their livelihood. A careful physical examination and an accurate diagnosis are key. The decision for elective phonosurgery should not be taken lightly, given the potential risks involved, and should always be preceded by maximized conservative, medical management.

17.18 Key Points

- Dysphonia and aphonia are markedly debilitating, affecting at least 28 million workers in the United States on a daily basis.
- Benign epithelial disease can and should be approached in a conservative manner. The very presence of a discrete lesion does not constitute a reason to operate.
- Prior to surgery, the physician must address relevant comorbidities and consider initiating an antireflux regimen and directed voice therapy, if indicated.
- Surgical excision is typically required for certain types of lesions, such as cysts, polyps, mature nodules, papilloma, and very large granulomas.
- More conservative management is the rule for most nodules and granulomas.
- The primary indication for surgical intervention for vascular ectasias is in the event of bleeding.
- Surgery is not curative for papilloma and therefore should not be overly aggressive.
- The ideal position for laryngoscopy is to put the patient into a "sniffing" position, with the head extended and neck flexed.
- Medialization thyroplasty is the primary means of addressing the laterally paralyzed vocal fold in a long-term fashion.
- Arytenoid adduction is useful in cases of a large posterior gap and in cases of a vocal fold-level mismatch.

References

[1] Hirano M. Morphological structure of the vocal cord as a vibrator and its variations. Folia Phoniatr (Basel) 1974; 26: 89–94

[2] Isshiki N, Morita H, Okamura H, Hiramoto M. Thyroplasty as a new phonosurgical technique. Acta Otolaryngol 1974; 78: 451–457

[3] Fujimura O. Body-cover theory of the vocal fold and its phonetic implications. In: Stevens KN, Hirano M, eds. Vocal Fold Physiology; 1980: 271

[4] Rubin A, Sataloff RT. General principles of microlaryngeal surgery. In: Merati AL, Bielamowicz SA, eds. Textbook of Laryngology; 2007: 167–188

[5] Verdolini K, Ramig LO. Review: occupational risks for voice problems. Logoped Phoniatr Vocol 2001; 26: 37–46

[6] Altman KW. Vocal fold masses. Otolaryngol Clin North Am 2007; 40: 1091–1108, viii

[7] Cohen SM, Garrett CG. Utility of voice therapy in the management of vocal fold polyps and cysts. Otolaryngol Head Neck Surg 2007; 136: 742–746

[8] Rosen CA. Benign vocal fold lesions and phonomicrosurgery. In: Bailey BJ, Johnson JT, Newland SD et al, eds. Head & Neck Surgery—Otolaryngology; 2006: 837–846

[9] Martins RHG, Santana MF, Tavares ELM. Vocal cysts: clinical, endoscopic, and surgical aspects. J Voice 2011; 25: 107–110

[10] Karkos PD, McCormick M. The etiology of vocal fold nodules in adults. Curr Opin Otolaryngol Head Neck Surg 2009; 17: 420–423

[11] Nakagawa H, Miyamoto M, Kusuyama T, Mori Y, Fukuda H. Resolution of vocal fold polyps with conservative treatment. J Voice 2012; 26: e107–e110

[12] Carroll TL, Gartner-Schmidt J, Statham MM, Rosen CA. Vocal process granuloma and glottal insufficiency: an overlooked etiology? Laryngoscope 2010; 120: 114–120

[13] Nasri S, Sercarz JA, McAlpin T, Berke GS. Treatment of vocal fold granuloma using botulinum toxin type A. Laryngoscope 1995; 105: 585–588

[14] Hoffman HT, Overholt E, Karnell M, McCulloch TM. Vocal process granuloma. Head Neck 2001; 23: 1061–1074

[15] Broekema FI, Dikkers FG. Side-effects of cidofovir in the treatment of recurrent respiratory papillomatosis. Eur Arch Otorhinolaryngol 2008; 265: 871–879

[16] Chhetri DK, Jahan-Parwar B, Hart SD, Bhuta SM, Berke GS, Shapiro NL. Local and systemic effects of intralaryngeal injection of cidofovir in a canine model. Laryngoscope 2003; 113: 1922–1926

[17] Koufman JA. Laryngoplasty for vocal cord medialization: an alternative to Teflon. Laryngoscope 1986; 96: 726–731

[18] Bielamowicz S, Berke GS, Gerratt BR. A comparison of type I thyroplasty and arytenoid adduction. J Voice 1995; 9: 466–472

[19] Chhetri DK, Gerratt BR, Kreiman J, Berke GS. Combined arytenoid adduction and laryngeal reinnervation in the treatment of vocal fold paralysis. Laryngoscope 1999; 109: 1928–1936

[20] Rosen CA, Simpson CB. Silastic medialization laryngoplasty for unilateral vocal fold paralysis. In: Operative Techniques in Laryngology; 2008: 242–251

[21] Isshiki N, Tanabe M, Sawada M. Arytenoid adduction for unilateral vocal cord paralysis. Arch Otolaryngol 1978; 104: 555–558

[22] Meyer T, Sulica L, Blitzer A. Vocal fold paralysis. In: Merati AL, Bielamowicz SA, eds. Textbook of Laryngology; 2007: 219–237

[23] Mortensen M. Laryngeal steroid injection for vocal fold scar. Curr Opin Otolaryngol Head Neck Surg 2010; 18: 487–491

[24] Gray SD, Bielamowicz SA, Titze IR, Dove H, Ludlow C. Experimental approaches to vocal fold alteration: introduction to the minithyrotomy. Ann Otol Rhinol Laryngol 1999; 108: 1–9

18 Voice Therapy

Linda M. Carroll

A clear, pleasing voice quality can be a tremendous personal asset. A pleasing voice allows social, academic, and professional pursuits to be successful. If the voice is dysphonic, the listener is distracted and communication becomes compromised. The concept of a "normal" voice may depend on age, sex, culture, personal demands, and environmental issues. Although many individuals experience brief dysphonia from overuse or as a secondary reaction to other health issues (colds, allergies), a voice disorder occurs when the dysphonia does not heal or recover in a normal manner or time period.

When an individual experiences a change in their voice quality or vocal function, they may be referred to a voice therapist. It is the role of the voice therapist to guide the patient from their current voice back to a functional voice that can meet the needs of their profession and social voice use.

The extent to which the voice can be returned to the premorbid state, or better than premorbid state, depends on several factors. Certainly, the severity of the pathology is a major factor. Also important are patient motivation, the therapist's ability to manipulate the patient's vocal production during the therapy sessions, changing a hoarse voice to a more focused voice, and the patient's ability to transfer use of voice exercises throughout the day to guide the laryngeal physiology to a positive compensation. With good compensatory measures, the vocal folds generally heal well, and heal rather quickly. At the end of each therapy session, the voice should feel and sound better than at the start of that therapy session.

Determining the necessary goals of voice therapy depends on the patient's daily voice activities, prior capacity and quality, and viable quality given the nature of the laryngeal structures. A skilled clinician can discern the premorbid voice quality from a brief amateur recording, such as a telephone announce message or audiovideo recording. The viable quality of voice must take into account the present laryngeal status as well as other subsystems and medications that can have an effect on voice.

In every course of therapy, there are counseling goals and education goals. Counseling goals include those for the patient and the patient's family (or principal communication environment). Counseling includes understanding etiologic factors that led to the voice disorder, and aspects of communication that challenge successful transfer of healthy, effective voice. Education includes an understanding of laryngeal anatomy and physiology, breath management, and transfer of acoustic energy to optimum voice quality, as well as management options and factors that can improve healing of the voice.

During the therapy session, which typically lasts 30 to 60 minutes, it is the responsibility of the clinician to create a safe, compassionate environment which, when coupled with the clinician's training and expert perceptual skills, can allow for improved voice function and understanding of the processes involved for the patient to gain that better voice. It is the responsibility of the patient to respect the appointment time and be open to trying new strategies to gain a better voice. Although there are some cases where the voice can be "fixed" in one session, effective voice therapy and transfer to functional voice use may take 4 to 10 sessions. More sessions are needed if there are complicating factors. Length of therapy depends on the ability to adapt to a healthy voice pattern in and out of the therapy room. The patient must get "hooked" to the new sound and sensation, and realize that a healthy voice may be a combination of his or her past voice and additional voice qualities.

Voice disorders may be acquired (nodules, cyst, polyp, scar, sulcus, vocal fold paralysis/paresis, contact ulcer, spasmodic dysphonia), congenital (laryngeal web, larnygomalacia, sulcus, vocal fold paralysis), traumatic (hemorrhage, arytenoid dislocation), inflammatory (larygneal sicca, gastroesophageal reflux disease, allergy), neoplastic (tumors), or behavioral (muscle tension dysphonia, laryngospasm, puberphonia, conversion disorder). The voice can be disturbed by more global disorders (Parkinson disease, cerebral palsy, Down syndrome), and may be triggered by other health aspects (hearing loss, thyroid imbalance, hormonal changes).

Some patients are very sensitive to changes in the vocal folds, while others seem to have little awareness. Similarly, some individuals have extraordinary compensatory skills; others have few skills to speak, or sing, around the pathology.

Because the voice is a combination of respiratory skill, laryngeal function, and acoustic transfer (resonance and articulation), individuals with a "great" upper vocal tract may produce a better voice than would be imagined. These same individuals with resonant voices are also acutely aware of laryngeal mucosa changes and may have a great deal of frustration. The skilled clinician with expert auditory and perceptual skills can decipher the dysphonic components in the voice production and guide the patient to better subsystem compensation and coordination, yielding a better voice.

18.1 Voice Therapy Techniques

18.1.1 Contact Ulcer and Granuloma

A contact ulcer or granuloma may be acquired from nonintubation or intubation irritation, and may occur at any age. The contact ulcer is a superficial ulceration on the arytenoid that may be unilateral or bilateral. Symptoms progress from vocal dryness, to throat tickle, to throat clearing (or coughing), to discomfort, to laryngeal pain. When the contact ulcer or granuloma resolves, the symptoms follow reverse order. Resolution of symptoms can take 3 to 4 times the length of development of the lesion, and strengthening of the voice can take an additional 3 to 6 months.

Key aspects to resolve the lesion are hydration (small sips of water every few minutes), optimum GERD management, avoidance of phonatory stress, and reduced voice use. If the granuloma is white, old, hard, and pedunculated, sharp cough techniques can be used in an attempt to "cough off" the lesion. In most cases, however, coughing is contraindicated, and smooth, reduced voice use with optimum hydration and reflux management is the standard course. Once the pathology has resolved, voice strengthening exercises are prescribed. Voice therapy can be crucial to reducing need for surgical intervention, and in reducing risk for recurrence.

18.1.2 Conversion Disorder

Some individuals develop aphonia (complete loss of voice) due to extreme stress. The stress trigger can be emotional or psychological, which causes a "massive automatic fight or flight reaction" at the larynx.[1] This strong muscular contraction causes an imbalance of the intrinsic and extrinsic laryngeal muscles, making phonation strained, or impossible. These individuals often exhibit abnormal breathing patterns as well, and may hold their breath during conversations, increasing laryngeal tension. Reflexive cough may be normal. Stress triggers are variable, from the death of a loved one (or beloved animal) to making a major appliance purchase. The trigger is not always so apparent to the individual, and the patient does not intend to have this reaction.

Treatment for conversion disorder is twofold: direct massage of the laryngeal musculature, and counseling for stress management. Direct circumlaryngeal massage can be highly effective, although initially quite painful for the patient. Educating the patient in advance that they have developed a "Charley horse" spasm at the larynx is helpful. During the massage, the patient is slowly guided toward using voicing (humming, lip flutters, sighs), which are then shaped into words and conversations. Even prolonged bouts of conversion aphonia can be resolved in only one session. It is remarkable and rewarding to see these distressed patients arrive with no voice, and leave laughing and chattering away.

18.1.3 Cyst

A vocal fold cyst is a benign encapsulated mass within the lamina propria of the vocal fold, typically unilateral, and often attributed to a glandular duct blockage. Although some cysts are congenital, most are phonotraumatic, like a rug-burn on the vocal fold, and may occur with excessive voice use, forceful breath, and dry laryngeal mucosa. Patients may be able to recall the injury event. Some individuals are cystic in nature during some period in their life, so a full medical history of possible cysts elsewhere in the body (especially for females) is helpful to differentiate these lesions from other elevated masses (nodules, polyps).

The classic symptoms of a vocal fold cyst include unpredictable voice quality, with the voice clear, then the voice quality becomes suddenly irregular, with no apparent change of technique by the patient. Voice fatigue is also present. Due to the encapsulated fluid within the cyst wall, vocal fold vibration can be in and out of sync with the affected fold. If the cyst is caught early (within 3 to 5 weeks) there is some chance to resolve the cyst through exercises focused on sustained diminuendo (lessening of vocal volume while maintaining support and optimum resonance), which changes the vocal fold edge contour from a broader contact to thinner contact edge. Once the cyst has developed a firm epithelial lining, phonosurgery is generally required. During surgery, it is important that the cyst be removed without fracture or collapse. If epithelial cells remain, the cyst can redevelop quickly. Some individuals will have a spontaneous collapse of the cyst (without phonosurgery), which can develop a mucosal bridge lesion, a sulcus, or mucosal deposits.

18.1.4 Gastroesophageal Reflux Disease and Laryngopharyngeal Reflux

Reflux laryngitis can cause significant irritation and inflammation to the laryngeal mucosa. Both gastroesophageal reflux disease (GERD) and laryngopharyngeal reflux (LPR) have the capacity to change the mechanics of phonation due to inflammation of the posterior glottis, and from inflammation and dryness of the membranous vocal fold. Because the arytenoids cannot close easily (or even fully in some individuals), greater stress is placed on the membranous folds. This is particularly problematic for singers who "anchor" the arytenoids to provide stability for their normal vocal fold vibratory tasks. When GERD or LPR is severe, contact ulcers can develop on the cartilagenous vocal fold, or elevated lesions can arise on the membranous vocal fold. Both GERD and LPR can be found across the lifespan, from infants to the elderly. Among children and women, there appears to be an increased risk of developing nodules when there is significant voice use in the presence of reflux.

Some individuals appear to be quite sensitive to even minor mucosal changes from GERD to LPR, while others appear to tolerate even moderate reflux without apparent voice breakdown. Patients with GERD may report heartburn symptoms, thick mucous, and hoarseness; patients with LPR typically report only hoarseness and thick mucous. Typical complaints include a lower pitched voice in the morning, or absence of voicing in the morning, increased roughness to the voice quality, and difficulty with vocal flexibility.

Diet and stress are often significant etiologic factors to GERD and LPR. Eating or drinking quickly can exacerbate reflux, and use of physical (or vocal exercise) after eating can increase reflux events. Most patients with GERD or LPR are placed on medications by their physician, and given specific food avoidances (chocolate, carbonated beverages, spicy foods). Therapy with a speech-language pathologist gives the patient another opportunity to receive information and counseling regarding diet and lifestyle modifications that could positively affect voice.

Voice therapy focuses on reducing laryngeal effort through use of tonal placement exercises (to reduce airflow resistance demands at the vocal fold level), voice exercises focused on changing the vocal fold edge contour (such as sustained soft–loud–soft, or small to moderate pitch changes with a constant vowel), as well as counseling and education to improve compliance with reflux management.

18.1.5 Idiopathic Parkinson Disorder

Dysphonia may be a primary or secondary feature that leads to the diagnosis of idiopathic Parkinson disorder (IPD). Voice symptoms include reduced vocal loudness, reduced pitch range flexibility, difficulty with rate of speaking, reduced voice clarity, or difficulty with breath management. In many ways, IPD can be thought of as a perceptual disorder. The patient does not try to speak (or walk) with reduced muscular force, but the resultant muscle activity is reduced.

Voice therapy focused on exaggerated movement (particularly of loudness and pitch) are quite beneficial. The Lee Silverman voice treatment (LSVT) is the most widely prescribed and effective management for IPD.[2] The LSVT motto of "think loud, think shout" focuses on intensive daily exercise to recalibrate the patient's use of voice. The resultant effect is a louder and more projected voice. The benefits of LSVT extend also to patients with other neurologic voice disorders such as stroke patients and multiple sclerosis. Clinicians using the LSVT receive additional certification beyond the required certification as a speech-language pathologist. Therefore, voice therapy referrals for a patient who could benefit from LSVT must be to a LSVT-certified clinician.

18.1.6 Laryngeal Sicca

Laryngeal sicca occurs when the laryngeal mucosa is exposed to a chemical or thermal irritant. The drying effects cause a "salt and pepper" appearance to the vocal folds and a sluggish vocal fold vibration. Patients with laryngeal sicca present with a low pitched, husky voice, poor projection, and voice fatigue. Laryngeal sicca is more common in adults than children. Triggers for laryngeal sicca may include heavy voice use in the presence of paint fumes, construction chemicals (including adhesives), low humidity in the work or home environment, medications with dehydrating effects, or generalized chemical exposure.

Improved vocal hygiene is essential to resolve laryngeal sicca, as well as frequent use of sustained diminuendo (gradual softening of vocal volume). Due to the severity of inflammation, resolution of laryngeal sicca can take 6 to 9 months, even with optimal management. The voice does return to normal clarity, range, and endurance; However, the patient must sip water frequently, take nonmedicated lozenges (hard candy), and use a humidifier to resolve the laryngeal sicca.

18.1.7 Laryngospasm

Involuntary adductory spasm at the glottis is the basis of laryngospasm. Triggers for spasms are typically chemical, temperature, sudden dryness, GERD or LPR, and/or stress. When laryngospasm is not accompanied by chronic cough, it resolves typically within several months, provided the triggers can be identified and eliminated. Elite-level swimmers may develop laryngospasm due to an allergic reaction to pool area chemicals and the stress of performance. Runners may develop laryngospasm from reflux events and respiratory challenges. Following the World Trade Center (WTC) attack in September 2001, many workers and volunteers at the WTC site developed laryngospasm several years later (as well as recalcitrant sinusitis and GERD).

Patient complaints include inability to breathe, hoarse voice, and tightness in the laryngeal or upper chest region. They also report shortness of breath when walking up stairs (or an incline), and when exposed to cleaning chemicals. These patients may be misdiagnosed with asthma, but a flattened inspiratory loop in pulmonary function testing can be helpful to diagnose this disorder. Laryngeal examination is remarkable for adduction of the vocal folds when the patient is instructed to inhale.

Therapy focuses on breathing exercises as well as airflow resistance exercises. Use of slower inhalation, especially when combined with high resistance to the inhalation (nares occlusion, or breathing through the mouth with lingual obstruction) can improve glottal abduction. In effect, higher resistance in the upper vocal tract can lower the resistance at the vocal fold level. Dry vocal folds can worsen symptoms, allowing the vocal folds to "stick together." For this reason, optimum hydration (small sips of water frequently) and optimum GERD or LPR management is important as well as management (or avoidance) of chemical and environmental triggers.

18.1.8 Musculoskeletal Tension Disorder

Normal vocal fold appearance in the absence of normal voice is a classic description of musculoskeletal tension disorder (MTD). During the laryngeal exam, there may be anteroposterior shortening during ascending pitch glides, or there may be visible compression of the false vocal folds against the true vocal folds. Some patients will have hypoadduction, with no nerve injury component, as a sign of MTD, but most patients exhibit hyperfunction with MTD. Palpation of the laryngeal region reveals discomfort or pain in the region of the thyroid cartilage and hyoid bone. In addition, there may be limited space between those structures. Palpation of extrinsic laryngeal muscles often reveals spasms in those regions as well. Musculoskeletal tension disorder can exist with only anterior laryngeal spasms, or only lateral and posterior neck tensions.

Typical patient complaints include loss of vocal loudness, reduced vocal range, reduced projection and voice discomfort. Triggers for MTD include stress, strained voice use, car accidents causing whiplash, and physical posture. Therapy focuses on rebalancing the muscular forces of the extrinsic and intrinsic laryngeal musculature, and reducing excessive thyroarytenoid or cricothyroid tension. Improved breath management and improved tonal placement can also be beneficial in reducing excessive laryngeal effort.

18.1.9 Nodules

Nodules are benign lesions that typically develop at the midmembranous point, or at the junction of the anterior one-third of the vocal fold and the posterior two-thirds of the vocal fold. They are commonly found in pairs. Nodules, or calluses, are more common for individuals who have extensive voice use (speaking and/or singing), projected voice use, and have dry vocal folds. Nodules arise because of increased frictional injury to the vocal fold edge. Nodular edema may be present with other elevated lesions (cysts, polyps). Nodules respond very well to voice therapy, and few individuals require surgery for these lesions.

Therapy for vocal nodules focuses on improving fluidity of voice use, improving vocal pacing, improving tonal placement (to redirect energy away from the vocal folds and place the vocal power demands on the resonance and articulatory structures), improving hydration, reducing risk for GERD or LPR, and counseling on adapting voice use patterns to allow the vocal fold to heal. Lip flutters ("raspberries") can be helpful because they require coordination of breath, phonation, and resonance. In addition, lip flutters require a dual vibratory source (lip vibration, vocal fold vibration) to a single air flow, thereby reducing demands at the vocal fold level during the voiced portion of lip flutters. For this reason, if the lip flutter is started unvoiced, abdominal-diaphragmatic support is established with the lips as the primary oscillator and when voicing is gently added to that sound, there is less trauma at the vocal fold level. Such exercises, when used with pitch glides and similar vocal massage slides, can be very effective in reducing phonotraumatic lesions. Staccato, and other brief-onset vocal patterns, should be avoided. Fluidity and improved range of motion is important, while using optimum resonance, articulatory assistance for projection, and balanced breath support. Breath inhalation should be silent and calm, helping avoid increased laryngeal dryness. Breath holding should be avoided due to potential compression at the laryngeal level, thereby increasing at-rest laryngeal strain.

In children, it is important to improve breath support and respiratory strength. In adults, it is important to optimize tonal placement and to monitor breath management. Voice rest without voice therapy is generally not effective because old muscle use patterns return following voice rest. Use of improved vocal range-of-motion is important, as well as monitoring of head and neck posture that can lead to vocal strain.

18.1.10 Papilloma

Recurring thickening of the epithelium combined with a fibrovascular core causes papilloma to be a particularly difficult laryngeal disorder. Because these epithelial growths can obscure the glottis, making breathing and voicing difficult, repeat phonosurgeries may be necessary.

The role of voice therapy for the papilloma patient is to establish the best voice quality between the necessary surgical and medical treatments, trying to reduce any minor scarring, and to provide counseling and education on the disease. If managed optimally by the surgeon, these patients may have a clear voice after the papilloma virus resolves, despite the necessary surgeries. Due to the length and complexity of management, this disease typically compromises professional voice use (speaking, singing).

18.1.11 Paresis and Paralysis

Weakness of the recurrent laryngeal nerve can cause significant dysphonia. Typically unilateral, the nerve injury can affect the membranous and/or cartilagnous vocal fold function. Because these nerve injuries affect glottal closure and compression skills, swallow may also be affected, causing the protective swallow to be weak or discoordinated.

Symptoms of recurrent nerve injury are vocal weakness, breathiness, loss of pitch stability, loss of pitch range, loss of projection, and a sense of the vocal folds "splaying" when phonation is initiated. It is not uncommon to have diplophonia due to difference in vocal fold thickness or level. If diagnosed early, medical management with steroids can be helpful.

Voice therapy should begin immediately to help strengthen the vocal folds. Laryngeal resistance exercises, vocal flexion exercises, and contrasting vocal register exercises (including vocal fry, which has a long closed phase sliding into higher register phonations), done frequently throughout the day, can return the voice to normal.

If the nerve injury is old, or severe, surgical management may be necessary. When laryngeal exercises are insufficient, improved attention to tonal placement (resonance and articulation) can be helpful for improved projection and quality. Because of the glottal weakness, it is important that the patient be guided to avoid excessive breath flow that can cause more vocal instability. Surgical management for the vocal fold is improving for both children and adults, but there is always a role for even brief voice therapy to optimize recovery of best voice.

18.1.12 Polyp

Polyps are highly variable in appearance, but all affect voice quality if they are located within the vibratory margin. These membranous lesions, located in the superficial layer of the lamina propria, are characteristically unilateral, and may trigger a contralateral lesion. Polyps arise from phonotrauma (excessive voice use, aggressive voice use, sharp sneeze, or cough), either to the cover of the vocal fold or to a blood vessel.

Polyps act as a weight on the affected vocal fold, causing pitch instability, and may be vascular (arising from a hemorrhage or varix), fibrous, fusiform, or pedunculated. Because of their fluid component, a common complaint is constant voice instability. If the lesion is pedunculated, there may be moments of sudden aphonia. Voice fatigue is present, largely due to excessive work at the laryngeal level in an effort to initiate and maintain voicing.

Voice therapy for polyps varies and the specific exercises depend on the type of polyp. A broad-based fluid polyp can respond well to voice therapy, but may still require surgery. The same is true for the hemorrhagic polyp, but depends on the appearance, location relative to the striking edge, and severity. Polyps that are more subcordal are difficult to manage, and have often arisen from excessive air flow. Fibrous polyps do not generally respond well to voice therapy, and require surgical management.

Soft, broad-based polyps near the striking edge can respond reasonably well to voice therapy. For these lesions, exercises focused on moderate-loud volume to soft sustained /u/ ("oo") can be helpful, as well as exercises that include onset of vocal fry (organized chaotic vibration of the vocal folds, avoiding pressed phonation) with the /a/ ("ah") vowel and then sliding up to higher pitches on /u/ ("oo") which uses the normal quasiperiodic vibration. Due to potential fatigue, it is unwise to use vocal fry exercises longer than about 5 minutes, even with supervision. It is also unwise to permit occasional interjections of vocal fry in general speaking tasks. However, vocal fry can firmly establish the clear resonances of the vocal tract, while establishing a lax adduction at the glottal level, and reduced air flow. These exercises manipulate the vocal fold edge, helping re-establish normal vibratory modes, and can improve coordination of airflow to phonation.

Hemorrhagic (vascular) polyps improved with sustained diminuendo exercises, use of fluid voice, and optimum resonance function. If the center of the hemorrhagic polyp is not in the immediate vibratory portion, and not subcordal, surgery can sometimes be avoided, but risks for repeat hemorrhage persist. Medical management can be helpful for these patients, but many often choose an in-office surgical intervention (such as pulsed dye or potassium titanyl phosphate laser) to resolve the lesion, if trial voice therapy does not establish adequate voice quality.

18.1.13 Puberphonia

During puberty, there are significant growth changes of the laryngeal cartilages and muscles. This creates vocal instability that is generally more severe in males. Puberphonia has continued use of the higher prepubescent voice despite the presence of the more mature laryngeal structures, and despite normal hormonal changes associated with puberty. A period of pitch instability is common and may persist for several months. In some individuals, however, they fail to adapt to the larger vocal structures. These individuals may exhibit a normal mature laugh, but speak in a light, higher pitched voice.

Voice therapy is the standard management for puberphonia, and a skilled clinician can usually guide the patient to use their new "mature" voice in the initial session. The initial voice breaking from puberphonia to "normal" is actually quite low in pitch, and may even be caught in vocal fry for a few weeks in severe cases. Over the period of several weeks, the voice range adapts for both pitch and loudness variation, and the patient is suddenly speaking in his "new voice."

The larger problem with resolving puberphonia is how the patient will explain the sudden pitch lowering and maturity of his voice to friends. Family members are characteristically delighted and in near shock hearing a sudden robust voice come from the patient, but classmates and teachers can add stress, making transfer a bit tenuous. It can be helpful for the patient to simply dismiss pointed questions, and just say "I don't know" and keep talking with the new voice.

18.1.14 Scar

There are several different kinds of scars and each carries different prognoses, which can depend on the location on the membranous vocal fold. Scar occurs as a result of injury. If the patient has a history of poor wound healing prior to phonosurgery, there may be increased risk for scarring, or a more prolonged recovery from the surgery. If a patient is unable, or unwilling, to use voice rest when prescribed by their physician, there is increased risk for scarring if there has been an injury to the mucosa (mucosal tear, hemorrhage, surgical incision).

Scars can be divided into two groups: those that are a general scar (flat or raised) and sulcus vocalis. A raised scar has a poor prognosis than a flat scar, although both soften over time. The flat scar is more likely to fully resolve. For these types of scars, gentle onset of voicing with lip flutters is helpful, and can be helpful as a general indicator of phonation threshold pressure.

Aerodynamic testing of the patient's softest /papapapapa/ yields the phonation threshold pressure (PTP). Phonation threshold pressure is a good indicator of how much effort the patient requires to initiate phonation. Normal PTP is 3 to 5 cm H_20,[3,4] and can be much lower in accomplished singers (2 cm H_2O).[5] Initiation of phonation is difficult to do when the vocal fold edge is stiff, and some patients may exhibit PTP as high as greater than 14 cm H_2O for softest modal voice. Therefore, it is no surprise that patients with vocal fold scar have fatigue and frustration. The initiation of voicing is unstable for pitch and quality, even in the voicing contrasts that occur in normal speech between some consonants and their adjoining vowels. For some patients, it can be beneficial to obtain aerodynamic measures to determine the extent of pressure necessary to initiate phonation, as well as the amount of air leakage during phonation.

Sulcus vocalis is a longitudinal furrow along the membranous vocal fold and may be acquired or congenital. Acquired sulci vocalis are often related to poor healing from a vocal fold hemorrhage. It is important to note that an acquired sulcus vocalis is usually a combination of poor healing skill (systemically) by the patient, and continued excessive, or sometimes aggressive, voice use following injury. Unfortunately, it is not always possible to know when a vocal fold trauma has occurred, making voice rest difficult to prescribe without a laryngeal exam. In general, if there is a sudden change in voice quality, range, or power, particularly following or during voice use, an examination by a qualified laryngologist is strongly recommended. Even in individuals with a history of poor healing, there may be ways to reduce abnormal healing if the injury is recognized early. Scars do soften with time, and most scars are more pliable at 12 months.

Ford et al[6] have defined three main forms of sulcus vocalis: type I (physiologic sulcus), type II (sulcus vergerture), and type III (sulcus vocalis proper). All three types reflect a permanent change in the microstructure of the lamina propria, compromising mucosal wave propagation.

The sulcus vocalis may be unilateral or bilateral, and cause stiffness to the vocal fold. The speaking voice is characteristically hoarse, husky, breathy, and rough. Some patients (tenors) may be able to sing quite well with a sulcus vocalis because the increased stiffness improves the mechanical properties necessary for singing sustained high pitches. However, most patients face significant loss of voice clarity for social and professional use.

Both traditional vocal fold scars and sulcus vocalis can improve with voice therapy. Poor prognosis is given to raised scar and sulcus vocalis type III. Smaller scars can respond well to lip flutters and laryngeal resistance exercises, even when the scar has been present for more than 12 months.

18.1.15 Spasmodic Dysphonia

Adductor spasmodic dysphonia, abductor spasmodic dysphonia (SD), and mixed spasmodic dysphonia are all focal laryngeal dystonias that have significant effects on initiation and maintenance of phonation. Patients with SD experience involuntary spasms at the laryngeal level, which cause compensatory tensions that further worsen voice quality and control. Once SD is present, timing and severity of spasms are unpredictable, and there may also be spasms in the upper vocal tract. This leads to significant phonation breakdown, with the patient struggling to begin words; it continues to worsen as the balance of laryngeal function and filter function (resonance and articulation) are further compromised. Symptoms are worse in the presence of stress.

Age of onset of SD is typically adult, although there have been some reported cases of childhood onset. Spasmodic dysphonia may be triggered by trauma, stress, or infection. Some individuals may have prior MTD, and years later they may develop SD. There are differences in the two disorders, however, and MTD does not typically lead to SD. However, nearly all SD patients have some aspect of MTD as a compensation for the involuntary spasms. Although MTD is curable, there is no present cure for

SD. Singers who develop SD often report their singing voice is more affected by spasms, while nonsingers report their singing voice is fairly adequate, but their speaking voice has lost stability and quality.

Management of SD is often a combination of paced botulinum toxin injections into the primary offending muscle, with voice therapy provided between injections to optimize effective compensation. Voice therapy strategies include improved fluidity of pitches, changing voice modes (chanting the intended verbal message rather than trying to speak the message), breath management exercises, and counseling for improved stress management.

18.1.16 Varix

A varix is an enlarged blood vessel on the membranous vocal fold that causes voice quality instability, mild turbulence, and breathiness. Because the blood vessels can enlarge with use (phonation), any varix that is within the vibratory margin places the voice user at higher risk for vocal fold hemorrhage, and the voice is often more unstable following voice use (particularly singing or lecturing). The vascular network is more fragile for women in the 2 days prior to menstruation and the first 2 days of menstruation. The fragility is worsened if anticoagulants (aspirin, alcohol, etc.) are used. There may be an isolated varix, or several varices present, and they may be unilateral of bilateral. Because there may be small bleeds from the varix, there may be regions of stiffness of the affected vocal fold.

Therapy focuses on improving control of vocal fold-edge contour (sustained diminuendo, slow pitch glides for small pitch intervals), optimizing control of voicing onset to reduce phonotrauma, and education on risk factors for exacerbation of the pathology and potential management options. There is some evidence that homeopathic medications such as horse chestnut extract and bromelain may be helpful in the management of varices, but many patients undergo surgical management with photoangiolytic laser to remove these troublesome lesions.

18.2 Counseling Issues

Panacea was the goddess of therapy in Greek mythology, and it is the voice clinician's responsibility to create a calm environment to elicit the best voice possible given the physiology available. To do this, the clinician must be compassionate to the problems the patient is facing, and must assure the patient that improved voice is possible and attainable. Fears, including grief over loss of their prior voice, may require referral to a stress-management specialist, but initial counseling can be started by the voice clinician.

It is important in counseling to view the glass as "half full," never "half empty." By focusing on the small positive steps and quality of voice, the patient is able to build a better voice. Counseling includes positive reinforcement for progress, even if only for the tonal placement of one sound.

Counseling needs to encourage the patient to self-monitor their own successes in voice function. When there is voice breakdown, it is important to recognize and discuss the myriad of factors that can influence breakdown.

18.3 Education Issues

It is important that the patient understand normal laryngeal anatomy and physiology, and to also understand how their pathology fits within the severity of others with the same diagnosis. For this reason, it is important that the voice clinician have available several reference texts that show photos of pathologies, and that the clinician tries to keep abreast of websites that offer reliable information. A laryngeal model is important to discuss anatomy. The clinician needs to be able to execute basic line drawings of the vocal fold edge so that the patient can understand the changes in vocal fold edge contour as a factor of fundamental frequency, intensity, register, muscle activation, and vowel interactions. Clinicians should be able to provide high-quality, effective therapy with only a pad and pencil and their ears, but having reference texts available is very important.

The patient should be educated on structures (and basic muscle function) within the respiratory organ, the structures and physiology of the larynx, and the structures and role of the supraglottic structures. They should be given basic information on sensory aspects of tonal placement, as well as an understanding of the transfer function from the source (larynx) to the resonance and articulatory structures. Patients need education on the difference in perception of voice quality (air conduction, bone conduction) as well as key acoustic features that signal voice distress versus voice success.

It is essential that the patient be educated on factors that led to their vocal demise so that risk for future pathologies is reduced, and the patient can understand their dysphonia. For example, nodules may arise from excessive voice use when sick with a cold or allergies. Nodules may arise from excessive voice use with emotional stress in a dry environment (physically dry environment, or systemically dry from lack of adequate hydration, or medication side effect). Nodules may arise from compensation for a mild vocal fold paresis. Nodules may develop from increased friction present during severe GERD or LPR. Therefore, nodules are not simple phonotraumatic lesions. They happen because of several factors. Car accidents happen daily, and the vocal folds have microtrauma every day. Fortunately, the tissues heal very quickly and very well: most of the time. For many pathologies, their development was "being in the wrong place at the wrong time." Resolving the dysphonia and the pathology requires an understanding of the positive compensatory exercises and strategies that can promote healing and development of the treasured clear voice.

18.4 The Team

The effective voice team is led by the laryngologist, with close collaboration by the speech-language pathologist with expertise in voice disorders, and with additional collaboration by singing teachers, voice trainers, psychologists, psychiatrists, vocal coaches, massage therapists, and acupuncture specialists. Each member should have an understanding of their key role in this patient management, and should also have some understanding of what the other team members do, think, and know.

There needs to be a close communication between the laryngologist and the speech pathologist. It is essential that the laryngologist communicate laryngeal status, primary and secondary diagnosis, and his or her initial thoughts of how they view the potential for the patient gaining a clear voice. A laryngeal photo and strobe exam copy can be invaluable to the speech pathologist (and other members of the team). For the speech pathologist, it allows direct education of the patient about their larynx, and the good and deficient aspects of appearance and function. Likewise, following the initial evaluation with the patient, it is important for the speech pathologist to communicate prognosis with the laryngologist and to discuss additional factors for dysphonia that may emerge during the history taking. Because the speech pathologist spends more time with the patient than most laryngology visits, the patient may disclose information to the speech pathologist that could impact the management plan.

18.5 Conclusion

Voice therapy plays an important role in the management of voice disorders. Many pathologies can resolve or be reduced with speech or voice therapy alone. For therapy to be effective, the voice clinician needs to be well trained in clinical management of diseases affecting the larynx, have a broad scope of knowledge related to factors that can influence dysphonia and perception of dysphonia, and have the capacity to relate to a wide variety of individuals who bring unique circumstances to typical pathologies.

With a strong voice-care team, the voice therapist can guide patients to better vocal choices to evoke improved laryngeal physiology, and help the patient find a better, functional voice through coordination of respiration, phonation, resonance, and articulation. Most pathologies respond to therapy within 4 to 10 sessions, but circumstances of the pathology and the patient preparedness can influence success.

It is the responsibility of the voice clinician to create a bit of "magic" in each therapy session, building and shaping better voice through sensation and perception. Through this approach, the patient can self-monitor their progress and expand their skills. Through counseling and education, the risk for repeat injury can be reduced, and recovery from the present dysphonia can be accomplished.

References

[1] Aronson A. Clinical Voice Disorders: An Interdisciplinary Approach. New York, NY: Thieme-Stratton; 1980: 130

[2] Ramig LO, Countryman S, O'Brien C, Hoehn M, Thompson L. Intensive speech treatment for patients with Parkinson's disease: short-and long-term comparison of two techniques. Neurology 1996; 47: 1496–1504

[3] Hertegård S, Gauffin J. Insufficient vocal fold closure as studies by inverse filtering. In: Gauffin J, Harrarberg B, eds. Vocal Fold Physiology: Acoustic, Perceptual and Physiological Aspects of Voice Mechanisms. San Diego, CA: Singular Publishing; 1991: 243–250

[4] Wilson JV, Leeper HA. Changes in laryngeal airway resistance in young adult men and women as a function of vocal sound pressure level and syllable context. J Voice 1992; 6: 235–245

[5] Carroll LM. Airflow Characteristics in Loud Singing during Register Transition among Highly Skilled Classical Singers [doctoral dissertation]. New York, NY: Columbia University; 2001

[6] Ford CN, Inagi K, Khidr A, Bless DM, Gilchrist KW. Sulcus vocalis: a rational analytical approach to diagnosis and management. Ann Otol Rhinol Laryngol 1996; 105: 189–200

19 Swallow Rehabilitation

William E. Karle and Cathy L. Lazarus

Swallow therapy is used for patients who are either experiencing dysphagia or who have potential to develop swallowing problems due to upcoming treatment. Dysphagia is associated with aspiration, malnutrition, dehydration, reduced quality of life, and social isolation.[1,2,3,4] Of specific concern is the potential for aspiration and subsequent aspiration pneumonia, which is a major cause of morbidity and mortality in this population.[3]

When designing a swallow therapy regimen, a clinician should aim to improve the patient's swallow safety, efficiency, and normalcy. This regimen should only be created after a thorough evaluation of the patient's swallow has been performed, optimally utilizing an instrumental assessment, such as a modified barium swallow (MBS) or flexible endoscopic evaluation of swallowing (FEES) exam. During this evaluation, it is it important to identify the underlying disorder and not the masking symptoms.

In this chapter, we provide information regarding the normal stages of deglutition and common swallowing disorders, as well as rehabilitation strategies to improve swallow safety and efficiency for dysphagic patients. These treatments include specific postures, maneuvers, diet modification, exercises, and sensory-enhancement techniques.

19.1 Stages of Deglutition

Swallowing is a complex process controlled by 31 paired striated muscles and innervated by either the ansa cervicalis or cranial nerves V_3, VII, IX, X, or XII.[5] The process of deglutition is often broken down into four separate phases: (1) oral preparatory, (2) oral, (3) pharyngeal, and (4) esophageal (▶ Fig. 19.1).[6] Although these phases are helpful to understand the process of deglutition, they are artificial demarcations that often blend or overlap with one another.[7] The esophageal phase occurs once the bolus has passed through the upper esophageal sphincter (UES) and ends once it has exited the lower esophageal sphincter (LES). There is little that can be behaviorally rehabilitated in the esophageal phase and management is typically medically based. The first three phases of this process are described in detail below.

19.1.1 Oral Preparatory Phase

The start of the swallow begins with the manipulation of the bolus within the oral cavity. As this phase is influenced by consistency, volume, and taste, the duration of this phase is under volitional/cortical control and there is no standard norm for duration of this phase.[8] This process starts once the bolus enters the oral cavity and ends once the tongue begins to propel it posteriorly.

Once the bolus is within the oral cavity, a labial seal must be maintained to prevent spillage out of the mouth. Simultaneously, another seal is formed with the soft palate resting anteriorly against the posterior portion of the tongue. This forms a glossopalatal sphincter to prevent spillage of the bolus into the pharynx prematurely and to allow nasal breathing.[9] With the oral cavity sealed, nasal breathing is performed with a relaxed and unprotected larynx. The lack of protection can lead to aspiration if the bolus prematurely spills into the pharynx.

The tongue is responsible for manipulation of the bolus during this phase and also acts as the major sensory input.[10] This sensory information helps modulate the cortical motor planning for the appropriate lingual gestures required to manipulate the bolus during mastication. When ingesting a liquid bolus, the only action required is positioning of the bolus on the dorsum of the tongue, maintaining the bolus on the tongue during elevation to the palate, and then sealing of the tongue against the hard palate.[11] However, with thicker consistencies or solids, chewing is required, involving lateral movement of the bolus between the teeth for mastication. This involves a lateral rotary movement of the mandible, as well as lateral motion of the tongue to position the food between the teeth for chewing and retrieving the food from the teeth for sealing the bolus against the palate. Contraction of the buccinator, adjacent to the lateral aspect of the teeth, prevents food from falling into the lateral sulci. During this process the tongue also mixes the food with saliva to prepare a cohesive bolus. While mastication is occurring, the glossopalatal sphincter is briefly disrupted as portions of the bolus are propelled posteriorly, collected in the valleculae and subsequently swallowed. A collection of material in the vallecular space prior to trigging of the swallow is only considered normal with solid boluses.[12,13]

19.1.2 Oral Phase

The normal duration of the oral phase is between one to two seconds and is under volitional/cortical control.[10,14] This phase begins once the leading edge of the bolus begins to move posteriorly and ends once the bolus head reaches the angle of the mandible. This movement is achieved through a stripping-type action performed by sequential contraction of the tongue against the hard palate.[15] The anterior two-thirds of the tongue contracts in a synchronous wave-like pattern from anterior to posterior applying pressure on the tail of the bolus.[11] During this process, the tip and lateral portions of the tongue maintain their tight apposition against the hard palate. It is also important for the labial seal to be maintained and a taut buccal musculature to prevent spillage of the bolus into the lateral sulci.

As the bolus is propelled toward the pharynx, the tongue base is pulled anteriorly and inferiorly, creating room for the bolus to enter the pharynx. When the bolus reaches the soft palate, the palate is elevated to open the glossopalatal sphincter. Concurrently, the palate is retracted against the posterior pharyngeal wall, sealing off any communication with the nasal cavity. This is achieved via contraction of the superior pharyngeal constrictors, forming a circular closure through apposition, preventing nasal regurgitation.

19.1.3 Pharyngeal Phase

Often described as the most complex of the four stages, it is also the most critical for prevention of aspiration and is a common area of dysfunction in patients with difficulty swallowing. The stage begins once the bolus head reaches the angle of the mandible and ends once the tail of the bolus has passed through the

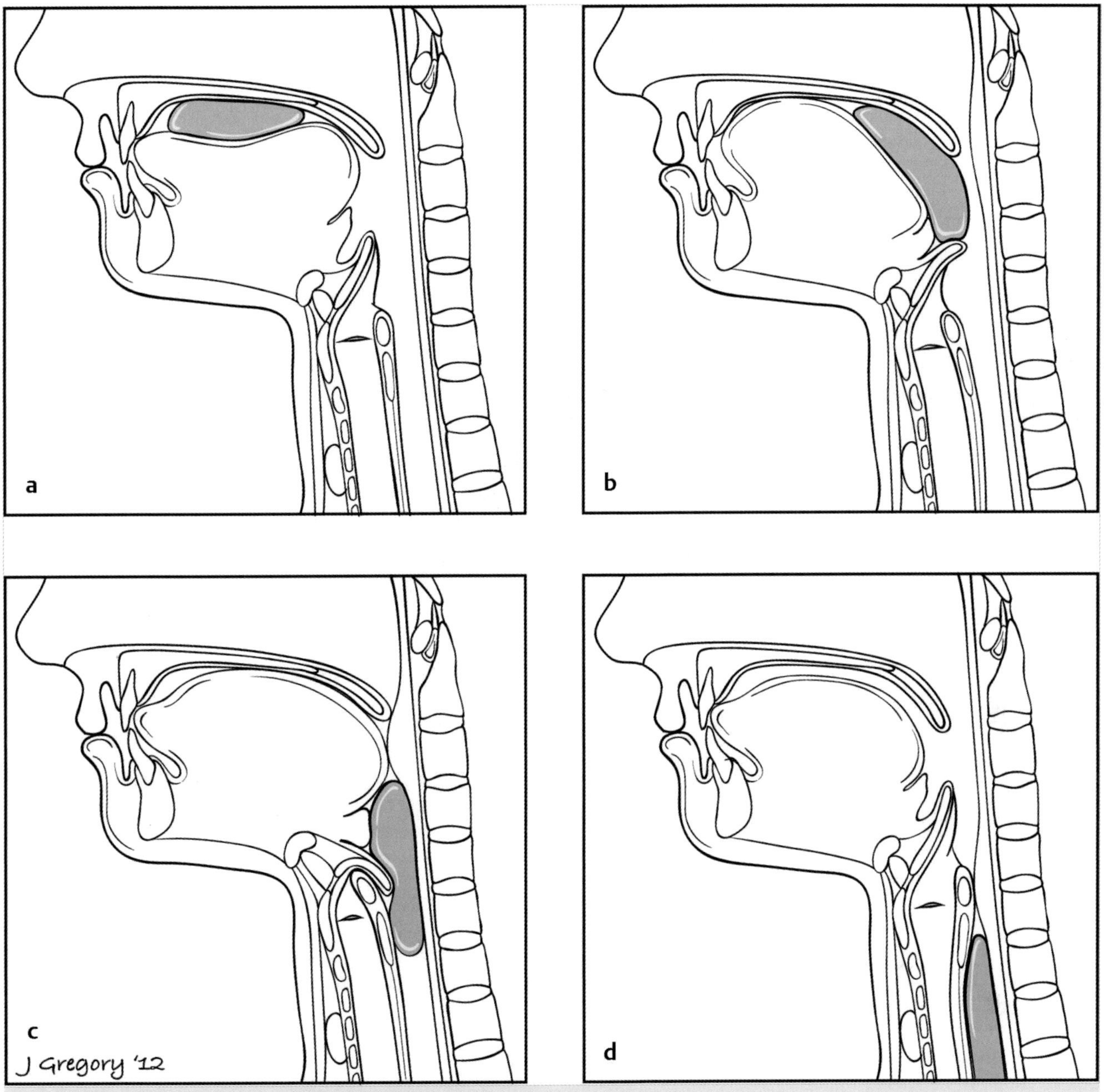

Fig. 19.1 Four stages of deglutition. (a) Oral preparatory phase. (b) End of oral phase. (c) Pharyngeal phase. (d) Esophageal phase.

UES. However, there is normal variability and the pharyngeal swallow can trigger when the bolus head is past this region or prior to reaching the angle of the mandible.[16] The main functions of this phase include (1) propulsion of the bolus through the pharynx by posterior motion of the base of tongue (BOT) and sequential constriction of the pharyngeal walls, (2) prevention of nasal regurgitation by maintenance of a velopharyngeal seal, (3) hyolaryngeal elevation, (4) protection of the airway (glottic and supraglottic), and (5) UES opening. The neuromuscular events that occur during the pharyngeal motor response happen fairly simultaneously; however, there is some variability and overlap in the timing of their onset.[16,7] These events are primarily under brainstem control, but the timing, extent, and duration of these events are modulated in response to the sensory input to the cortex.[10] The pharyngeal swallow is most likely triggered by a combination of stimulation to the posterior region of the tongue and pharyngeal wall, with control maintained by the swallowing center within the brainstem.[5,17] This entire process should occur within one second.[10]

Once the swallow is initiated, medialization and anterior tilting of the arytenoids begin the process of airway protection.[18] This is immediately followed by contraction of the suprahyoid muscles, which leads to the elevation and anterior pulling of the hyoid bone. Due to muscular attachments between the hyoid, thyroid, and cricoid, the larynx is simultaneously pulled anteriorly and superiorly causing the introitus of the larynx to tilt forward and down, with apposition of the arytenoids to the epiglottic base. This change in position aids in airway protection, expands the hypopharynx for bolus accommodation, and provides mechanical anterior traction on the UES. This movement also causes the epiglottis to move from a vertical to horizontal position. Subsequently, contraction of the aryepiglottic and thyroepiglottic muscles causes the free tip of the epiglottis to bend inferiorly (retroflex) to seal the vestibule. The process of airway protection is completed with the adduction of the true and false vocal folds.[19]

While the airway is in the process of closing, the bolus is propelled through the pharynx with the aid of a posterior tongue thrust and caudally orientated sequential contraction of the superior, middle, and inferior pharyngeal constrictors.[9] Elevation and retraction of the palate form the velopharyngeal sphincter to prevent regurgitation into the oral or nasal cavities. The "piston-like" retraction of the BOT to the anteriorly bulging posterior pharyngeal wall in combination with sequential pharyngeal constrictor contraction results in pharyngeal shortening and provides the pressure needed to drive the bolus through the UES.[20] As the bolus is passing through the pharynx, it often separates midline once it has reached the epiglottis and flows into either one or both of the pyriform sinuses laterally before reaching the UES.

The UES is tonically contracted except during the pharyngeal motor response, at which point it relaxes and becomes compliant for approximately half a second during cessation of neural input.[21] In addition, hyolaryngeal elevation and anterior motion of the larynx and cricoid cartilage provide mechanical traction and opening of the UES region. There is further dilation of this region as a result of the pressure exerted by the incoming bolus (i.e., intrabolus pressures).[22]

19.2 Variation in Swallowing

Although the oropharyngeal swallow occurs in a fairly systematic fashion, normal swallowing is modulated by various factors. Bolus volume and viscosity can result in alteration of the oropharyngeal swallow in terms of timing, extent, and duration of structural movement as well as bolus flow. As previously mentioned, a solid bolus typically collects in the valleculae during chewing, which is considered pathologic for other bolus consistencies. The amount of oral and pharyngeal pressures applied to a bolus will also vary, with greater pressures for larger bolus volumes and more viscous consistencies.[23,24] In addition, bolus volume can alter the timing and duration of structural movement, such as shorter duration of tongue base contact to the pharyngeal wall on larger bolus volumes. Larger boluses also often result in overlapping of the oral and pharyngeal phases to ensure adequate airway protection.[10] Longer airway closure and longer UES opening durations are also observed with larger bolus volumes.[25,26] Normal swallowing is also dependent on age, with the elderly demonstrating longer oropharyngeal swallow duration, as well as less swallow flexibility and reserve.[27,28,29] Finally, any phase of the oropharyngeal swallow can be altered under voluntary control by a compensatory or direct strategy, as discussed below.

19.3 Specific Dysphagias

Dysphagia can be caused by a wide range of etiologies. When prescribing the appropriate treatment for a patient's swallow impairment, it is important to understand the underlying cause and not simply the symptoms. Dysphagia can occur secondary to either anatomical or neurologic dysfunction, disturbing either the physiology or structural organization of the swallow.[10] Abnormal swallow physiology can result in reduced bolus clearance through the oral cavity and pharynx, resulting in residue within common locations (▶ Fig. 19.2). In addition, abnormal structural movement can result in bolus misdirection into the oral and/or nasal cavities, and airway (▶ Fig. 19.3). Aspiration can occur prior to, during, or after the swallow, based on the specific swallowing defect (▶ Fig. 19.4). The following include many of the more common swallowing disorders as well as the symptoms and fluoroscopic findings with which they often present.

19.3.1 Oral Preparation and Oral Phase Dysphagia

Reduced Labial Closure

With this disorder, patients complain about food or liquids spilling out of the mouth. The cause is most commonly labial dysfunction, but also may be the result of being unable to perform nasal breathing. Range-of-motion and labial strengthening exercises are usually indicated for this disorder.

Delayed Oral Initiation

This dysfunction is seen in patients who experience oral apraxia or reduced oral sensation. This can occur in patients who have undergone oral radiation therapy or cancer resection with reconstruction using nonsensate tissue. This is also seen in patients with dementia or cortical damage after traumatic brain injury or stroke.[30,31,32] For patients who experience reduced sensory awareness, it is often helpful to use stronger stimuli such as a sour or spicy bolus.[33]

Reduced Range of Motion, Reduced Control, and Reduced Strength in the Oral Cavity

Patients with impaired tongue function demonstrate difficulty manipulating a bolus, which can result in longer oral transit times. In addition, residue may result within the oral cavity, commonly on the dorsum of the oral tongue or coating the surface of the hard palate, particularly if lingual strength is a problem. Due to inability to control a bolus within the oral cavity, patients may experience spillage into the anterior and lateral sulci or premature spillage into the pharynx, the latter of which can cause aspiration before the swallow. In addition, aspiration can occur after the swallow with poor oral tongue control, as oral residue may slip into the pharynx and airway after the swallow.

For those patients with difficulty maintaining a lingual-palatal seal, a palatal augmentation prosthesis is often used to improve bolus clearance through the oral cavity.

Reduced Buccal Tension

Buccal tension is required to prevent foods and liquids from falling into the lateral sulci during oral preparatory and oral phases of swallowing. Patients with this disorder will often

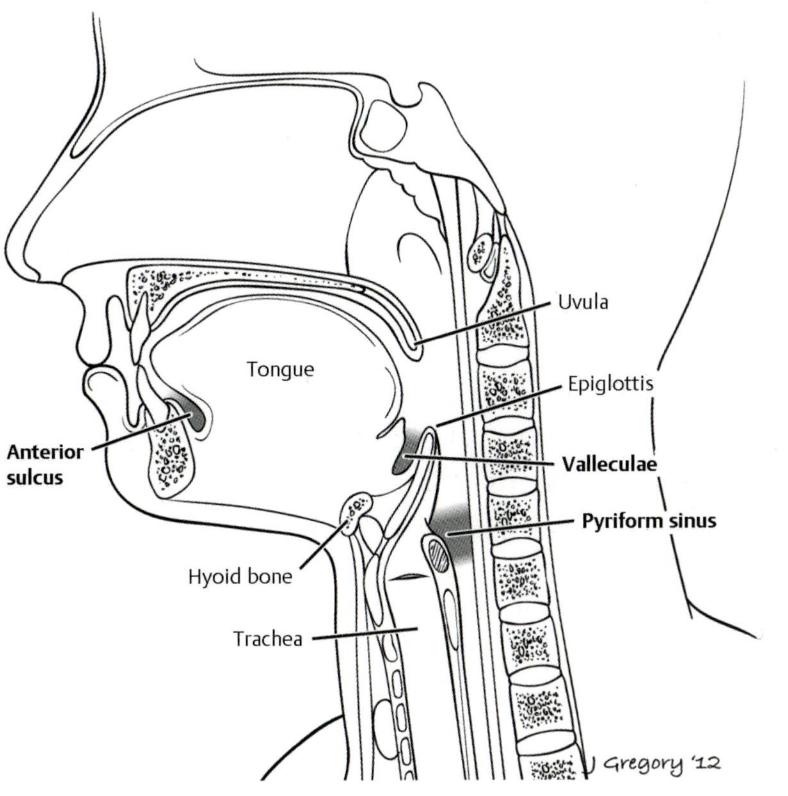

Fig. 19.2 Common areas of bolus residue. It is very common in different swallowing disorders for residue to be located in the anterior sulcus, vallecula, or piriform sinuses as shown here.

avoid foods that require chewing. External pressure can be applied to the cheek to prevent food from spilling into the lateral sulcus on the affected side, as well as use of a head tilt to the unimpaired side.

19.3.2 Pharyngeal Phase Dysphagia

Absent or Delayed Triggering of Pharyngeal Swallow

This is a common problem seen in patients who have undergone radiation therapy, have had oral or oropharyngeal surgery, or have suffered damage to the medulla or the peripheral nervous system. The pharyngeal motor response is either absent or delayed. The bolus is propelled into the pharynx, but if the motor response is late or absent, aspiration can occur before the swallow triggers. A lack of laryngeal sensation has also been shown to increase the incidence of premature spillage, pharyngeal residue, and laryngeal penetration for all bolus consistencies.[34] Patients with this impairment are best treated with thermal-tactile stimulation.[35]

Reduced Velopharyngeal Closure

This is commonly seen in patients who have had a resection of part or all of their soft palate or who have denervation to the palate. Patients may experience nasal regurgitation during the swallow or hypernasal speech. This may also cause a reduction in pressures on the bolus within the pharynx, resulting in residue within this cavity.

Reduced BOT Posterior Movement

This swallowing disorder can result in residue within the valleculae, requiring repeat dry swallows to clear. This residue can be aspirated after the swallow.

Reduced Pharyngeal Contraction

This may present as unilateral or bilateral involvement of the pharyngeal constrictors. When the impairment is unilateral, residue is observed on the weaker/affected side of the pharynx. For a bilateral deficit, residue typically coats the entire pharyngeal wall. To help identify the specific impairment, an MBS exam should include an anteroposterior view. A FEES exam will also identify the locus of impairment and residue. These patients can also aspirate this residue after a swallow.

Upper Esophageal Sphincter Dysfunction

This disorder can be caused by either a failure of the cricopharyngeus muscle to relax, reduced hyo-laryngeal elevation, or reduced pharyngeal pressures upon the bolus. Residue is commonly found within the pyriform sinuses, which can lead to aspiration after the swallow.[36]

Reduced Laryngeal Elevation

Laryngeal elevation and anterior movement are needed for airway protection and to aid in UES opening. Inadequate laryngeal motion can result in impaired laryngeal vestibule closure and

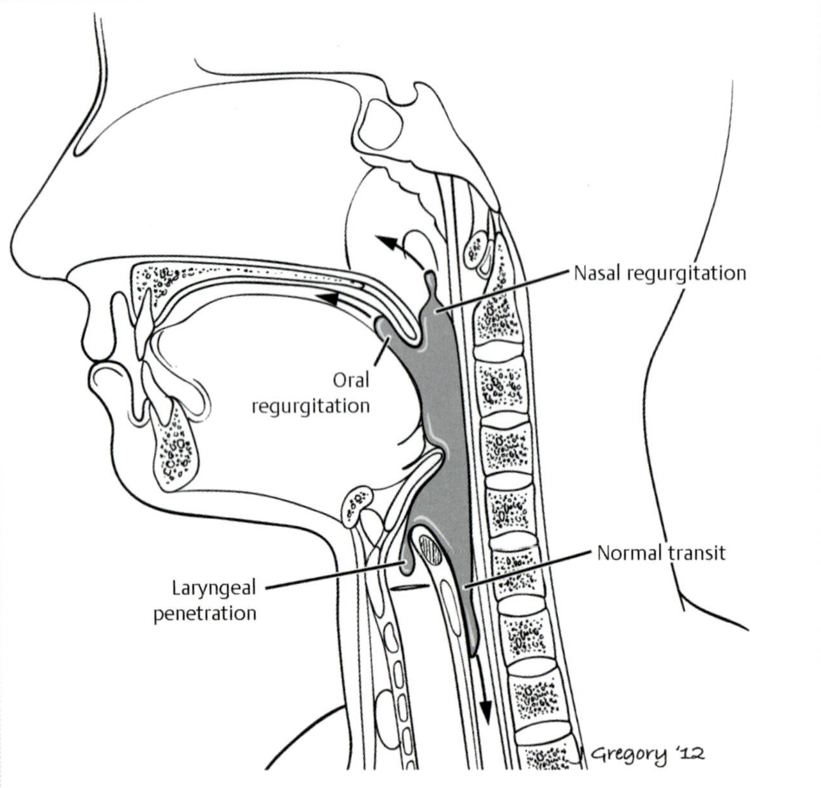

Fig. 19.3 Abnormal bolus transit. If swallowed improperly, a bolus may enter the airway or be regurgitated into the oral or nasal cavities.

penetration of material into the airway entrance, with resultant aspiration after the swallow.[37] If airway entrance and glottic closure are reduced, aspiration will occur during the swallow.[38]

Cervical Osteophytes

Cervical osteophytes are bony outgrowths of cervical vertebrae often seen in older patients with degenerative bone disease.[39] These may protrude into the pharynx causing it to narrow and making it difficult for larger more viscous boluses to pass. Surgical treatment can include removal/shaving of the osteophytes by orthopedic or neurosurgical colleagues.

Dysphagia in Head and Neck Cancer Patients

Patients with head and neck cancer may experience dysphagia as a direct result of the tumor or its treatment, including surgery and radiation. These patients should be managed with a multidisciplinary team involving the surgeon, radiation oncologist, medical oncologist, radiologist, speech-language pathologist, prosthodontist, and social worker.[40] Prior to any treatment, the patient's swallow should be evaluated. It is important to establish a baseline for the patient and to diagnose any swallowing disorders that may have already manifested. Previous studies have shown that more than 25% of head and neck cancer patients suffer from dysphagia prior to the start of cancer treatment.[41] It has also been demonstrated that patients who suffer from dysphagia prior to treatment are more likely to have chronic swallowing issues following any therapy.[42] If the patient cannot be seen prior to treatment, at the very least, counseling over the phone should be provided. Patients should be prescribed appropriate exercises based on the targeted area of surgery or radiation. It is important that these exercises be performed throughout and following their treatment. Patients should be re-evaluated after treatment. As with the initial assessment, an instrumental examination utilizing the MBS or FEES procedures should be conducted.

Head and neck cancer patients who undergo radiation or chemoradiation are at a high risk of developing pharyngeal phase swallow impairment. It has been demonstrated that these patients are more likely to develop reduced tongue base posterior retraction, delayed laryngeal vestibular closure, and reduced laryngeal elevation during swallowing.[43] Unlike other modes of therapy, these patients may first experience swallowing problems during, after, or long after their treatment has been completed. During, or shortly after treatment, patients may experience transient mucositis, pain, or erythema. Patients may later experience skin thickening, increased density of subcutaneous fat, thickening of the epiglottis, and tissue fibrosis.[40] These changes may also cause altered tactile sensation, altered taste sensation, reduced dental sensation, bone changes, reduced appetite, and xerostomia. A direct dose-effect relationship between radiation to specific pharyngeal structures and swallowing difficulties has been demonstrated, and the amount of radiation a patient receives should be monitored in expectation of swallowing impairment.[44]

Patients who undergo surgery for head and neck cancer also suffer from swallowing disorders after their surgery. The swallowing issue experienced by these patients is usually directly related to the size of the resection, as well as any anatomical or neurologic insults that occur.[45] Oral cancer surgery can result in both oral preparatory and oral phase impairment, with reduced ability to manipulate and propel a bolus into the pharynx. These patients also demonstrate pharyngeal phase impairment,

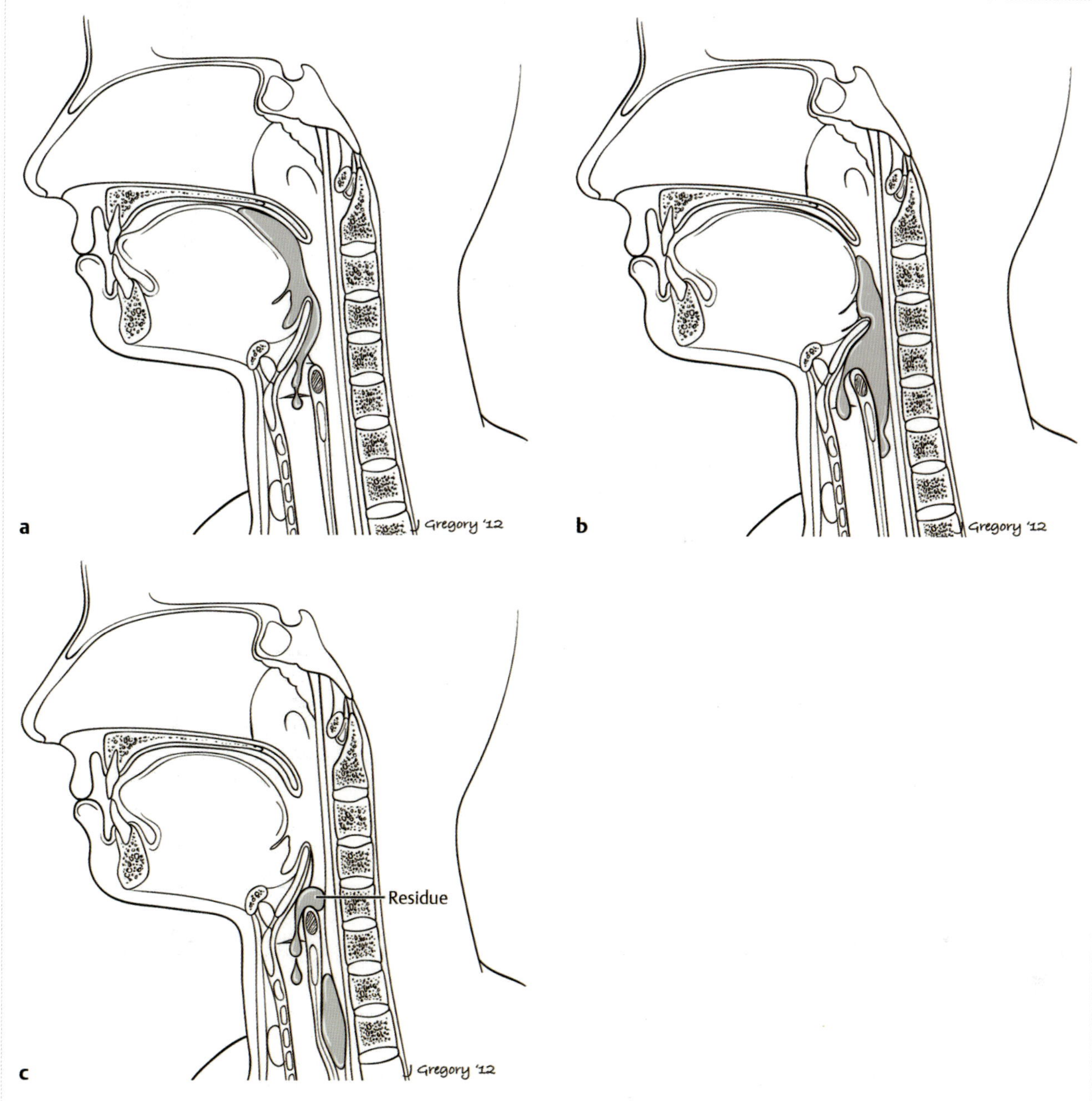

Fig. 19.4 Aspiration. (**a**) Before the swallow. (**b**) During the swallow. (**c**) After the swallow.

often with reduced tongue base motion, reduced pharyngeal contraction and impaired hyolaryngeal motion, depending on the specific structures resected.[46] Partial laryngectomy often results in airway closure problems.[47] Total laryngectomy patients experience difficulty with pressure generation within the pharynx, often requiring a softer diet.[48]

19.4 Compensatory Treatments for Swallowing Disorders

The following strategies are provided to alter bolus flow through the oral cavity and pharynx.[49] Compensatory strategies and swallow therapy are considered first-line measures that should be attempted prior to more aggressive treatments. These strategies are designed to maintain oral feeding, prevent aspiration, and improve efficiency for each swallow. Before using these compensatory treatments, a patient's swallow should be thoroughly examined to uncover the specific anatomical and physiologic dysfunctions that are present. Optimally, this will be done with a MBS exam using videofluoroscopy, but may also include ultrasound, manometry, or fiberoptic endoscopic evaluation of swallowing (FEES).[50] It is also important to perform this assessment to determine the efficacy and safety of a prescribed posture or maneuver. Because the MBS exam exposes patients to radiation, it is important to prioritize the postures or maneuvers that are most likely to target the specific swallowing disorder to minimize exposure time. All compensatory treatments and swallow therapies are influenced by patients' underlying medical conditions including general physical condition, psychosocial aspects, mental status, cognitive ability, and language fluency.[51]

Compensatory swallowing strategies should begin with postures, followed by sensation techniques, maneuvers, and lastly, adjustment of bolus texture and size.[52] The order in which these are prescribed should be adjusted based on patient comfort and the expertise of the clinician. The compensatory swallowing strategies including postures and diet modification are outlined below.

19.4.1 Postures

Swallowing postures are deigned to alter bolus flow during the swallow. These postures alter either the dimensions of the pharynx or the direction in which gravity pulls the bolus. They are especially useful for pediatric or neurologically/cognitively impaired patients who may find the directions involved with maneuvers or swallow exercises too complex. Several studies have shown that aspiration of liquids can be eliminated in the majority of patients who use the appropriately prescribed posture.[53,54] Head immobility or spinal disease are potential contraindications to using postures, and should be identified before starting a regimen, especially in the elderly.

Chin Tuck

The chin tuck posture is used for patients with difficulty triggering the pharyngeal swallow, demonstrates reduced airway entrance closure, or demonstrates reduced posterior movement of the BOT.[55] This posture widens the vallecular space allowing the bolus to be caught within the vallecula, preventing it from entering the airway. The chin tuck also protects against aspiration by reducing the size of the airway introitus by manipulating the arytenoids closer to the epiglottic base. It also tilts the epiglottis in a more protective position and adjusts the base of tongue to be in closer apposition to the posterior pharyngeal wall.[56] To perform this posture, the patient is instructed to lower his or her chin to the chest.

Head Back

This posture is used for patients who have tongue mobility issues and experience difficulty propelling the bolus posteriorly into the pharynx.[53] The head back posture uses gravity to pull the bolus from the oral cavity into the pharynx. Following the placement of the bolus within the patient's mouth, they are instructed to retroflex the neck. It is important to note that this posture can pose a serious risk to patients due to the increased likelihood of aspiration. Therefore, patients are often instructed to maintain a breath hold (i.e., supraglottic swallow, to be discussed below) to prevent aspiration from occurring before the swallow. This posture should not be used on patients who demonstrate severe pharyngeal phase disorders or have difficulty protecting their airway. This posture should be assessed using videofluoroscopy or FEES before being prescribed to a patient.

Head Rotation

This posture is used for patients with unilateral pharyngeal or vocal fold weakness, as well as those with reduced cricopharyngeal opening.[57] When presented with unilateral weakness, the patient is instructed to turn their head toward the weaker or impaired side. The patient is instructed to turn their head as far as comfortably possible, directing the bolus down the stronger side by collapsing the pharyngeal side towards which the head is turned and improving pressure generation within the pharynx. This posture also causes extrinsic pressure on the thyroid cartilage helping the vocal folds approximate to one another.[58] Rotating the head also pulls the cricoid cartilage away from the posterior pharyngeal wall, which can result in a reduction in UES resting pressure.[57]

Head Tilt

The head tilt is prescribed to patients with unilateral tongue or pharyngeal weakness.[59] The patient is instructed to tilt the head towards the nondamaged side. With this posture, the bolus is directed by gravity along the stronger side of the oral cavity and pharynx. For this posture, the patient is asked to bend their head to the side bringing their ear as close to their shoulder as possible.

Side Lying

This posture is used for patients with reduced pharyngeal clearance leading to pharyngeal residue and potential aspiration following a swallow.[60] Side lying will pull residue within the pharynx laterally along the pharyngeal wall, rather than entering the airway. This posture requires the patient to lie on their side with their head elevated slightly. The patient should also be instructed to perform several dry swallows after each swallow to clear any residue from the lateral pharyngeal wall. It is important to note that this posture should only be used after all other postures and maneuvers have been found ineffective. Although the posture is effective, it is difficult for patients to be relegated to lying on their side during meals and makes eating in public impractical.

19.4.2 Changes in Diet

Restricting a patient's diet should only be done after all other strategies have been attempted. When making any change to the types of food or liquids a patient may ingest, it is important to ensure that they are maintaining a full nutritional diet. Within the chart below are some of the more common swallowing disorders and the changes in bolus consistency that might be required (▸ Table 19.1).

19.5 Therapy for Swallowing Disorders

Unlike the aforementioned compensatory procedures, therapy techniques are designed to alter the physiology of a patient's swallow. The goal of therapy should be to slow the decline in

Table 19.1 Changes in bolus consistency

Swallowing disorder	Best	Worst
Reduced lingual ROM or control	Thin/thick liquids	Solid food
Reduced tongue-base posterior movement	Liquids	Solid food
Reduced UES opening	Thin liquids	Solid food
Reduced strength pharyngeal wall	Thin liquids	Solid food
Delayed pharyngeal swallow	Thick liquids/ solid food	Thin liquids
Reduced airway closure	Thick liquids/ solid food	Thin liquids

Abbreviations: ROM, Range of motion; UES, upper esophageal sphincter.

swallow function or aid in its recovery. As described previously, a patient's swallowing disorder and anatomical defects should be fully explored prior to attempting treatment. The following therapy techniques are described in detail: (1) swallow maneuvers, (2) sensory enhancement techniques, (3) sensory–motor integration, and (4) muscle exercises.

19.5.1 Swallow Maneuvers

Swallow maneuvers are designed to alter the pharyngeal phase of the swallow, specifically, alter the timing, extent, and duration of structural movement, thereby improving swallowing efficiency and safety.[61,62] This includes the movement of oral, pharyngeal, or laryngeal structures. These maneuvers are designed to place specific aspects of the swallow under volitional control. Unlike postures, maneuvers are often viewed as more socially acceptable and can often go unnoticed while eating in public; however, there are certain disadvantages to these techniques. Performing swallow maneuvers may prove too difficult for some pediatric (or neurologically or cognitively-impaired) patients. Maneuvers also require increased effort during the swallow, which may tire patients and may prevent their use, particularly in progressive neurologic populations such as Parkinson disease or amyotrophic lateral sclerosis (ALS).

Supraglottic

The supraglottic maneuver provides airway protection in patients who are aspirating either during or before the pharyngeal swallow due to glottic closure problems.[63] This maneuver results in early closure of the true vocal folds before and during the swallow (▶ Fig. 19.5). Examination of this maneuver

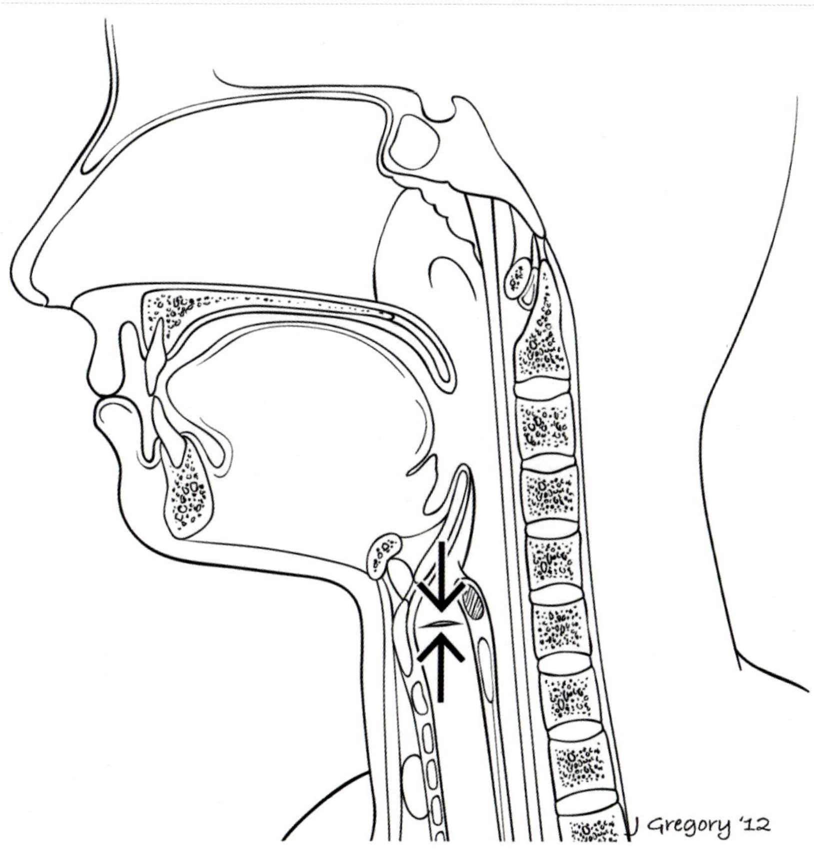

Fig. 19.5 Supraglottic swallow. Performing this maneuver will cause the closure of the true vocal folds before and during the swallow.

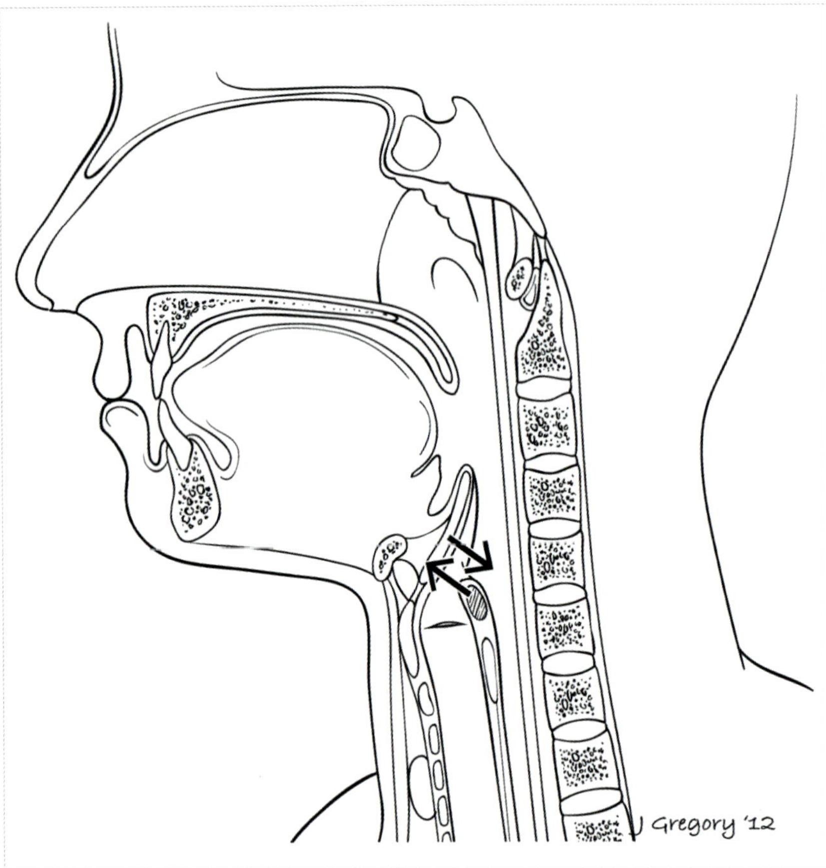

Fig. 19.6 Supersupraglottic swallow. Performing this maneuver causes approximation of the true and false vocal cords. It also forces the arytenoid cartilage to tilt anteriorly towards the base of the epiglottis and the base of the epiglottis to move posteriorly.

using fluoroscopy or FEES will ensure that a patient is correctly maintaining a breath hold, ensuring vocal fold closure and not simply immobilizing the chest with an open airway.[18]

Patient Instructions

Patients are instructed to take a normal breath, exhale a small amount, and proceed to hold their breath. If a tracheostomy tube is present, the patient must occlude the tube. The patient should be instructed to continue to hold their breath through the swallow. Immediately after the swallow, the patient is instructed to cough out, to ensure that any residue on the vocal folds or in the laryngeal vestibule will be expelled. After the cough, they may resume normal breathing.

Supersupraglottic

This swallow maneuver is very similar to the supraglottic maneuver. However, this maneuver requires more effort, but provides better airway protection. The supersupraglottic maneuver causes approximation of the true and false vocal cords and results in the arytenoid cartilages tilting anteriorly toward the base of the epiglottis (▶ Fig. 19.6).[18,56,64] These actions result in laryngeal vestibule closure larynx and also aids in laryngeal elevation. This maneuver is most often used for patients who have undergone a supraglottic laryngectomy.[65] However, it is useful for any patient who demonstrates reduced airway closure during the swallow.

Patient Instructions

Patients are provided the same instructions as those for the supraglottic swallow. However, during the breath hold, patients are instructed to bear down with the abdominal muscles.

Effortful Swallow

This maneuver is helpful for patients with reduced posterior movement of the BOT that may result in residue in the valleculae, BOT, or posterior pharyngeal wall.[66] The effortful swallow is designed to increase contact between the base of tongue and the posterior pharyngeal wall during the pharyngeal phase of the swallow to improve bolus clearance past this region during the swallow. This maneuver increases the posterior movement of the base of tongue as well as the anterior movement of the posterior pharyngeal wall (▶ Fig. 19.7).[51,67]

Patient Instructions

Patients should be instructed to "swallow as hard as you can" or "squeeze your throat muscles with as much force as possible" while swallowing. They are often instructed to swallow as if they are eating a big piece of meat, requiring as much effort as possible.

Mendelsohn Maneuver

The Mendelsohn maneuver has the combined effect of increasing excursion and prolonging duration of laryngeal elevation and of increasing the width and duration of cricopharyngeal

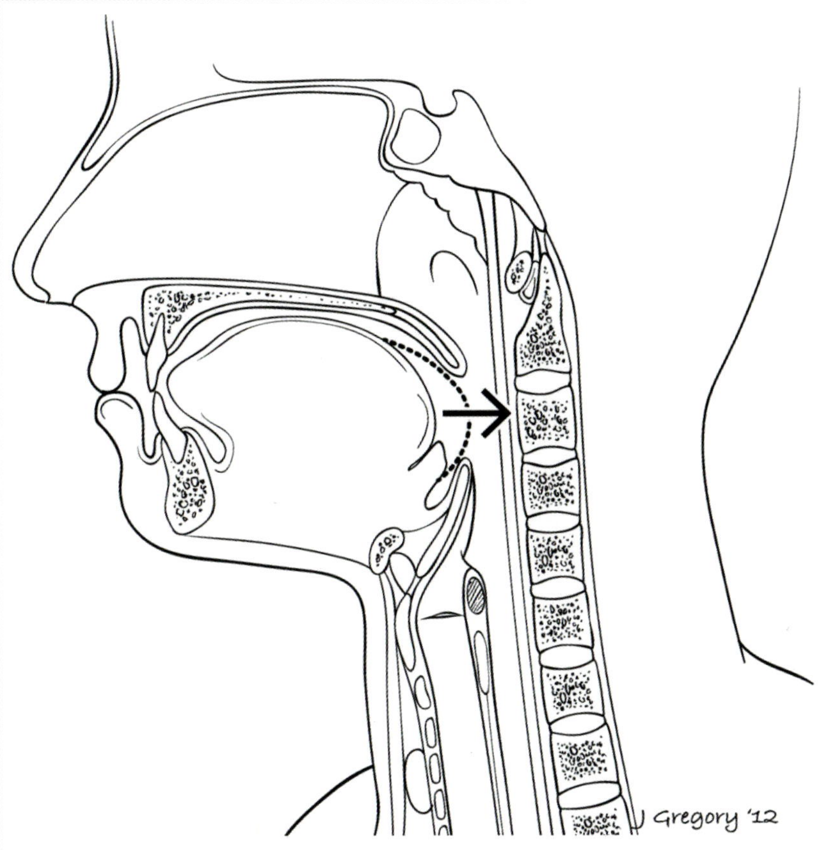

Fig. 19.7 Effortful swallow. Performing this maneuver increases the posterior movement of the tongue base and the anterior movement of the posterior pharyngeal wall during the pharyngeal phase of the swallow.

opening (▶ Fig. 19.8).[68] This maneuver is helpful for patients with UES dysfunction, something that is very common in patients suffering from a brainstem stroke. This technique involves modifying the swallow physiology, specifically, modifying the pharyngeal motor response, with prolongation of the swallow at the height of laryngeal excursion and a resultant improvement in UES opening width and duration. This maneuver will also improve the coordination of the swallow.[69,70]

Patient Instructions

This maneuver is often difficult for patients to grasp. This maneuver is more easily achieved if the clinician demonstrates the maneuver, while the patient palpates the clinician's thyroid cartilage. The patient is asked to feel the clinician's Adam's apple go up and down. Then, the clinician performs the Mendelsohn maneuver, cuing the patient to feel the "Adam's apple" go up, stay up a while, then come down. Then, the clinician palpates the patient's thyroid cartilage and cues the patient to maintain the laryngeal lift during the swallow. The instructions are to swallow normally, then, in the middle of the swallow when they feel the Adam's apple lift, to try to prolong the swallow, keeping the Adam's apple up, squeezing with the throat and tongue. When the clinician palpates the thyroid cartilage and feels the start of the swallow, the clinician says "hold!" to get the patient to try to maintain the laryngeal elevation. Then after about 2 seconds, the clinician instructs the patient to relax. If the larynx palpably descends, the patient has done the maneuver correctly. This may take a few tries for the patient to accurately perfrorm the maneuver. But patients typically can perform this maneuver if they palpate the larynx while the clinician is performing the maneuver.

Tongue-Hold Maneuver (Masako Maneuver)

This exercise is designed to increase the anterior motion of the pharyngeal constrictors to improve the contact between the BOT and PPW during a normal swallow, thus improving pharyngeal pressure exerted on a bolus and improving bolus clearance through this region.[67] Specifically, muscular attachments between the BOT and PPW cause increased resistance on the middle and superior pharyngeal constrictors when the tongue is displaced anteriorly (▶ Fig. 19.9).[71] The patient is instructed to place the tongue tip between the teeth (or lips, if edentulous), and anchor it there while swallowing. Unlike other maneuvers, this maneuver should only be used as an exercise in therapy with dry swallows, and should not be performed with boluses of liquids or foods.

Combining Postures

Many times the effectiveness of a posture or maneuver can be enhanced when coupling it with another synergistic posture or maneuver. The combined chin tuck–head turn is probably the most common of these pairings. This combined posture is often prescribed to patients with unilateral pharyngeal weakness, reduced tongue-base clearance, and/or reduced airway closure. For this combined posture, the head should be turned to the weaker side. Combining the head tilt and head back postures is useful for patients with a unilateral oral deficit and difficulty pro-

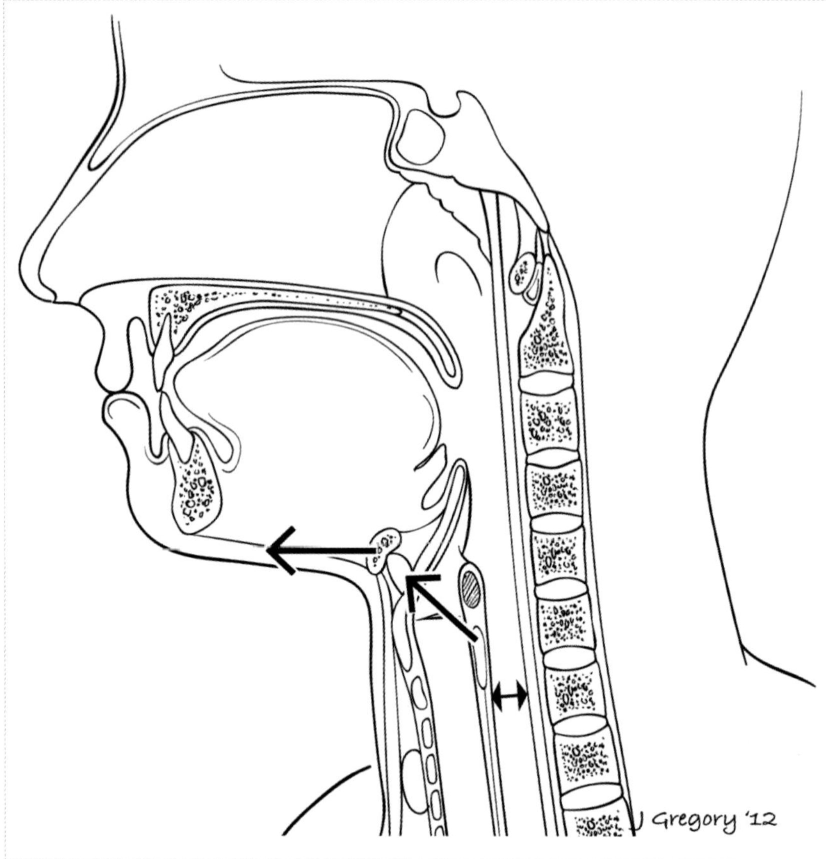

Fig. 19.8 Mendelsohn maneuver. Performing this maneuver causes an increase and prolonging of laryngeal elevation as well as increasing and prolonging UES relaxation.

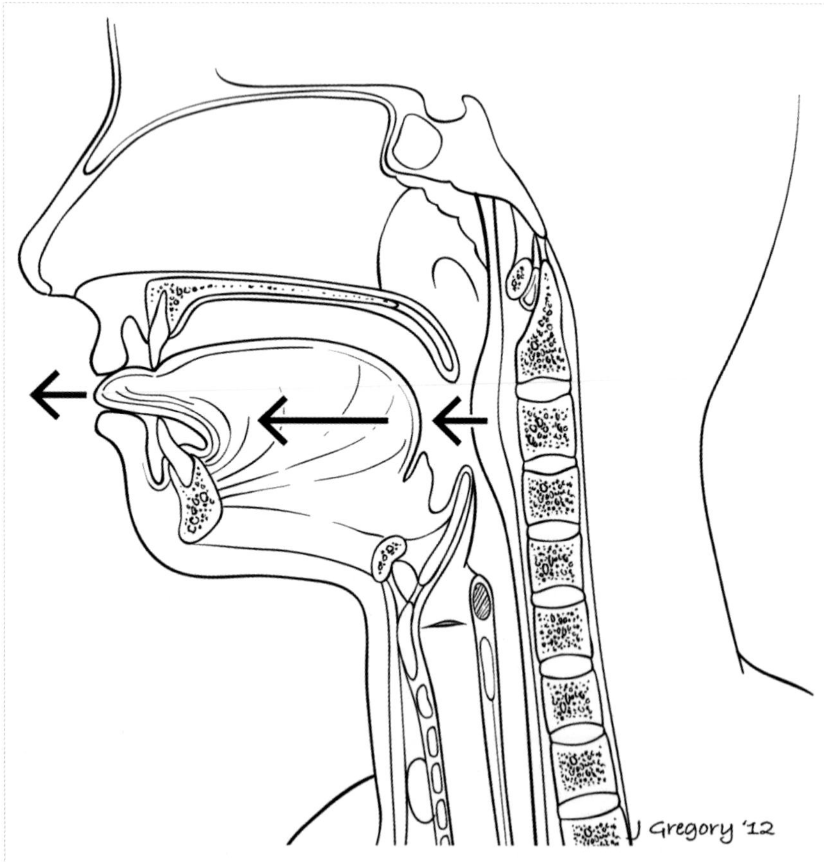

Fig. 19.9 Tongue-hold maneuver. Performing this maneuver causes the tongue base to move anteriorly and pull the posterior pharyngeal wall along with it.

pelling the bolus posteriorly through the oral cavity. This is designed to aid bolus transit and clearance through the oral cavity. The chin tuck and supersupraglottic swallow is useful for patients who cannot achieve adequate airway closure with the chin-down posture alone. Finally, the chin tuck and effortful swallow combination is useful for patients who have difficulty maintaining or achieving BOT to posterior pharynxgeal wall apposition and demonstrate reduced bolus clearance past this region.

19.6 Sensory-Enhancement Techniques

These techniques are designed for patients who demonstrate reduced oral sensation, oral apraxia, or a delay in triggering of the pharyngeal swallow. Each acts as a sensory stimulus prior to initiating the swallow. These techniques do not trigger a swallow, but rather lower the sensory threshold required by a bolus to stimulate a motor response. A benefit of these techniques over other swallow therapies is that they do not require active participation by the patient and thus can be employed for low-level patients. Examples of these techniques include pressure on the dorsum of the tongue with a spoon, introducing different strong tastes (e.g., sour), using a cold bolus, changing the texture, using large volumes, use of carbonation, and thermal-tactile stimulation.[62,72] All of these procedures can be used to increase oral awareness and lower the threshold to trigger a pharyngeal swallow.

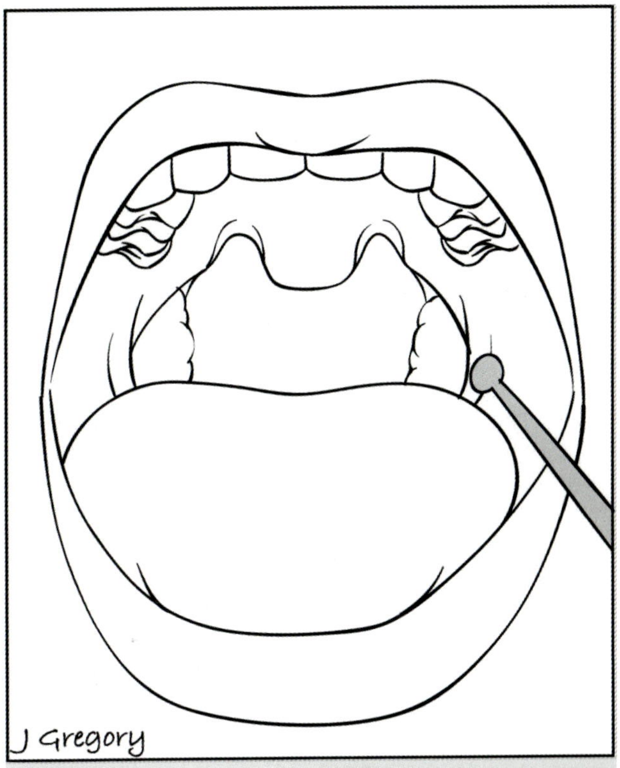

Fig. 19.10 Thermal-tactile stimulation using laryngeal mirror. Rubbing a cold, size-00 laryngeal mirror vertically along the anterior faucial arches.

19.6.1 Thermal–Tactile Stimulation

This is the most commonly prescribed sensory technique used for patients who have difficulty triggering the pharyngeal swallow. The sensory stimulation (i.e., tactile and cold) generated from this technique is relayed to the swallowing center within the brainstem (i.e., reticular formation of the medulla) where the threshold needed to trigger the swallow is altered.

Instructions

This technique involves cooling a size-00 laryngeal mirror in ice and then stroking the mirror along the anterior faucial arches (▶ Fig. 19.10).[35] If the patient experiences unilateral swallow impairment or has undergone flap reconstruction, the laryngeal mirror should be placed against the faucial arch of the unaffected side.

19.6.2 Sensory–Motor Integration Procedures

These procedures use sensory feedback to alter the degree and timing of neuromuscular activity for swallowing. This can be accomplished either through visual feedback or by electrical stimulation, although the data differ regarding the efficacy of this latter technique.

Neuromuscular Electric Stimulation

Neuromuscular electric stimulation (NMES) is a relatively new treatment used for swallowing disorders; there have been no large randomized controlled trials examining its efficacy. The theory behind its use is that electrical stimulation will either provide strengthening to the suprahyoid musculature or will provide enhancement of signaling pathways to and from these muscles.[73,74] To elicit this response, electrodes are placed either transcutaneously or intramuscularly on/in the muscles of the anterior neck and submental region, which emit a low-level electrical current to effect contraction of the muscles. This electrical signal is released in short pulses and has been found to be most efficacious when combined with a swallow or swallow maneuver.[75] Data have demonstrated that NMES can inhibit the response, as well as place the airway entrance in a more compromised position, potentially leading to aspiration.[76,77] More research is needed to determine the efficacy of this treatment technique to improve swallowing.

Biofeedback

This strategy involves direct visualization or a visual representation of a patient's muscular contraction during swallowing. This is an excellent strategy to teach patients swallow maneuvers. This technique is used in real time to provide the patient with volitional control over the deglutitive process. Swallow maneuvers and the resultant muscle contraction can be visualized on camera during an ultrasound, videonasendoscopy, or with electromyography (EMG) biofeedback by allowing the patient to watch the screen during swallowing. Ultrasound is useful to visualize tongue movements. Videonasendoscopy can be helpful to assist patients is performing the supersupraglottic swallow, by providing a good view of airway entrance closure. With EMG, the patient can watch the monitor to view the amplitude and duration of the action potential created by the swallow. These electrodes can be placed on the lips for labial closure or in the submental or thyrohyoid regions to measure muscle contraction generated while performing the effortful and Mendelsohn maneuvers, respectively. Patients are coached to achieve a more forceful swallow or to perform a swallow maneuver, as appropriate.

19.7 Muscle Exercises

Swallowing exercises can include nonswallow exercises, using range-of-motion (ROM), resistance, or fine motor control. These exercises are designed to improve the function of the muscle being targeted. These can be performed by any patient who can follow commands. Contraindications include those who experience muscle fatigue, or those with inadequate tissue. These exercises can be used with patients who are not yet able to take oral nutrition, but are also useful for those on oral diets.

19.7.1 Range-of-Motion Exercises

Range-of-motion exercises are indicated for patients who experience reduced motion of any structure involved in deglutition, including the lips, tongue, tongue base, pharyngeal constrictors, larynx, and vocal folds. These are commonly prescribed for patients who have head and neck cancer, weakness secondary to neurologic insult or deconditioning, or fibrosis caused by radiation treatment. Described below are some ROM exercises that can be used for the tongue or lips. Tongue ROM exercises are designed to improve lingual range of motion on protrusion, lateralization, and elevation. The dosage, frequency, and duration of these exercises has not been well studied; however, repetition during the day (i.e., 3–5 times) and throughout the week (i.e., 3–5 times per week), has been suggested, as is recommended in the exercise literature.[51]

Lip Range-of-Motion Exercises

These are useful for those patients with deficits in labial range of motion due to facial paralysis and/or head and neck surgical procedures, including resection or mandibulotomy. The focus of treatment is to improve range on protrusion, retraction, and closure.

19.7.2 Resistance Exercises

These exercises are designed to strengthen an intended muscle through active resistance. Below are some of the more commonly used techniques.

Tongue Resistance

Patients are instructed to resist against a tongue depressor or other flat object on protrusion, elevation, and lateral movements. Tongue exercises have been shown to improve swallow function in healthy young, elderly, oral cancer, and stroke patients.[78,79,80,81]

19.7.3 Vocal Folds Bear Down

This exercise can be useful for any patient experiencing aspiration during the swallow. The patient is instructed to hold their breath and bear down for one second and then release to achieve tighter vocal fold closure.

19.7.4 Base of Tongue Movement

The patient should be instructed to pull the tongue base as far as possible toward the pharynx. The instruction to dry gargle (no liquids) has been found to be useful for patients to perform this exercise.[82]

19.7.5 Laryngeal Elevation (Falsetto Exercise)

The patient is instructed to produce the highest pitch on a slide upward and maintain the high pitch for about 3 to 4 seconds. Although there are no data to support the use of this specific exercise, data have shown that inability to raise pitch is predictive of aspiration in dysphagic patients.[83]

19.7.6 Pharyngeal Constrictor Movement

The pharyngeal squeeze has been advocated to improve muscle contraction of the constrictor musculature. Increased pharyngeal contraction has been observed with this technique.[84] Patients are instructed to produce a high-pitched "eee" for a few seconds and the pharyngeal constrictor activity can be visualized endoscopically.[84]

19.7.7 Shaker Exercises

These exercises are designed to increase the strength of the suprahyoid muscles to improve hyolaryngeal elevation.[85] With improvement in laryngeal motion, width and duration of UES opening have been found to increase with this technique in healthy and in dysphagic neurologically impaired patients[86,87] This technique involves a head lift exercise, with the patient lying flat on his or her back.

Lingual Control Exercises

These exercises are prescribed for patients who have difficulty with bolus manipulation due to reduced tongue control. This is especially helpful for patients who have undergone a partial glossectomy or a stroke resulting in lingual weakness. This exercise involves manipulating a gauze or licorice stick within the mouth, with focus on sealing the gauze or licorice against the palate, moving it laterally to the teeth, and moving it up and backwards, as if to propel for swallowing (while holding the outer portion by the patient or clinician to prevent possible choking).

19.8 Conclusion

Swallow rehabilitation is of paramount importance for patients with dysphagia. Before a specific therapy can be tailored to a patient, clinicians must have a thorough understanding of the nature of the swallowing disorder and any anatomical abnormalities before therapeutic strategies can be implemented. Through the use of postures, maneuvers, exercise, sensory-enhancement techniques, and diet modification, patients are more likely to maintain adequate nutrition, while reducing the likelihood of aspiration or discomfort.[88,89,90,91,92] These noninvasive techniques should be considered prior to medical and surgical management. Swallow management requires a team effort through a combined multidisciplinary approach, with good communication among health professionals, as well as good communication with the patient.

References

[1] Altman KW, Yu GP, Schaefer SD. Consequence of dysphagia in the hospitalized patient: impact on prognosis and hospital resources. Arch Otolaryngol Head Neck Surg 2010; 136: 784–789

[2] Lovell SJ, Wong HB, Loh KS, Ngo RY, Wilson JA. Impact of dysphagia on quality-of-life in nasopharyngeal carcinoma. Head Neck 2005; 27: 864–872

[3] Marik PE, Kaplan D. Aspiration pneumonia and dysphagia in the elderly. Chest 2003; 124: 328–336

[4] Palmer JB, Drennan JC, Baba M. Evaluation and treatment of swallowing impairments. Am Fam Physician 2000; 61: 2453–2462

[5] Steele CM, Miller AJ. Sensory input pathways and mechanisms in swallowing: a review. Dysphagia 2010; 25: 323–333

[6] Dodds WJ, Stewart ET, Logemann JA. Physiology and radiology of the normal oral and pharyngeal phases of swallowing. AJR Am J Roentgenol 1990; 154: 953–963

[7] Martin-Harris B, Michel Y, Castell DO. Physiologic model of oropharyngeal swallowing revisited. Otolaryngol Head Neck Surg 2005; 133: 234–240

[8] Palmer JB, Hiiemae KM, Matsuo K, Haishima H. Volitional control of food transport and bolus formation during feeding. Physiol Behav 2007; 91: 66–70

[9] Dodds WJ, Taylor AJ, Stewart ET, Kern MK, Logemann JA, Cook IJ. Tipper and dipper types of oral swallows. AJR Am J Roentgenol 1989; 153: 1197–1199

[10] Logemann JA. Swallowing disorders. Best Pract Res Clin Gastroenterol 2007; 21: 563–573

[11] Kahrilas PJ, Lin S, Logemann JA, Ergun GA, Facchini F. Deglutitive tongue action: volume accommodation and bolus propulsion. Gastroenterology 1993; 104: 152–162

[12] Palmer JB, Rudin NJ, Lara G, Crompton AW. Coordination of mastication and swallowing. Dysphagia 1992; 7: 187–200

[13] Hiiemae KM, Palmer JB. Food transport and bolus formation during complete feeding sequences on foods of different initial consistency. Dysphagia 1999; 14: 31–42

[14] Martin RE, MacIntosh BJ, Smith RC et al. Cerebral areas processing swallowing and tongue movement are overlapping but distinct: a functional magnetic resonance imaging study. J Neurophysiol 2004; 92: 2428–2443

[15] Ono T, Hori K, Nokubi T. Pattern of tongue pressure on hard palate during swallowing. Dysphagia 2004; 19: 259–264

[16] Dantas RO, Kern MK, Massey BT et al. Effect of swallowed bolus variables on oral and pharyngeal phases of swallowing. Am J Physiol 1990; 258: G675–G681

[17] Jean A. Brain stem control of swallowing: neuronal network and cellular mechanisms. Physiol Rev 2001; 81: 929–969

[18] Martin BJ, Logemann JA, Shaker R, Dodds WJ. Normal laryngeal valving patterns during three breath-hold maneuvers: a pilot investigation. Dysphagia 1993; 8: 11–20

[19] Van Daele DJ, McCulloch TM, Palmer PM, Langmore SE. Timing of glottic closure during swallowing: a combined electromyographic and endoscopic analysis. Ann Otol Rhinol Laryngol 2005; 114: 478–487

[20] Kahrilas PJ, Logemann JA, Lin S, Ergun GA. Pharyngeal clearance during swallowing: a combined manometric and videofluoroscopic study. Gastroenterology 1992; 103: 128–136

[21] Doty RW, Bosma JF. An electromyographic analysis of reflex deglutition. J Neurophysiol 1956; 19: 44–60

[22] Ren J, Massey BT, Dodds WJ et al. Determinants of intrabolus pressure during esophageal peristaltic bolus transport. Am J Physiol 1993; 264: G407–G413

[23] Rademaker AW, Pauloski BR, Colangelo LA, Logemann JA. Age and volume effects on liquid swallowing function in normal women. J Speech Lang Hear Res 1998; 41: 275–284

[24] Reimers-Neils L, Logemann J, Larson C. Viscosity effects on EMG activity in normal swallow. Dysphagia 1994; 9: 101–106

[25] Jacob P, Kahrilas PJ, Logemann JA, Shah V, Ha T. Upper esophageal sphincter opening and modulation during swallowing. Gastroenterology 1989; 97: 1469–1478

[26] Logemann JA, Kahrilas PJ, Cheng J et al. Closure mechanisms of laryngeal vestibule during swallow. Am J Physiol 1992; 262: G338–G344

[27] Logemann JA, Pauloski BR, Rademaker AW, Kahrilas PJ. Oropharyngeal swallow in younger and older women: videofluoroscopic analysis. J Speech Lang Hear Res 2002; 45: 434–445

[28] Logemann JA, Pauloski BR, Rademaker AW, Colangelo LA, Kahrilas PJ, Smith CH. Temporal and biomechanical characteristics of oropharyngeal swallow in younger and older men. J Speech Lang Hear Res 2000; 43: 1264–1274

[29] Shaker R, Ren J, Bardan E et al. Pharyngoglottal closure reflex: characterization in healthy young, elderly and dysphagic patients with predeglutitive aspiration. Gerontology 2003; 49: 12–20

[30] Lazarus C, Logemann JA. Swallowing disorders in closed head trauma patients. Arch Phys Med Rehabil 1987; 68: 79–84

[31] Robbins J, Levin RL. Swallowing after unilateral stroke of the cerebral cortex: preliminary experience. Dysphagia 1988; 3: 11–17

[32] González-Fernández M, Daniels SK. Dysphagia in stroke and neurologic disease. Phys Med Rehabil Clin N Am 2008; 19: 867–888, x

[33] Logemann JA, Pauloski BR, Colangelo L, Lazarus C, Fujiu M, Kahrilas PJ. Effects of a sour bolus on oropharyngeal swallowing measures in patients with neurogenic dysphagia. J Speech Hear Res 1995; 38: 556–563

[34] Sulica L, Hembree A, Blitzer A. Swallowing and sensation: evaluation of deglutition in the anesthetized larynx. Ann Otol Rhinol Laryngol 2002; 111: 291–294

[35] Lazzara G, Lazarus C, Logemann JA. Impact of thermal stimulation on patients with swallowing disorders. Dysphagia 1986; 1: 73–77

[36] Cook IJ. Cricopharyngeal function and dysfunction. Dysphagia 1993; 8: 244–251

[37] Morton R, Minford J, Ellis R, Pinnington L. Aspiration with dysphagia: the interaction between oropharyngeal and respiratory impairments. Dysphagia 2002; 17: 192–196

[38] Kahrilas PJ, Lin S, Rademaker AW, Logemann JA. Impaired deglutitive airway protection: a videofluoroscopic analysis of severity and mechanism. Gastroenterology 1997; 113: 1457–1464

[39] Carlson ML, Archibald DJ, Graner DE, Kasperbauer JL. Surgical management of dysphagia and airway obstruction in patients with prominent ventral cervical osteophytes. Dysphagia 2011; 26: 34–40

[40] Lazarus CL. Management of swallowing disorders in head and neck cancer patients: optimal patterns of care. Semin Speech Lang 2000; 21: 293–309

[41] Logemann JA, Rademaker AW, Pauloski BR et al. Site of disease and treatment protocol as correlates of swallowing function in patients with head and neck cancer treated with chemoradiation. Head Neck 2006; 28: 64–73

[42] Lewin JS. Dysphagia after chemoradiation: prevention and treatment. Int J Radiat Oncol Biol Phys 2007; 69 Suppl: S86–S87

[43] Logemann JA, Pauloski BR, Rademaker AW et al. Swallowing disorders in the first year after radiation and chemoradiation. Head Neck 2008; 30: 148–158

[44] Feng FY, Kim HM, Lyden TH et al. Intensity-modulated radiotherapy of head and neck cancer aiming to reduce dysphagia: early dose-effect relationships for the swallowing structures. Int J Radiat Oncol Biol Phys 2007; 68: 1289–1298

[45] Raber-Durlacher JE, Brennan MT, Verdonck-de Leeuw IM et al. Dysphagia Section, Oral Care Study Group, Multinational Association of Supportive Care in Cancer (MASCC)/International Society of Oral Oncology (ISOO). Swallowing dysfunction in cancer patients. Support Care Cancer 2012; 20: 433–443

[46] Kronenberger MB, Meyers AD. Dysphagia following head and neck cancer surgery. Dysphagia 1994; 9: 236–244

[47] Rademaker AW, Logemann JA, Pauloski BR et al. Recovery of postoperative swallowing in patients undergoing partial laryngectomy. Head Neck 1993; 15: 325–334

[48] Manikantan K, Khode S, Sayed SI et al. Dysphagia in head and neck cancer. Cancer Treat Rev 2009; 35: 724–732

[49] Lazarus CL. Management of dysphagia. In: Bailey BJ, ed. Head and Neck Surgery-Otolaryngology. Vol 1. Philadelphia, PA: Lippincott Williams & Wilkins; 2006: 713–720

[50] Logemann JA. Behavioral management for oropharyngeal dysphagia. Folia Phoniatr Logop 1999; 51: 199–212

[51] Logemann JA. Evaluation and Treatment of Swallowing Disorders. 2nd ed. Austin, TX: Pro-Ed; 1997

[52] Logemann JA. Evaluation of swallowing disorders. In: Evaluation and Treatment of Swallowing Disorders. Vol 2. Austin, TX: Pro-Ed; 1998: 135–185
[53] Rasley A, Logemann JA, Kahrilas PJ, Rademaker AW, Pauloski BR, Dodds WJ. Prevention of barium aspiration during videofluoroscopic swallowing studies: value of change in posture. AJR Am J Roentgenol 1993; 160: 1005–1009
[54] Logemann JA, Gensler G, Robbins JA et al. A randomized study of three interventions for aspiration of thin liquids in patients with dementia or Parkinson's disease. J Speech Lang Hear Res 2008; 51: 173–183
[55] Logemann JA. Manual for the Videofluroscopic Study of Swallowing. 2nd ed. Austin, TX: Pro-Ed; 1993
[56] Carrau RL. Therapeutic intervention for swallowing disorders. In: Comprehensive Management of Swallowing Disorders. San Diego, CA: Singular Publishing; 1999: 243–248
[57] McCulloch TM, Hoffman MR, Ciucci MR. High-resolution manometry of pharyngeal swallow pressure events associated with head turn and chin tuck. Ann Otol Rhinol Laryngol 2010; 119: 369–376
[58] Ohmae Y, Ogura M, Kitahara S, Karaho T, Inouye T. Effects of head rotation on pharyngeal function during normal swallow. Ann Otol Rhinol Laryngol 1998; 107: 344–348
[59] Logemann JA. Noninvasive approaches to deglutitive aspiration. Dysphagia 1993; 8: 331–333
[60] Drake W, O'Donoghue S, Bartram C, Lindsay J, Greenwood R. Eating in sidelying facilitates rehabilitation in neurogenic dysphagia. Brain Inj 1997; 11: 137–142
[61] McCabe D, Ashford J, Wheeler-Hegland K et al. Evidence-based systematic review: Oropharyngeal dysphagia behavioral treatments. Part IV—impact of dysphagia treatment on individuals' postcancer treatments. J Rehabil Res Dev 2009; 46: 205–214
[62] Lazarus CL. Management of swallowing disorders in head and neck cancer patients: optimal patterns of care. Semin Speech Lang 2000; 21: 293–309
[63] Logemann JA. Approaches to management of disordered swallowing. Baillieres Clin Gastroenterol 1991; 5: 269–280
[64] Logemann JA, Kahrilas PJ, Cheng J et al. Closure mechanisms of laryngeal vestibule during swallow. Am J Physiol 1992; 262: G338–G344
[65] Logemann JA, Gibbons P, Rademaker AW et al. Mechanisms of recovery of swallow after supraglottic laryngectomy. J Speech Hear Res 1994; 37: 965–974
[66] Witte U, Huckabee ML, Doeltgen SH, Gumbley F, Robb M. The effect of effortful swallow on pharyngeal manometric measurements during saliva and water swallowing in healthy participants. Arch Phys Med Rehabil 2008; 89: 822–828
[67] Lazarus C, Logemann JA, Song CW, Rademaker AW, Kahrilas PJ. Effects of voluntary maneuvers on tongue base function for swallowing. Folia Phoniatr Logop 2002; 54: 171–176
[68] Ding R, Larson CR, Logemann JA, Rademaker AW. Surface electromyographic and electroglottographic studies in normal subjects under two swallow conditions: normal and during the Mendelsohn manuever. Dysphagia 2002; 17: 1–12
[69] Bodén K, Hallgren Å, Witt Hedström H. Effects of three different swallow maneuvers analyzed by videomanometry. Acta Radiol 2006; 47: 628–633
[70] Hoffman MR, Mielens JD, Ciucci MR, Jones CA, Jiang JJ, McCulloch TM. High-resolution manometry of pharyngeal swallow pressure events associated with effortful swallow and the Mendelsohn maneuver. Dysphagia 2012; 27: 418–426
[71] Doeltgen SH, Witte U, Gumbley F, Huckabee ML. Evaluation of manometric measures during tongue-hold swallows. Am J Speech Lang Pathol 2009; 18: 65–73
[72] Logemann JA. The role of the speech language pathologist in the management of dysphagia. Otolaryngol Clin North Am 1988; 21: 783–788
[73] Clark H, Lazarus C, Arvedson J, Schooling T, Frymark T. Evidence-based systematic review: effects of neuromuscular electrical stimulation on swallowing and neural activation. Am J Speech Lang Pathol 2009; 18: 361–375
[74] Ludlow CL. Electrical neuromuscular stimulation in dysphagia: current status. Curr Opin Otolaryngol Head Neck Surg 2010; 18: 159–164
[75] Humbert IA, Poletto CJ, Saxon KG, Kearney PR, Ludlow CL. The effect of surface electrical stimulation on vocal fold position. Laryngoscope 2008; 118: 14–19
[76] Humbert IA, Poletto CJ, Saxon KG et al. The effect of surface electrical stimulation on hyolaryngeal movement in normal individuals at rest and during swallowing. J Appl Physiol 2006; 101: 1657–1663
[77] Power M, Fraser C, Hobson A et al. Changes in pharyngeal corticobulbar excitability and swallowing behavior after oral stimulation. Am J Physiol Gastrointest Liver Physiol 2004; 286: G45–G50
[78] van der Molen L, van Rossum MA, Burkhead LM, Smeele LE, Rasch CR, Hilgers FJ. A randomized preventive rehabilitation trial in advanced head and neck cancer patients treated with chemoradiotherapy: feasibility, compliance, and short-term effects. Dysphagia 2011; 26: 155–170
[79] Robbins J, Gangnon RE, Theis SM, Kays SA, Hewitt AL, Hind JA. The effects of lingual exercise on swallowing in older adults. J Am Geriatr Soc 2005; 53: 1483–1489
[80] Lazarus C, Logemann JA, Huang CF, Rademaker AW. Effects of two types of tongue strengthening exercises in young normals. Folia Phoniatr Logop 2003; 55: 199–205
[81] Robbins JA, Kays SA, Gangnon RE et al. The effects of lingual exercise in stroke patients with dysphagia. Arch Phys Med Rehabil 2007; 88: 150–158
[82] Veis S, Logemann JA, Colangelo L. Effects of three techniques on maximum posterior movement of the tongue base. Dysphagia 2000; 15: 142–145
[83] Malandraki GA, Hind JA, Gangnon R, Logemann JA, Robbins J. The utility of pitch elevation in the evaluation of oropharyngeal Dysphagia: preliminary findings. Am J Speech Lang Pathol 2011; 20: 262–268
[84] Fuller SC, Leonard R, Aminpour S, Belafsky PC. Validation of the pharyngeal squeeze maneuver. Otolaryngol Head Neck Surg 2009; 140: 391–394
[85] Easterling C, Grande B, Kern M, Sears K, Shaker R. Attaining and maintaining isometric and isokinetic goals of the Shaker exercise. Dysphagia 2005; 20: 133–138
[86] Shaker R, Easterling C, Kern M et al. Rehabilitation of swallowing by exercise in tube-fed patients with pharyngeal dysphagia secondary to abnormal UES opening. Gastroenterology 2002; 122: 1314–1321
[87] Mepani R, Antonik S, Massey B et al. Augmentation of deglutitive thyrohyoid muscle shortening by the Shaker exercise. Dysphagia 2009; 24: 26–31
[88] Speyer R, Baijens L, Heijnen M, Zwijnenberg I. Effects of therapy in oropharyngeal dysphagia by speech and language therapists: a systematic review. Dysphagia 2010; 25: 40–65
[89] Tang Y, Shen Q, Wang Y, Lu K, Wang Y, Peng Y. A randomized prospective study of rehabilitation therapy in the treatment of radiation-induced dysphagia and trismus. Strahlenther Onkol 2011; 187: 39–44
[90] Rofes L, Arreola V, Almirall J et al. Diagnosis and management of oropharyngeal dysphagia and its nutritional and respiratory complications in the elderly. Gastroenterol Res Pract 2011; 2011: 1–13
[91] Crary MA, Carnaby GD, LaGorio LA, Carvajal PJ. Functional and physiological outcomes from an exercise-based dysphagia therapy: a pilot investigation of the McNeill Dysphagia Therapy Program. Arch Phys Med Rehabil 2012; 93: 1173–1178
[92] Wheeler-Hegland K, Ashford J, Frymark T et al. Evidence-based systematic review: oropharyngeal dysphagia behavioral treatments. Part II—impact of dysphagia treatment on normal swallow function. J Rehabil Res Dev 2009; 46: 185–194

20 Tracheotomy

Bradley A. Schiff

Tracheotomy is one of the core procedures in otolaryngology–head and neck surgery. Although the procedure itself is relatively straightforward, the indications and nuances of tracheotomy are more intricate, and can vary greatly from institution to institution. In addition, the medical and surgical complexities intrinsic to many patients requiring tracheotomy make facility with this procedure essential for otolaryngologists–head and neck surgeons.

20.1 History

Although the first tracheotomy was referenced 3500 years ago, making it one of the earliest recorded surgical procedures, it was not until 1909, when Chevalier Jackson first described the procedure, that the details of tracheotomy technique were formally presented. Dr. Jackson's technique became the standard of care and was similar to the technique performed today; therefore, he is considered by many to be the father of the modern tracheotomy.[1,3] Over the past 30 years, there have been significant variations employed in the procedure. After the introduction of percutaneous tracheotomy in the 1980s, the optimal technique has become a controversial issue, and a number of excellent recent studies have again made tracheotomy an important topic of investigation.

20.2 Anatomy

Although the anatomy of the trachea is relatively straightforward compared to other parts of the upper aerodigestive tract, knowledge of this anatomy is an essential component of tracheotomy management (▶ Fig. 20.1). The trachea is comprised of 18 to 22 semicircular rings of cartilage anteriorly and laterally, with a membranous portion abutting the esophagus on the posterior tracheal wall. The flat posterior membranous portion

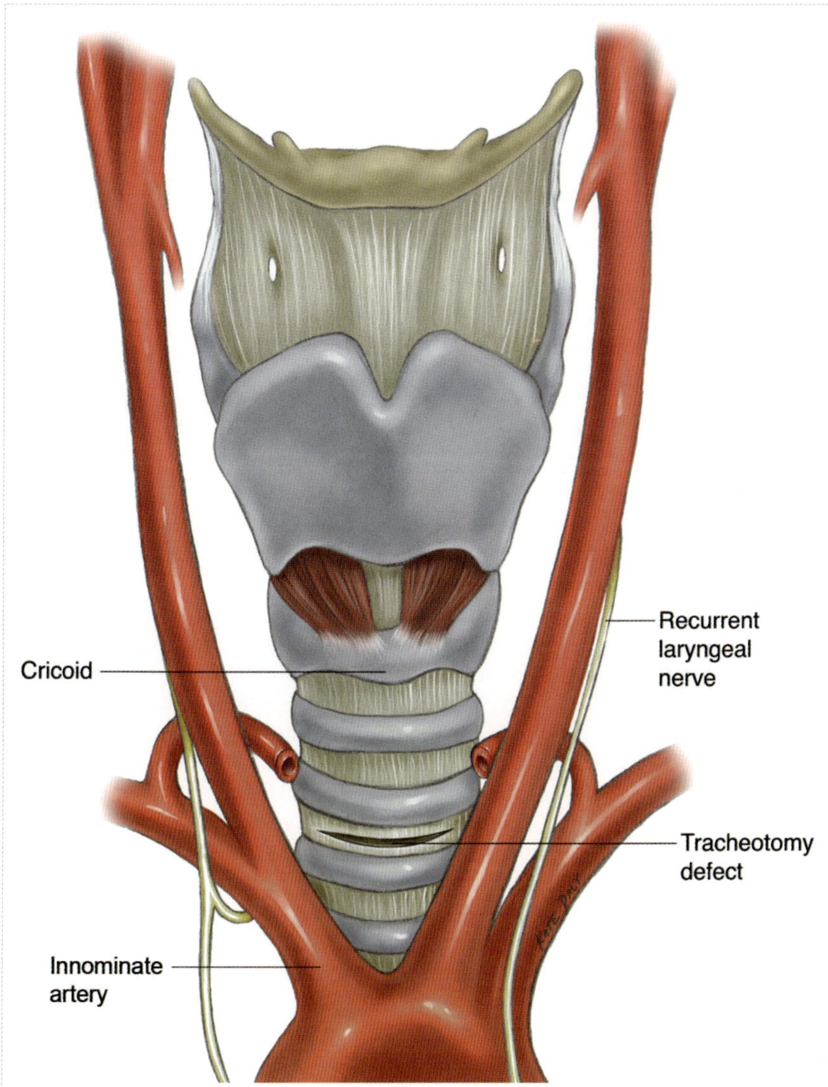

Fig. 20.1 Relationship of tracheotomy site to surrounding anatomical structures.

is made up of a smooth muscle, the trachealis. The C-shaped tracheal rings help provide the support necessary to ensure tracheal patency. The cricoid is the only complete cartilaginous ring of the trachea and is essential in the maintenance of the diameter of the tracheal lumen. The average width of the trachea is 2.3 cm from left to right, and 1.8 cm from the posterior membrane to the anterior cartilaginous aspect.[4] The length of the average adult trachea is approximately 11 cm in length, and ranges from 10 to 13 cm.

The cricoid cartilage lies just superior to the first tracheal ring and is attached to the first tracheal ring by the cricotracheal ligament. Superiorly, the cricoid is attached to the thyroid cartilage by the median cricothyroid ligament. The trachea extends from the cricoid (at approximately the sixth cervical vertebrae) and ends at the fourth or fifth thoracic vertebrae, where it divides into the left and right mainstem bronchi. The trachea is covered by the pretracheal layer of the deep cervical fascia. This extends from the inferior portion of the hyoid into the thorax. The pretracheal fascia includes a muscular part, which encompasses the strap muscles, and a visceral part that surrounds the thyroid, trachea and esophagus.

The innominate (brachiocephalic) artery runs from left to right anterior to the trachea, and typically lies beneath the sternal notch (although it can be more cephalad in some patients placing it at risk for injury during a tracheotomy). The thyroid gland lies anterior and lateral to the trachea with the isthmus in the center most commonly over tracheal rings 2 to 4. The recurrent laryngeal nerves can be found in the tracheoesophageal grooves, lateral to the trachea and posteromedial to the thyroid lobes. Overlying the thyroid gland are the sternohyoid and sternothyroid muscles. The carotid artery, vagus nerve, and internal jugular vein all are lateral to the thyroid.

The blood supply of the lateral and anterior tracheal walls is a complex network of arteries derived from numerous arteries including the inferior thyroid, subclavian, supreme intercostals, internal thoracic, innominate, and superior and middle bronchial arteries. Branches from each of these vessels contribute to two lateral longitudinal vascular anastomoses that run parallel to the trachea. These longitudinal vessels provide the blood supply to the transverse segmental vessels that run in the soft tissues between the tracheal rings. The transverse vessels in turn supply the submucosal capillary network that runs beneath the endotracheal mucosa and provides the blood supply to the lateral and anterior tracheal walls. The posterior membranous portion of the trachea derives its blood supply from the esophageal arteries and their subdivisions.[5]

20.3 Definitions

The words tracheotomy and tracheostomy are often used interchangeably, but each word has a distinct meaning, and the correct use of these words is important to many otolaryngologists. The term tracheotomy refers to the surgical creation of an opening in the anterior tracheal wall to create an airway. The term tracheostomy refers to the formation of an opening in the trachea in which a permanent stoma is created, or to the stoma itself.[2]

20.4 Indications

The indications for tracheotomy have evolved throughout the history of the procedure. With improved understanding of the disease processes affecting the airway, the indications have become more standardized and rigorous in recent years.

Today there are numerous indications recognized in the adult population. These indications were defined by the American Academy of Otolaryngology and Head and Neck Surgery in the 2010 Clinical Indicators Compendium (see the box "Indications for tracheotomy as defined by the American Academy of Otolaryngology–Head and Neck Surgery in the 2010 Clinical Indicators Compendium (p. 206)").[7]

Indications for tracheotomy as defined by the American Academy of Otolaryngology–Head and Neck Surgery in the 2010 Clinical Indicators Compendium

- Upper airway obstruction with any of the following:
  - Stridor
  - Air hunger
  - Retractions
  - Obstructive sleep apnea with documented arterial desaturation
  - Bilateral vocal fold paralysis
  - Previous neck surgery or throat trauma
  - Previous irradiation to the neck
- Prolonged or expected prolonged intubation
- Inability of patient to manage secretions, including aspiration or excessive bronchopulmonary secretions
- Facilitation of ventilation support
- Inability to intubate
- Adjunct to manage head and neck surgery
- Adjunct to manage significant head and neck trauma

The indications for tracheotomy fall into four broad categories: to relieve a mechanical obstruction (or potential obstruction), to manage aspiration (and promote improved pulmonary toilet), to provide long-term ventilation (and avoid the complications of long-term translaryngeal intubation), and to promote weaning from the ventilator.

Tracheotomy can be used to relieve many different types of mechanical airway obstruction. Tracheotomy is frequently used to bypass obstructive lesions of the upper respiratory tract and/or alimentary tract, most commonly neoplastic lesions. However, if a patient has a nonobstructive lesion that might be predispose him to future airway obstruction, either from growth of the lesion or from edema secondary to future interventions (such as radiation), a tracheotomy is often performed prior to the treatment to ensure protection of the airway. It is also frequently performed in head and neck surgical procedures involving a free flap in the oral cavity, oropharynx, hypopharynx or larynx, where postsurgical edema could lead to obstruction and reintubation might prove difficult and/or potentially damaging to the newly placed free flap.

Tracheotomy is occasionally necessary to bypass edema secondary to infection of the glottis, supraglottis, or oral cavity. This was a much more common use of tracheotomy before the widespread use of the influenza vaccine, which has drastically reduced the incidence of epiglottitis. Tracheotomy is also occasionally used in patients when severe angioedema of the upper aerodigestive tract prevents safe intubation. Laryngeal or maxillofacial trauma may lead to an inadequate respiratory lumen and thus require a tracheotomy for adequate control of the airway. Vocal cord paralysis or paresis may require a tracheotomy if the patient is unable to maintain an adequate glottic aperture. Finally, tracheotomy is the gold standard for curing patients with extreme cases of obstructive sleep apnea recalcitrant to other therapies.

The stability of the airway is considerably improved with a tracheotomy compared to endotracheal intubation; thus, it is often used for patients with a tenuous airway. The notion that the tracheotomy is a more stable airway than the endotracheal tube (ET) is supported by the decreased risk of accidental extubation in tracheotomy patients. Intubated patients are noted to have an 8 to 21% incidence of accidental extubation, compared with a 1% incidence in patients with a surgical airway.[8] In a patient who is a difficult or impossible intubation and is at risk for accidental extubation, a precautionary tracheotomy can be a lifesaving procedure.

For some patients with excessive brochopulmonary secretions or chronic aspiration, tracheotomy can be considered to assist in pulmonary toilet by providing improved access to tracheal secretions and aspirated fluids.[9] Although tracheotomy has traditionally been used to treat patients with chronic aspiration pneumonia, it should be used with caution, as tracheotomy placement has also been associated with an increased risk of aspiration.[9,10] Between 20 and 80% of patients with a chronic tracheotomy experience at least one episode of aspiration every 48 hours.[10] Inflating the cuff, a maneuver many nonotolaryngologists feel decreases aspiration, may actually increase the risk of aspiration because the inflated cuff can hinder swallowing by compressing the esophagus, thus leading to increased secretions.[10] Related studies have shown that patients with increased secretions in the presence of a tracheotomy tube are at higher risk of aspiration.[15] Furthermore, a deflated cuff allows air to pass around the tube during feeding, which may assist in the clearance of any food that does penetrate the glottis. Previous studies suggested that the tracheotomy tube prevents normal upward movement of the larynx during swallowing and hinders glottis closure[10] (presumably increasing aspiration), but recent studies do not support these findings.[11,12,13,14]

Tracheotomy is also frequently used to facilitate weaning from a ventilator. The inner diameter of the tracheotomy tube commonly varies from 4 to 9 mm and is the essential variant determining airway resistance in tracheotomy patients. At these diameters, a tracheotomy tube does not cause a significant amount of airflow resistance. The work of breathing for patients after extubation is significantly decreased in patients with a tracheotomy compared to patients without a tracheotomy,[4,16] as airflow resistance of the normal upper airway constitutes between 50 and 80% of total airway resistance[4] and a tracheotomy tube bypasses this resistance. Tracheotomy tubes may also reduce dead space up to 100 mL when compared with spontaneous breathing.[4,16]

More importantly, tracheotomy tubes have the potential to decrease the work of breathing compared to endotracheal tubes. Tracheotomy tubes are shorter, more rigid, and easier to keep clean (thus decreasing secretions that cause turbulent airflow and increase resistance). When compared to endotracheal intubation, tracheotomy is associated with a trend toward lower resistive work of breathing, and reductions in elastic work of breathing, intrinsic positive end-expiratory pressure (PEEP), and pressure time product.[4] Although not all studies show physiologic advantage of tracheotomy compared with endotracheal intubations,[4] tracheotomy has been shown to decrease tidal volumes, respiratory rate, and minute ventilation[17] compared to endotracheal intubation,[16,17] ultimately resulting in a decreased mechanical workload in ventilator-dependent patients. Although the clinical significance of this remains controversial, the existing evidence suggests that patients with borderline pulmonary status may benefit from the improvement in airway resistance noted.[8] Finally, patients with tracheotomies can be placed on and off the ventilator without any significant risk to the patient. This may allow earlier extubation in patients with marginal respiratory status because potential future respiratory distress can easily be managed by reattaching the ventilator.

The most common indication for tracheotomy in the patient in the intensive care unit (ICU) is the need for long-term mechanical ventilation. Patients often require ventilatory support secondary to numerous causes, with pulmonary failure, cardiac failure, and neurologic defects being most common. It is generally accepted that tracheotomy improves comfort level when compared with translaryngeal intubation. Supporting this hypothesis, it has been noted that patients with tracheotomies required less intravenous (IV) sedation, spent less time heavily sedated, and achieved self-sufficiency earlier than intubated patients.[18] After a tracheotomy is performed, patients have improved mobility secondary to a more stable airway. Patients also have improved tracheal suctioning, oral care, and improved ability to take oral nutrition and articulate speech[19,20] compared to intubated patients.

Finally, tracheotomy eliminates the oropharyngeal and laryngeal trauma caused by the endotracheal tube. Long-term orotracheal and nasotracheal tubes can produce ulcerative and erosive lesions anywhere along the course of the tube. These lesions can lead to laryngeal web formation, vocal cord paralysis or fixation, posterior glottic stenosis, and granulation tissue formation (which in turn can progress to granuloma formation or interarytenoid adhesions).[10]

20.5 Timing

The optimal timing for a tracheotomy depends on the patient and the situation. For patients requiring an airway secondary to tracheal or laryngeal obstruction, emergency tracheotomy or cricothyroidotomy may be necessary. However, there is significant controversy regarding the timing of surgery for patients undergoing an elective tracheotomy after intubation.

Physicians in the 1960s promoted the placement of early tracheotomy tubes, as high-pressure cuffs and rigid endotracheal tubes led to significant complication rates.[8] With the arrival of the more flexible ETs with low-pressure cuffs in the 1970s, combined with the reported high complication rate of tracheotomy, delayed tracheotomy, 3 to 4 weeks after intubation, became the rule. Since the mid-1980s, with the introduction of percutaneous tracheotomy and the decreased complication rates associated with open tracheotomy, there has been a shift toward earlier tracheotomy placement.

The ideal time for tracheotomy in ventilated patients has not been established, despite the many studies addressing this topic. Translaryngeal intubation is recognized to cause oral and labial damage, laryngeal and tracheal damage, sinusitis and otitis, subglottic stenosis, increased rates of accidental extubation, and possibly increased rates of ventilator-associated pneumonia.[8,21] These risks must be weighed in relation to the risks of the procedure, which are discussed later in this chapter. The timely placement of a tracheotomy tube can minimize ET-related complications.[22]

There are many studies examining the appropriate timing for tracheotomy.[23] Earlier recommendations were that tracheotomy be performed in patients requiring mechanical ventilation for more than 21 days.[20] More recent guidelines advise that translaryngeal intubation be used only for patients requiring less than 10 days of artificial ventilation, and that tracheotomy be performed for those requiring artificial ventilation for greater than 21 days. The decision is left to the physician for those patients falling between 10 and 21 days.[24]

A common method of determining the need for and timing of a tracheotomy is the "anticipatory approach." This involves initially stabilizing the patient and treating the primary disease process. If extubation is felt to be possible in the first several days of mechanical ventilation, then tracheotomy is not considered necessary. If after a week of translaryngeal intubation the patient is felt (1) likely to benefit from a tracheotomy, and (2) likely to require extended intubation (more than an additional 7 days), then a tracheotomy should be performed.[8,25] As the clinician's ability to predict the duration of intubation improves, even earlier tracheotomy can be considered.

Some studies advocate tracheotomy earlier than 7 days in patients who appear certain to require prolonged intubation. A recent study by Tong et al, looking at almost 600 patients, demonstrated decreased days of mechanical ventilation, decreased length of ICU stay, and shorter hospital stays in patients receiving an early tracheotomy 7 days or less from intubation, compared to patients trached after 7 days.[94] Another recent systematic review and meta-analysis of the literature concluded that early tracheotomy in critically ill adult patients who require prolonged mechanical ventilation may shorten the duration of artificial ventilation and decrease the length of stay in the ICU.[21,24,27,28] Other studies demonstrate that early tracheotomy is associated with improved survival and decreased resource utilization.[29,30] Unfortunately, the definition of early tracheotomy varies among studies and can include tracheotomies done anywhere from day 0 to day 7. Current guidelines support an individualized approach to tracheotomy that recognizes the potential benefits of early tracheotomy.[26]

While previous research has been equivocal regarding the benefit of early tracheotomy to decrease ventilator-associated pneumonia (VAP),[10,21] recent studies, although significantly limited by their methodology, support the relationship between lower rates of VAP and decreased mortality in patients undergoing an early procedure.[31,32] Further prospective randomized studies are needed to draw definitive conclusions on the relationship between VAP and early tracheotomy.

20.6 Technique

The technique used to perform a tracheotomy has evolved throughout its history. Initial tracheotomies were placed high in the trachea because of the speed and ease of this approach. In 1921 this practice was altered because of the recognition of the increased rates of subglottic stenosis[1] in patients receiving high tracheotomies. Tracheotomy continues to be performed with many variations in technique. The techniques can be divided into two broad categories: the open surgical approach and percutaneous tracheotomy. Several variations exist within each category.

20.6.1 The Open Surgical Tracheotomy

The open surgical tracheotomy can be performed in the operating room or at the bedside in the ICU. The procedure is most commonly performed under general anesthesia with the patient previously intubated. Occasionally, it is necessary to perform the procedure under local anesthesia and to maintain spontaneous respiration for those patients with a tenuous airway.

The technical aspects of a tracheotomy are relatively simple and straightforward and the procedure itself is usually relatively bloodless and quick. However, despite the relative ease of the procedure, the potential for significant morbidity and mortality is always present, as even relatively short-term loss of the airway can lead to significant morbidity or even death. The key to performing tracheotomy safely and successfully over time is to take the precautions necessary to avoid potential complications. Careful and thoughtful preoperative planning is essential. Because many tracheotomy patients have a multitude of medical problems, a thorough preoperative evaluation is always needed. In addition, a complete physical examination, checking for anatomical abnormalities such as a goiter or a high-riding innominate artery, is also important. Before starting the case, the surgeon must ensure that all necessary instruments and materials (including multiple tracheotomy tubes) are present. Intraoperatively, meticulous hemostasis and dissection along natural tissue planes help the surgeon avoid situations where the airway can become tenuous. Finally, the surgeon must always remember that performing successful tracheotomies is a team effort involving the surgeon, assistant, and other involved medical personnel. Good communication among all team members is a key component of avoiding complications when performing tracheotomies.

The operation begins with the palpation of the landmarks of the neck, including the thyroid cartilage, the cricoid cartilage, and the sternal notch. A marking pen can be used to indicate the position of each. The importance of this step should not be underestimated, as the patient's anatomy can vary greatly, and starting dissection in the proper location is a key element in avoiding complications. Palpation for other anatomical abnormalities, such as an enlarged thyroid or a high-riding innominate artery, should also be performed at this time. A shoulder roll is placed under the patient's shoulder to help elevate the larynx and expose the trachea. The skin is then prepped and the patient draped.

A 2- to 3-cm incision is carried out in a vertical or horizontal fashion, depending on the preference of the surgeon. The horizontal incision theoretically provides a more aesthetically pleasing postoperative scar, as it follows relaxed skin tension lines and can easily be converted to a longer incision if needed. The cosmetic benefits of a horizontal incision, however, decrease significantly the longer a tracheotomy remains in place. Vertical incisions help to avoid damage to the anterior jugular venous system and are the standard of care in emergent tracheotomies, so familiarity with this method during routine tracheotomy may increase one's facility during emergency procedures. For these reasons, the vertical incision is generally my incision of choice. Vertical incisions are typically made with the superior aspect of the incision at or just below the cricoid, whereas horizontal incisions are usually made between the cricoid and the sternal notch, typically over the second or third tracheal rings. The incision site is sometimes injected with lidocaine with epinephrine to promote hemostasis, although I and others prefer making the incision with the Bovie on a setting of cut and blend to prevent bleeding.

A #15 blade or an electrocautery is then used to extend the incision down through the subcutaneous tissues. Upward traction on the subcutaneous tissue with forceps or Aliss clamps facilitates this dissection. The dissection continues until the strap muscles are identified. Care should be taken while dissecting through the subcutaneous tissues due to the proximity of the anterior jugular veins. If encountered, the anterior jugular veins should be lateralized if possible, or cauterized or ligated as needed. Once the level of the strap muscles is identified, the midline raphe between the pairs of sternothyroid and sternohyoid muscles is incised, and the cricoid exposed. I and many others use the cricoid as an important safety landmark. Because it is the hardest of the tracheal rings and easily palpable, dissection onto the cricoid itself directs the surgeon toward a safe plane at the level of the trachea. There are often some blood vessels associated with the thyroid gland at the level of the cricoid and I prefer to coagulate these vessels before dissecting onto the cricoid.

The thyroid gland can be manipulated in a number of ways. Depending on the location of the thyroid isthmus, the isthmus can be either retracted (superiorly or inferiorly) or divided to expose the second and third tracheal rings. Kirchner[33] advocated division and ligation of the isthmus to minimize complication rates. One potential advantage of division of the thyroid gland is that if the thyroid is retracted away from the stoma and the tracheotomy tube falls out, the thyroid could move back to its original location and obstruct the stoma, making replacement of the tracheotomy tube difficult. If the thyroid is divided, many people use suture ligation to achieve hemostasis, but I and others prefer using a Bovie without sutures to divide the thyroid and have not noticed an increase in postoperative or intraoperative bleeding. A clamp can be utilized to develop the plane between the thyroid and the trachea. Care must be taken to perform this dissection in the fascial plane between the trachea and the thyroid, as dissection into the thyroid will lead to bleeding. Once the trachea is adequately exposed, the second and third tracheal rings can be identified. The pretracheal fascia can be removed from the anterior trachea using a peanut; a cricoid hook is often placed beneath the cricoid and retracted superiorly to elevate the trachea and improve exposure.

The tracheal incision is typically located between the second and third tracheal rings for an elective tracheotomy (▶ Fig. 20.2). Higher incisions, which may be appropriate for tracheotomy done prior to a planned total laryngectomy, have an increased incidence of subglottic stenosis; lower incisions place the innominate artery at greater risk.[34]

The type of incision into the trachea can vary significantly. Although some surgeons prefer a single horizontal incision between tracheal rings (usually made with a #11 blade), other surgeons prefer an H-type incision or make a tracheal window by removing a portion of the second or third cartilage. The method of incising the trachea does not appear to have a significant impact on the development of tracheal stenosis in clinical and laboratory studies.[35,36,37] The Bjork flap is another method commonly used when entering the trachea. In this technique, an incision is made between the second and third tracheal rings and the third tracheal ring is divided laterally, on both sides. The flap is then hinged using the connective tissue linking the third and fourth tracheal rings and is sutured to the skin. The suture can be either absorbable or nonabsorbable. If nonabsorbable sutures are used, they are typically removed at the

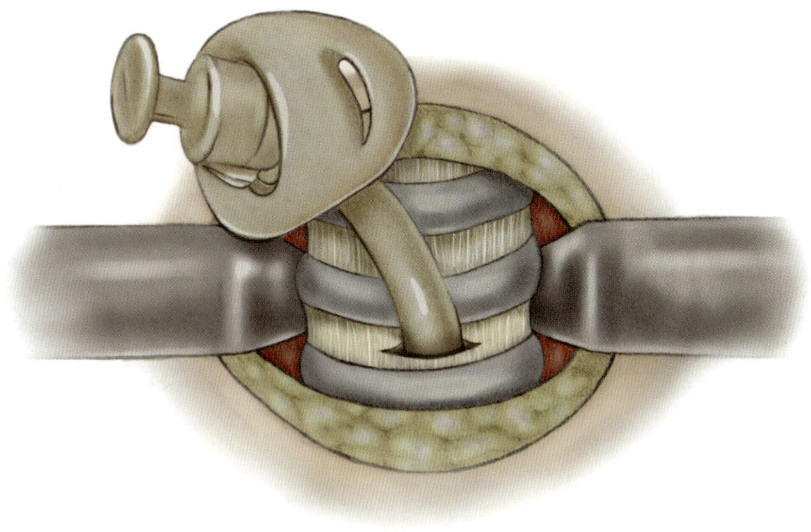

Fig. 20.2 Tracheotomy tube insertion.

time of the first tracheotomy change (most commonly 3–7 days posttracheotomy). Many physicians believe this flap allows improved ability to reinsert the tracheotomy tube if accidental decannulation occurs shortly after the procedure; therefore, it is more commonly utilized in obese patients, in whom reinsertion of the tracheotomy tube after accidental decannulization can be difficult. The concern of increased risk of tracheocutaneous fistula or clinical tracheal stenosis when using the Bjork flap prevents its common use. Although there are few data in the literature supporting the benefits of the Bjork flap, a study by Malata et al[38] suggests that there is no greater risk of tracheal stenosis or tracheocutaneous fistula in patients receiving Bjork flaps.

Once the trachea is entered, a tracheotomy dilator can be used to further expose the tracheal lumen, although this is usually not a necessary step and should be used with caution because excess use of the dilator can cause trauma to the tracheal rings. Once the endotracheal tube is visualized, the anesthesiologist is asked to retract the endotracheal tube superiorly until the posterior tracheal wall is visualized. After the endotracheal tube is retracted superior to the newly created opening in the tracheotomy, the tracheotomy tube can be placed into the tracheal lumen under direct visualization. Finally, the cuff should be inflated and the anesthesia circuit attached and carbon dioxide (CO_2) return noted. The endotracheal tube should be left in the airway until CO_2 return is noted by the anesthesiologist so that if the tracheotomy tube has been placed into a false passage, the ET can be advanced back into place prior to subsequent attempts at tracheotomy placement. In addition, any retractors and cricoid hooks used during placement of the trach should be left in place until CO_2 is confirmed. The tracheotomy tube is then sutured into place with nonabsorbable sutures (preferably monofilament) through the phalanges, and further secured with a tracheotomy tie around the patient's neck.

20.6.2 Percutaneous Dilation Tracheotomy

The percutaneous tracheotomy is a relatively new procedure. It was initially developed by Shelden in 1955 and Toye and Weinstein in 1969[2] and was reintroduced by Ciaglia in 1985.[39] Since its introduction in the mid-1980s, it has continued to gain popularity, largely because it is considered a rapid, easy to learn, cost-effective alternative to the open tracheotomy. Additionally, the ability to perform the procedure in the ICU further adds to its appeal. Initially, there was significant controversy regarding the relative safety of the procedure compared to the open technique, but several meta-analyses have shown it to be a safe and cost-effective alternative to the open tracheotomy in a subset of patients.[40,41,42,43,44,45,46,47,48,49,50,51,52,53,54,55,56,57,58,59]

Traditionally, contraindications to the procedure have included patients with morbid obesity, obscure cervical anatomy, inability to extend the neck, an enlarged thyroid gland or other midline neck mass, short thick neck, uncorrectable coagulopathy, previous tracheotomy or neck surgery, active cervical infection, heavily calcified tracheal rings, and cervical trauma.[2,8,60,61] Percutaneous tracheotomy is also not indicated for emergent tracheotomy or for pediatric patients. Recently, however, several of these contraindications have come under further examination and may soon exist only as relative contraindications. Specifically, the safety of percutaneous dilation tracheotomy (PDT) in patients with varying neck length,[62] obesity,[63,64,65] coagulopathies,[63] and previous tracheotomy[66] has been demonstrated in the literature.

Three commonly practiced techniques exist for the percutaneous placement of a tracheotomy tube: the Griggs procedure, also known as the forceps-dilation technique, the Fanconi translaryngeal technique, and the Ciaglia or modified Ciaglia technique.

The Ciaglia technique is the most commonly performed PDT technique. The technique is a modified Seldenger technique and was created using a percutaneous nephrostomy–Amplatz renal dilator set.[39] After palpation of the thyroid and cricoid cartilages, lidocaine with epinephrine is injected subcutaneously. A 1- to 2-cm transverse or vertical incision is made immediately below the cricoid. A needle is passed into the trachea after the existing tracheal tube has been deflated and withdrawn above the incision site. Air is then aspirated into the syringe, confirming proper position within the trachea. A flexible fiberoptic bronchoscopy is often carried out at this time to visually confirm proper placement of the needle. The initial procedure did not describe simultaneous bronchoscopy, but subsequent studies have shown improved safety with this method.[60,67,68,69] Once the needle is in the appropriate position, xylocaine is instilled into the tracheal lumen. The syringe is then removed and a guidewire is passed through the needle, toward the carina. The needle is then removed and the flexible J-wire guide remains in place. Multiple dilators are then threaded over the guidewire and used to dilate the stoma. Finally, the tracheotomy tube is passed over the guidewire and the tracheotomy is sutured into place.

Since the introduction of this technique in 1986, several modifications to the Ciaglia technique have improved its safety and rapidity. As discussed, the introduction of flexible bronchoscopy allows direct visualization of the inserted needle, guidewire, and subsequent dilators and improves patient safety. Additional modifications employ the use of only a single dilator,[60] decreasing the time of the procedure.

The Griggs forceps-dilation technique is performed in a similar fashion to the Ciaglia technique described above, with the exception of the method of dilation. In this technique, a forceps dilator is used and the tracheal cannula is inserted over the guidewire.[70]

Finally, the Fanconi translaryngeal technique involves insertion of a guidewire through a needle similar to the technique described above. In the Fanconi technique, the guidewire is directed toward the larynx and ultimately through the mouth. The guidewire is then attached to a device made of a flexible plastic cone with a pointed metal tip attached to a tracheal cannula. The device is then retracted through the oral cavity and larynx, until it eventually perforates trachea and anterior neck. Once extruded through the neck, the cannula is separated from the cone and metal tip. The tracheal cannula is initially straightened perpendicular to the skin until the tip remaining in the trachea can be rotated caudally.[71]

20.6.3 Bedside Open-Surgical Tracheotomy

Bedside open surgical tracheotomy is typically performed in a similar manner to a surgical tracheotomy performed in the operating room (OR). Bedside tracheotomy allows for timely scheduling and avoids the risks of transporting the patient to the OR. Bedside tracheotomy requires an intubated patient in a monitored setting and significant preoperative planning and intraoperative communication to ensure patient safety. The team must include the surgeons, respiratory therapists (or anesthesiologist) to manage the airway, and an intensivist or the equivalent to manage sedation and any medical issues that arise, as well as an ICU nurse experienced in tracheotomy. A well-planned and well-stocked tracheotomy cart containing duplicates of all necessary equipment, including trach trays, electric cautery, sutures, multiple tracheotomy tubes, and a headlight, helps ensure all equipment needed is close at hand. Once the setup is complete, the procedure should proceed exactly the same as a tracheotomy done in an OR, including patient identification measures and performing a time out.

Similar to percutaneous tracheotomy, bedside open-surgical tracheotomy has been shown to be safe[72,73,74] when restricted to a subset of patients. Massick[72] utilized three eligibility criteria for bedside tracheotomy, including palpable cricoid at least 3 cm above the sternal notch (with the neck extended), history of uneventful/uncomplicated translaryngeal intubation, and positive end-expiratory pressure requirement of less than 10 cm H_2O. A separate study uses the ability to palpate the cricoid as a sole selection criterion for bedside tracheotomy.[75] Selection criteria vary greatly from surgeon to surgeon depending on the comfort of the surgeon and the experience of the airway team.

A recent study by Yoo et al comparing 150 patients receiving open bedside tracheotomy with 150 patients receiving open tracheotomy in the OR showed that the group receiving bedside tracheotomy had significantly decreased time from consult to tracheotomy (3.24 days vs. 1.48 days) and a cost savings of US $4,575.00 per patient without any increase in complications.[96] One of the most commonly cited benefits of PDT is the decreased costs of the procedure compared to the open-surgical tracheotomy performed in the OR. This cost saving seems to disappear when compared with the bedside open tracheotomy, and in fact several studies have argued that bedside open tracheotomy is more cost effective than PDT.[55,72,74,76,77]

20.6.4 Cricothyroidotomy

Cricothyroidotomy is the preferred technique if minimizing the time to establishing the airway is critical (such as in an emergency airway). It has also been noted to be useful for patients with maxillofacial trauma, altered cervical anatomy, and cervical spine injury.[78] It has been supported for use by health care professionals without surgical training in need of an emergency surgical airway because of the relative ease with which this procedure can be performed.[79] In a cricothyroidotomy, the landmarks (tracheal and cricoid cartilage) are rigid, easily palpable, and relatively superficial, making the approach to the airway faster and more straightforward than conventional approaches.

Cricothyriodotomy, however, has a significantly higher long-term complication rate than tracheotomy, and therefore should only be used in emergency situations. Studies demonstrate a 0 to 52% complication rate, with 0 to 32% incidence of voice dysfunction and an increased incidence of subglottic stenosis with cricothyroidotomy compared to tracheotomy.[78,80,81] It is generally believed that patients receiving an emergency crycothyroidotomy should be stabilized and converted to a standard tracheotomy within 48 to 72 hours,[8] although it has been argued that in selected patient populations crycothyroidotomy may not require conversion to a tracheotomy and may be considered an alternative to tracheotomy. However, sufficient data to fully support this concept are still lacking.[78,82]

20.7 Types of Tracheotomy Tubes

Many different types and makes of tracheotomy tubes exist, and the choice of tube depends partially on the comfort and familiarity of the surgeon. Tracheotomy tubes can be characterized by the combination of four main categories: cuffed versus uncuffed, single lumen versus double lumen, metal versus plastic, and fenestrated versus unfenestrated.

Cuffed tubes are mostly used in a patient who is on, or may soon be on, a ventilator. The cuff provides a seal in the trachea allowing the delivery of a constant amount of pressurized air. All fresh tracheotomy tubes should be cuffed, even in patients not anticipated to need ventilation. Changing a tracheotomy tube before the stoma is well formed can be difficult, and if a patient requires ventilatory support in the immediate postoperative period, and does not have a cuffed tracheotomy tube in place, the airway can become tenuous.

Double-lumen tubes have an inner cannula and an outer cannula. The dual lumen provides the ability to remove the inner cannula for cleaning or replacement if a patient obstructs the tube with mucus or blood, making ventilation difficult. Single lumen tracheotomy tubes, in contrast to double-lumen tubes, provide the benefit of an increased inner diameter compared to outer diameter. Thus, with a single-lumen tracheotomy tube, a smaller tube can be placed while still providing an equivalent inner diameter. However, single-lumen tubes should be used with caution, as complete removal of the tube may be required if a single-lumen tube becomes obstructed with blood or mucous.

Fenestrated tracheotomy tubes are used to allow egress of air from the distal airway below the tube to the proximal airway above the tube, improving phonation. In patients with a small tracheotomy tube and a large trachea, fenestrated tubes may not be needed for phonation, but in a patient with a smaller trachea, either due to anatomy, edema, or stenosis, a fenestrated tube may be the only way for a patient to phonate. Fenestrated tubes should be used with care as the fenestrated portion of the tube can promote suprastomal granulation tissue.

Metal tracheotomy tubes have become less common. Historically, metal tracheotomy tubes were commonly used for long-term tracheotomy patients. The advantages of metal tubes were increased durability, the ability to be sterilized and reused, and increased inner diameter compared to outer diameter when compared to plastic tubes.

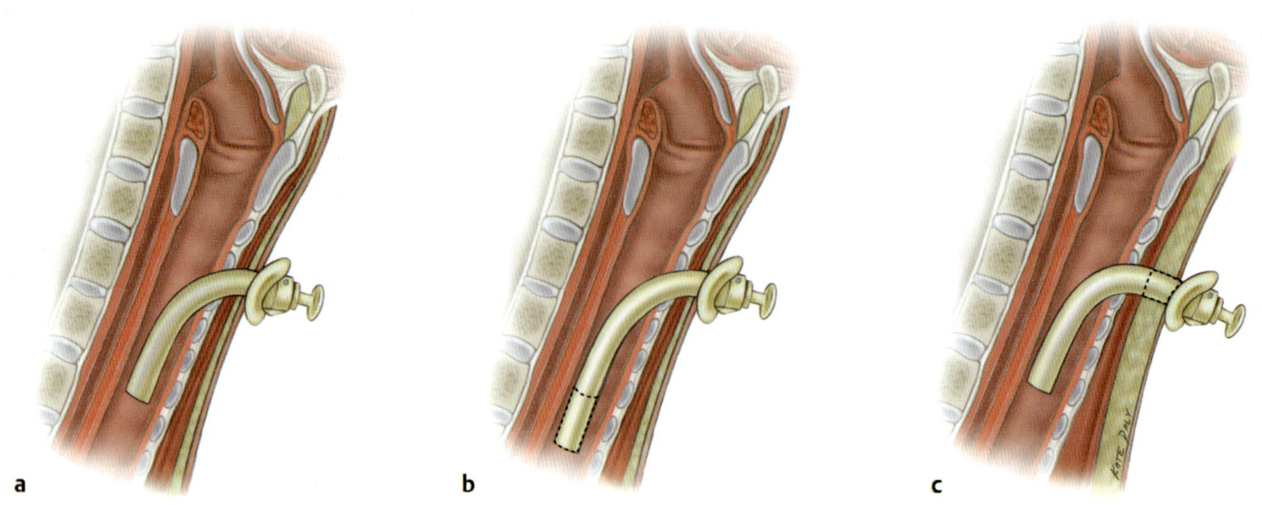

Fig. 20.3 (a) Standard, (b) distal, and (c) proximal extended-length tracheotomy tubes. The distal extended-length tube has a longer vertical length within the trachea when compared to the standard tube, and the proximal extended-length tube has a longer horizontal length between neck skin and tracheal lumen when compared to the standard tube.

Finally, many different sizes and makes of tracheotomy tubes exist, including custom-made tubes. One common specialty tube that all otolaryngologists should be familiar with is the extended-length tracheotomy tube, commonly either a proximal or distal extended-length tube (▶ Fig. 20.3). The proximal extended-length tubes have an elongated portion in the area of the tracheotomy tube going from the stoma, through the tissues of the neck, into the trachea. This is most commonly used in obese patients. Distal extended-length tubes are used when tracheal stenosis or obstruction in the distal aspect of the trachea would not be bypassed with a normal tube. Having immediate access to a variety of sizes and types of extended-length tubes is essential to providing comprehensive tracheotomy care.

20.8 Management Practices

There is little consensus among otolaryngologists regarding posttracheotomy management. A recent survey answered by 478 members of the American Academy of Otolaryngology-Head and Neck Surgery highlighted the significant variability in posttracheotomy management.[97] On average, responding otolaryngologists follow a fresh tracheotomy daily for 6 days, then monthly for 3 months, then every 4 months indefinitely. However, there was considerable variability in follow-up between otolaryngologists. Many practitioners change the tracheotomy tube at the end of their initial surveillance period. The duration of time to tracheotomy change varies greatly between otolaryngologists and upon the ventilator status of the patient. The time to initial tracheotomy tube change after tracheotomy averaged 3.8 days in patients who did not require a ventilator after tracheotomy, 6.2 days in those patients weaned from the ventilator postoperatively, and 8.3 days in patients who remained ventilator dependent.[98] The benefits of changing the tracheotomy before signing off on the patient are that it ensures a formal examination of the tracheotomy site, ensures removal of tracheotomy sutures, and establishes whether the stoma is sufficiently formed to constitute a stable airway, giving the surgeon appropriate information to decide whether the patient is stable enough to hand over the care to the primary team. For a patient under long-term surveillance, tracheotomy tubes were changed on an average of every 2 months.

Although no formal decannulation algorithm exists in the literature, approximately 70% of otolaryngologists utilize a decannulation algorithm. A recent survey was unable to quantify standard practices and again highlighted the disparity in management between different otolaryngologists. The decannulation algorithms ranged from 2 weeks of tracheotomy capping followed by endoscopic examination in the OR, followed by overnight admission to the hospital to capping the tracheotomy during the day for 3 days and then overnight prior to extubation. The key in all algorithms is to balance the risk of decannulation with the benefit of removing the tracheotomy tube. A patient's ability to manage the capping and uncapping of a tracheotomy tube varies greatly depending on the physical and mental abilities of the patient; therefore, an algorithm that may be safe for one patient may be extremely risky in another. If decannulation is to be done on an outpatient, it is paramount that the patient understands the mechanism of uncapping and capping the tracheotomy and demonstrates the ability to do so with comfort and ease.

20.9 Complications

Many of the changes in the techniques and indications for tracheotomy are derived from the impetus to lower the high morbidity and mortality initially associated with the procedure. In 1833, Trousseau reported a 75% mortality rate for tracheotomy patients, compared with current mortality rates of approximately 1%.[1,34,83] Today, although tracheotomy is a relatively safe procedure, complications still occur. A recent study looking at 113,653 tracheotomies performed in the United States in 2006 showed a 3.2% complication rate and 0.6% mortality rate.[95] Another recent study showed that the intraoperative complication rate is 0.39% when the tracheotomy is performed by otolaryngologists and 3.5% when performed by nonotolaryngologists.[98] In the same study, the surgeons performing the fewest tracheotomies demonstrated the highest complication rates. Tracheotomy-related complications can be divided into three categories, intraoperative, early postoperative, and late postoperative (see the box Tracheotomy complications). Several studies exist that attempt to quantify the incidence of complications, including multiple meta-analyses comparing the complication rates of open and percutaneous tracheotomies.[46,47,48,54,84]

Tracheotomy complications

- Intraoperative
  - Hemorrhage
  - Damage to adjacent structures
  - Creation of a false passage
  - Airway fire
  - Premature airway obstruction
  - Anesthesia related
- Early postoperative
  - Hemorrhage
  - Infection
  - Subcutaneous emphysema
  - Pneumothorax
  - Pneumomediastinum
  - Tube displacement
  - Obstruction
- Late postoperative
  - Hemorrhage
  - Tracheal stenosis
  - Tracheoesophageal fistula
  - Tracheocutaneous fistula
  - Tracheomalacia
  - Dysphagia

20.9.1 Intraoperative Complications

Intraoperative complications include hemorrhage, damage to adjacent structures, creation of a false passage, airway fire, premature airway obstruction, and anesthesia-related complications. Such complications are rare and are often well controlled in the operative setting.

Inability to ventilate immediately after placement of a tracheotomy tube is a common occurrence and suggests that the tube may be in a false passage. False passages most commonly occur anterior to the trachea because the fascial plane anterior to the trachea can be easily dissected with pressure. If incorrect placement of the tracheotomy tube is not recognized, and ventilation begins, the patient can develop subcutaneous emphysema and possibly pneumomediastinum or a pneumothorax. Passing a soft suction catheter through the trach tube immediately after tracheotomy tube placement can help confirm the proper placement of the tube and help prevent the complications that might occur if incorrect trach placement is not recognized. Keeping all retractors and the cricoid hook in place until the anesthesiologist notes CO_2 return can help minimize the time required to properly place a misplaced tube.

Intraoperative hemorrhage is most commonly the result of injury to the anterior jugular veins. Massive bleeding is usually rare but can occur from a high-riding innominate artery if the dissection is carried inferiorly. Damage to the recurrent laryngeal nerve is also very rare and is more common in emergent cricothyroidotomies or tracheotomies. Superior laryngeal nerve injury is also more commonly associated with cricothyroidotomy than tracheotomy.[85] Airway fires are fortunately both rare and preventable. Airway fires during tracheotomies are usually the result of use of electric cautery near high concentrations of oxygen. Care should be taken after entering the airway not to use the electric cautery if concentrated oxygen is being used for ventilation. Evidence supports that a concentration of greater than 50% FIO_2 is necessary to support combustion in the OR.[86]

Premature airway obstruction is a potential complication for patients undergoing tracheotomy for upper airway obstruction and may occur prior to intubation or during an awake tracheotomy. The best means of preventing complications from premature airway obstruction is proper planning and coordination of operating room personal and equipment. Flexible and rigid laryngoscopy and bronchoscopy equipment must be readily available, and transtracheal jet ventilation equipment should be accessible as well. Cooperation between the surgeon and anesthesiologist is essential for managing difficult airways safely.

20.9.2 Early Postoperative Complications

Early postoperative complications occur hours to days after the procedure. They include hemorrhage, infection, subcutaneous emphysema, pneumothorax, pneumomediastinum, tube displacement, and obstruction of the tracheotomy tube. Postoperative hemorrhage can occur early or late and can be the result of erosion of nearby vessels, bleeding from granulation tissue, or simply elevation of blood pressure in the previously hypotensive patient.[83] One meta-analysis reports the incidence of clinically relevant bleeding at 5.7%.[84] A more recent study showed bleeding to be the most common early postoperative complication occurring in 2.6% of cases.[95] Wound infection was noted to occur at a rate of 6.6% by Delaney, but it can be difficult to define.[47,48]

Subcutaneous emphysema, pneumothorax, and pneumomediastinum may all result from excessive surgical cervical dissection. Dissection of air along the pretracheal fascia can occur with tube dislodgement, tube obstruction in association with positive-pressure ventilation, and/or tight wound closure.[87] The incidence of subcutaneous emphysema and pneumothorax ranges from 0 to 9% and 0 to 4%, respectively.[83] A recent large series looking at 1,130 tracheotomy patients found the incidence of subcutaneous emphysema and pneumothorax to be less than 1% each.[83] The complications of subcutaneous emphysema are usually self-limited and resolve with recognition and correction of the cause, but if untreated and unrecognized can cause significant morbidity or even mortality.

The tracheotomy tube may become obstructed secondary to mucous plugging, blood clots, or tube displacement in the postoperative period. Rigorous tracheostomy care is essential in the postoperative period and includes frequent suctioning and irrigation of the tracheotomy tube as well as the use of humidified oxygen. The use of a tracheotomy tube with an inner cannula facilitates care of the tube in the postoperative period when secretions and bleeding are increased. If a tube with an inner cannula does plug in the immediate postoperative period, simply removing the inner cannula removes the plug. If a patient with a single-lumen tracheotomy tube has a plug in the postoperative period, the entire trach may need to be changed—a potentially dangerous situation if the tracheotomy tract is not yet well formed. In this situation, it may be necessary to temporarily place an endotracheal tube through the stoma or translaryngeally until the patient can be stabilized and the tracheotomy tube can be replaced under controlled conditions.

20.9.3 Late Postoperative Complications

Late postoperative complications include hemorrhage, tracheal stenosis, tracheoesophageal fistula, tracheocutaneous fistula, tracheomalacia, and dysphagia. A tracheoinnominate fistula is the most feared tracheotomy complication. The two main etiologies of a tracheoinnominate fistula are either tracheal necrosis caused by the cuff of a trach tube, allowing direct contact of the cuff with the artery, or direct pressure of the tracheostomy tube itself on the innominate artery (usually secondary to a high innominate artery or a low tracheotomy). Tracheoinnominate fistula often presents as a sentinel bleed, but it can present as massive life-threatening hemoptysis. The reported incidence of tracheoinnominate fistula is approximately 0.7%,[88] and the mortality ranges from 80 to 100%.[83] All brisk, bright red, tracheal bleeding should be evaluated thoroughly to make sure a tracheoinnominate fistula is not present.

Tracheal and subglottic stenosis are also well recognized complications of tracheotomy and have been reported in some studies to be the most common late complication, occurring in 1.7% of cases,[95] although other studies report a range of anywhere from 0.6 to 21%.[83] Tracheal stenosis is categorized as suprastomal, stomal, or infrastomal. Suprastomal or subglottic stenosis is usually secondary to damage to the cricoid. Stomal stenosis is secondary to cartilage damage and occurs at an increased rate in patients with postoperative tracheal wound infections.[89,90] Infrastomal stenosis results from tracheal damage secondary to direct pressure from the cuff or tracheotomy tube. Tracheal stenosis is considered clinically relevant when the tracheal diameter is reduced by greater than 50% of its original diameter.[89,91] Ragjuaman suggests that stenosis secondary to PDT occurs earlier and is more commonly subglottic in nature (and therefore may be more difficult to treat a stenosis caused by surgical tracheotomy).[91] He attributed this finding to the tracheal puncture site occurring more superiorly in patients with PDT than open tracheotomies.

Tracheoesophageal fistula also occurs secondary to pressure necrosis of the posterior tracheal wall, either by pressure from an overinflated cuff or direct pressure from the tracheotomy tube. The presence of a nasogastric or orogastric tube in the esophagus can increase the risk of tracheoesophageal fistula formation. Tracheoesophageal fistula can also occur secondary to surgical laceration of the posterior tracheal wall. These fistulas can present with copious secretions, dyspnea, or aspiration of food contents. Furthermore, chest radiographs with evidence of an air-filled esophagus or gastric distention may suggest a tracheoesophageal fistula. Tracheoseophageal fistulas are associated with high mortality.

Tracheocutaneous fistulas occur with the overgrowth of the skin epithelial layer up to the mucosa of the tracheal wall and occur in 3.3 to 29% of patients.[92,93] Tracheocutaneous fistula can lead to increased respiratory infections, poor aesthetic appearance, decreased voice quality, and limitations of daily activities (bathing and swimming). The incidence of tracheocutaneous fistula is directly related to the duration of cannulation, but it can be influenced by other factors, such as the patient's nutritional status, history of radiation exposure, and level of stomal care.[92,93]

20.10 Conclusion

Although a tracheotomy is a simple procedure, the management of a patient requiring tracheotomy can be challenging. The medical complexities of these patients, and the occasional urgency of the procedure, make understanding the nuances of tracheotomy essential to the otolaryngologist–head and neck surgeon.

References

[1] Borman J, Davidson JT. A history of tracheostomy: si spiritum ducit vivit (Cicero). Br J Anaesth 1963; 35: 388–390

[2] Ferlito A, Rinaldo A, Shaha AR, Bradley PJ. Percutaneous tracheotomy. Acta Otolaryngol 2003; 123: 1008–1012

[3] Grillo HC. Development of tracheal surgery: a historical review. Part 1: Techniques of tracheal surgery. Ann Thorac Surg 2003; 75: 610–619

[4] Epstein SK. Anatomy and physiology of tracheostomy. Respir Care 2005; 50: 476–482

[5] Salassa JR, Pearson BW, Payne WS. Gross and microscopical blood supply of the trachea. Ann Thorac Surg 1977; 24: 100–107

[6] Cawthorne T. Two historical tracheostomies. Proc R Soc Med 1968; 61: 1169–1176

[7] Archer SM, Baugh RF, Nelms CR, et al. Tracheostomy: Clinical indicators compendium. Am Aca Otolaryngol Head Neck Surg; 2000: 45

[8] Heffner JE. Tracheotomy application and timing. Clin Chest Med 2003; 24: 389–398

[9] Hafidh MA, Young O, Russell JD. Intractable pulmonary aspiration in children: which operation? Int J Pediatr Otorhinolaryngol 2006; 70: 19–25

[10] Heffner JE, Hess D. Tracheostomy management in the chronically ventilated patient. Clin Chest Med 2001; 22: 55–69

[11] Goldsmith T. Evaluation and treatment of swallowing disorders following endotracheal intubation and tracheostomy. Int Anesthesiol Clin 2000; 38: 219–242

[12] Leder SB, Joe JK, Ross DA, Coelho DH, Mendes J. Presence of a tracheotomy tube and aspiration status in early, postsurgical head and neck cancer patients. Head Neck 2005; 27: 757–761

[13] Leder SB. Incidence and type of aspiration in acute care patients requiring mechanical ventilation via a new tracheotomy. Chest 2002; 122: 1721–1726

[14] Terk AR, Leder SB, Burrell MI. Hyoid bone and laryngeal movement dependent upon presence of a tracheotomy tube. Dysphagia 2007; 22: 89–93

[15] Donzelli J, Brady S, Wesling M, Theisen M. Secretions, occlusion status, and swallowing in patients with a tracheotomy tube: a descriptive study. Ear Nose Throat J 2006; 85: 831–834

[16] Davis K, Campbell RS, Johannigman JA, Valente JF, Branson RD. Changes in respiratory mechanics after tracheostomy. Arch Surg 1999; 134: 59–62

[17] Diehl JL, El Atrous S, Touchard D, Lemaire F, Brochard L. Changes in the work of breathing induced by tracheotomy in ventilator-dependent patients. Am J Respir Crit Care Med 1999; 159: 383–388

[18] Nieszkowska A, Combes A, Luyt CE et al. Impact of tracheotomy on sedative administration, sedation level, and comfort of mechanically ventilated intensive care unit patients. Crit Care Med 2005; 33: 2527–2533

[19] Heffner JE. The role of tracheotomy in weaning. Chest 2001; 120 Suppl: 477S–481S
[20] Plummer AL, Gracey DR. Consensus conference on artificial airways in patients receiving mechanical ventilation. Chest 1989; 96: 178–180
[21] Clum SR, Rumbak MJ. Mobilizing the patient in the intensive care unit: the role of early tracheotomy. Crit Care Clin 2007; 23: 71–79
[22] Esteller-Moré E, Ibañez J, Matiñó E, Ademà JM, Nolla M, Quer IM. Prognostic factors in laryngotracheal injury following intubation and/or tracheotomy in ICU patients. Eur Arch Otorhinolaryngol 2005; 262: 880–883
[23] Groves DS, Durbin CG. Tracheostomy in the critically ill: indications, timing and techniques. Curr Opin Crit Care 2007; 13: 90–97
[24] Griffiths J, Barber VS, Morgan L, Young JD. Systematic review and meta-analysis of studies of the timing of tracheostomy in adult patients undergoing artificial ventilation. BMJ 2005; 330: 1243
[25] Heffner JE. Timing tracheotomy: calendar watching or individualization of care? Chest 1998; 114: 361–363
[26] De Leyn P, Bedert L, Delcroix M et al. Belgian Association of Pneumology and Belgian Association of Cardiothoracic Surgery. Tracheotomy: clinical review and guidelines. Eur J Cardiothorac Surg 2007; 32: 412–421
[27] Arabi Y, Haddad S, Shirawi N, Al Shimemeri A. Early tracheostomy in intensive care trauma patients improves resource utilization: a cohort study and literature review. Crit Care 2004; 8: R347–R352
[28] Freeman BD, Borecki IB, Coopersmith CM, Buchman TG. Relationship between tracheostomy timing and duration of mechanical ventilation in critically ill patients. Crit Care Med 2005; 33: 2513–2520
[29] Armstrong PA, McCarthy MC, Peoples JB. Reduced use of resources by early tracheostomy in ventilator-dependent patients with blunt trauma. Surgery 1998; 124: 763–766, discussion 766–767
[30] Flaatten H, Gjerde S, Heimdal JH, Aardal S. The effect of tracheostomy on outcome in intensive care unit patients. Acta Anaesthesiol Scand 2006; 50: 92–98
[31] Möller MG, Slaikeu JD, Bonelli P, Davis AT, Hoogeboom JE, Bonnell BW. Early tracheostomy versus late tracheostomy in the surgical intensive care unit. Am J Surg 2005; 189: 293–296
[32] Nseir S, Di Pompeo C, Jozefowicz E et al. Relationship between tracheotomy and ventilator-associated pneumonia: a case control study. Eur Respir J 2007; 30: 314–320
[33] Kirchner JA. Avoiding problems in tracheotomy. Laryngoscope 1986; 96: 55–57
[34] Heffner JE, Miller KS, Sahn SA. Tracheostomy in the intensive care unit. Part 2: Complications. Chest 1986; 90: 430–436
[35] Whitley R, Castillo N, Hassett JM, Banyas J, Luchette FA. Early tracheostomal healing in rabbits with use of various tracheal incisions. Wound Repair Regen 1997; 5: 323–328
[36] Natvig K, Olving JH. Tracheal changes in relation to different tracheostomy techniques. (An experimental study on rabbits.) J Laryngol Otol 1981; 95: 61–68
[37] Lin ZM, Chen PR, Chou AS, Hsu LP. Tracheal incision for elective tracheotomy in oral cavity cancer. Oral Oncol 2007; 43: 15–19
[38] Malata CM, Foo IT, Simpson KH, Batchelor AG. An audit of Björk flap tracheostomies in head and neck plastic surgery. Br J Oral Maxillofac Surg 1996; 34: 42–46
[39] Ciaglia P, Firsching R, Syniec C. Elective percutaneous dilatational tracheostomy. A new simple bedside procedure; preliminary report. Chest 1985; 87: 715–719
[40] Gysin C, Dulguerov P, Guyot JP, Perneger TV, Abajo B, Chevrolet JC. Percutaneous versus surgical tracheostomy: a double-blind randomized trial. Ann Surg 1999; 230: 708–714
[41] Kaylie DM, Andersen PE, Wax MK. An analysis of time and staff utilization for open versus percutaneous tracheostomies. Otolaryngol Head Neck Surg 2003; 128: 109–114
[42] Heikkinen M, Aarnio P, Hannukainen J. Percutaneous dilational tracheostomy or conventional surgical tracheostomy? Crit Care Med 2000; 28: 1399–1402
[43] MacCallum PL, Parnes LS, Sharpe MD, Harris C. Comparison of open, percutaneous, and translaryngeal tracheostomies. Otolaryngol Head Neck Surg 2000; 122: 686–690
[44] Silvester W, Goldsmith D, Uchino S et al. Percutaneous versus surgical tracheostomy: a randomized controlled study with long-term follow-up. Crit Care Med 2006; 34: 2145–2152
[45] Porter JM, Ivatury RR. Preferred route of tracheostomy—percutaneous versus open at the bedside: a randomized, prospective study in the surgical intensive care unit. Am Surg 1999; 65: 142–146
[46] Dulguerov P, Gysin C, Perneger TV, Chevrolet JC. Percutaneous or surgical tracheostomy: a meta-analysis. Crit Care Med 1999; 27: 1617–1625
[47] Oliver ER, Gist A, Gillespie MB. Percutaneous versus surgical tracheotomy: an updated meta-analysis. Laryngoscope 2007; 117: 1570–1575
[48] Higgins KM, Punthakee X. Meta-analysis comparison of open versus percutaneous tracheostomy. Laryngoscope 2007; 117: 447–454
[49] Freeman BD, Isabella K, Cobb JP et al. A prospective, randomized study comparing percutaneous with surgical tracheostomy in critically ill patients. Crit Care Med 2001; 29: 926–930
[50] Bowen CP, Whitney LR, Truwit JD, Durbin CG, Moore MM. Comparison of safety and cost of percutaneous versus surgical tracheostomy. Am Surg 2001; 67: 54–60
[51] Angel LF, Simpson CB. Comparison of surgical and percutaneous dilational tracheostomy. Clin Chest Med 2003; 24: 423–429
[52] Anderson JD, Rabinovici R, Frankel HL. Percutaneous dilational tracheostomy vs. open tracheostomy. Chest 2001; 120: 1423–1424
[53] Koitschev A, Simon C, Blumenstock G, Mach H, Graumueller S. Surgical technique affects the risk for tracheostoma-related complications in post-ICU patients. Acta Otolaryngol 2006; 126: 1303–1308
[54] Freeman BD, Isabella K, Lin N, Buchman TG. A meta-analysis of prospective trials comparing percutaneous and surgical tracheostomy in critically ill patients. Chest 2000; 118: 1412–1418
[55] Levin R, Trivikram L. Cost/benefit analysis of open tracheotomy, in the OR and at the bedside, with percutaneous tracheotomy. Laryngoscope 2001; 111: 1169–1173
[56] Grover A, Robbins J, Bendick P, Gibson M, Villalba M. Open versus percutaneous dilatational tracheostomy: efficacy and cost analysis. Am Surg 2001; 67: 297–301, discussion 301–302
[57] Goldenberg D, Golz A, Huri A, Netzer A, Joachims HZ, Bar-Lavie Y. Percutaneous dilation tracheotomy versus surgical tracheotomy: our experience. Otolaryngol Head Neck Surg 2003; 128: 358–363
[58] Bacchetta MD, Girardi LN, Southard EJ et al. Comparison of open versus bedside percutaneous dilatational tracheostomy in the cardiothoracic surgical patient: outcomes and financial analysis. Ann Thorac Surg 2005; 79: 1879–1885
[59] Crofts SL, Alzeer A, McGuire GP, Wong DT, Charles D. A comparison of percutaneous and operative tracheostomies in intensive care patients. Can J Anaesth 1995; 42: 775–779
[60] Kost KM. Endoscopic percutaneous dilatational tracheotomy: a prospective evaluation of 500 consecutive cases. Laryngoscope 2005; 115: 1–30
[61] Bhatti N, Tatlipinar A, Mirski M, Koch WM, Goldenberg D. Percutaneous dilation tracheotomy in intensive care unit patients. Otolaryngol Head Neck Surg 2007; 136: 938–941
[62] Tabaee A, Geng E, Lin J et al. Impact of neck length on the safety of percutaneous and surgical tracheotomy: a prospective, randomized study. Laryngoscope 2005; 115: 1685–1690
[63] Blankenship DR, Kulbersh BD, Gourin CG, Blanchard AR, Terris DJ. High-risk tracheostomy: exploring the limits of the percutaneous tracheostomy. Laryngoscope 2005; 115: 987–989
[64] Heyrosa MG, Melniczek DM, Rovito P, Nicholas GG. Percutaneous tracheostomy: a safe procedure in the morbidly obese. J Am Coll Surg 2006; 202: 618–622
[65] Mansharamani NG, Koziel H, Garland R, LoCicero J, Critchlow J, Ernst A. Safety of bedside percutaneous dilatational tracheostomy in obese patients in the ICU. Chest 2000; 117: 1426–1429
[66] Meyer M, Critchlow J, Mansharamani N, Angel LF, Garland R, Ernst A. Repeat bedside percutaneous dilational tracheostomy is a safe procedure. Crit Care Med 2002; 30: 986–988
[67] Jefferson P, Ball DR. Endoscopy is useful during percutaneous tracheostomy. BMJ 2002; 324: 977–978
[68] Oberwalder M, Weis H, Nehoda H et al. Videobronchoscopic guidance makes percutaneous dilational tracheostomy safer. Surg Endosc 2004; 18: 839–842
[69] Berrouschot J, Oeken J, Steiniger L, Schneider D. Perioperative complications of percutaneous dilational tracheostomy. Laryngoscope 1997; 107: 1538–1544
[70] Griggs WM, Worthley LI, Gilligan JE, Thomas PD, Myburg JA. A simple percutaneous tracheostomy technique. Surg Gynecol Obstet 1990; 170: 543–545
[71] Fantoni A, Ripamonti D. A non-derivative, non-surgical tracheostomy: the translaryngeal method. Intensive Care Med 1997; 23: 386–392
[72] Massick DD, Yao S, Powell DM et al. Bedside tracheostomy in the intensive care unit: a prospective randomized trial comparing open surgical tracheostomy with endoscopically guided percutaneous dilational tracheotomy. Laryngoscope 2001; 111: 494–500

[73] Van Natta TL, Morris JA, Eddy VA et al. Elective bedside surgery in critically injured patients is safe and cost-effective. Ann Surg 1998; 227: 618–624, discussion 624–626

[74] Wease GL, Frikker M, Villalba M, Glover J. Bedside tracheostomy in the intensive care unit. Arch Surg 1996; 131: 552–554, discussion 554–555

[75] Husein OF, Massick DD. Cricoid palpability as a selection criterion for bedside tracheostomy. Otolaryngol Head Neck Surg 2005; 133: 839–844

[76] Van Natta TL, Morris JA, Eddy VA et al. Elective bedside surgery in critically injured patients is safe and cost-effective. Ann Surg 1998; 227: 618–624, discussion 624–626

[77] Wang SJ, Sercarz JA, Blackwell KE, Aghamohammadi M, Wang MB. Open bedside tracheotomy in the intensive care unit. Laryngoscope 1999; 109: 891–893

[78] Schroeder AA. Cricothyroidotomy: when, why, and why not? Am J Otolaryngol 2000; 21: 195–201

[79] Boyle MF, Hatton D, Sheets C. Surgical cricothyrotomy performed by air ambulance flight nurses: a 5-year experience. J Emerg Med 1993; 11: 41–45

[80] Bennett JD. High tracheostomy and other errors—revisited. J Laryngol Otol 1996; 110: 1003–1007

[81] Heffner JE. Percutaneous dilatational vs standard tracheotomy: a meta-analysis but not the final analysis. Chest 2000; 118: 1236–1238

[82] François B, Clavel M, Desachy A, Puyraud S, Roustan J, Vignon P. Complications of tracheostomy performed in the ICU: subthyroid tracheostomy vs surgical cricothyroidotomy. Chest 2003; 123: 151–158

[83] Goldenberg D, Ari EG, Golz A, Danino J, Netzer A, Joachims HZ. Tracheotomy complications: a retrospective study of 1130 cases. Otolaryngol Head Neck Surg 2000; 123: 495–500

[84] Delaney A, Bagshaw SM, Nalos M. Percutaneous dilatational tracheostomy versus surgical tracheostomy in critically ill patients: a systematic review and meta-analysis. Crit Care 2006; 10: R55

[85] Gleeson MJ. Cricothyroidotomy: a satisfactory alternative to tracheostomy? Clin Otolaryngol Allied Sci 1984; 9: 1–2

[86] Thompson JW, Colin W, Snowden T, Hengesteg A, Stocks RM, Watson SP. Fire in the operating room during tracheostomy. South Med J 1998; 91: 243–247

[87] Heffner JE, Miller KS, Sahn SA. Tracheostomy in the intensive care unit. Part 2: Complications. Chest 1986; 90: 430–436

[88] Scalise P, Prunk SR, Healy D, Votto J. The incidence of tracheoarterial fistula in patients with chronic tracheostomy tubes: a retrospective study of 544 patients in a long-term care facility. Chest 2005; 128: 3906–3909

[89] Sue RD, Susanto I. Long-term complications of artificial airways. Clin Chest Med 2003; 24: 457–471

[90] Sarper A, Ayten A, Eser I, Ozbudak O, Demircan A. Tracheal stenosis after tracheostomy or intubation: review with special regard to cause and management. Tex Heart Inst J 2005; 32: 154–158

[91] Raghuraman G, Rajan S, Marzouk JK, Mullhi D, Smith FG. Is tracheal stenosis caused by percutaneous tracheostomy different from that by surgical tracheostomy? Chest 2005; 127: 879–885

[92] Stanton DC, Kademani D, Patel C, Foote JW. Management of post-tracheotomy scars and persistent tracheocutaneous fistulas with dermal interpositional fat graft. J Oral Maxillofac Surg 2004; 62: 514–517

[93] Lee UJ, Goh EK, Wang SG, Hwang SM. Closure of large tracheocutaneous fistula using turn-over hinge flap and V-Y advancement flap. J Laryngol Otol 2002; 116: 627–629

[94] Tong CCL, Kleinberger AJ, Paolino J, Altman KW. Tracheotomy timing and outcomes in the critically ill. Otolaryngol Head Neck Surg 2012; 147: 44–51

[95] Shah RK, Lander L, Berry JG, Nussenbaum B, Merati A, Roberson DW. Tracheotomy outcomes and complications: a national perspective. Laryngoscope 2012; 122: 25–29

[96] Yoo DB, Schiff BA, Martz S et al. Open bedside tracheotomy: impact on patient care and patient safety. Laryngoscope 2011; 121: 515–520

[97] Zhu H, Das P, Brereton J, Roberson D, Shah RK. Surveillance and management practices in tracheotomy patients. Laryngoscope 2012; 122: 46–50

[98] Halum SL, Ting JY, Plowman EK et al. A multi-institutional analysis of tracheotomy complications. Laryngoscope 2012; 122: 38–45

21 Pediatric Laryngology

Christopher Hartnick and Jennifer Setlur

Pediatric laryngology is a less-developed discipline than adult laryngology. One reason is that a young child is often more difficult to examine than an adult, which can impede our ability to make an accurate diagnosis. Another is the lack of knowledge about the fine structure and development of the vocal fold as a child grows. Furthermore, outcome-based results have not previously existed for treatments of common pediatric vocal fold pathologies. As the field of pediatric laryngology moves forward, there is a need to understand the particular issue of anatomical and structural development as it relates to evaluating a child. Clinicians also have to keep in mind that children are not "small adults." One should consider the child's current developmental and emotional conditions, as well as his or her desires and motivations, along with those of the parents. These may well change as they mature and develop.

It is the authors' goal in this chapter to shed some light on these issues. Common pediatric laryngeal pathologies are discussed.

21.1 Patient Evaluation

Examination of the child with a primary laryngeal symptom or complaint begins with obtaining a thorough history from the child's caregiver. Particularly important are questions about airway complaints (noisy breathing, retractions, cyanotic episodes, apneas), voice quality (breathiness, hoarseness, pitch breaks, for example) and any related problems with swallowing (gastroesophageal reflux, coughing when eating, and chronic cough). A birth history and any prior airway manipulation should also be recorded.

Most patients presenting with an upper airway complaint warrant a flexible fiberoptic laryngoscopy in the office. Digital fiberoptic scopes as small as 2.9 mm in diameter allow for improved physical examination of pediatric patients, but there are nondigital scopes that are even smaller and can still be used.[1] Ideally, these examinations should be recorded, as a real-time view of the larynx can be limited, particularly in the pediatric patient population, and video recording allows for repeated reviewing and slow-motion playback, which may offer a better assessment. In addition, videos can also be archived for pre- and posttreatment comparisons. The exam can usually be performed in the office on the youngest of patients.

There are still rare occasions when a child cannot be fully evaluated in the office, such as the infant who appears in distress or the infant with significant cardiac history, which may make office examination unsafe. For these children, a direct laryngoscopy in the operating room with the aid of a microscope or telescope is necessary. The advantages of this technique are that the surgeon has a clear view of the larynx, the ability to palpate the lesion, and the opportunity to obtain a biopsy sample for diagnosis. The disadvantages are that the child requires general anesthetic and there can be no dynamic evaluation of the vocal folds.

21.2 Voice-Related Quality of Life

For patients who present with a primary voice complaint, specific subjective and objective voice measures should be obtained. A complete evaluation by our voice therapy colleagues is extremely important. The aerodynamic profile allows for subjective measurement of voice changes following therapy. A second method for obtaining subjective measurements is administering quality-of-life surveys. The Pediatric Voice-Related Quality of Life Questionnaire (PVRQoL) is a validated instrument that is simple to administer and complete and is responsive to changes in voice-related quality of life.[2] It can be used in the general pediatric patient population and is a 10-question survey that is scored on a scale of 0 to 100 (see the box "Pediatric Voice-Related Quality of Life Survey (p. 217)"). Lower scores reflect less impact on quality of life than higher scores. The Pediatric Voice Handicap Index (pVHI) is the other commonly cited vocal quality-of-life instrument, and has been validated in children (see the box "Pediatric Voice Handicap Index (p. 218)").[3] Scores range from 0 to 120 points with higher scores representing worse perceived quality of life. The pVHI is used to differentiate between the different areas in a child's life that a voice disorder can affect, but can take more time than the PVRQoL to complete.

Pediatric Voice-Related Quality of Life Survey

Please answer these questions based on what your child's voice (your own voice if you are a teenage respondent) has been like over the past 2 weeks. Considering both how severe the problem is when you get it, and how frequently it happens, please rate each item below on how bad it is (that is, the amount of each problem that you have). Use the following rating scale:

1 = None, not a problem
2 = A small amount
3 = A moderate amount
4 = A lot
5 = Problem is "as bad as it can be"
6 = Not applicable

Because of my child's voice, how much of a problem is this?

1. My child has trouble speaking loudly or being heard in noisy situations.

   1 2 3 4 5 6

2. My child runs out of air and needs to take frequent breaths when talking.

   1 2 3 4 5 6

3. My child sometimes does not know what will come out when he or she begins speaking.

   1 2 3 4 5 6

4. My child is sometimes anxious or frustrated (because of his or her voice).

   1 2 3 4 5 6

5. My child sometimes gets depressed (because of his or her voice).

 1 2 3 4 5 6

6. My child has trouble using the telephone or speaking with friends in person.

 1 2 3 4 5 6

7. My child has trouble doing his or her job or schoolwork (because of his or her voice).

 1 2 3 4 5 6

8. My child avoids going out socially (because of his or her voice).

 1 2 3 4 5 6

9. My child has to repeat himself or herself to be understood.

 1 2 3 4 5 6

10. My child has become less outgoing (because of his or her voice).

 1 2 3 4 5 6

Pediatric Voice Handicap Index

0 = Never
1 = Almost never
2 = Sometimes
3 = Almost always
4 = Always

Part I—Functional

1. My child's voice makes it difficult to hear him/her.

 1 2 3 4

2. People have difficulty understanding my child in a noisy room.

 1 2 3 4

3. At home, we have difficulty hearing my child when he or she calls through the house.

 1 2 3 4

4. My child tends to avoid communicating because of his or her voice.

 1 2 3 4

5. My child speaks with friends, neighbors, or relatives less often because of his or her voice.

 1 2 3 4

6. People ask my child to repeat himself or herself when speaking face-to-face.

 1 2 3 4

7. My child's voice difficulties restrict personal, educational, and social activities.

 1 2 3 4

Part II—Physical

8. My child runs out of air when talking.

 1 2 3 4

9. The sound of my child's voice changes throughout the day.

 1 2 3 4

10. People ask, "What's wrong with your child's voice?"

 1 2 3 4

11. My child's voice sounds dry, rasp, and/or hoarse.

 1 2 3 4

12. The quality of my child's voice is unpredictable.

 1 2 3 4

13. My child uses a great deal of effort to speak (e.g., straining).

 1 2 3 4

14. My child's voice is worse in the evening.

 1 2 3 4

15. My child's voice "gives out" while speaking.

 1 2 3 4

16. My child has to yell in order for others to hear him or her.

 1 2 3 4

Part III—Emotional

17. My child appears tense when talking to others because of his or her voice.

 1 2 3 4

18. People seem irritated with my child's voice.

 1 2 3 4

19. I find that other people don't understand my child's voice problem.

 1 2 3 4

20. My child is frustrated by his or her voice problem.

 1 2 3 4

21. My child is less outgoing because of his or her voice problem.

 1 2 3 4

22. My child is annoyed when people ask him or her to repeat.

 1 2 3 4

23. My child is embarrassed when people ask him or her to repeat.

 1 2 3 4

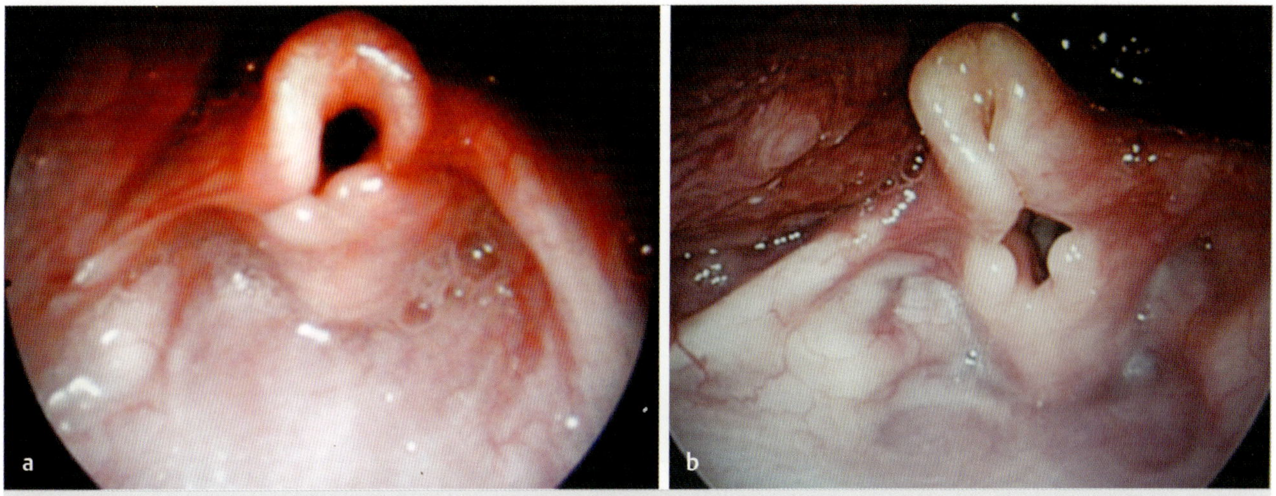

Fig. 21.1 (a) Prolapse of the arytenoids into the airway in laryngomalacia. (b) Infolding of the immature epiglottis.

Further patient evaluation depends on the specific complaint and differential diagnosis and is discussed as it pertains to each specific pathology.

21.3 Laryngomalacia

Laryngomalacia represents a delay of maturation of the supporting structures of the larynx and is both the most common cause of congenital stridor and the most common congenital lesion of the larynx. It may affect the epiglottis, the arytenoid cartilages, or both. When the epiglottis is involved, it is often elongated, and the walls fold in on themselves (▶ Fig. 21.1a). The epiglottis in cross section resembles an omega, and the lesion has been referred to as an omega-shaped epiglottis. If the arytenoid cartilages are involved, they appear enlarged (▶ Fig. 21.1b). In either case, the cartilage is floppy and is noted to prolapse over the larynx during inspiration, resulting in inspiratory stridor.

Infants with laryngomalacia have a higher incidence of gastroesophageal reflux, presumably a result of the more negative intrathoracic pressures necessary to overcome the inspiratory obstruction.[4] Conversely, children with significant reflux may have pathologic changes similar to laryngomalacia, especially enlargement and swelling of the arytenoid cartilages. Some of the swelling of the arytenoid cartilages and of the epiglottis may be secondary to reflux.

Evaluation of the symptomatic child should begin with flexible laryngoscopy. This allows for assessment of dynamic airway collapse, as well as other causes of stridor, such as vocal fold immobility or vocal fold lesions. Further evaluation with airway fluoroscopy may be helpful to look for distal airway lesions.

In the majority of cases, observation is the only treatment necessary. As the laryngeal cartilage matures, symptoms improve and resolve by 2 years of age. If the baby has normal cry, normal weight gain, normal development, and purely inspiratory noise that developed within the first 2 months of life, then no further workup may be necessary. Parents may be told that laryngomalacia is the most likely diagnosis, and they can be assured of its natural history. In severe cases in which the laryngomalacia results in dysphagia, persistent or recurrent hypoxia, or failure to thrive, surgery is indicated.[5] Most patients improve with a supraglottoplasty to reduce airway obstruction. This can be done in a staged fashion if there are multiple components of laryngomalacia contributing to upper airway obstruction. Cold dissection to divide the aryepiglottic folds or to debulk redundant arytenoid mucosa can be performed, or a laser may be used to accomplish the same results (▶ Fig. 21.2). Details of the procedure depend on the surgeon's preference and the nature of the laryngomalacia.[6]

21.4 Vocal Fold Immobility

Vocal fold immobility (VFI) may present in the neonate or young child as stridor in up to 70% of patients, but it can also present as respiratory distress, poor feeding, weak cry, cyanosis, and aspiration. Hoarseness and poor vocal projection are more often the chief complaints in older children and adolescents. Unilateral VFI (UVFI) and bilateral VFI (BVFI) are different pathophysiologic and clinical entities with distinct symptoms and etiologies.[7,8] Unilateral VFI is most commonly due to iatrogenic injury, such as cardiothoracic surgery, which carries a risk of recurrent laryngeal nerve injury. Pediatric procedures like ligation of a patent ductus arteriosus are being performed with increasing frequency, thereby leading to a growing number of children with UVFI postoperatively.[9] Congenital BVFI is the most common presentation of BVFI, with various etiologies, such as neurologic or idiopathic.[10] It is important to distinguish unilateral (UVFI) from bilateral (BVFI) dysfunction. Though the two have an almost equal occurrence, their management options are dramatically different.[11]

Diagnosis is made with flexible fiberoptic laryngoscopy, although imaging may also be needed to evaluate the course of the vagus nerve and to assess for any intracranial abnormalities (▶ Fig. 21.3). The question then becomes how and when to treat the symptomatic child. Many children are able to compensate without surgical intervention. If aspiration is a problem in the very young child, alternate means of giving nutrition should be

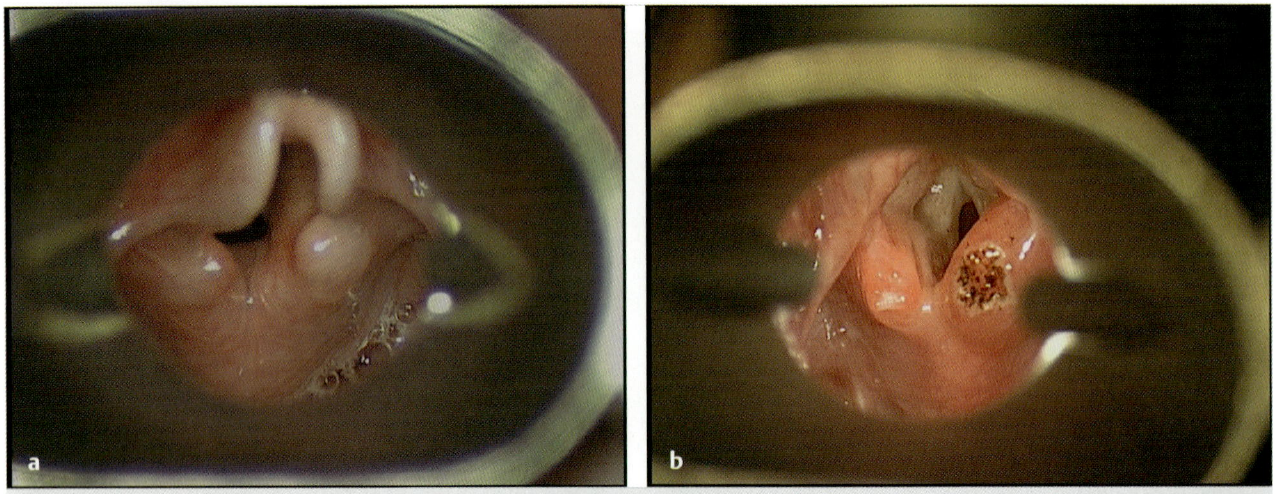

Fig. 21.2 (a) Suspension laryngoscopy in preparation for supraglottoplasty. (b) Carbon dioxide laser treatment of redundant arytenoid mucosa bilaterally.

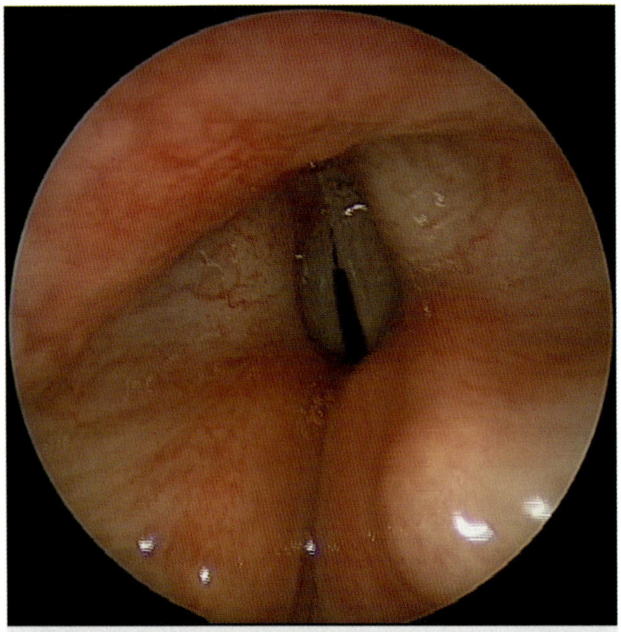

Fig. 21.3 Concave left true vocal fold after left recurrent laryngeal nerve injury.

sought, such as a thickened diet if proven safe on a modified barium swallow study. If this is not possible, feeding tubes or gastrostomy tubes are other options.

It has been generally accepted in the adult literature to wait at least 1 year before performing more permanent procedures for VFI. This period has been extended even further in children because the literature has suggested that vocal fold function may return many years later.[11,12] There is no simple test or procedure to help predict return of vocal fold function. In adult patients, laryngeal electromyography (LEMG) has been used to help guide management decisions and is gaining interest as a diagnostic tool in children. Intraoperative LEMG is a safe method for determining the likelihood of recurrent laryngeal nerve function return in children who have undergone patent ductus arteriosus ligation, in children with centrally correctable lesions, and in children with idiopathic VFI. A recent investigation by Maturo et al looked at the use of LEMG to predict the return of vocal fold function.[13] In children who had VFI due to PDA ligation, if there are no normal-appearing motor unit action potentials (MUAPs) by 6 months, then it is highly unlikely that vocal fold function will recover. In this study, 5 patients who had LEMG before 6 months all had LEMG findings showing no normal MUAPs, and none recovered function. This group also suggested that performing serial EMGs may not be needed, as children can be followed with office-based flexible laryngoscopy.

In the child with BVFI, treatment will focus on maintaining a patent airway. This can range from a tracheotomy for the severely obstructed child to a cordotomy or arytenoidectomy for the child who is moderately symptomatic.[7] It is possible for children with BVFI to improve over time; therefore, only supportive care is needed with close airway monitoring.

For children with UVFI, the management options are numerous and vary with patient age and symptoms. The two most common symptoms associated with UVFI for which parents seek help are aspiration and dysphonia (or a combination of both).[9] In patients who are older than 4 years and who have continued symptoms from UVFI for at least 9 months, surgical treatment should be considered. A frequently used and relatively low-risk treatment is injection laryngoplasty with either autologous fat or synthetic material.[14] This allows for immediate results, but they are short term and the child may need repeated injections to remain symptom-free. Another option is a medialization thyroplasty, which is most suitable for the adolescent patient who can tolerate a procedure under light sedation and local anesthesia. This allows the medialization to be fine-tuned for improved dysphonia, as the patient can phonate during the procedure while the surgeon manipulates the implant.[15] The benefit is a definitive procedure that limits the need for future intervention. Finally, a neurorrhaphy can be performed between the affected recurrent laryngeal nerve and the ansa cervicalis to achieve reinnervation and restore tone to the immobile vocal fold, the results of which are maintained long-term.[16] Results of the neurorrhaphy are not immediate, and injection laryngoplasty can be used until reinnervation has occurred. Choosing between a medialization thyroplasty and a reinnervation procedure, as both are long-term solutions, depends on the individual case and the experience of the surgeon.

21.5 Vocal Fold Nodules

True vocal fold nodules are the most common cause for prolonged hoarseness in the pediatric age group.[17] They are considered to be the result of phonatory trauma and consist of subepithelial fibrovascular depositions (in the superficial layer of the lamina propria) along the membranous vocal fold.[18,19] Generally they are symmetric and are located at the junction of the anterior and middle one-third of the vocal fold; in other words, at the midpoint of the membranous vocal fold (▶ Fig. 21.4). Videostroboscopy can sometimes be used to differentiate nodules from intracordal lesions and polyps. The mucosal wave can be present or decreased with nodules, depending on their size. The wave is often present or increased when a polyp is present. Finally, the mucosal wave is usually asymmetric with vocal fold cysts.[20]

The etiology of vocal fold nodules is likely multifactorial and includes genetic predisposition, behavioral factors, and environmental factors, such as exposure to laryngopharyngeal reflux (LPR).[17] Laryngopharyngeal reflux has not been studied extensively in the pediatric population as a potential causative factor. Kuhn and colleagues have been the only group to objectively measure the presence of reflux using a triple pH probe. They found in a group of 11 adult patients with nodules that pharyngeal reflux was more prevalent in these patients than in a group of control patients. They suggested a contributory role in the pathogenesis of nodules.[21]

The largest published series of pediatric patients with vocal fold nodules involved 254 children over a 7-year period. This study revealed that the majority of nodules were found in boys (72%) and that the average age at presentation was 7.7 years. Hyperfunction was noted in 75% and laryngoesophageal reflux in only 25% (only a subjective assessment was made, based on endoscopic findings). Acoustic measurements seemed to correlate with the size of the nodules. Treatment options and outcomes were not evaluated.[22]

Most would agree that children with nodules should first be treated with maximal medical management. The first step involves voice therapy with a speech-language pathologist, although there is currently no standard technique for therapy nor is there a preset duration of therapy. The treatment of pediatric vocal cord nodules with voice therapy is an active area of research. In most cases, improvement can be expected within 4 weeks; if there is no improvement, further examination is required. In addition, good vocal hygiene should be stressed and gastroesophageal reflux treated if it is thought to exist. Vocal hygiene includes reducing vocal fold trauma by limiting abusive behaviors (e.g., talking in a noisy environment, screaming, throat clearing), limiting risk factors for reflux, and keeping well hydrated. Initial therapy teaches both the child and the parents techniques of breath control and muscle relaxation. The parents play an important role in continuing therapy in the home environment and must take an active role if the child is to get the maximum benefit. The endpoint of therapy is patient and family satisfaction with voice and maintenance of good vocal hygiene.[23]

If conservative therapy fails, surgical excision appears to be a viable treatment option. However, only a very small minority of cases require surgery before puberty. Only children or parents who complain about difficulty with being able to communicate should be considered for surgical excision. Some believe that children should be over the age of 7 or 8 years because this is when the trilaminar structure of the vocal fold appears to be completely developed (▶ Fig. 21.5).[24]

On the other hand, it is important not to do surgery until the child is mature enough to comply with a course of voice rest postoperatively, which is usually recommended for 1 week afterward.[25] In addition, if surgery is considered, one should be

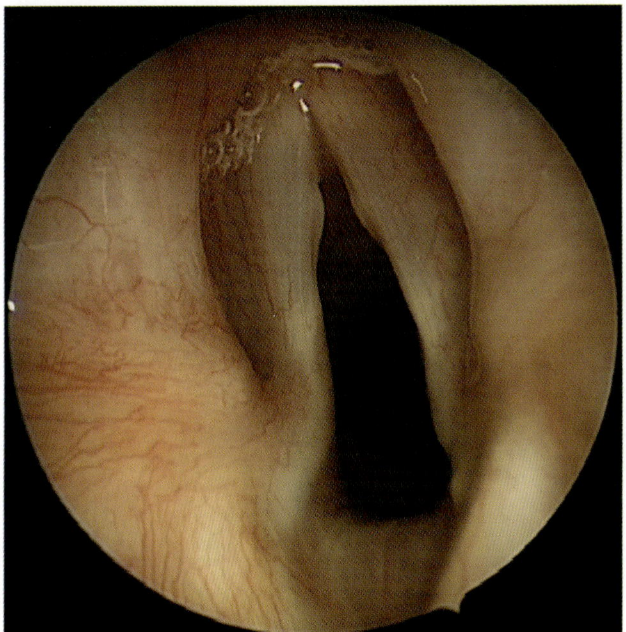

Fig. 21.4 Bilateral true vocal fold nodules.

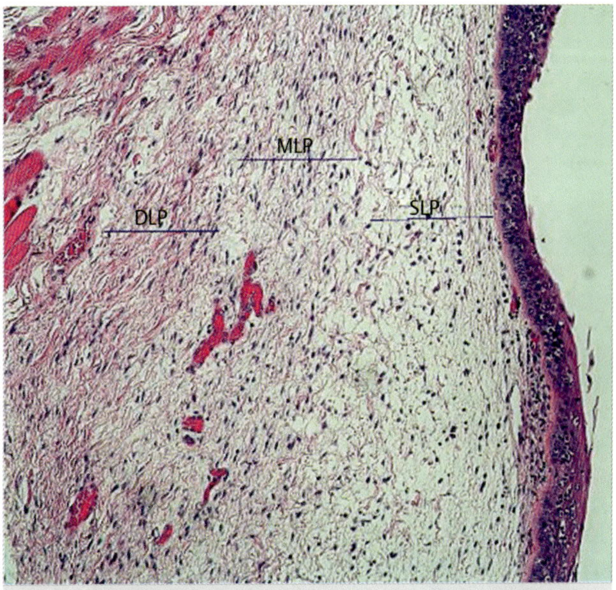

Fig. 21.5 Trilaminar structure of mature vocal fold. LP, deep lamina propria; MLP, middle lamina propria; SLP, superficial lamina propria

relatively certain that the traumatic vocal pattern that produced the nodules has been corrected preoperatively. This fact also limits the role for surgery at a younger age because young children are often unable to comply with good vocal hygiene. The surgeon must carefully counsel both child and parent to choose the best management option.

Currently, there are no published data on pre- and postsurgery voice outcomes for pediatric patients with vocal nodules. Zeitels has published the largest series on surgical outcomes in the adult population. His was a single-arm, noncontrolled study that included 185 patients with 201 nodules that were excised. Four of these patients developed recurrent nodules and required a second operation. A subepithelial microdissection technique was employed in each case, with the epithelial cordotomy being performed either immediately superior or lateral to the lesion. Overall, 182 out of 185 patients had a subjectively improved performing voice (of note is that not all of the patients had nodules; nodules made up 201 of the 365 benign vocal fold lesions removed from this population). All objective acoustic measurements for those patients who returned to the office were within normal limits.[26]

21.6 Papillomas

Juvenile-onset recurrent respiratory papillomatosis (JORRP) is a disease caused by the human papillomavirus (HPV) and is considered to be juvenile in onset when it occurs before the age of 5 years. Warty growths in the upper airway may cause significant airway obstruction or voice change (▶ Fig. 21.6). Juvenile-onset recurrent respiratory papillomatosis is caused by peripartum transmission of the virus from an infected mother. Vaginal delivery is a risk factor, but cesarean delivery is not completely protective.[27] Although more than 20 types of HPV can cause genital warts, only two of these, HPV-6 and HPV-11, cause the vast majority of cases of JORRP. The disease associated with HPV-11 is more severe.[28]

In general, papillomas may develop anywhere in the respiratory tract, from the nose to the lung; however, 95% of cases involve the larynx. The sites of respiratory system involvement have been described more completely for juvenile-onset RRP; 52% of children have isolated laryngeal involvement. The trachea is the next most commonly involved site. However, 31.8% of children have papillomas in areas outside of the trachea and larynx (e.g., oropharynx, nasopharynx, mouth, bronchi, lung parenchyma).[28] Because the larynx is the most frequently affected site, symptoms of upper airway obstruction predominate. Upper airway obstruction may be life threatening and may be the presenting symptom. Hoarseness is the most common presenting symptom, but patients may have a range of symptoms, including stridor, globus sensation, dysphagia, and cough.

Diagnosis of JORPP in patients presenting with hoarseness or voice change requires visualization of the vocal cords. Because laryngeal involvement occurs in more than 95% of patients, direct or indirect laryngoscopy reveals the characteristic warty growths. Rarely, the trachea is involved without laryngeal lesions, and bronchoscopy may be required for evaluation. Obtaining a biopsy specimen of visualized lesions is essential for histologic confirmation of respiratory papillomatosis and to rule out malignancy. The specimen should also be sent for HPV subtyping. The majority of patients will enter remission around the time of puberty. In 3 to 5% of patients, respiratory papillomas may undergo malignant degeneration to squamous cell carcinoma, and the prognosis for patients with these cancers is quite poor.

Standard treatment is primarily surgical debulking of lesions to produce and maintain a patent airway. Tracheotomy should be avoided in these patients, as this will generally result in seeding of the tracheostoma and tract with papilloma due to the squamous epithelial lining. In the setting of acute airway compromise and an inability to obtain airway access via endotracheal intubation, a tracheotomy may be unavoidable. Therefore, the goal of intervention is not cure, but to improve symptoms until the time of remission. Microdebridement can be employed for large bulky lesions as it offers the advantage of shorter operative times, potential for outpatient surgery, decreased risk to personnel, and avoidance of the risk of airway

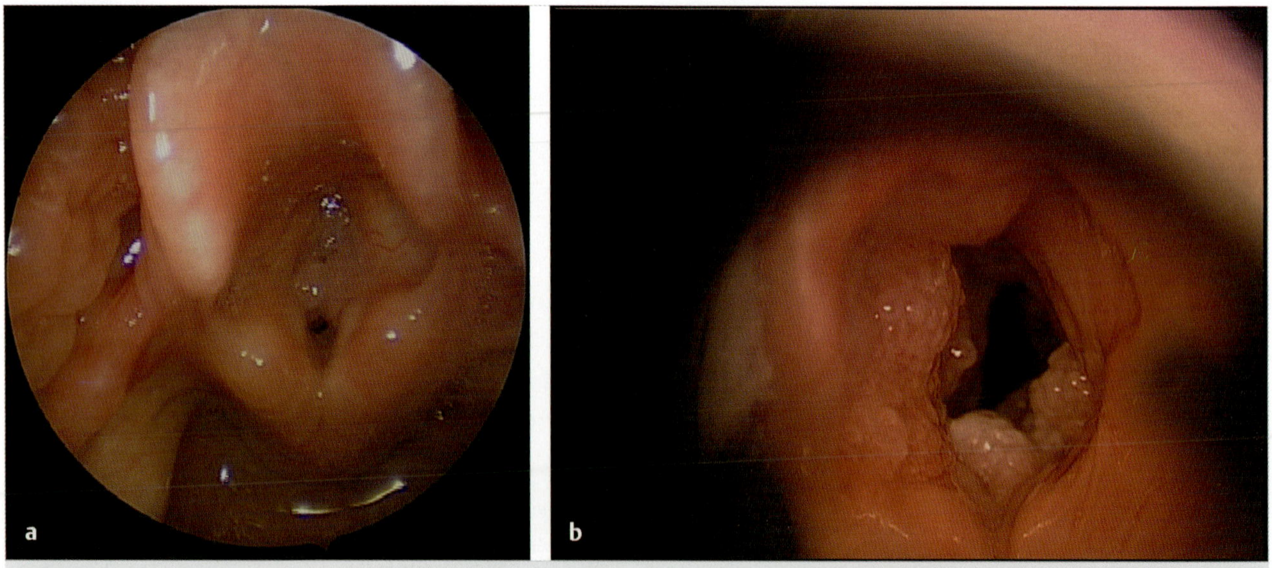

Fig. 21.6 (a) Papillomatosis seen on direct laryngoscopy. (b) Papillomatosis seen on suspension laryngoscopy.

burns. Many surgeons prefer to use the CO_2 laser because it affords good hemostasis and minimizes potential thermal injury of surrounding healthy tissues. Laryngeal coblator offers similar advantages. For small lesions or sessile papillomatous changes, angiolytic laser may be an option as well.

Resection may also be augmented with adjuvant treatments that aim to slow the regrowth of lesions; none have been demonstrated to be curative to date. Adjuvant therapies are appropriate when patients need more than six procedures in one year for RRP. They include intralesional cidofovir, oral indole-3-carbinol, interferon, and photodynamic therapy.[29,30,31,32,33] Agents that demonstrate variable effect include acyclovir and retinoic acid.[34,35]

Of recent interest has been the use of photoangiolytic laser treatment combined with sublesional injections of the antiangiogenic agent bevacizumab (Avastin, Genentech, South San Francisco, CA). A prospective open-label investigation was conducted by Zeitels in 20 adult patients with bilateral vocal fold RRP.[36] The patients underwent planned 532-nm pulsed KTP (potassium titanyl phosphate) laser photoangiolysis of bilateral glottal disease four times, with an approximately 6-week interval between procedures. At each planned laser procedure, the vocal fold that on initial presentation had a greater volume of disease also underwent serial sublesional bevacizumab injections, and the contralateral cord was injected with saline as a control. No local or systemic complications were noted. After four injections, three of the 20 patients had no discernible disease in either vocal fold. Of the remaining 17 patients, 16 had less disease in the bevacizumab-treated vocal fold despite starting with more disease. Only one of the 17 had more disease in the bevacizumab-treated vocal fold after four injections. Moreover, seven of the 20 patients (35%) did not require a laser procedure in the vocal fold that had received four bevacizumab injections, as compared with three of the 20 vocal folds (15%) that were treated with laser alone. Combining bevacizumab with KTP laser photoangiolysis is encouraging and it is under investigation in the pediatric population to determine its efficacy and safety.

21.7 Laryngeal Stenosis

Congenital laryngeal stenosis results from failure of the laryngeal lumen to recanalize. During normal development, the laryngeal lumen is obliterated to give rise to the epithelial lamina, which later recanalizes. By the 10th week of gestation, the laryngeal lumen is re-established following recanalization. Incomplete recanalization results in various degrees of glottic and/or subglottic stenosis. Laryngeal atresia represents the most severe end of the spectrum of disease, arising from failed recanalization. Atresia can be diagnosed prenatally based on ultrasound by identifying signs of congenital high airway obstruction syndrome (CHAOS). Glottic and supraglottic atresia require immediate tracheotomy at the time of delivery. Prenatal diagnosis of CHAOS allows for the use of the ex utero intrapartum treatment (EXIT) procedure to evaluate and secure the airway at birth.[37] Laryngotracheal reconstruction to repair the atresia is necessary at a later stage.

Congenital laryngeal webs account for about 5% of congenital laryngeal anomalies (▶ Fig. 21.7). Seventy-five percent of these are at the glottic level. Treatment varies depending on the nature of the web and associated symptoms, ranging from division of thin membranous webs, staged dilations following incision, keel placement, open laryngotracheal reconstruction, and tracheostomy.[38] Laryngeal webs often involve both the glottis and subglottis and may rarely involve the supraglottis. Glottic stenosis may also result from impaired vocal cord mobility, or rarely, complete fusion of the true vocal folds.

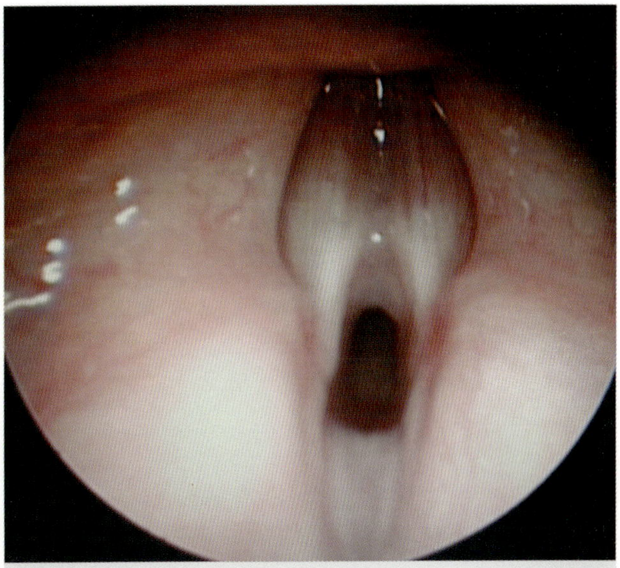

Fig. 21.7 Congenital anterior laryngeal web.

Congenital subglottic stenosis is defined as an airway smaller than 4 mm in diameter or 3.5 mm in the premature infant. It is diagnosed where subglottic narrowing exists with no history of intubation or surgical trauma. Distinguishing congenital from acquired stenosis once a child has been intubated is difficult, but the suspected incidence is 5%. Congenital stenosis can be a contributing factor in acquired laryngeal stenosis (▶ Fig. 21.8a). It is generally divided into two types: membranous (fibrosis, submucous gland hyperplasia, granulation tissue) and cartilaginous; membranous stenosis is more common than cartilaginous stenosis. Most commonly, membranous stenoses are circumferential and symmetric and may extend upward to include the true vocal cords. Cartilaginous stenosis is a deformity of the cricoid cartilage or tracheal ring projecting into the lumen. It may be symmetric (small but normal-shaped cricoid or a nondistensible complete first tracheal ring trapped inside the cricoid) or asymmetric (elliptic or oval-shaped cricoid, isolated enlargement of either the anterior or posterior cricoid lamina, or laryngeal cleft). Severity of stenosis is based on the Myer-Cotton grading system.[39]

Acquired laryngeal stenosis occurs secondary to instrumentation of the airway (▶ Fig. 21.8b). Ninety percent of acquired subglottic stenoses in infants and children are due to endotracheal intubation. The incidence of subglottic stenosis after intubation is reported to be 1 to 10%. Other factors that are associated with an increased risk of stenosis following intubation include traumatic intubation, prolonged duration of intubation, multiple extubations and reintubations, use of an oversized endotracheal tube for intubation, motion of the patient or the tube, gastroesophageal reflux, and local infection. In the pediatric population, because the pediatric subglottis is the

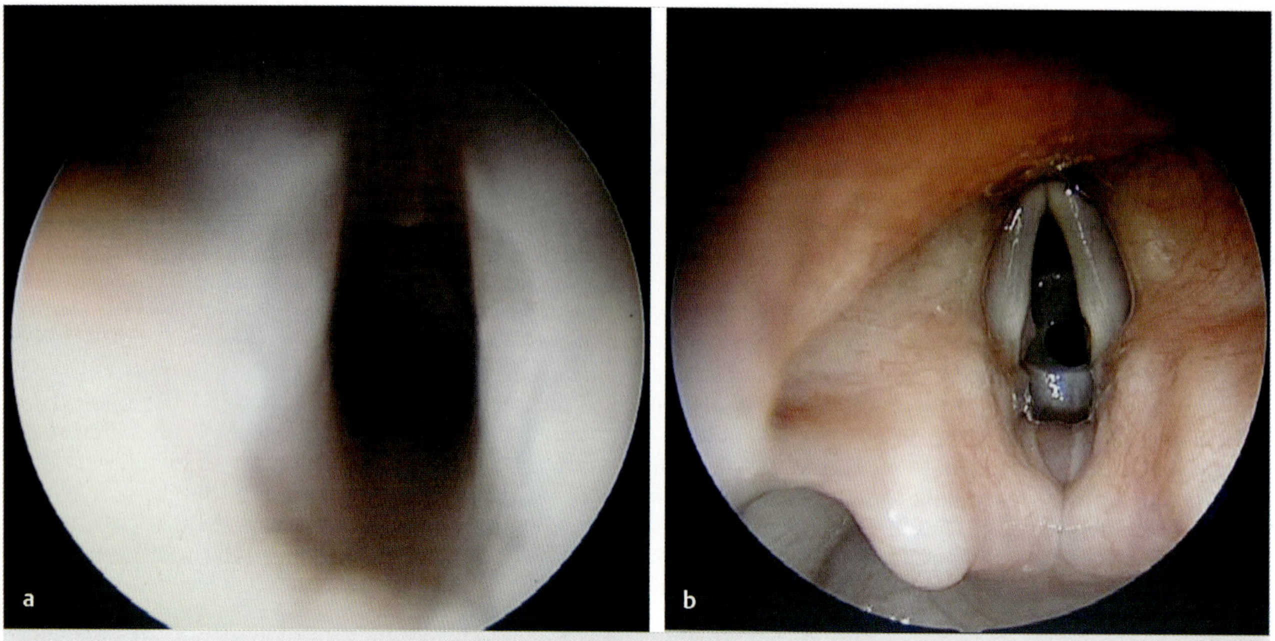

Fig. 21.8 (**a**) Elliptical congenital subglottic stenosis. (**b**) Acquired subglottic stenosis following endotracheal intubation.

narrowest portion of the airway, it is predisposed to injury by intubation. The above-mentioned extrinsic factors lead to such changes as submucosal edema and granulation tissue deposition from fibroblast proliferation. Ulceration due to pressure or trauma (i.e., from endotracheal or nasogastric tube) can progress perichondritis or chondritis with associated scar formation and/or arytenoid fixation.

The history should include an assessment of dyspnea and stridor, including the characteristics of the stridor, time of onset, and relieving and aggravating factors. Voice quality should also be assessed. History should also include questions to identify possible etiological factors, such as a history of prolonged intubation, prior surgery (airway or otherwise), trauma, or caustic ingestion. In general, though anterior glottic scarring results in dysphonia, posterior glottic scarring tends to present with dyspnea. Acquired posterior glottic stenosis usually presents as difficulty on extubation or tracheotomy dependence.

Diagnosis should include flexible fiberoptic laryngoscopy in the awake patient is performed to assess for supraglottic and glottic pathology such as vocal cord paralysis and laryngomalacia. Next, direct laryngoscopy and bronchoscopy with the patient under general anesthesia is performed. This allows careful evaluation of each segment of the airway: supraglottis, glottis, subglottis, and trachea. The outer diameter of the largest bronchoscope that can pass through the stenosis should be noted as well as the length of the stenotic segment, its location, thickness, and composition. The size of the airway should be determined as the largest endotracheal tube that permits an air leak at less than 30 cm of water pressure. This size should be compared to the age-appropriate size tube ([age + 16]/4) to calculate the degree of stenosis.

Treatment is individualized and varies greatly with the severity of stenosis, etiology, and specific shape and location of stenosis. Mild cases of stenosis (grade I) are typically managed with a conservative approach consisting of regular follow-up care and aggressive medical management of upper respiratory infections. Most patients with greater than 50% obstruction are likely to require some surgical intervention. These include both endoscopic (dilation, laser resection) and external approaches to cricoid expansion. Laser resection and dilation are rarely effective if the stenosis is cartilaginous. Patients with a need for ventilatory support are generally poor surgical candidates. Pulmonary status must be maximized prior to any airway intervention. Infants and children with a history of bronchopulmonary dysplasia may need to demonstrate a season without hospitalization for severe respiratory illness before consideration for reconstruction. A tracheotomy for airway control may be necessary until pulmonary reserve is optimized.

21.8 Voice after Laryngotracheal Reconstruction

The primary goal of laryngotracheal reconstruction (LTR) is to re-establish a patent laryngeal and subglottic airway. For those children who are tracheotomy dependent, this includes the ability to decannulate these patients. A secondary goal of surgical reconstruction is to improve the ability of these children to communicate. Unfortunately, it is often difficult to determine how successful we have been when it comes to postoperative voice results. Many of these children have tracheotomies at a very young age prior to reconstructive surgery and therefore never had a "normal" preoperative voice. Therefore, it has been difficult to determine whether the voice is improved following surgery. In addition, most of the published data on post-LTR voice have included a heterogenous group of patients. Many have had prior open and endoscopic airway surgery, some included patients who had had stents placed, and the subjective results often have relied on nonvalidated caregiver questionnaires. Thus, it is difficult to form definitive conclusions.

However, all of the published studies report a high incidence of abnormal voice following LTR.

Zalzal was the first to publish on post-LTR voice. He noted in a group of 16 patients that 12 had a functional voice postoperatively, as compared to only six preoperatively. However, 15 of the 16 patients had "abnormal" voices, as evidenced by low pitch, breathiness, and hoarseness.[40] These findings were further substantiated by Smith et al in 1993, who documented postoperative voice in a group of eight patients. Videostroboscopic findings revealed that two patients had glottal insufficiency, three had vocal fold asymmetry and stiffness, and three exhibited phonation with supraglottic structures.[41] MacArthur et al found similar results among a small sample of patients. They examined speech samples in six patients and found 100% had decreased vocal quality, 50% had decreased intelligibility, 100% had decreased volume, and 80% had a low fundamental frequency and increased jitter.[42] Finally, in the largest reported series of 50 patients, Bailey reported that 52% had an "acceptable" voice following airway reconstruction. The assessment consisted of a parental questionnaire, voice analysis, video nasendoscopy and videostroboscopy, and pulmonary function tests.[43]

Although it might be impossible to determine absolute change in voice after LTR because many children have no voice prior to surgery, there are several observations that can be made. The first is that when the anterior commissure is divided, it is more likely that the voice will be altered. The ability of the surgeon to reapproximate the true vocal folds in the correct anatomical position is crucial in determining how much voice will be affected (▶ Fig. 21.9).

A second important consideration is that use of stents that sit above the level of the true vocal folds can cause granulation tissue and scarring to form on the vocal folds. If this were to occur, there would obviously be an adverse effect on voice. Future surgical considerations may include limiting the need to divide the anterior commissure. This may be a more practical consideration in older children because their larger airway may allow for better visualization to place the cartilage graft without the additional exposure that dividing the vocal folds affords. In addition, the development of new techniques to stabilize cartilage grafts without the need for stenting should prove helpful. Finally, it is important to continue to gather data on these children, particularly prior to them undergoing their first airway procedure. This should include gathering objective data from aerodynamic voice analysis and qualitative information using validated voice instruments.

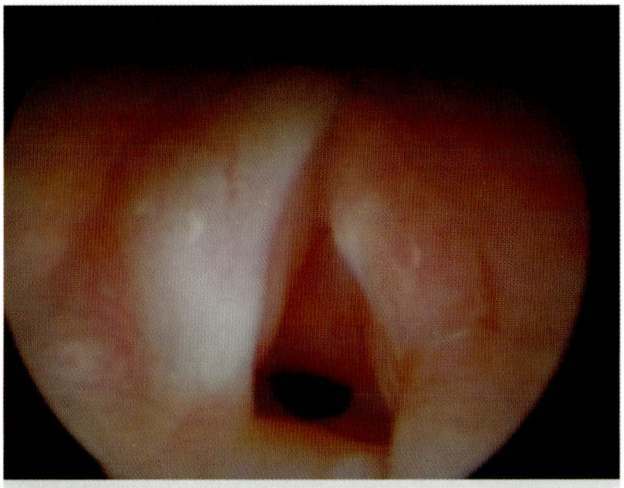

Fig. 21.9 Uneven vocal folds after laryngofissure and airway reconstruction.

21.9 Reflux

Gastroesophageal reflux disease (GERD) is a relatively common problem encountered by otolaryngologists. Symptoms in the adult population include throat clearing, chronic throat irritation, chronic hoarseness, and chronic cough.[44] Infants, on the other hand, often present initially with complaints of frequent "spitting up" during feeds. Others have a more worrisome history that includes failure to thrive, hematemesis, anemia, or recurrent pneumonia.[45]

The true incidence of GERD in children is difficult to ascertain, as many infants can spit up without any untoward complications. Premature infants, however, seem to have a higher likelihood of having reflux than other children. Marino found that in a group of 75 such patients, 63% had GERD.[46] The good news is that the majority of these patients improve as they grow. It appears that 55% have resolution of their symptoms by 10 months of age and an additional 16% improve by 18 months.[47]

The source of GERD in children is multifactorial, and thorough evaluation includes consultation with a pediatric gastroenterologist. Though transient relaxation of the lower esophageal sphincter may be the major causative factor, other causes, such as hiatal hernia should, also be considered. Large fluid boluses during infant feeds and placement in the supine position following feeding are also likely causes.

Children under the age of 12 months with failure to thrive, weight loss, pulmonary disease, and/or an apparent life-threatening episode warrant further work-up. For those over the age of 12 months, persistent spitting up is adequate to pursue further testing.[48] The diagnostic process can include an upper gastrointestinal series, pH probe testing, impedance monitoring, and endoscopy. Referral to a pediatric gastrointestinal physician is warranted.

Operative endoscopy of the aerodigestive tract can be extremely useful when trying to make the diagnosis of GERD, particularly in those that have failed medical management.

This group of children includes those with failure to thrive, chronic cough, and airway symptoms (including those with recurrent croup, pneumonias, and/or suspicion for aspiration). The laryngeal airway should be examined first to look for signs of pharyngeal reflux, such as erythema and/or intra-arytenoid or true vocal fold edema. Also, care is taken to inspect for a laryngeal cleft, as this could be the underlying cause for aspiration.

Bronchoscopy should then be performed. A cobblestone appearance of the tracheal wall is a visual clue on endoscopy that the child may be aspirating (▶ Fig. 21.10). A bronchoalveolar lavage should be performed to confirm a suspicion of aspiration. Specifically, 100 macrophages are collected and stained with oil red O to test for lipid. Lipid-laden macrophages become positive approximately 6 hours after a reflux episode and remain positive for up to 3 days.[49] Upper gastrointestinal

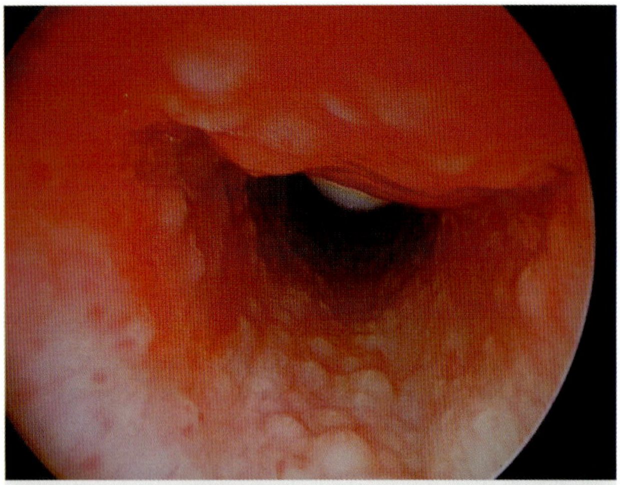

Fig. 21.10 Cobblestoning of the tracheal mucosa, as seen in the setting of aspiration. This patient also has a tracheostomy tube in place.

endoscopy should be performed by a gastroenterologist and biopsies should be taken. The specimens are examined for evidence of Barrett esophagus or eosinophils, which would suggest chronic reflux or allergic esophagitis. An endoscopic finding of "trachealization" or ringed appearance of the esophageal mucosal can be suggestive of esosinophilic esophagitis (▶ Fig. 21.11).

Once the diagnosis of GERD is made, the usual first step in treatment is conservative management. Techniques like formula changes (when allergy is suspected), thickening of feeds, smaller feeding size, suggestions for burping techniques, and positioning after feeds should all be entertained prior to beginning treatment with medications.[45,48] When necessary, medical treatment is successful in approximately 80% of cases.[50] If more severe GERD is suspected, proton-pump blockers have become an important therapeutic option and generally include a 6- to 8-week course minimum. The addition of histamine receptor-2 antagonists and prokinetic agents may also be needed if initial medication fails. For the child with disease refractory to medical management, consultation with a pediatric surgeon for a fundoplication should be considered.

21.10 Tracheomalacia

Tracheomalacia is an abnormal collapse of the tracheal walls. Most cases are related to a developmental defect in the cartilage of the tracheal wall; typically, symptoms resolve by 3 years of age (in many before age 1 year). However, tracheomalacia can be found in combination with other lesions that cause compression or damage of the airway, such as tracheoesophageal fistula postrepair, mediastinal masses, vascular slings, and vascular rings (▶ Fig. 21.10). If the lesion is extrathoracic, the collapse and airway sounds occur primarily during inspiration. If the lesion is intrathoracic, the collapse and airway sounds occur primarily during exhalation. Because most of the trachea is intrathoracic, exhalatory collapse accounts for most cases of tracheomalacia.

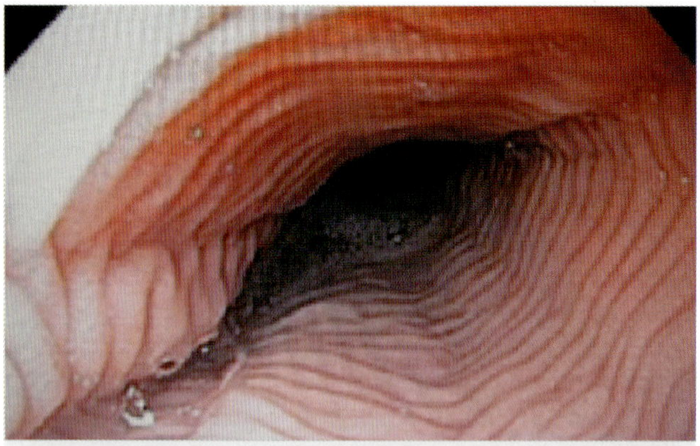

Fig. 21.11 Trachealization of the esophagus.

The history of a patient with tracheomalacia typically includes a wheeze that usually begins when the individual is age 4 to 8 weeks. Although the congenital lesion is present before this time, airflow is apparently insufficient during the first few weeks of life to generate abnormal sounds. The wheeze generally increases with activity and colds and decreases during quiet periods. Unlike most infants with asthma or cystic fibrosis, infants with tracheomalacia are described as "happy wheezers" (i.e., they maintain normal oxygenation and disposition and grow and develop normally, despite the chronic airway noises).[51]

As far as tracheomalacia is understood, most cases are isolated and idiopathic. A recent study proposed a possible neurologic etiology for tracheomalacia. This group was caring for a child with increased intracranial pressure. When the pressure was elevated, the child developed tracheomalacia. When the pressure was relieved, the tracheomalacia remitted. This scenario recurred, although the pathophysiology for increased intracranial pressure causing tracheomalacia is unknown.[52]

The definitive method of diagnosis is bronchoscopy. Rigid bronchoscopy is used to assess for static airway changes or anatomical abnormalities, but dynamic tracheal wall movement is best seen with flexible bronchoscopy. If there is concern for compression secondary to vascular anomaly, imaging may be needed to further define thoracic anatomy. Patients with vascular anomalies may suffer from esophageal compression and dysphagia in addition to tracheomalacia; these patients will benefit from esophagoscopy to assess for obstruction or compression of the digestive tract.

Depending on the severity of symptoms and operative findings, treatment can be observation, conservative management, or surgical intervention. If cartilaginous immaturity is to blame, time will allow for tissue maturation. Chest physiotherapy can assist with cough and clearance of secretions in the meantime. If there is mild collapse with minimal symptoms, noninvasive positive pressure may be beneficial. One group showed that positive expiratory pressure during an illness improved the cough flow rates in children with tracheomalacia, making the chest physical therapy and cough itself more effective.[53] Continuous positive airway pressure or bilevel positive airway pressure provided by means of a tight-fitting face or nasal mask, endotracheal tube, or tracheotomy tube can provide relief from severe obstruction. Medications like bronchodilators should generally be avoided as they act as smooth-muscle relaxers that can lead to worsened collapse. For the child with failure to thrive, recurrent pneumonias, or a need for long-term airway support due to severe tracheomalacia, surgery should be considered. Tracheotomy can be performed to allow for ventilation in very young infants. This allows the child to grow and develop until the problem potentially resolves. Other children may benefit from aortopexy to improve the tracheal airway. For other infants, placement of a tracheal stent may be warranted.[54] Children with vascular compression need treatment of the anomaly to resolve compression.

21.11 Conclusion

Laryngeal pathology in children is diverse, owing to the presence of both congential and acquired problems. Diagnosis relies heavily on caregiver history and endoscopy, which is at times supplemented by imaging. Treatment options are growing in sophistication and variety, offering the surgeon multiple options to care for the patient. Although some information can be extrapolated from experience in adults, most information will come directly from working with children to understand their airway complexity.

21.12 Key Points

- Children present with a variety of laryngeal pathologies, which may be congenital or acquired.
- Diagnostic techniques should take into account the pathology suspected, patient's age and cooperation, and airway safety during the examination.
- For the child with dysphonia, quality-of-life surveys are important in determining the severity of disease and for monitoring treatment effects.
- Treatment of laryngeal problems in children may not always be surgical, and the usefulness of noninvasive therapies should not be underestimated.

References

[1] Hartnick CJ, Zeitels SM. Pediatric video laryngo-stroboscopy. Int J Pediatr Otorhinolaryngol 2005; 69: 215–219

[2] Boseley ME, Cunningham MJ, Volk MS, Hartnick CJ. Validation of the pediatric voice-related quality of life survey. Arch Otolaryngol Head Neck Surg 2006; 132: 717–720

[3] Zur KB, Cotton S, Kelchner L, Baker S, Weinrich B, Lee L. Pediatric Voice Handicap Index (pVHI): a new tool for evaluating pediatric dysphonia. Int J Pediatr Otorhinolaryngol 2007; 71: 77–82

[4] Manning SC, Inglis AF, Mouzakes J, Carron J, Perkins JA. Laryngeal anatomic differences in pediatric patients with severe laryngomalacia. Arch Otolaryngol Head Neck Surg 2005; 131: 340–343

[5] Richter GT, Thompson DM. The surgical management of laryngomalacia. Otolaryngol Clin North Am 2008; 41: 837–864

[6] Whymark AD, Clement WA, Kubba H, Geddes NK. Laser epiglottopexy for laryngomalacia: 10 years' experience in the west of Scotland. Arch Otolaryngol Head Neck Surg 2006; 132: 978–982

[7] Chen EY, Inglis AF. Bilateral vocal cord paralysis in children. Otolaryngol Clin North Am 2008; 41: 889–901, viiiviii.

[8] Berkowitz RG. Natural history of tracheostomy-dependent idiopathic congenital bilateral vocal fold paralysis. Otolaryngol Head Neck Surg 2007; 136: 649–652

[9] Boseley ME, Bloch I, Hartnick CJ. Charcot-Marie-Tooth disease type 1 and pediatric true vocal fold paralysis. Int J Pediatr Otorhinolaryngol 2006; 70: 345–347

[10] Daya H, Hosni A, Bejar-Solar I, Evans JN, Bailey CM. Pediatric vocal fold paralysis: a long-term retrospective study. Arch Otolaryngol Head Neck Surg 2000; 126: 21–25

[11] Miyamoto RC, Parikh SR, Gellad W, Licameli GR. Bilateral congenital vocal cord paralysis: a 16-year institutional review. Otolaryngol Head Neck Surg 2005; 133: 241–245

[12] Maturo SC, Braun N, Brown DJ, Chong PST, Kerschner JE, Hartnick CJ. Intraoperative laryngeal electromyography in children with vocal fold immobility: results of a multicenter longitudinal study. Arch Otolaryngol Head Neck Surg 2011; 137: 1251–1257

[13] Parikh SR. Pediatric unilateral vocal fold immobility. Otolaryngol Clin North Am 2004; 37: 203–215

[14] Umeno H, Shirouzu H, Chitose S, Nakashima T. Analysis of voice function following autologous fat injection for vocal fold paralysis. Otolaryngol Head Neck Surg 2005; 132: 103–107

[15] Sipp JA, Kerschner JE, Braune N, Hartnick CJ. Vocal fold medialization in children: injection laryngoplasty, thyroplasty, or nerve reinnervation? Arch Otolaryngol Head Neck Surg 2007; 133: 767–771

[16] Smith ME, Roy N, Stoddard K. Ansa-RLN reinnervation for unilateral vocal fold paralysis in adolescents and young adults. Int J Pediatr Otorhinolaryngol 2008; 72: 1311–1316

[17] Gray SD, Smith ME, Schneider H. Voice disorders in children. Pediatr Clin North Am 1996; 43: 1357–1384

[18] Hirano M. Structure and vibratory behavior of the vocal folds. In: Sawashima M, Franklin S, eds. Dynamic Aspects of Speech Production. Tokyo, Japan: University of Tokyo Press; 1977:13–30

[19] Hirano M. Structure of the vocal fold in normal and disease states: anatomical and physical studies. ASHA Rep. 1981; 11: 11–30

[20] Johns MM. Update on the etiology, diagnosis, and treatment of vocal fold nodules, polyps, and cysts. Curr Opin Otolaryngol Head Neck Surg 2003; 11: 456–461

[21] Kuhn J, Toohill RJ, Ulualp SO et al. Pharyngeal acid reflux events in patients with vocal cord nodules. Laryngoscope 1998; 108: 1146–1149

[22] Shah RK, Woodnorth GH, Glynn A, Nuss RC. Pediatric vocal nodules: correlation with perceptual voice analysis. Int J Pediatr Otorhinolaryngol 2005; 69: 903–909

[23] Wohl DL. Nonsurgical management of pediatric vocal fold nodules. Arch Otolaryngol Head Neck Surg 2005; 131: 68–70, discussion 71–72

[24] Hartnick CJ, Rehbar R, Prasad V. Development and maturation of the pediatric human vocal fold lamina propria. Laryngoscope 2005; 115: 4–15

[25] Behrman A, Sulica L. Voice rest after microlaryngoscopy: current opinion and practice. Laryngoscope 2003; 113: 2182–2186

[26] Zeitels SM, Hillman RE, Desloge R, Mauri M, Doyle PB. Phonomicrosurgery in singers and performing artists: treatment outcomes, management theories, and future directions. Ann Otol Rhinol Laryngol Suppl 2002; 190: 21–40

[27] Kosko JR, Derkay CS. Role of cesarean section in prevention of recurrent respiratory papillomatosis—is there one? Int J Pediatr Otorhinolaryngol 1996; 35: 31–38

[28] Armstrong LR, Derkay CS, Reeves WC. Initial results from the national registry for juvenile-onset recurrent respiratory papillomatosis. RRP Task Force. Arch Otolaryngol Head Neck Surg 1999; 125: 743–748

[29] Derkay C Multi-Disciplinary Task Force on Recurrent Respiratory Papillomas. Cidofovir for recurrent respiratory papillomatosis (RRP): a re-assessment of risks. Int J Pediatr Otorhinolaryngol 2005; 69: 1465–1467

[30] Lee AS, Rosen CA. Efficacy of cidofovir injection for the treatment of recurrent respiratory papillomatosis. J Voice 2004; 18: 551–556

[31] Rosen CA, Bryson PC. Indole-3-carbinol for recurrent respiratory papillomatosis: long-term results. J Voice 2004; 18: 248–253

[32] Healy GB, Gelber RD, Trowbridge AL, Grundfast KM, Ruben RJ, Price KN. Treatment of recurrent respiratory papillomatosis with human leukocyte interferon. Results of a multicenter randomized clinical trial. N Engl J Med 1988; 319: 401–407

[33] Shikowitz MJ, Abramson AL, Freeman K, Steinberg BM, Nouri M. Efficacy of DHE photodynamic therapy for respiratory papillomatosis: immediate and long-term results. Laryngoscope 1998; 108: 962–967

[34] Endres DR, Bauman NM, Burke D, Smith RJ. Acyclovir in the treatment of recurrent respiratory papillomatosis. A pilot study. Ann Otol Rhinol Laryngol 1994; 103: 301–305

[35] Lippman SM, Donovan DT, Frankenthaler RA et al. 13-Cis-retinoic acid plus interferon-alpha 2a in recurrent respiratory papillomatosis. J Natl Cancer Inst 1994; 86: 859–861
[36] Zeitels SM, Barbu AM, Landau-Zemer T et al. Local injection of bevacizumab (Avastin) and angiolytic KTP laser treatment of recurrent respiratory papillomatosis of the vocal folds: a prospective study. Ann Otol Rhinol Laryngol 2011; 120: 627–634
[37] DeCou JM, Jones DC, Jacobs HD, Touloukian RJ. Successful ex utero intrapartum treatment (EXIT) procedure for congenital high airway obstruction syndrome (CHAOS) owing to laryngeal atresia. J Pediatr Surg 1998; 33: 1563–1565
[38] Amir M, Youssef T. Congenital glottic web: management and anatomical observation. Clin Respir J 2010; 4: 202–207
[39] Myer CM, O'Connor DM, Cotton RT. Proposed grading system for subglottic stenosis based on endotracheal tube sizes. Ann Otol Rhinol Laryngol 1994; 103: 319–323
[40] Zalzal GH, Loomis SR, Derkay CS, Murray SL, Thomsen J. Vocal quality of decannulated children following laryngeal reconstruction. Laryngoscope 1991; 101: 425–429
[41] Smith ME, Marsh JH, Cotton RT, Myer CM. Voice problems after pediatric laryngotracheal reconstruction: videolaryngostroboscopic, acoustic, and perceptual assessment. Int J Pediatr Otorhinolaryngol 1993; 25: 173–181
[42] MacArthur CJ, Kearns GH, Healy GB. Voice quality after laryngotracheal reconstruction. Arch Otolaryngol Head Neck Surg 1994; 120: 641–647
[43] Bailey CM, Clary RA, Pengilly A, Albert DM. Voice quality following laryngotracheal reconstruction. Int J Pediatr Otorhinolaryngol 1995; 32 Suppl: S93–S95
[44] Koufman JA. The otolaryngologic manifestations of gastroesophageal reflux disease (GERD): a clinical investigation of 225 patients using ambulatory 24-hour pH monitoring and an experimental investigation of the role of acid and pepsin in the development of laryngeal injury. Laryngoscope 1991; 101 Suppl 53: 1–78
[45] Tsou VM, Bishop PR. Gastroesophageal reflux in children. Otolaryngol Clin North Am 1998; 31: 419–434
[46] Marino AJ, Assing E, Carbone MT, Hiatt IM, Hegyi T, Graff M. The incidence of gastroesophageal reflux in preterm infants. J Perinatol 1995; 15: 369–371
[47] Khalaf MN, Porat R, Brodsky NL, Bhandari V. Clinical correlations in infants in the neonatal intensive care unit with varying severity of gastroesophageal reflux. J Pediatr Gastroenterol Nutr 2001; 32: 45–49
[48] Sutphen JL. Pediatric gastroesophageal reflux disease. Gastroenterol Clin North Am 1990; 19: 617–629
[49] Zalzal GH, Tran LP. Pediatric gastroesophageal reflux and laryngopharyngeal reflux. Otolaryngol Clin North Am 2000; 33: 151–161
[50] Andze GO, Brandt ML, St Vil D, Bensoussan AL, Blanchard H. Diagnosis and treatment of gastroesophageal reflux in 500 children with respiratory symptoms: the value of pH monitoring. J Pediatr Surg 1991; 26: 295–299, discussion 299–300
[51] Boogaard R, Huijsmans SH, Pijnenburg MW, Tiddens HA, de Jongste JC, Merkus PJ. Tracheomalacia and bronchomalacia in children: incidence and patient characteristics. Chest 2005; 128: 3391–3397[Medline]
[52] Jamal N, Bent JP, Vicencio AG. A neurologic etiology for tracheomalacia? Int J Pediatr Otorhinolaryngol 2009; 73: 885–887
[53] Yalçin E, Doğru D, Ozçelik U, Kiper N, Aslan AT, Gözaçan A. Tracheomalacia and bronchomalacia in 34 children: clinical and radiologic profiles and associations with other diseases. Clin Pediatr (Phila) 2005; 44: 777–781
[54] Vinograd I, Keidar S, Weinberg M, Silbiger A. Treatment of airway obstruction by metallic stents in infants and children. J Thorac Cardiovasc Surg 2005; 130: 146–150

22 Cough and the Unified Airway

Manikandan Sugumaran and Kenneth W. Altman

Cough is a common problem encountered by many specialties that is significant to our public health system and daily living. It is the single leading diagnosis for outpatient visits to physicians (other than a general medical examination) and supports an over-the-counter pharmaceutical industry approaching US $3.6 billion annually. However, with a prevalence from 9 to 33% worldwide, it is not uncommon for it to be overlooked as a minor detail in a patient's history.[1] The complaint of cough can apply to a wide spectrum of problems. On an individual level, it may equate to embarrassment during coughing episodes, interference with one's occupation, or the sentinel symptom of a life-threatening process. On a global level, it may be a reflection of environmental triggers, dietary trends, or an infectious epidemic.

Cough is often categorized by duration of symptoms, which are addressed later in this chapter. Although the acute cough (< 3 weeks) and subacute cough (3–8 weeks) carry similar concerns as chronic cough (> 8 weeks), patients with the latter are those who seek medical attention more often. As the cough becomes chronic, it is not uncommon for other symptoms to become noticed in a "cause and effect" model. These symptoms include but are not limited to: globus, hoarseness, dyspnea, emesis, postnasal drip, laryngospasm, etc. However, it may be unclear whether the cough is the "cause" or the "effect." For this reason, patients see a variety of physicians to help them, including primary care physicians, pulmonologists, gastroenterologists, otolaryngologists, and allergists. It would not be uncommon for one of these physicians to diagnose and treat the patient adequately. Conversely, chronic cough is often multifactorial and isolating the source of the cough to one cause can lead to frustration from the physician and disappointment from the patient. The causes of cough along with an appreciation of their interrelatedness is depicted in ▶ Fig. 22.1.

As otolaryngologists, we have the unique ability to champion and coordinate the care of these complicated issues.[1] Due to the increasing cost of health care, there have been recent strides to improve outcomes, lower cost, and increase the value of care provided.[2,3] This is sometimes best served in a coordinated team approach termed *integrated practice units*. These have been employed in the treatment of cancer and cleft palate management, where a multidisciplinary team is needed. Management of complicated patients with cough can be best accomplished with these teams. The decision to involve other specialties through consultation is discussed in this chapter. As otolaryngologists, we are in position to have a comprehensive view of the problem and need to appreciate which patients would be best served with the help of other specialties.

The requisite of a variety of specialties to appreciate the total picture involved with cough is a demonstration of the unified airway, and appreciating it is an integral component to understanding and treating cough.[4] The unified airway is a model that has evolved from previous proposed mechanisms and has

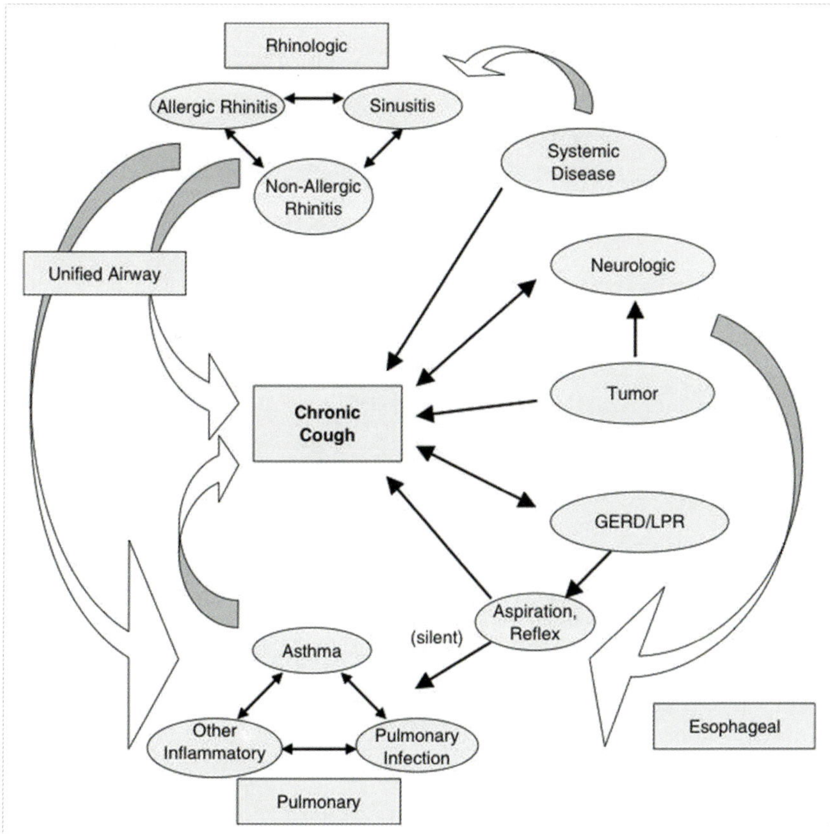

Fig. 22.1 Flow diagram showing the different contributing factors to chronic cough and their relationships. GERD, gastroesophageal reflux disease; LPR, laryngopharyngeal reflux.

been described as the presence and severity of disease processes within the upper and lower airway that are linked closely, with exacerbations of the disease in one component of the airway likely encouraging worsening of airway disease diffusely.[5]

Throughout this chapter, the importance of the unified airway will be readily evident as an underlying theme. Over the past decade, there has been increasing awareness of the relationships between inflammatory diseases of the upper and lower airway. Data suggest the entire respiratory tract, from the eustachian tubes through the nose and paranasal sinuses to the lower pulmonary trees, behaves as a unit. Although the gastrointestinal tract is not part of the unified airway, there is a clear implication that it can alter the airway environment. The larynx serves as a bridge between the two main divisions of the unified airway. Potential explanations for the effects on the larynx that lead to symptoms of cough and dysphonia could (1) direct airway inflammation in the laryngeal structures, (2) manifestations of the trafficking of materials through this anatomic region, or (3) the development of secondary edema as a result of the cough.[4]

Our goal in this chapter is to guide the otolaryngologist through the care of patients with cough. The chapter will highlight the important points of the history and physical exam, describe many of the most common diagnoses in the differential, evaluate the myriad ancillary tests, guide the physician when other specialist input may be beneficial, and explore the treatment options.

22.1 History and Physical Examination

The initial encounter with a patient who seeks attention for cough can be challenging because it is a nonspecific symptom that can be associated with a broad spectrum of diagnoses. An organized approach must be employed, with an initial focus on the duration of the cough. A lack of efficiency and effectiveness in the evaluation of the cough can negatively impact patient satisfaction, worsen their sense of helplessness, and lower the quality of life.[6] Guidelines have been published in several countries to help diagnose and manage cough. The common features shared by these guidelines are discussed in this chapter, and the discussion focues on immunocompetent adult patients with cough.

22.1.1 Individualizing Cough

The physiologic mechanism of cough is simple. The cough reflex serves as a protective mechanism and important component of respiratory clearance, especially when the normal mucocilliary transport mechanism is inadequate or overwhelmed.[7] The reflex manifests itself as a coordinated release of air, with intrathoracic pressures as high as 300 mm Hg and air velocities up to 500 miles per hour. The toll on the body after repeated vigorous coughing is often the reason why patients seek help. It is important to appreciate this toll while interviewing patients. Profiling the impact of cough on a patient dictates the tone and goals of the visit. Some seek confirmation that the cough is not a sign of a life-threatening disease. Others seek a remedy for a long-term issue that has plagued them with conditions like broken ribs, syncope, and public embarrassment. Understanding patient goals and motivation leads to higher patient satisfaction.

22.1.2 Taking a Focused History

The stratification of cough based on the duration of symptoms helps to narrow the differential diagnoses and is the basis behind many guidelines for management of cough.[8,9] Cough is categorized as acute (i.e., lasting < 3 weeks), subacute (lasting 3–8 weeks); or chronic (> 8 weeks). A list of causes based on duration of symptoms can be seen in ▶ Table 22.1 and will be discussed in depth. There should be an emphasis on detecting "red flag" symptoms. These are symptoms or details that are indicative of a serious life-threatening condition or reflect the severe nature of the cough. They include, but are not limited to, the following: syncope, rib fracture, pneumonia, hemoptysis, stridor, and palpitations. These symptoms may dictate that the patient receive acute care and bypass the routine cough management paradigm. Recent illnesses, such as upper respiratory infections (URI), are an important detail to elicit during the history, along

Table 22.1 Common causes of cough based on duration

Cough classification	Most common causes
Acute: < 3 weeks	Viral upper respiratory tract infection (URTI) Exacerbation of underlying lung disorder (chronic obstructive pulmonary disorder, asthma) Acute environmental exposure to irritant Acute cardiopulmonary disease (e.g., pneumonia, pulmonary embolism)
Subacute: 3–8 weeks	Postinfectious cough (URTI, pertussis) Non-postinfectious cough (chronic cough)
Chronic: > 8 weeks	Active cigarette smoking or chronic irritant use Angiotensin-converting enzyme inhibitor use Radiographic apparent disease process of the lung With normal chest radiograph: • Upper airway cough syndrome • Asthma • Nonasthmatic eosinophilic bronchitis • Gastroesophageal reflux disease

Source: Adapted from Madison JM, Irwin RS. Cough: a worldwide problem. Otolaryngologic Clinics of North America. 2010;43(1):1–13, vii.

with associated symptoms. The common cold is the most common cause of acute cough, and subacute cough is frequently the result of a lingering URI that resolves prior to 8 weeks. The timing of the cough may also help with diagnosis. Cough with eating and postprandial cough may indicate a reflux-associated cough, or an acute onset of cough with choking episode may point to a foreign body aspiration. The productive nature of a cough lacks specificity for exact diagnoses, but studies have shown that a productive cough is more likely associated with a pulmonary etiology.[10]

The social history plays a large role in the evaluation of cough. The living and working environment can be a major contributing factor to cough. Reviewing any changes in the patient's living environment or addition of pets may identify undiagnosed allergies that contribute to the cough. Cough may also be irritant-induced by dust, chemicals, or debris. Finally, exposure to tobacco smoke is an obvious cause of cough. The smoking history of the patient and a history of smoke exposure must be obtained. A review of medications should be performed to ensure there are none being taken that cause cough, and no medication changes have been correlated with the duration of the cough.

At this juncture, a review of the potential diagnoses must then be considered, and history taking and review of systems should be geared toward supporting one or multiple diagnoses. Remember, it is relatively common to have multiple causes for cough, especially for the patient with chronic cough. Each diagnosis requires certain evidence to either support or oppose the likelihood of it being a cause. A recommended approach is to "clinically profile" the patients into common diagnoses. Rhinosinus disease, gastroesophageal reflux disease (GERD), asthma, and noneosinophilic bronchitis are four common causes of chronic cough that will fit a clinical profile based on questioning.[11]

There are potential pitfalls that may interfere with the care of the chronic cough patient. Twenty-three percent of patients referred to a cough specialist have been misdiagnosed with psychogenic cough due to a lack of convincing history of the common differential diagnoses.[12] Narrowing the etiology to one source can also lead to failure in management. Up to 93% of troublesome coughs have more than one cause.[13] Patients will fail to get better when clinicians do not acknowledge the common causes for cough and treatment is initiated for another "more obvious cause." For example, a smoker may have cough from the irritant effect of tobacco smoke. However, unless there is cessation with resolution of cough, smoking cannot be ascertained as the only source of cough. The patient is still likely to suffer from other common causes of cough.

22.1.3 Physical Examination

The physical examination of a patient presenting with cough should consist of a routine otolaryngology exam with a focus on the upper airway, laryngoscopy, and auscultation of the lungs. The routine otolaryngology exam can pick up other manifestations of the common causes of cough. It should be conducted in a systematic manner to avoid missing those manifestations. Systemic diseases that may play a role in cough, such as sarcoidosis or granulomatosis with polyangitis (formerly, Wegener granulomatosis), can be picked up by more obvious findings on routine exam. Otologic exam may reveal manifestations of allergies, with retracted tympanic membranes or serous otitis. The neck exam may reveal lymphadenopathy, suggesting infection or malignancy. Neurologic exam may detect weakness, which can be indicative of vocal fold palsy. The examination of the upper airway for cough is best performed with a flexible fiberoptic scope. Although a Hopkins rod 70-degree telescope will provide excellent visualization of the larynx and surrounding area, it fails to provide a "bird's-eye view" of the laryngeal environment. It can miss sinus and nasopharyngeal contributions to inflammation and cough. The recent advances in distal chip technology have made these scopes readily available for office use. However, a true color match is better with a traditional fiberoptic scope. For this reason, it is recommended to use a quality traditional fiberoptic scope with direct visualization through the eyepiece.[14]

Although there may be a tendency to focus on the laryngeal findings with a fiberoptic scope, a comprehensive exam should include examination of both sides of the nasal cavity, nasopharynx, oropharynx, and hypopharynx as well. Some findings will be readily apparent, such as signs of infection, tumors, or motility issues. However, most of the time, the findings will prove to be vague, but they can paint a picture and trail of inflammation or irritation. The clinician should pay special attention to the color, vascularity, and presence of edema on the mucosal lining from nasal cavity to the larynx. Lymphoid hyperplasia and cobblestoning are also common signs of chronic inflammation, particularly in the oropharynx. Mucus secretion and clearance play a crucial role in primary physical defenses. Overproduction of phlegm and mucus is a hallmark of infectious and chronic inflammatory airway disease and should be noted during the exam.[15]

The laryngeal examination is most efficacious when done in a systematic manner as well. Once again, mucus secretions, mucosal lining, and patterns of erythema and edema should be inspected. The clinician should appreciate pooling of secretions and/or laryngeal penetration, which may be warning signs for aspiration. The laryngeal anatomy can be broken into subsites to help objectively document findings. Each site should be scrutinized for any benign- or malignant-appearing growths. A complete laryngeal examination should include active phonation and quiet breathing. Ulcerations and erythema can be hidden when the glottis is closed during phonation. Mobility, symmetry, and closure of the true vocal folds are best appreciated during phonation. The subglottis can be appreciated in a cooperative patient with proper positioning. Although this is not a routine means of evaluating the subglottis, it can provide a glimpse at the laryngeal subsite.

22.2 Differential Diagnoses

Once the history and physical have been completed, the differential diagnoses for the patient should start to take shape. As mentioned, the duration of the cough will serve as the primary means of narrowing the differential. There are also causes of cough that should be immediately included or excluded in your differential based on simple questioning. These exclusionary diagnoses are discussed first, followed by the common causes of acute, subacute, and chronic cough. It should also be noted that as otolaryngologists, the majority of patients seen in our offices will present with chronic cough. Most acute cough and even subacute cough is either resolved prior to the patient's seeking medical advice or is addressed by a primary care physician. One study has shown that 20% of visits to a primary care physician are for acute cough, making it one of the most common causes for consultation in primary care.[16] Only a fraction of these patients will require evaluation by an otolaryngologist.

22.2.1 Exclusionary Diagnoses

Angiotensin-Converting Enzyme Inhibitors

In 2010, angiotensin-converting enzyme (ACE) inhibitors were the fifth most commonly prescribed drug class in the United States, accounting for 168 million prescriptions.[17] They have replaced beta-blockers and diuretics as first-line treatment for hypertension. Otolaryngologic side effects include angioedema and cough. The incidence of cough has been reported anywhere from 0.2 to 33%.[12] The cough is usually described as "dry" or "tickly" and is not dose dependent.[18] The time of onset can be unpredictable, with cough potentially occurring from the first dose to years after initiation of treatment. It should not be assumed that all patients taking an ACE inhibitor have cough, but it needs consideration. If medically reasonable, replacing the ACE inhibitor with an angiotensin II receptor antagonist should be considered prior to performing extensive diagnostic testing. Switching between two different ACE inhibitors is not adequate, as the side effect is of the drug class. Once the drug is discontinued, adequate time should be allotted for resolution of the cough. The median time for resolution of the cough has been shown to be 26 days.[18]

Chronic Bronchitis: Smoke and Other Inhaled Irritants

Environmental irritants are obvious causes of cough that should be elicited during the history, smoke exposure being the most common irritant. The common presentation is cough that is worse in the morning, with phlegm production. Cough secondary to smoke or other environmental irritant exposure is termed *chronic bronchitis*. In the absence of smoke exposure or environmental irritants, patients who have cough–phlegm syndrome should not be diagnosed as having chronic bronchitis because it does not meet the definition.[19] Workers with exposure to low-molecular-weight particles have been shown to have an increased incidence of cough.[16] And community studies have shown that active smoking is associated with a two- to threefold increase and passive smoking a 1.3-fold to 1.6-fold increase in prevalence of cough. These studies have been shown the effect to be dose dependent. They have also shown a return to near normal prevalence in exsmokers.[20,21,22] When active cigarette smoking is the lone etiology of cough, 94% of patients notice improvement in symptoms after abstinence for at least 4 weeks. However, there is an initial short-term increase in cough sensitivity prior to resolution. Patients with cough and irritant exposure may suffer from multiple other causes, but removal of the irritant should be the initial step in management. Once a reasonable amount of time has been allotted with no resolution of cough, further workup is warranted.

22.2.2 Acute Cough: Less than Three Weeks

Upper Respiratory Tract Infections

Upper respiratory tract infections (URTI), such as the common cold, are the most common cause of acute cough. The common viral pathogens are influenza, parainfluenza, adenovirus, rhinovirus, and respiratory syncytial virus. The frequency of acute cough due to URTI in a population is correlated with the incidence of influenza. The cough associated with untreated URTIs is most prevalent in the first 48 hours, at 83%, and over the course of the next 2 weeks, the prevalence diminishes to 26%.[23] The clinical presentation is predictable for otherwise healthy patients, with cough being part of the constellation of symptoms associated with the URTI. The symptoms predominantly originate from the nasal passages: nasal obstruction, rhinorrhea, sneezing, increased lacrimation, etc. Acute dyspnea is uncommon and is a red flag for a more severe process. Fever may or may not be associated with the symptoms. Examination of the nasal cavity usually demonstrates clear watery discharge with edematous mucosal lining of the turbinates. Mucosal discharge that is green or yellow, thicker, or foul smelling may be indicative of a bacterial component of the infection. Exam findings distal to the nasal cavity will likely show increased secretions, mild edema, and erythema in the posterior glottis associated with the severity of the cough. Auscultation of the lung fields is usually normal. Rarely is hospital admission or further workup for URTI-associated cough required, and they should be reserved for immunocompromised patients. Even preliminary testing, such as a chest x-ray has a low yield, with 97% being normal.[24] Cough associated with a UTRI is almost always benign and should therefore be managed conservatively. Prescription medications are usually regarded as unnecessary, and most patients report benefit from over-the-counter preparations, commonly antihistamines and decongestants, despite little evidence of specific pharmacologic effect.[9] Central modulation of the cough reflex has been shown to be a simple means of controlling the acute cough. Effective agents include dextromethorphan, morphine, and codeine. Some of these agents should be used with caution due to their abuse potential. Additionally, agents like mucolytics may aid in the symptomatic relief of cough. A list of these medications and others, with their influences on cough, is shown in ▶ Table 22.2.[9,25,26]

Other Causes of Acute Cough

Acute cough is also associated with exacerbations of chronic diseases like asthma, chronic obstructive pulmonary disease, allergies, and the initial catarrhal stages of *Bordetella pertussis*. An increased suspicion should be raised with patients having a prior diagnosis or risk factors noted during the history. The history and physical will also highlight red flags, which may point to more serious causes of acute cough. Although rarely an isolated symptom, acute cough can present in patients with pneumonia, congestive heart failure, and even pulmonary embolism. It is the responsibility of the clinician to determine when patients may be suffering from the aforementioned life-threatening diagnoses or the more common URTI-associated cough and to conduct further evaluation and management.

Table 22.2 Antitussive agents

Agent	Mechanism	Comments
Codeine	Opioid	May serve purpose in spontaneous cough; however, ineffective in common cold and cough associated with chronic obstructive pulmonary disease.
Morphine	Opioid	40% decrease in cough in patients with cough refractory to specific therapy; significant side effects and abuse potential.
Dextromethorphan	Nonopioid	No effect on chronic irritant cough (i.e., smoking); slight improvement with cough due to upper airway disorders.
N-acetylcysteine	Mucolytic, possible antioxidant	Significant alleviation in patients with chemical injury to lungs; decreases mucus viscosity to allow easier clearance.
Erdosteine	Possible antioxidant	Potentiates cough suppressant effect of antibiotics during infection
First-generation antihistamine	Sedative	Suppresses cough; however, sedative effect causes drowsiness; consider for nocturnal cough

22.2.3 Subacute Cough: Lasting Three to Eight Weeks

Categorizing cough based on duration of symptoms has a catch; all chronic cough started as an acute cough that extended beyond 3 weeks. However, the diagnostic group of chronic cough would be diluted if it included all cough that lingered past 3 weeks but ended prior to 8 weeks. This specific diagnostic group, where the cough has lasted 3 to 8 weeks, is known as subacute cough. The main diagnostic distinction that should be made in this group is whether the cough is postinfectious or not. Patients who have a noninfectious etiology for their cough, but have symptoms between 3 and 8 weeks, are likely to have cough triggered by the causes of chronic cough which can often be multifactorial.[7]

Postinfectious cough is classified as a cough lasting between 3 to 8 weeks, with a chest x-ray ruling out pneumonia. The pathogenesis of subacute postinfectious cough is not completely understood, but it has been thought to be due to the extensive disruption of epithelial integrity and widespread airway inflammation of the upper and/or lower airways with or without transient hyperresponsiveness.[27] An additional mechanism may be that the increased secretions produced secondary to the level of inflammation continue to stimulate the cough reflex.[23] It is also worth mentioning that gastroesophageal reflux may play a role in subacute cough. This is not to say that the cough causes reflux, but the repeated forceful cough causes increases in abdominal pressure that may aggravate pre-existing reflux disease.[27]

Bordetella pertussis or "whooping cough" is a unique cause of postinfectious cough and is highly contagious. The diagnosis of *B. pertussis* is suggested by recent infections in the community, contact with a known case, a cough with biphasic course, or a characteristic "whoop" or cough–vomit syndrome.[27] It is important to distinguish a biphasic cough from the two first exacerbations of chronic lung disease. The timeline for pertussis is an initial 1 to 3 week incubation period, a catarrhal period that may include conjunctivitis, rhinorrhea, fever, and cough, and a paroxysmal period that features worsening of the cough. This clinical profile is the cornerstone of the diagnosis. Laboratory or serological testing is variable and often performed 2 weeks after infection, when cultures of the nasopharynx are usually negative. The organism is extremely contagious; one active case has the potential of infecting 70 to 100% of the household and 50 to 80% school contacts. Although the dTap vaccine has caused an initial decline in pertussis, there has been a recent resurgence.[28] Potential explanations may be the waning effectiveness of the immunization over time, the decrease in adults who gained immunity from a natural infection, or that the immunization is not protective for all children. *Bordetella parapertussis* infection can produce similar symptoms as regular pertussis; however, it does not produce pertussis toxin and is not covered by the standard dTap vaccine.

Suspected pertussis should be managed immediately and not delayed for confirmation with diagnostic testing. Erythromycin (or trimethoprim/sulfamethoxazole for patients who cannot tolerate a macrolide) is recommended. Patients should avoid exposure to the public and isolate themselves during the first 5 days of treatment to avoid spread of the infection.[27] Treatment initiated during the paroxysmal stage has been shown to be somewhat effective, but the benefit is limited.[29] Symptomatic control of the paroxysmal cough with beta-agonist, corticosteroids, and antihistamines has been shown to have no benefit for these patients and is not recommended.[27]

22.2.4 Chronic Cough

Chronic cough, defined as cough lasting longer than 8 weeks, can be a very frustrating problem for the patient and clinician. Much of this frustration stems from the fact that a significant portion (25%) of these patients will have multiple causes for the cough.[12] One or more of these causes may have been treated during the treatment course for these patients; yet, the patient may still have cough because another cause has been overlooked during the treatment plan. After completion of the focused history and physical, chronic systemic disease, tumors, or neurologic conditions should be apparent as contributing to the cough. If these more obvious diagnoses have been excluded, the next important step in the evaluation process is a chest x-ray. Any findings on the chest x-ray should be addressed first as a potential cause of the cough.[8] It is during this period that a consultation by a pulmonologist should be considered. These causes are pulmonary related and include, but are not limited to, interstitial lung disease, bronchiectasis, or bronchogenic carcinoma. Disease-specific treatment should be initiated by a pulmonologist, and the patient's symptoms should be followed to

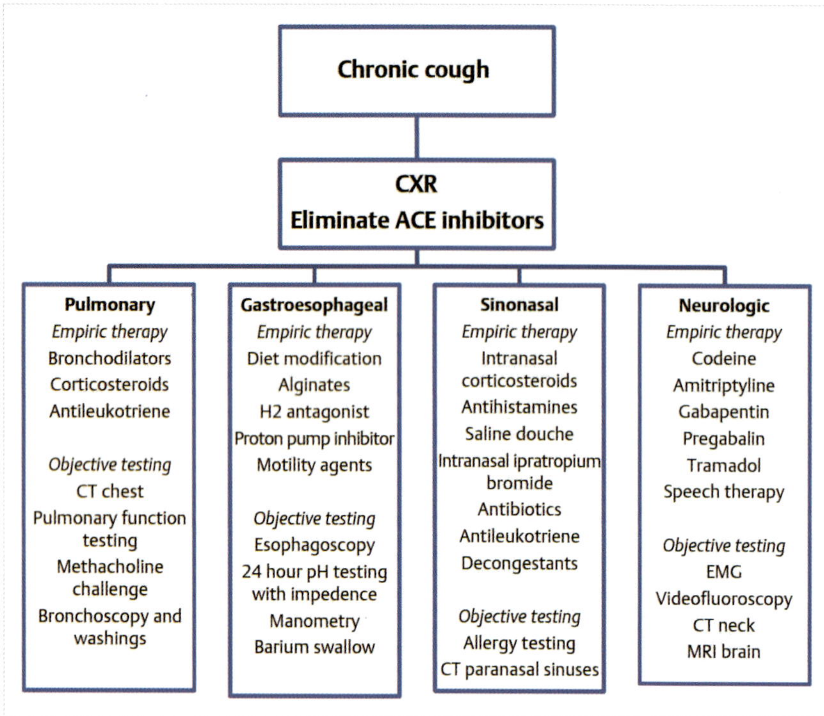

Fig. 22.2 Management algorithm for chronic cough in adult patients. ACE-I, angiotensin-converting enzyme inhibitor; A/D, antihistamine/decongestant; BD, bronchodilator; HRCT, high-resolution computed tomography scan; ICS, inhaled corticosteroid; LTRA, leukotriene receptor antagonist; PPI, proton pump inhibitor. Section 26 referred to in the figure begins on page 2065 of the American College of Chest Physicians cough guidelines. (Data from Pratter MR, Brightling CE, Boulet L-P et al. An empiric integrative approach to the management of cough: ACCP evidence-based clinical practice guidelines. Chest 2006; 129:225S)

the end of the treatment course. If the patient's cough is not completely relieved, the otolaryngologist should then consider that other more common causes of chronic cough might be contributing simultaneously.[7] According to the American College of Chest Physicians (ACCP) evidence-based clinical practice guidelines, these common causes of chronic cough are upper airway cough syndrome (UACS), asthma, nonasthmatic eosinophilic bronchitis (NAEB), and GERD. The management algorithm for chronic cough is shown in ▶ Fig. 22.2.[30]

Upper Airway Cough Syndrome

Upper airway cough syndrome (UACS) is the preferred nomenclature for cough attributable to what is commonly known as "postnasal drip." By itself or in combination with other conditions, UACS has been found to be the most common cause of chronic cough.[31] These rhinosinus conditions may be of irritant, infectious, or allergic etiology and represent a true reflection of the unified airway model. A modified model proposed by Krouse[4] to illustrate the effects of irritants as well as indolent sinus disease involves three primary components in cases of chronic rhinogenic laryngitis and cough.

1. Inflammatory effects occur at all levels of the respiratory tract, leading to mediator release and increased edema and mucus production in the nose, sinuses, pharynx, and lungs.
2. This increased mucus is transported throughout the respiratory tract, both upstream and downstream, and results in increased mucus at the level of the larynx.
3. Increased mucus and irritation in the larynx and pharynx lead to compensatory behaviors, including throat clearing and coughing, which result in anatomical and histological changes to the laryngeal mucosa, with observable, discrete laryngeal pathologies, such as edema and irregularities, which may play a role in cough.

The reason postnasal drip has been replaced by UACS is because the former term implies that a "drip" is felt by the patient. When felt, it is described as the sensation of fluid dripping down on to their throats from the back of the nose, frequently requiring a cough or clearing of the throat. On exam, the nasopharynx or oropharynx may show mucoid/mucopurulent secretions or cobblestoning of the mucosa to indicate chronic inflammation.[32] However, it is important to know that patients may not always feel the drip sensation, and the above-stated clinical picture is neither sensitive nor specific.[7] Furthermore, cough may be the only manifestation of this complicated process. Further frustration in this picture comes from the fact that there is no objective means of proving the rhinosinus etiology of cough. Computed tomography (CT) scans of the sinuses may be useful in the diagnosis of patients with sinusitis, but clinicians must ultimately use their judgment based on the history and physical exam findings to place the patient in a clinical profile that most likely fits and will dictate management. Appropriate management with resolution of cough is the only means of diagnosing UACS.

The specific upper airway disease that is inciting the irritation and compensatory cough dictates the treatment options for UACS. When there is an allergic rhinitis component, avoidance of the allergen is ideal, but often not realistic. Nasal steroids, antihistamines, and/or cromolyn are usually the initial drug choices for the treatment of cough due to allergic rhinitis.[33] Allergic immunotherapy for desensitization is also a viable option, but not for immediate results. It may be reasonable to treat acute sinusitis initially with antihistamines and decongestants. If the infection does not show signs of resolution, it is best to start antibiotic therapy directed at the most likely bacteria implicated. These are commonly *Streptococcus pneumoniae, Haemophilus influenza, Staphylococcus aureus,* and some anaerobes. Included with the antibiotic should be an intranasal steroid and possibly a nasal decongestant, such as oxymetazoline. There is a role for surgery for patients suffering from chronic rhinosinusitis (CRS) or allergic fungal sinusitis (AFS). Physically removing the irritants in AFS, allowing the sinus to process mucus better in CRS, and providing better aeration of the sinuses may sometimes be a required therapeutic intervention when medical management has failed.

Gastroesophageal Reflux Disease

Understanding the causative relationship between GERD and laryngopharyngeal reflux (LPR) with cough is still in evolution. In fact, LPR as a separate diagnosis from GERD is a relatively recent idea. Laryngopharyngeal reflux is the diagnosis given for manifestations in the pharynx and larynx secondary to the backflow of stomach contents, and diagnosis is commonly made by an otolaryngologist.[34] This is an important concept to understand by all members of the treatment team. Mixed messages given to the patient regarding their diagnosis and results of diagnostic testing can be confusing and frustrating. For the purposes of this chapter, the distinctions between the two diagnoses will be bypassed to focus on their contribution to chronic cough. The pathophysiology behind reflux-associated cough is related to the retrograde flow of gastric contents past the lower esophageal sphincter (LES). The LES reserves the ability to allow retrograde flow for instances such as emesis or release of gas, and pathologic reflux may be a byproduct of this capability.[35] There is variability in reflux episodes and severity from patient to patient, which can be related to intra-abdominal and intrathoracic pressures, fluctuations in LES tone, and the composition of gastric contents. The contents are not limited to acid and include bile[36] and pepsin,[37] which have been implicated in laryngeal irritation. An esophageal–bronchial reflex in the mucosa of the distant esophagus may also play a role in stimulating chronic cough.[38] Hence, the use of the term "acid reflux" may be confusing and misleading when describing chronic cough caused by GERD/LPR.

The prevalence of GERD-related chronic cough based upon favorable response with empiric treatment has increased from 10% in 1981 to 36% in 1998 based on prospective studies published by Irwin et al.[39] Similar to UACS, alone or in combination, it is one of the most common causes of chronic cough. Reflux should be suspected in patients with daily heartburn and regurgitation[38] but is often present in only about half of patients. Cough in the morning, cough after eating, and cough with phonation are common scenarios associated with cough secondary to reflux. However, it is important to know that there is rarely anything about the timing or severity of reflux-associated cough that makes it unique from any other causes. Risk factors for GERD include medications like alendronate, beta-2 agonists, calcium channel blockers, anticholinergics, and inhaled corticosteroids, which may influence both LES tone and gastric contents. Certain foods have also been proven to increase the irritating effect, such as chocolate, tomatoes, and citric acid-containing foods.[39] Although it is difficult to quantify each risk factor in terms of contribution to the cough, it can be assumed that removing such risk factors would be a component in the management of these patients. The clinical profile recommended by the ACCP for these patients has been proven to be highly predictive that the cough will respond to antireflux management. However, when examined carefully, it is a profile that simply rules out the other most common cause of chronic cough. For this reason, empiric treatment with improvement or resolution of cough is the only means to confirm a diagnosis of cough secondary to reflux.

The neck should not be overlooked during physical examination. Patients may describe pain, discomfort, or even a globus sensation at the level of the cricoid. Tenderness on palpation around the larynx may be indicative of reflux or complications of reflux, such as vocal granulomas. A mass in the neck should raise suspicion for malignancy. The fiberoptic exam and laryngeal findings have been the topic of debate because such findings have been felt to be neither sensitive nor specific, leading to overdiagnosis of reflux. However, the findings of erythema and edema of the true folds, interarytenoid mucosa, the medial aspect of the arytenoid, and posterior pharyngeal wall have been shown to be associated with reflux.[40,41] During the exam, one must also consider that these findings are associated with the trauma from cough itself. Regardless of the source, the findings have been shown to improve with empiric treatment.[41]

Further diagnostic testing should be performed when a patient's history or physical point to a more complicated clinical picture or severe symptoms or findings. In the case of the more severe or atypical symptoms, involving a gastrointestinal (GI) consultation may prove to be prudent. Common diagnostic testing that may be conducted with your GI colleague includes barium esophagram, esophagoscopy, and pH probe testing with or without impedance testing. These studies should not be used to diagnose cough due to reflux, rather they should be employed to explore the severity or other complicating factors of reflux. Barium esophagram is a good study to understand dysmotility, strictures, and some esophageal lining disease. In regard to reflux, the study approaches a sensitivity as low as 33% in some studies.[42] Esophagoscopy for subjectively examining the esophageal lining can be useful in the diagnosis of esophagitis, Barrett esophagus, and esophageal malignancy. Esophagitis can be seen in patients with GERD; however, studies have shown that the incidence is quite variable. Cough is also a common symptom seen in patients with carcinoma of the esophagus, which can be screened for with esophagoscopy. Twenty-four-hour pH testing with impedance should be recommended for a patient when empiric treatment has not improved symptoms or there is need to escalate therapy. Testing with impedance can distinguish between acid and nonacid reflux and how it correlates with symptomatic cough. Studies have shown that acidic events are associated with more symptoms, but nonacidic events have influenced symptoms for a larger time span surrounding the event.[43,44]

Treatment of chronic cough due to reflux is started with eliminating the risk factors associated with disease. Lifestyle changes, such as weight loss and diet modification, should also be explored with the patient. Proton pump inhibitor (PPI) is currently the mainstay of treatment for reflux-induced cough. A trial for 8 weeks is the usual treatment duration to monitor for improvement of symptoms. Although there has been a consensus that PPI treatment has a positive impact on reflux cough, its effects are not universal. This appears to be due in part to the multifactorial influence from nonacid reflux, misdiagnosis, fluctuations, risk factors, and variable compliance. Patients taking a PPI should be advised on risks of decreased calcium absorption, interactions with other medication, and gastric adenomas with long-term use. Alginate available in the form of Gaviscon (GlaxoSmithKline, London, England) shows promise for improving cough secondary to nonacid reflux. It functions by forming a barrier on top of gastric contents and preventing reflux past the LES. Prokinetic medications, such as metoclopramide and domperidone (not sold in the United States), have been shown to control cough and hoarseness when combined with PPI in the majority of patients.[35] The lack of availability of domperidone in the United States and the poor side effect profile of metoclopramide has limited their use. Antireflux surgery should be discussed with the patient when the following four criteria are met: (1) the findings of a 24-h esophageal pH study are positive; (2) the patient fits the clinical profile that reflux disease is the most likely cause of his or her cough; (3) cough has not improved with a minimum of 3 months of intensive therapy; and (4) the patient expresses that cough has not allowed him or her to have a satisfactory quality of life.[39] When these criteria are met, a consultation should be made to the appropriate surgeon for management.

Asthma, Cough-Variant Asthma, and Nonasthmatic Eosinophilic Bronchitis

Asthma accounts for 24 to 29% of chronic cough in nonsmoking adults.[12] The presentation of asthma is typically with the common symptoms of dyspnea and wheezing. Cough may be a sentinel symptom for newly diagnosed asthma, and in a subset of patients with asthma, cough may be the dominant or only symptom.[45] This subset has been classified as having cough-variant asthma (CVA). Although the presentations may be different, the management of both entities is the same. The cough reflex in CVA patients is stronger than in patients with asthma, and the bronchial hyperresponsiveness to methacholine is less. This may explain the discrepancy in symptoms. Nonasthmatic eosinophilic bronchitis (NAEB) is defined as cough with no symptoms or objective findings of airflow obstruction, normal airway hyperresponsiveness, and sputum eosinophilia (> 3% nonsquamous sputum eosinophils).[46] The etiology of asthma and NAEB is unknown, but it can be associated with exposure to inhaled aeroallergen or an occupational sensitizer.[47] On a microscopic level, there are increased mast cell numbers in the smooth muscle of asthmatic patients and in the mucosa of NAEB patients. The different pathways of immunologic airway inflammation for these two entities translate to the contrasting clinical manifestations.

For most patients, the diagnosis of asthma has often already been made, and an associating cough can often be made with a good history. The usual history associated with typical asthma is wheezing, dyspnea, reversible clinical nature, and possibly an identified trigger. Conversely, CVA or cough as the initial presenting symptom for typical asthma can have a limited history and nondiagnostic findings on exam and spirometry. It is recommended by the ACCP that patients with nondiagnostic findings undergo methacholine inhalation challenge (MIC). Although a positive MIC is merely consistent with CVA, and not diagnostic, the very high negative predictive value for a negative MIC essentially rules out asthma as the etiology of cough.[48] If a MIC is unable to be performed, then empiric treatment of asthma should be started. Response to treatment without performing a MIC does not rule out NAEB.[49] Partial response may be achieved within one week with an inhaled bronchodilator, but complete resolution of cough may require up to 8 weeks of treatment with inhaled corticosteroids.[50,51] It is during this process that involvement of a pulmonologist should be considered. For patients with symptoms refractory to treatment or severe symptoms, titration to stronger anti-inflammatory medications may be indicated. Prior to this, bronchoscopy with bronchoalveolar lavage or induced sputum may help identify patients who may benefit from more aggressive treatment.

Patients with chronic cough from suspected NAEB may present with an even more frustrating history and exam findings. These patients frequently present with cough as their sole presenting symptom. In addition to a nondiagnostic exam and normal chest x-ray, patients will exhibit no objective evidence of variable airflow obstruction, or evidence of airway hyperresponsiveness (i.e., a provocative concentration of methacholine producing a 20% decrease in FEV_1 of > 16 mg/mL).[52] At this point, involvement from a pulmonology consultation should be employed. The diagnosis of NAEB is confirmed by the presence of airway eosinophilia with sputum induction or bronchial wash fluid obtained with bronchoscopy. According to the ACCP, > 3% nonsquamous cell sputum eosinophil count is indicative of NAEB.[52] When NAEB is suspected, like other diagnoses for chronic cough, it is confirmed with improvement with treatment. It should be noted that NAEB might be related to a casual allergen or occupational sensitizer. If this is the case, avoidance is the best treatment. Otherwise, inhaled corticosteroid is the first-line treatment. Currently, there is no data available to recommend an inhaled corticosteroid at a certain dose and duration to gain optimal results.[52] If control of symptoms is not resolved, oral corticosteroids may be required. However, if symptoms are reluctant to resolve, it is important to revisit the other common and uncommon causes of chronic cough.

22.3 Conclusion

Treating patients with cough of any duration can be frustrating. The number of potential sources of cough is a very long list, and this is made exponentially longer by the fact that multiple causes are often at play. A systematic way of filtering out the more obvious diagnoses such as cancer, and aspiration, neurogenic, and systemic diseases by taking a careful history and physical exam is a good place to start. Eliminating obvious sources such as ACE inhibitor use or smoking should be prioritized. Stratification of the cough based on duration will then allow focusing on a smaller list of potential diagnoses. It is prudent, as the physician, to explain the process of determining the etiology of the cough to the patient. Matching the patient to a clinical profile and starting empiric treatment may seem like guessing to some patients: especially when the patient returns with limited or no change in symptoms. The patient with chronic cough should understand that a definitive diagnosis is made when there is improvement of symptoms with treatment. It is also important for patients to understand that it is very common to have multiple causes of cough, and this can create a prolonged process in achieving resolution of the cough. Diagnosis and treatment of cough is optimal with the patient's understanding and a collective effort from a multidisciplinary team. As otolaryngologists, it is our role to co-ordinate and champion this systematic approach.

22.4 Key Points

- Cough is best categorized based on the duration of symptoms: acute (< 3 weeks), subacute (3–8 weeks), and chronic (> 8 weeks).
- Understand the patient's goals in seeking your help in the management of their cough.
- As otolaryngologists, we have a unique global perspective of the common etiologies for cough; we should use this perspective to guide the diagnosis and management in a multidisciplinary approach when needed.
- The initial assessment should elicit obvious sources of cough, such as smoking or ACE inhibitor use, which can be eliminated before proceeding with a more extensive workup, and identify any red flags that should require expedited diagnosis and/or management.
- Identifying the cause of chronic cough is often done by empiric treatment for the common etiologies. However, it is not uncommon to have multiple causes, which is an important concept to explain to the patient.
- Further diagnostic testing should be performed when there is a worsening of or failure to improve symptoms after adequate treatment, the severity or profile of symptoms are concerning enough to forgo an extended empiric trial, or if the symptom of cough appears to be a part of a larger problem such as an autoimmune or neurologic disease.

References

[1] Altman KW, Irwin RS. Cough: a new frontier in otolaryngology. Otolaryngol Head Neck Surg 2011; 144: 348–352

[2] Porter ME. A strategy for health care reform—toward a value-based system. N Engl J Med 2009; 361: 109–112

[3] Bohmer RMJ, Lee TH. The shifting mission of health care delivery organizations. N Engl J Med 2009; 361: 551–553

[4] Krouse JH, Altman KW. Rhinogenic laryngitis, cough, and the unified airway. Otolaryngol Clin North Am 2010; 43: 111–121, ix–x

[5] Krouse JH. The unified airway—conceptual framework. Otolaryngol Clin North Am 2008; 41: 257–266, vv.

[6] Kuzniar TJ, Morgenthaler TI, Afessa B, Lim KG. Chronic cough from the patient's perspective. Mayo Clin Proc 2007; 82: 56–60

[7] Madison JM, Irwin RS. Cough: a worldwide problem. Otolaryngol Clin North Am 2010; 43: 1–13, viivii.

[8] Irwin RS, Baumann MH, Bolser DC et al. American College of Chest Physicians (ACCP). Diagnosis and management of cough executive summary: ACCP evidence-based clinical practice guidelines. Chest 2006; 129 Suppl: 1S–23S

[9] Morice AH, McGarvey L, Pavord I British Thoracic Society Cough Guideline Group. Recommendations for the management of cough in adults. Thorax 2006; 61 Suppl 1: i1–i24

[10] Cerveri I, Accordini S, Corsico A et al. ISAYA Study Group. Chronic cough and phlegm in young adults. Eur Respir J 2003; 22: 413–417

[11] Irwin RS, Madison JM. The persistently troublesome cough. Am J Respir Crit Care Med 2002; 165: 1469–1474

[12] Irwin RS, Curley FJ, French CL. Chronic cough. The spectrum and frequency of causes, key components of the diagnostic evaluation, and outcome of specific therapy. Am Rev Respir Dis 1990; 141: 640–647

[13] Irwin RS, Boulet LP, Cloutier MM et al. Managing cough as a defense mechanism and as a symptom. A consensus panel report of the American College of Chest Physicians. Chest 1998; 114 Suppl Managing: 133S–181S

[14] Eller R, Ginsburg M, Lurie D, Heman-Ackah Y, Lyons K, Sataloff R. Flexible laryngoscopy: a comparison of fiber optic and distal chip technologies-part 2: laryngopharyngeal reflux. J Voice 2009; 23: 389–395

[15] Rubin BK. Mucus and mucins. Otolaryngol Clin North Am 2010; 43: 27–34, vii–viii

[16] Morice AH. Epidemiology of cough. Pulm Pharmacol Ther 2002; 15: 253–259

[17] 2010_Top_Therapeutic_Classes_by_RX.pdf. imshealth.com. Available at: http://www.imshealth.com/deployedfiles/ims/Global/Content/Corporate/Press%20Room/Top-line%20Market%20Data/2010%20Top-line%20Market%20Data/2010_Top_Therapeutic_Classes_by_RX.pdf. Accessed January 4, 2012

[18] Lacourcière Y, Brunner H, Irwin R et al. Losartan Cough Study Group. Effects of modulators of the renin-angiotensin-aldosterone system on cough. J Hypertens 1994; 12: 1387–1393

[19] Pavord ID, Wardlaw AJ. The A to E of airway disease. Clin Exp Allergy 2010; 40: 62–67

[20] Jansen DF, Schouten JP, Vonk JM et al. Smoking and airway hyperresponsiveness especially in the presence of blood eosinophilia increase the risk to develop respiratory symptoms: a 25-year follow-up study in the general adult population. Am J Respir Crit Care Med 1999; 160: 259–264

[21] Janson C, Chinn S, Jarvis D, Zock JP, Torén K, Burney P European Community Respiratory Health Survey. Effect of passive smoking on respiratory symptoms, bronchial responsiveness, lung function, and total serum IgE in the European Community Respiratory Health Survey: a cross-sectional study. Lancet 2001; 358: 2103–2109

[22] Larsson ML, Loit HM, Meren M et al. Passive smoking and respiratory symptoms in the FinEsS Study. Eur Respir J 2003; 21: 672–676

[23] Curley FJ, Irwin RS, Pratter MR et al. Cough and the common cold. Am Rev Respir Dis 1988; 138: 305–311

[24] Diehr P, Wood RW, Bushyhead J, Krueger L, Wolcott B, Tompkins RK. Prediction of pneumonia in outpatients with acute cough—a statistical approach. J Chronic Dis 1984; 37: 215–225

[25] Bolser DC. Pharmacologic management of cough. Otolaryngol Clin North Am 2010; 43: 147–155, xixi.

[26] Pavord ID, Chung KF. Management of chronic cough. Lancet 2008; 371: 1375–1384

[27] Braman SS. Postinfectious cough: ACCP evidence-based clinical practice guidelines. Chest 2006; 129 Suppl: 138S–146S

[28] Rohani P, Drake JM. The decline and resurgence of pertussis in the US. Epidemics 2011; 3: 183–188

[29] Hoppe JE The Erythromycin Study Group. Comparison of erythromycin estolate and erythromycin ethylsuccinate for treatment of pertussis. Pediatr Infect Dis J 1992; 11: 189–193

[30] Irwin RS. Unexplained cough in the adult. Otolaryngol Clin North Am 2010; 43: 167–180, xi–xiixi–xii.

[31] Smyrnios NA, Irwin RS, Curley FJ, French CL. From a prospective study of chronic cough: diagnostic and therapeutic aspects in older adults. Arch Intern Med 1998; 158: 1222–1228

[32] Pratter MR. Chronic upper airway cough syndrome secondary to rhinosinus diseases (previously referred to as postnasal drip syndrome): ACCP evidence-based clinical practice guidelines. Chest 2006; 129 Suppl: 63S–71S

[33] Naclerio RM. Allergic rhinitis. N Engl J Med 1991; 325: 860–869

[34] Koufman JA. Laryngopharyngeal reflux is different from classic gastroesophageal reflux disease. Ear Nose Throat J 2002; 81 Suppl 2: 7–9

[35] Merati AL. Reflux and cough. Otolaryngol Clin North Am 2010; 43: 97–110, ixix.

[36] Adhami T, Goldblum JR, Richter JE, Vaezi MF. The role of gastric and duodenal agents in laryngeal injury: an experimental canine model. Am J Gastroenterol 2004; 99: 2098–2106

[37] Johnston N, Dettmar PW, Bishwokarma B, Lively MO, Koufman JA. Activity/stability of human pepsin: implications for reflux attributed laryngeal disease. Laryngoscope 2007; 117: 1036–1039

[38] Irwin RS, French CL, Curley FJ, Zawacki JK, Bennett FM. Chronic cough due to gastroesophageal reflux. Clinical, diagnostic, and pathogenetic aspects. Chest 1993; 104: 1511–1517

[39] Irwin RS. Chronic cough due to gastroesophageal reflux disease: ACCP evidence-based clinical practice guidelines. Chest 2006; 129 Suppl: 80S–94S

[40] Hanson DG, Jiang J, Chi W. Quantitative color analysis of laryngeal erythema in chronic posterior laryngitis. J Voice 1998; 12: 78–83

[41] Park W, Hicks DM, Khandwala F et al. Laryngopharyngeal reflux: prospective cohort study evaluating optimal dose of proton-pump inhibitor therapy and pretherapy predictors of response. Laryngoscope 2005; 115: 1230–1238

[42] Richter JE, Castell DO. Gastroesophageal reflux. Pathogenesis, diagnosis, and therapy. Ann Intern Med 1982; 97: 93–103

[43] Sifrim D, Dupont L, Blondeau K, Zhang X, Tack J, Janssens J. Weakly acidic reflux in patients with chronic unexplained cough during 24 hour pressure, pH, and impedance monitoring. Gut 2005; 54: 449–454

[44] Agrawal A, Roberts J, Sharma N, Tutuian R, Vela M, Castell DO. Symptoms with acid and nonacid reflux may be produced by different mechanisms. Dis Esophagus 2009; 22: 467–470

[45] Corrao WM, Braman SS, Irwin RS. Chronic cough as the sole presenting manifestation of bronchial asthma. N Engl J Med 1979; 300: 633–637

[46] Brightling CE, Ward R, Goh KL, Wardlaw AJ, Pavord ID. Eosinophilic bronchitis is an important cause of chronic cough. Am J Respir Crit Care Med 1999; 160: 406–410

[47] Berry MA, Hargadon B, McKenna S et al. Observational study of the natural history of eosinophilic bronchitis. Clin Exp Allergy 2005; 35: 598–601

[48] Crapo RO, Casaburi R, Coates AL et al. Guidelines for methacholine and exercise challenge testing-1999. This official statement of the American Thoracic Society was adopted by the ATS Board of Directors, July 1999. Am J Respir Crit Care Med 2000; 161: 309–329

[49] Dicpinigaitis PV. Chronic cough due to asthma: ACCP evidence-based clinical practice guidelines. Chest 2006; 129 Suppl: 75S–79S

[50] Cheriyan S, Greenberger PA, Patterson R. Outcome of cough variant asthma treated with inhaled steroids. Ann Allergy 1994; 73: 478–480

[51] Irwin RS, French CT, Smyrnios NA, Curley FJ. Interpretation of positive results of a methacholine inhalation challenge and 1 week of inhaled bronchodilator use in diagnosing and treating cough-variant asthma. Arch Intern Med 1997; 157: 1981–1987

[52] Brightling CE. Chronic cough due to nonasthmatic eosinophilic bronchitis: ACCP evidence-based clinical practice guidelines. Chest 2006; 129 Suppl: 116S–121S

23 Office-Based Laryngeal Surgery

Sunil P. Verma and Seth H. Dailey

The field of laryngeal surgery has undergone a full circle of development since its inception in 1855.[1] Mirror laryngoscopy initially allowed for evaluation of the larynx and pharynx and later became the tool that enabled office-based laryngeal surgery.[2,3] The 20th century bore witness to the era of direct laryngoscopy, which, as techniques of general anesthesia were refined, allowed for the performance of laryngeal surgery almost entirely in the operating room.

In the 1980s and 1990s, laryngology began to undergo another shift returning to its roots of office-based laryngeal surgery.[4,5] The flexible fiberoptic laryngoscope was recognized as a tool for in-office endoscopy and instrumentation.[4,5] During the turn of the 21st century the distal-chip flexible laryngoscope was introduced, which permitted higher quality endoscopic views of the larynx and pharynx. This, combined with other technological advances including development of fiber-based lasers and an increase in the number of vocal fold injectables, led to a proliferation of office-based laryngeal surgery suites.

Office-based laryngeal surgery (OBLS) includes the performance of endoscopy including tracheobronchoscopy and esophagoscopy, as well as interventions, including biopsy, vocal fold injection, and laser surgery. Office-based laryngeal surgery is performed as an outpatient procedure without the need for intraveneous medication or cardiopulmonary monitoring. Patients are able to drive themselves to and from the appointment because no sedatives or narcotics are administered during the procedure. With a lack of prolonged operating room "turnover" time between surgical cases, physicians are able to introduce increased efficiency into their practices. An additional advantage of OBLS includes decreased cost as there are no fees with operating room time and anesthesiology.[6,7,8]

23.1 Equipment

Office-based laryngeal surgery is performed in an otolaryngology clinic suite, which consists of a powered otolaryngology examination chair and a video tower with photodocumentation capability. For optimal visualization, distal chip endoscopes and rigid angled telescopes are used. The ideal armamentarium includes a flexible distal chip endoscope, a channeled flexible distal chip endoscope, a flexible esophagoscope, and a 70-degree rigid angled telescope. An alternative to these include the use of a disposable sheath over a flexible fiberoptic laryngoscope coupled to a camera. This allows for administration of medication and tools such as biopsy forceps through the collapsible channel within the sheath.

Injections are performed using either standard 25- or 27-gauge needles, or a curved orotracheal injector (Medtronic, Jacksonville, FL). Tools for biopsy include transoral laryngeal biopsy forceps and flexible endoscopic biopsy forceps. Laser surgery is typically performed with a fiber based 585-nm pulsed dye laser, 532-nm KTP (potassium titanyl phosphate) laser, or a carbon dioxide (CO_2) laser.

23.2 Anesthesia

The principles of anesthesia include

1. The upper airway is protective.
2. The reactive mechanisms are powerful and easily triggered by physical stimuli.
3. The reactivity of those mechanisms is increased with increased circulating adrenaline.
4. Pain, stress, and anxiety all increase circulating adrenaline.
5. High levels of circulating adrenaline also perpetuate long-term memory production.
6. Once the protective mechanisms are activated, they will not return to their preactivation baselines. They will be more easily activated with additional stimulus.
7. Stress and anxiety can be reduced with specific behavioral approaches.
8. Behavioral approaches can target both psychological and physical targets.
9. Behavioral approaches are temporary, giving a window of time for any upper airway procedure.
10. The time and effort taken by the physician to encourage behavioral approaches that reduce anxiety and stress are inherently beneficial.
11. Pain can be reduced with topical anesthetics.
12. Pain and stress/anxiety coaugment each other.

The rise of OBLS is due in large part to the ease of performing surgery using only local anesthesia. To work within these confines, an understanding of the nature of the upper airway is important. The upper airway is largely a protective system, designed to direct ingested materials into the pharynx and esophagus and air to be breathed into the larynx and trachea. When there is a risk of these pathways being misdirected then the body reacts strongly and closes down in a dramatic fashion with intrinsic and extrinsic muscles rapidly contracting until control is regained. Furthermore, the reactivity of the system is modulated by stress and anxiety with circulating adrenaline being the lynchpin.

Thus, the success of unsedated office-based procedures requires limited adrenaline levels. High circulating adrenaline induces increased reactivity of the patient and a likelihood of durable traumatic memories for the patient. This latter point is particularly important given that many procedures are performed more than once for patients with chronic upper airway disorders such as laryngeal papillomatosis or premalignant vocal fold epithelium. Increased patient reactivity and long-term memory production are both influenced by levels of circulating catecholamines. The higher the levels of adrenaline, the more reactive a patient will be and the more likely they will be to form long-term memories. So, a pre-emptive approach to prevent high levels of circulating catecholamines has been developed to mitigate this effect. This approach uses techniques to lower adrenaline levels by addressing psychological and physical factors that induce stress. For example, the strangeness of the experience of an unsedated procedure tends to induce uncertainty-related stress. Stress is an obvious source for increased adrenaline. A lengthy explanation of steps of the procedure reduces uncertainty, particularly when coupled with details about anticipated sensations. For example, a helpful notion to share with the patient is "This is what is going to happen and this is how it may make you feel. I'm going to spray some lidocaine into your mouth three times. It may make your mouth and throat feel odd and sometimes makes people feel like they can't swallow right. If you feel this, it is normal and will go away in 40 minutes or so." In addition to the explanation, the reassurance is helpful in relieving stress. Not to be underestimated is the mere fact of explaining the steps and sensations represents an act of caring by the treating otolaryngologist, which individuals in our fast-paced world universally appreciate.

Careful review of the informed consent including the nature, purpose, risks, benefits, and alternatives of the procedure also tends to reduce rather than augment stress because the unknowns are made explicit. A procedural "time out" similar to a "time out" performed in the operating room also underscores the team's dedication to the patient's safety and good outcome. Empowering the patient to participate in a manner helpful to his or her own good outcome tends to reduce a feeling of being "acted upon" and being helpless. These include slow "yoga-type" breathing, and maintenance of an "eyes-open" position because closing the eyes tends to lead to a mental place of uncertainty like a haunted house. Encouragement to relax the more powerful muscles of the head and neck such as the muscles of mastication, the forehead musculature, the trapezius, and tongue muscles helps reduce tension and adrenaline. Clearly, topical anesthesia is important to reduce the adrenaline related to feeling pain. Within this construct, an important concept is that of avoiding significant spikes in circulating adrenaline. This concept is crucial because the patient will not return to a prestimulus adrenaline level after a meaningful rise in their adrenaline such as an acute pain event. This notion has been called "waking the dog" referring to the notion that a guard dog, once awoken, is extremely unlikely to go back to sleep anytime soon.

Depending on the approach used, appropriate anesthesia should be employed. All or any combination of the following may be indicated.

23.2.1 Nasal Anesthesia

For any approach involving a transnasal flexible endoscope the nasal cavity should be appropriately decongested and anesthetized. First, anterior rhinoscopy is performed to assess for septal deviation, turbinate hypertrophy and to determine which nasal passage is more patent. For endoscopes smaller than 4 millimeters (mm) it is adequate to pretreat the patient's nasal cavity with an aerosolized mixture of 50/50 oxymetazoline/4% lidocaine. For endoscopes larger than 4 mm, which includes most channeled endoscopes, both a nasal spray and placement of cottonoids with the same solution into the nasal cavity is beneficial. Nasal anesthesia should be given at least 5 minutes to take effect, and the flexible scope should be lubricated with 2% lidocaine jelly to permit smooth passage through the nasal cavity as well as to provide additional topical anesthesia.

23.2.2 Oral Cavity Anesthesia

The transoral approach for vocal fold injection or laryngopharyngeal biopsy requires topical anesthesia. Three atomized sprays of 4% lidocaine are applied to the patient's tonsillar fossa, soft palate, posterior pharyngeal wall, and base of tongue.

23.2.3 Laryngeal Anesthesia

For procedures involving the vocal folds such as glottic biopsy, vocal fold injection, and glottic laser surgery, topical 4% lidocaine is satisfactory to obtain adequate anesthesia. This may be applied through the channel of a flexible endoscope or through the channel on a sheath of an endoscope. The endoscope is placed transnasally and suspended approximately 1 centimeter (cm) superior to the larynx.

The technique of obtaining laryngeal anesthesia is the same regardless of conduit used. If the transnasal route is used, then the flexible endoscope is passed through the nasal cavity and suspended 1 cm above the larynx. The patient is asked to phonate and 1 milliliter of 4% lidocaine is dripped on the laryngeal surface of the epiglottis and the glottis. As the patient phonates, the lidocaine distributes along the false vocal folds, epiglottis, arytenoids, and piriform sinus. This is repeated twice. Each time the patient will be able to phonate for a longer period of time as the larynx becomes progressively more anesthetized. This is known as a *laryngeal gargle*.[9]

A laryngeal gargle may also be completed transorally. To do this, the patient holds his or her tongue out of the oral cavity with a 4 × 4 gauze. The surgeon may use a transnasal flexible endoscope or a rigid angled telescope to visualize the larynx. The Abraham cannula is placed transorally along the lingual sulcus and is suspended above the larynx. The laryngeal gargle is similarly completed with three separate applications of lidocaine.

23.2.4 Laryngotracheal Anesthesia

A nebulizer is an excellent tool to deliver anesthesia from the oral cavity to the tracheobronchial tree. Preceding procedures such as tracheobronchoscopy, laryngopharyngeal biopsy, and laser surgery, the patient is instructed to inhale 5 cc of 4% nebulized lidocaine. This takes approximately 5 minutes to complete. ▶ Fig. 23.1 demonstrates the clinical se-up for the above topical anesthesia applications.

23.3 Patient Selection

Most patients are good candidates for OBLS as there are no absolute medical contraindications for OBLS. However, patients who are unable to come off anticoagulation may be better treated under general anesthesia should hemorrhage occur.

Patients with tight nasal vaults due to septal deviation or turbinate hypertrophy are generally not good candidates for transnasal procedures. The transoral approach for instrumentation should be avoided for the patient with a small mandible, large tongue, retroflexed epiglottis, trismus, or a strong gag reflex.

As previously described the success of OBLS relies heavily on patient participation. The ideal patient is able to communicate well with the physician and follow instructions. A patient with severe anxiety also may be better managed under general anesthesia.

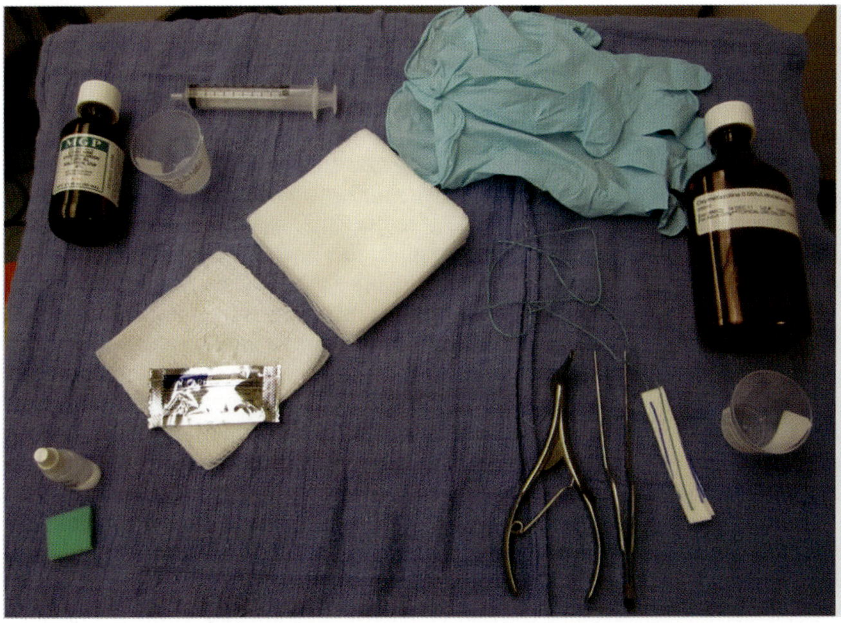

Fig. 23.1 Preparation setup for office-based surgery anesthesia application.

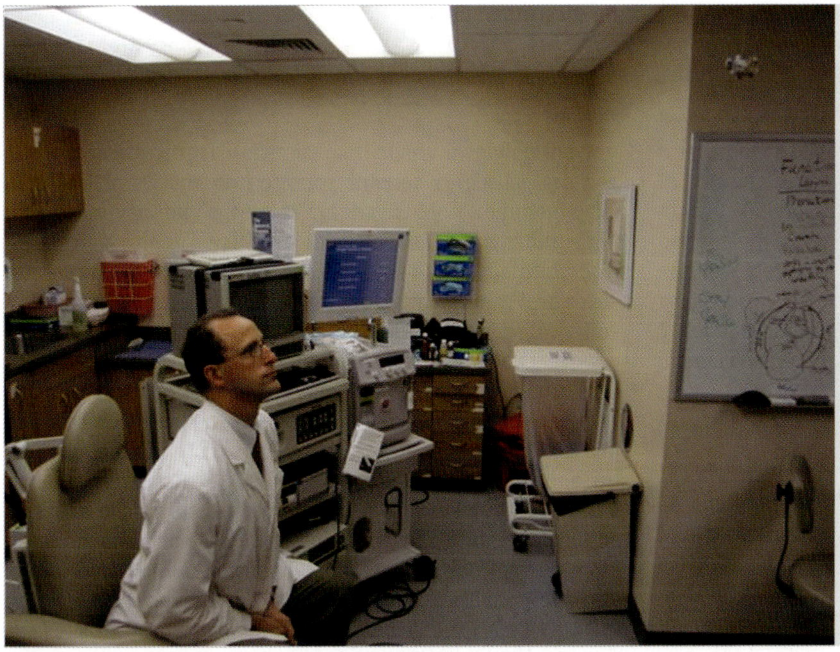

Fig. 23.2 Photograph of correct "sniffing" position for office-based laryngeal surgery.

23.4 Patient Positioning

Proper patient positioning is important during OBLS. The preferred positioning for patients is seated with hips back in the chair, knees together, and torso bent forward at the waist. Ideally, the patient should sit with the thin chin extended in a "sniffing position" (▶ Fig. 23.2). This serves to position the larynx optimally for examination and intervention.

23.5 Risks

In general, OBLS is very safe. However, risks of OBLS include

1. Epistaxis: This may occur in a patient with a tight nasal vault, and is more likely to occur when using a larger bore endoscope such as an esophagoscope.
2. Bleeding: This may result from a laceration caused by a needle, laser, or biopsy forceps.

3. Inadvertent placement of injectate: During vocal fold injection a filler may be placed in the incorrect portion of the vocal fold.
4. Nausea and vomiting: Some individuals may have a prominent gag reflex that is not overcome with local anesthesia.
5. Laryngospasm: This may occur in a patient with an inadequately anesthetized larynx.
6. Airway obstruction: During a vocal fold injection, this may result from a hematoma or less likely from overinjection of filler or medication. During laser surgery or biopsy, this may result from displacement of a mass.
7. Esophageal perforation: This may occur during standard esophagoscopy, but is more likely to occur during biopsy or instrumentation. Although there are no reports of perforation following office-based transnasal esophagoscopy, the risk should still be mentioned to the patient.

23.6 Tracheoscopy and Bronchoscopy

Evaluation of the tracheobronchial tree has historically been performed under sedation or general anesthesia. However, with the improvement of in-office endoscopy equipment this procedure can be quickly performed under local anesthesia.[9,10,11,12,13,14,15,16]

Indications include:

1. Evaluation of stridor
2. Planning for endoscopic or open airway surgery
3. Postoperative monitoring of endoscopic or open airway intervention
4. Pandendoscopy for head and neck cancer
5. Evaluation of the airway prior to tracheotomy tube decannulation

Transnasal tracheoscopy and bronchoscopy is performed using a channeled laryngoscope or esophagoscope. Nasal anesthesia is achieved as previously described. Laryngotracheal anesthesia is achieved using inhaled lidocaine through an atomizer as previously described as well. A channeled endoscope coated in viscous 2% lidocaine is placed within the nasal cavity and advanced to the laryngopharynx.

The endoscope is then passed to the larynx and advanced through the vocal folds, while the patient inspires. The endoscope is advanced through the trachea and into the main stem bronchi as indicated. If a tracheotomy tube is present this may be removed during the examination intermittently to assess the airway.

23.7 Esophagoscopy

Transnasal esophagoscopy was introduced in 2001.[17,18,19,20] The advent of the transnasal esophagoscope revolutionized the ability to evaluate patients with dysphagia.

The commonest indications for this procedure include

1. Dysphagia
2. Globus
3. Panendoscopy for head and neck cancer
4. Cough
5. Acid reflux

Esophagoscopy may safely be performed for patients under local anesthesia.

Nasal anesthesia is achieved as previously described. An esophagoscope coated in viscous 2% lidocaine is placed within the nasal cavity and advanced to the laryngopharynx. The esophagoscope is advanced to the patient's piriform sinus and the patient is asked to take a hard swallow. While the patient swallows, the esophagoscope is gently passed into the esophagus.

Occasional insufflation of air may be used to dilate the esophagus as the esophagoscope is advanced. While the esophagoscope is passed through the body of the esophagus, three normal narrowings will be noted.[20] Twenty-four centimeters from the nasal tip on the left anterior-lateral wall the aortic compression is noted. At approximately 26 cm the left mainstem bronchus produces an anterior compression. The final compression is noted at 41 cm and is created by the diaphragm. The patient may be instructed to sniff to open the diaphragm to help in identifying this landmark.

The esophagogastric junction is evaluated for presence of esophagitis, hiatal hernia, and Barrett metaplasia. The esophagoscope is advanced into the stomach and retroflexed upon itself to evaluate the hiatus of the stomach. The body of the stomach is evaluated and prior to removal of the esophagoscope, air is suctioned out of the stomach. The esophagoscope is gently withdrawn.

Pathologies that the endoscopist should be familiar with include esophagitis, hiatal hernia, stricture, and Barrett esophagus.

23.8 Vocal Fold Injection

Vocal fold injections account for a large percentage of the laryngopharyngeal interventions performed in-office. Vocal fold injection may be performed for augmentation or for delivery of therapeutic substances such as botulinum toxin or steroids.

Vocal fold augmentation is performed for patients with glottic insufficiency including causes such as vocal fold paralysis, vocal fold paresis, presbylarynges, and scar. Although augmentation does not improve vocal fold mobility, it medializes the vocal fold allowing for the contralateral fold to better oppose it.

Botulinum toxin is typically used for patients with spasmodic dysphonia or tremor, and steroids are typically applied to inflammatory lesions such as scar and granuloma.

Proper placement of the injectate is paramount to obtain excellent voice results during injection laryngoplasty. Ideally, the injectate should be applied in the lateral portion of the glottis within the body of the thyroarytenoid muscle or within the paraglottic space (▶ Fig. 23.3; ▶ Fig. 23.4). The depth of the injection should be approximately 4 to 6 mm deep and directed towards the infraglottic aspect of the vocal fold. An injection that is placed too superficial will inhibit the mucosal wave and negatively affect a patient's voice.

Care should also be taken to place the injectate along the posterior half of the vocal fold. An injection that is placed too anterior will cause a "pressed" voice.

Proper placement of injectate presents a challenge during OBIL because the patient is able to move during the procedure. During suspension microlaryngoscopy under general anesthesia, the injectate can be precisely placed. If the injectate is misapplied during general anesthesia it can be removed in the same setting. However, a large advantage of OBIL is the ability to titrate the injection based on a patient's voice. Additionally, a patient is able to cough during the procedure to help adequately distribute the injectate prior to termination of the procedure.

For augmentation purposes, there are currently several products that are approved by the Federal Drug Administration: calcium hydroxyapatite (Radiesse Voice, Merz Aesthetics, San Mateo, CA), carboxymethylcellulose (Radiesse Voice Gel, Merz Aesthetics, San Mateo, CA), and micronized dermis (Cymetra, Lifecell Corp, Branchburg, NJ). A number of injectates are used off-label as well. Depending on the injectate used, the vocal fold should be intentionally overinjected to account for injectate absorption. Cadaveric studies demonstrate that approximately 0.5 to 0.6 cc of injectate are necessary to medialize the vocal fold.[21]

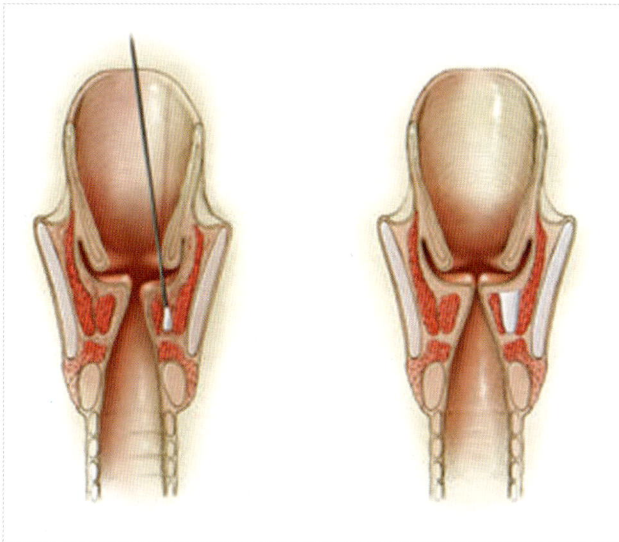

Fig. 23.3 Depth and location of injection material within the vocal fold.

As with all office-based procedures excellent visualization is paramount to obtain excellent results. Regardless of approach it is important that the entire surgical field be visualized adequately.

The decision as to whether to perform an injection through a transcutaneous or transoral route is largely based upon surgeon preference. The transcutaneous approach requires at least two persons, whereas the transoral approach may be performed with one person or two people.

23.8.1 Transcutaneous Approaches

There are three transcutaneous approaches: the transthyrohyoid membrane approach, the transthyroid cartilage approach, and the transcricothyroid membrane approach. In all of these approaches an assistant holds an endoscope transnasally while the surgeon directs placement of the injection through the skin into the larynx. Prior to performing the procedure, the hyoid bone, thyroid cartilage, and cricoid cartilage are outlined in the midline with a skin marker. The nasal cavity is anesthetized as previously described. Laryngeal anesthesia is obtained with a laryngeal gargle of 4% lidocaine.

23.8.2 Transthyrohyoid Membrane Approach

The skin overlying the thyroid notch is anesthetized with 1% lidocaine. Approximately two cc of anesthesia is applied to the skin to create a wheal and passed deeper to anesthetize the preepiglottic space. An assistant passed an endoscope transnasally and a laryngeal gargle is performed. The larynx is visualized.

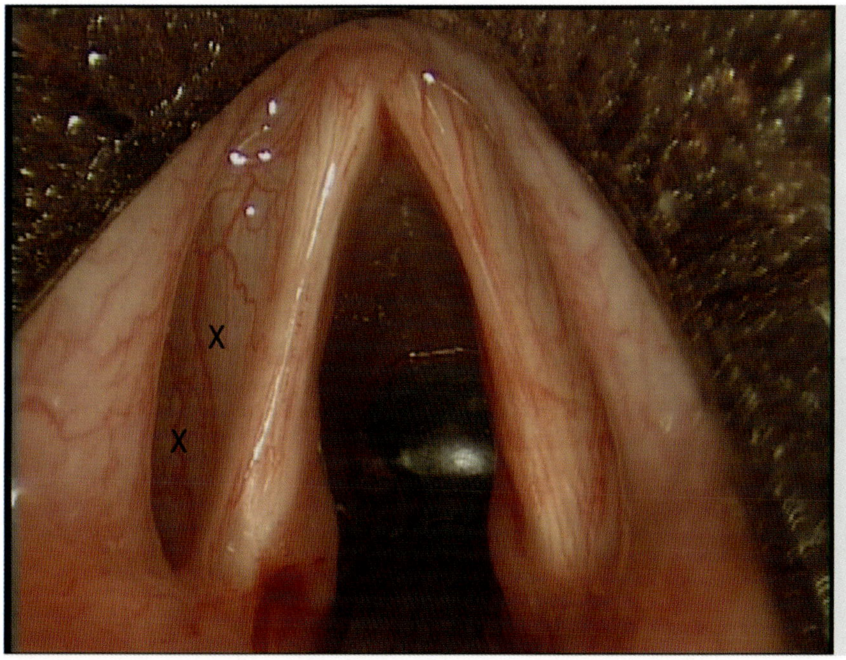

Fig. 23.4 Ideal location of needle entrance for injection laryngoplasty.

A syringe filled with augmentation material with a 25-gauge needle is passed superior to the thyroid notch through the skin, subcutaneous tissue, and pre-epiglottic space, superior to the vocal folds, into the airway.[22] The needle is passed steeply through the skin in a plane almost perpendicular to the vocal fold.[23] The needle enters the airway through the petiole of the epiglottis in the midline. Once the needle enters the airway, it can be visualized with the flexible laryngoscope and is directed laterally into the paraglottic space of the vocal fold.

23.8.3 Transthyroid Cartilage Approach

This approach is best used in younger patients before the thyroid cartilage has ossified. In this approach, the vocal fold is approached laterally and the needle is passed through the skin and thyroid cartilage and then into the vocal fold.

The thyroid prominence and lower thyroid cartilage border are marked in the midline with a skin marking pen. The level of the vocal fold is midway between these two points and travels in a plane perpendicular to this line.

The skin overlying this area is anesthetized. The needle is passed through the skin and felt to touch the thyroid cartilage. The skin, subcutaneous tissue, and strap muscles are anesthetized with approximately 2 cc of 1% lidocaine.

An assistant passed an endoscope transnasally and a laryngeal gargle is performed. The larynx is visualized with the endoscope. A 25-gauge needle, attached to a syringe filled with augmentation material, is passed through the lateral thyroid cartilage into the vocal fold in a horizontal plane. The needle is passed through the outer and inner lamina of the thyroid cartilage and aimed towards the arytenoid cartilage. Movement of the needle is seen with the flexible laryngoscope deep to the vocal fold mucosa. Injectate is slowly applied into the paraglottic space as the needle is withdrawn.

23.8.4 Transcricothyroid Membrane Approach

In this approach, the needle enters the airway through the subglottis below the level of the vocal fold.[24] The cricothyroid membrane is located inferior to the vocal folds between the thyroid and cricoid cartilages.

The position of the thyroid and cricoid cartilages is marked on the skin with a skin-marking pen. The skin overlying the midline cricothyroid membrane is injected with 1% lidocaine. An assistant passed an endoscope transnasally and a laryngeal gargle is performed. The larynx including the subglottis is visualized.

A 27-gauge needle attached to a syringe filled with augmentation material is passed through the skin overlying the cricothyroid membrane. The needle is directed superoposteriorly through the cricothyroid membrane to enter the airway. It is then directed towards the infraglottic aspect of the vocal fold. Injectate is deposited within the paraglottic space.

23.8.5 Transoral Approach

Vocal fold injections may also be performed transorally. The oral cavity is anesthetized with topical lidocaine spray applied with an atomizer as previously described. The patient is asked to assume the "sniffing" position and directed to hold his tongue with gauze. Visualization of the laryngopharynx is obtained with either a transnasal flexible laryngoscope held by an assistant, or with a transoral rigid 70-degree angled telescope held by the surgeon. The view from the scope is transmitted to a screen on the video tower.

An Abraham cannula (▶ Fig. 23.5) attached to a syringe with 4% lidocaine is placed along the patient's lingual sulcus and directed over the larynx. A laryngeal gargle is performed with 4% lidocaine. The surgeon then advances a syringe with injectate attached to an orotracheal injector needle along the patient's lingual sulcus and directs it to the larynx. The needle may be used to lateralize the patient's false vocal fold. The needle is inserted through the superior surface of the vocal fold into its body. Injectate is applied within the paraglottic space.

23.9 Therapeutic Vocal Fold Injection

Using the same techniques for delivery of anesthesia and injection as OBIL, therapeutic injection to the vocal folds can be performed as well. For example, steroids may be injected to inflammatory lesions such as scar and granuloma, and cidofivir may be injected for management of recurrent respiratory papillomatosis.

23.10 Laryngopharyngeal Biopsy

Lesions of the base of tongue, hypopharynx, and larynx are amenable to in office-biopsy. For a number of patients performance of biopsy in-office allows for patients to receive

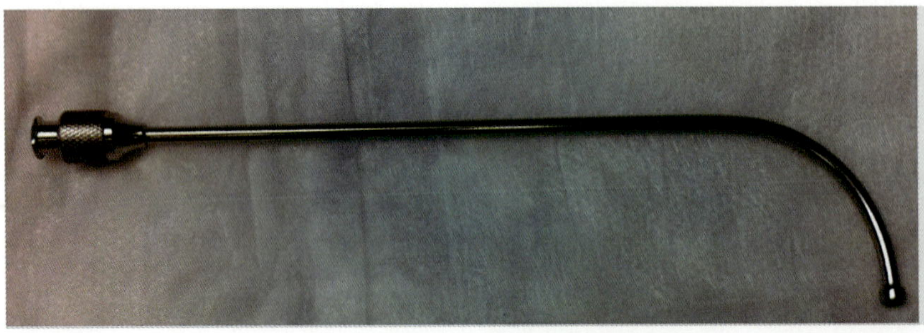

Fig. 23.5 Abraham cannula.

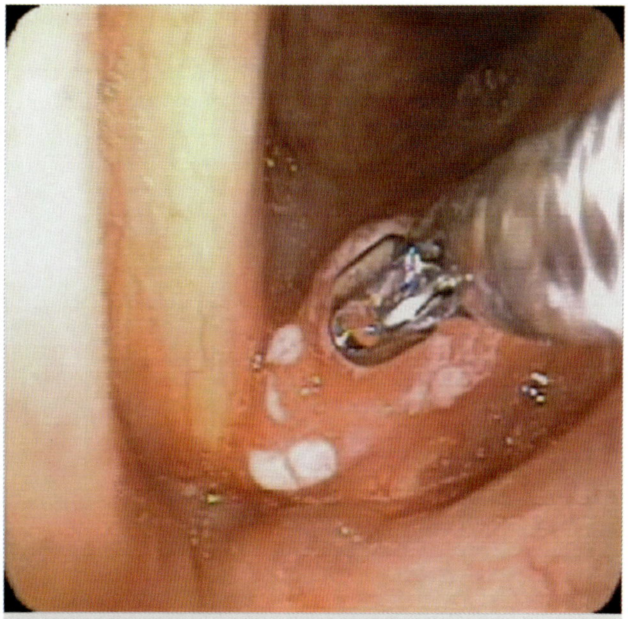

Fig. 23.6 Biopsy of left true vocal fold mass with a flexible fiberoptic laryngoscope with a side channel.

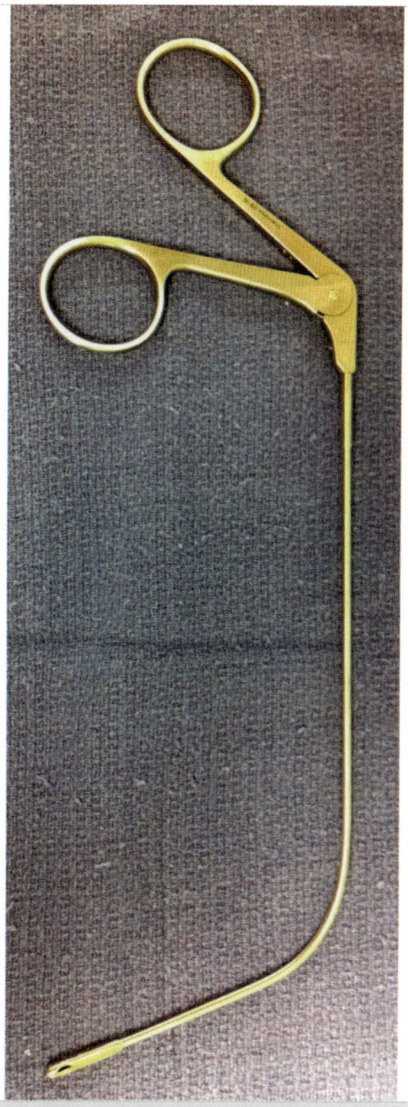

Fig. 23.7 A transoral biopsy forcep.

a diagnosis easily without need to be placed under general anesthesia. In-office biopsy is especially helpful for patients with bulky lesions who may not be intubated easily and would require a tracheotomy to be placed under general anesthesia. For some patients with head and neck cancer, an in-office biopsy, bronchoscopy, and esophagoscopy completes the "panendoscopy" that was traditionally performed in the operating room.

Biopsy may be performed with the patient unsedated using only topical anesthesia. The procedure may be performed through an entirely transnasal or transoral approach.

23.10.1 Transnasal Approach

Nasal anesthesia is obtained as previously described. Nebulized lidocaine is administered. A channeled flexible endoscope is placed within the nasal cavity and advanced to the laryngopharynx. Four-percent lidocaine is distributed over the lesion and a laryngeal gargle is performed as previously described. Additional topical lidocaine may be placed along the lesion.

A channeled endoscope is advanced through the nasal cavity, suspended above the lesion, and an assistant passes the biopsy forceps through the channel.

The forceps are opened and are used to grasp a portion of the lesion (▶ Fig. 23.6). The endoscopist then advances the endoscope to touch the tissue being biopsied. The person holding the forceps pulls firmly using the endoscope against the tissue to provide countertraction. The forceps are removed from the endoscope and the tissue is carefully removed from the forceps. While the tissue is removed from the biopsy forceps, the endoscope is kept within the patient's nasal passage and suspended in the oropharynx. Suction is intermittently applied throughout the procedure as necessary. Two to four biopsies are applied to ensure adequate amount of specimen.

23.10.2 Transoral Approach

The patient is first instructed to inhale neublized lidocaine as previously described. For additional oropharyngeal anesthesia an atomizer used to apply 4% lidocaine to the oropharynx. The patient is asked to assume the "sniffing" position (▶ Fig. 23.2) and directed to hold his tongue with gauze. Visualization of the laryngopharynx is obtained with either a transnasal flexible laryngoscope held by an assistant, or with a transoral rigid 70-degree angled telescope held by the surgeon. The view from the scope is transmitted to a screen on the video tower.

An Abraham cannula attached to a syringe with 4% lidocaine is placed along the patient's lingual sulcus and directed over the lesion.[5] Three 1-cc aliquots of 4% lidocaine are distributed over the lesion. A transoral biopsy forcep (▶ Fig. 23.7) is then inserted into the oral cavity, placed superior to the lesion, and used to grasp the lesion.

23.11 Laser Surgery

Indications for laser surgery include recurrent respiratory papillomatosis, dysplasia, Reinke edema, and vocal process granulomas.[25] Although the CO_2 laser has been in use in laryngology since the 1970s, it was the advent of the fiber-based laser that promoted the in-office use of lasers. Today there are four lasers that are commonly used in-office for laryngeal surgery. They include the 585-nm pulsed dye laser,[26,27,28,29] the 532- nm KTP laser,[30] the CO_2 laser,[29] and the thulium laser.[29,31] The first two lasers are considered photoangiolytic lasers; the latter two are classified as cutting/ablative lasers.

Photoangiolytic laser energy is preferentially absorbed by oxyhemoglobin, while cutting/ablative laser energy is preferentially absorbed by water. The photoangiolytic lasers are used in a pulsed mode to treated vascular lesions such as recurrent respiratory papillomatosis, dysplasia, and ectasias.

To perform office-based laser surgery, the nasal cavity is anesthetized as previously described. Nebulized lidocaine is used to obtain laryngopharyngeal anesthesia. After this a channeled endoscope is placed transnasally and a laryngeal gargle is performed to complete laryngeal anesthesia.

The door to the room is closed and signage to alert potential in-comers of laser use is placed on the door. Personnel in the room are distributed appropriate laser-safe eye wear. The laser fiber is passed through the channel of the endoscope and suction is connected. The laser fiber is placed approximately 3 to 5 mm superior to the lesion to be treated. Laser energy is applied while suction is maintained to evacuate smoke.

Patients are typically able to tolerate 10 minutes of procedural time, although this may vary.

23.12 Conclusion

Office-based laryngeal surgery is an extremely exciting field within laryngology. The benefits of decreased cost, fast turnover, and avoidance of general anesthesia are very attractive to physicians and patients alike. However, limitations including equipment cost and a steep learning curve some procedures such as injection may prevent applicability in all otolaryngologic practices. However, because there are so few contraindications for OBLS, most patients who may undergo general anesthesia are excellent candidates for equivalent office-based procedures.

23.13 Key Points

- Excellent preparation is paramount for successful performance of office-based laryngeal surgery.
- Patients should have procedures explained to them in detail prior to the procedure. The surgeon should have all equipment ready prior to initiating a procedure.
- Laryngotracheal anesthesia can be reliably achieved using topical lidocaine.
- Laryngeal procedures can be performed as outpatient procedures without need for cardiac monitoring.
- The laryngeal surgeon should be familiar with all approaches for injection laryngoplasty to enable the maximum number of patients being treated.

References

[1] Green H. Observations of the human voice. Proc R Soc Lond 1855; 7: 397–410
[2] Mackenize M. The Use of the Laryngoscope in Diseases of the Throat with an Appendix on Rhinoscopy. London: J & A Churchill; 1865: 121–128
[3] Elsberg L. Laryngoscopal Medication or the Local Treatment of the Diseases of the Throat, Larynx, and Neighboring Organs, Under Sight. New York, NY: William Wood & Co. 1864
[4] Bastian RW, Collins SL, Kaniff T, Matz GJ. Indirect videolaryngoscopy versus direct endoscopy for larynx and pharynx cancer staging. Toward elimination of preliminary direct laryngoscopy. Ann Otol Rhinol Laryngol 1989; 98: 693–698
[5] Bastian RW, Delsupehe KG. Indirect larynx and pharynx surgery: a replacement for direct laryngoscopy. Laryngoscope 1996; 106: 1280–1286
[6] Andrade Filho PA, Carrau RL, Buckmire RA. Safety and cost-effectiveness of intra-office flexible videolaryngoscopy with transoral vocal fold injection in dysphagic patients. Am J Otolaryngol 2006; 27: 319–322
[7] Rees CJ, Postma GN, Koufman JA. Cost savings of unsedated office-based laser surgery for laryngeal papillomas. Ann Otol Rhinol Laryngol 2007; 116: 45–48
[8] Bové MJ, Jabbour N, Krishna P et al. Operating room versus office-based injection laryngoplasty: a comparative analysis of reimbursement. Laryngoscope 2007; 117: 226–230
[9] Hogikyan ND. Transnasal endoscopic examination of the subglottis and trachea using topical anesthesia in the otolaryngology clinic. Laryngoscope 1999; 109: 1170–1173
[10] Hartzell LD, Richter GT, Glade RS, Bower CM. Accuracy and safety of tracheoscopy for infants in a tertiary care clinic. Arch Otolaryngol Head Neck Surg 2010; 136: 66–69
[11] Lindstrom DR, Book DT, Conley SF, Flanary VA, Kerschner JE. Office-based lower airway endoscopy in pediatric patients. Arch Otolaryngol Head Neck Surg 2003; 129: 847–853
[12] Morris LG, Zeitler DM, Amin MR. Unsedated flexible fiberoptic bronchoscopy in the resident clinic: technique and patient satisfaction. Laryngoscope 2007; 117: 1159–1162
[13] Amin MR, Simpson CB. Office evaluation of the tracheobronchial tree. Ear Nose Throat J 2004; 83 Suppl 2: 10–12
[14] Simpson CB, Amin MR, Postma GN. Topical anesthesia of the airway and esophagus. Ear Nose Throat J 2004; 83 Suppl 2: 2–5
[15] Halum SL, Postma GN. Office-based examinations in laryngology—including TNE, FEES, FEESST. In: Merati AL, Bielamowicz SA, eds. Textbook of Laryngology. San Diego, CA: Plural Publishing; 2007; 135–146
[16] Verma SP, Smith ME, Dailey SH. Transnasal tracheoscopy. Laryngoscope 2012; 122: 1326–1330
[17] Aviv JE, Takoudes TG, Ma G, Close LG. Office-based esophagoscopy: a preliminary report. Otolaryngol Head Neck Surg 2001; 125: 170–175
[18] Belafsky PC, Postma GN, Daniel E, Koufman JA. Transnasal esophagoscopy. Otolaryngol Head Neck Surg 2001; 125: 588–589
[19] Belafsky PC, Postma GN, Koufman JA. Normal transnasal esophagoscopy. Ear Nose Throat J 2001; 80: 438
[20] Postma GN, Belafsky PC, Aviv JE. Atlas of Transnasal Esophagoscopy. Philadelphia, PA: Lippincott Williams & Wilkins; 2007: xi, 108
[21] Mau T, Courey MS. Influence of gender and injection site on vocal fold augmentation. Otolaryngol Head Neck Surg 2008; 138: 221–225
[22] Amin MR. Thyrohyoid approach for vocal fold augmentation. Ann Otol Rhinol Laryngol 2006; 115: 699–702

[23] Damrose EJ. Transthyroid membrane injection. In: Dailey SP, Verma, SH. eds. Laryngeal dissection and surgical guide. New York, NY: Thieme Medical Publishers; 2012; 64–66

[24] Ward PH, Hanson DG, Abemayor E. Transcutaneous Teflon injection of the paralyzed vocal cord: a new technique. Laryngoscope 1985; 95: 644–649

[25] Clyne SB, Halum SL, Koufman JA, Postma GN. Pulsed dye laser treatment of laryngeal granulomas. Ann Otol Rhinol Laryngol 2005; 114: 198–201

[26] Zeitels SM, Franco RA, Dailey SH, Burns JA, Hillman RE, Anderson RR. Office-based treatment of glottal dysplasia and papillomatosis with the 585-nm pulsed dye laser and local anesthesia. Ann Otol Rhinol Laryngol 2004; 113: 265–276

[27] Mouadeb DA, Belafsky PC. In-office laryngeal surgery with the 585 nm pulsed dye laser (PDL). Otolaryngol Head Neck Surg 2007; 137: 477–481

[28] Rees CJ, Halum SL, Wijewickrama RC, Koufman JA, Postma GN. Patient tolerance of in-office pulsed dye laser treatments to the upper aerodigestive tract. Otolaryngol Head Neck Surg 2006; 134: 1023–1027

[29] Koufman JA, Rees CJ, Frazier WD et al. Office-based laryngeal laser surgery: a review of 443 cases using three wavelengths. Otolaryngol Head Neck Surg 2007; 137: 146–151

[30] Zeitels SM, Akst LM, Burns JA, Hillman RE, Broadhurst MS, Anderson RR. Office-based 532-nm pulsed KTP laser treatment of glottal papillomatosis and dysplasia. Ann Otol Rhinol Laryngol 2006; 115: 679–685

[31] Zeitels SM, Burns JA, Akst LM, Hillman RE, Broadhurst MS, Anderson RR. Office-based and microlaryngeal applications of a fiber-based thulium laser. Ann Otol Rhinol Laryngol 2006; 115: 891–896

Index

Note: Page numbers set **bold** or *italic* indicate headings or figures, respectively.

A

B

M

N

O

P

Q

R

S

T

U

V

W

X

Z